A Practical Approach to Anesthesia Equipment

Jerry A. Dorsch, MD
Associate Professor Emeritus
Mayo Medical School
Mayo Clinic
Jacksonville, Florida

Susan E. Dorsch, MD
Jacksonville, Florida

Wolters Kluwer | Lippincott Williams & Wilkins
Health
Philadelphia • Baltimore • New York • London
Buenos Aires • Hong Kong • Sydney • Tokyo

Acquisitions Editor: Brian Brown
Product Manager: Nicole Dernoski
Production Manager: Bridgett Dougherty
Senior Manufacturing Manager: Benjamin Rivera
Marketing Manager: Angela Panetta
Design Coordinator: Doug Smock
Production Service: Aptara, Inc.

© 2011 by LIPPINCOTT WILLIAMS & WILKINS, a WOLTERS KLUWER business
Two Commerce Square
2001 Market Street
Philadelphia, PA 19103 USA
LWW.com

All rights reserved. This book is protected by copyright. No part of this book may be reproduced in any form by any means, including photocopying, or utilized by any information storage and retrieval system without written permission from the copyright owner, except for brief quotations embodied in critical articles and reviews. Materials appearing in this book prepared by individuals as part of their official duties as U.S. government employees are not covered by the above-mentioned copyright.

Printed in China

Library of Congress Cataloging-in-Publication Data

Dorsch, Jerry A., 1941-
A practical approach to anesthesia equipment / Jerry A. Dorsch, Susan E. Dorsch.
p. ; cm.
Includes bibliographical references.
Summary: "This paperback, full-color book is ideally suited for anesthesiologists, residents, and nurse anesthetists who need a concise, practical, easily accessible reference on anesthesia equipment. Written by the authors of the definitive text Understanding Anesthesia Equipment, A Practical Approach to Anesthesia Equipment covers the most commonly used machines and devices and addresses common problems and pitfalls that affect clinical situations. The book is written in outline format and thoroughly illustrated with full-color photographs and line drawings"–Provided by publisher.
ISBN 978-0-7817-9867-9 (pbk.)
1. Anesthesiology–Apparatus and instruments–Outlines, syllabi, etc.
I. Dorsch, Susan E., 1942- II. Title.
[DNLM: 1. Anesthesiology–instrumentation–Handbooks. WO 231 D717p 2011]
RD78.8.D666 2011
617.9'6–dc22

2010023256

Care has been taken to confirm the accuracy of the information presented and to describe generally accepted practices. However, the authors, editors, and publisher are not responsible for errors or omissions or for any consequences from application of the information in this book and make no warranty, expressed or implied, with respect to the currency, completeness, or accuracy of the contents of the publication. Application of the information in a particular situation remains the professional responsibility of the practitioner.

The authors, editors, and publisher have exerted every effort to ensure that drug selection and dosage set forth in this text are in accordance with current recommendations and practice at the time of publication. However, in view of ongoing research, changes in government regulations, and the constant flow of information relating to drug therapy and drug reactions, the reader is urged to check the package insert for each drug for any change in indications and dosage and for added warnings and precautions. This is particularly important when the recommended agent is a new or infrequently employed drug.

Some drugs and medical devices presented in the publication have Food and Drug Administration (FDA) clearance for limited use in restricted research settings. It is the responsibility of the health care provider to ascertain the FDA status of each drug or device planned for use in their clinical practice.

To purchase additional copies of this book, call our customer service department at (800) 638-3030 or fax orders to (301) 223-2320. International customers should call (301) 223-2300.

Visit Lippincott Williams & Wilkins on the Internet: at LWW.com. Lippincott Williams & Wilkins customer service representatives are available from 8:30 am to 6 pm, EST.

10 9 8 7 6 5 4 3

CCS1214

❖

This text is dedicated to the trainees in all phases of anesthesia practice who are striving to provide high-quality care for all their patients.

Preface

The fifth edition of *Understanding Anesthesia Equipment* was published in 2008. It contains a great deal of detail on the subjects covered. Unfortunately, the size of the text intimidates many trainees. Since students are not the decision makers in their departments, there is a great deal of information that is not yet useful to them. This text is aimed to give trainees basic information about the equipment they employ on a daily basis. We have tried to focus on equipment use as well as problems that could occur. We have introduced the concept of clinical moments that highlight certain situations related to equipment use that trainees need to know.

A chapter about the basics of ultrasound, which is rapidly gaining popularity and likely will have a great impact on the anesthesia of the future, has also been added.

The fifth edition of *Understanding Anesthesia Equipment* will continue to be available. We hope that this text will stimulate enough interest among readers to cause them to want greater detail on its subjects and that when the training period is over, they will maintain a strong interest in equipment.

Jerry A. Dorsch
Susan E. Dorsch

Acknowledgments

The support of manufacturers is essential when writing a textbook on equipment. This included providing technical information, copies of user and service manuals, and photographs. We thank all these companies.

Our profound gratitude to Christian Robards, Roy Greengrass, and Timothy Shine of Mayo Clinic, Jacksonville, for lending us their expertise for the chapter on ultrasound equipment.

The medical library at Mayo Clinic provided stellar service in helping obtain the references we needed.

As always, special thanks to Billy Atkins, a great guy, for keeping our computers functioning throughout this project.

Contents

V. EQUIPMENT RELATED TO ENVIRONMENTAL SITUATIONS

Gas Supply and Distribution Systems

1 Medical Gas Sources

ANESTHESIA PROVIDERS ARE RESPONSIBLE FOR providing the correct gases, especially oxygen, to the patient. It is therefore important that they know about gas sources and how to deal with malfunctions in the supply system.

I. Definitions

A. Psi, Psig, Psia

1. Psi stands for pounds per square inch. Psig stands for pounds per square inch gauge, which is the difference between the measured pressure and the surrounding atmospheric pressure. Most gauges are constructed to read zero at atmospheric pressure. Psia stands for pounds per square inch absolute. Absolute pressure is based on a reference point of zero pressure for a perfect vacuum. Psia is psig plus the local atmospheric pressure. For example, at sea level, the atmospheric pressure is 0 psig but 14.7 psia.
2. **Table 1.1** shows some units of pressure and their conversion factors.

Table 1.1 Units of Pressure

kPa	Kilopascal
cm H_2O	Centimeters of water
psi	Pounds per square inch
mbar	Millibar
mm Hg	Millimeters of mercury
100 kPa = 1000 mbar = 760 mm Hg = 1030 cm H_2O = 14.7 psi = 1 atmosphere	
Therefore,	
1 kPa = 10.3 cm H_2O	1 cm H_2O = 0.098 kPa
1 kPa = 0.147 psi	1 psi = 6.8 kPa
1 kPa = 7.6 mm Hg	1 mm Hg = 0.13 kPa
1 kPa = 10 mbar	1 mbar = 0.1 kPa
1 mbar = 1.03 cm H_2O	1 cm H_2O = 0.97 mbar
1 mbar = 0.76 mm Hg	1 mm Hg = 1.32 mbar
1 mbar = 0.0147 psi	1 psi = 68 mbar

B. Nonliquefied Compressed Gas

A nonliquefied compressed gas is a gas that does not liquefy at ordinary ambient temperatures regardless of the pressure applied. Examples include oxygen, nitrogen, air, and helium. These gases do become liquids at very low temperatures, at which point they are referred to as cryogenic liquids.

C. Liquefied Compressed Gas

A liquefied compressed gas is one that becomes liquid to a large extent in containers at ambient temperature and at pressures from 25 to 1500 psig (172 to 10,340 kPa). Examples include nitrous oxide and carbon dioxide.

II. Cylinders

Gases such as oxygen, nitrous oxide, carbon dioxide, and air are supplied in cylinders (tanks). Cylinders vary in size. Sizes A through E are frequently attached to an anesthesia machine to back up the pipeline system or for use when a pipeline system is unavailable. G and H cylinders are often used in banks to supply or back up the pipeline system and sometimes to supply the anesthesia machine (1).

A. Cylinder Body

1. Most medical gas cylinders are made of steel, with various alloys added. In recent years, manufacturers have moved away from traditional steel cylinders toward steel carbon fiber cylinders. These can hold more gas than their older steel counterparts and are lighter in weight. Cylinders made from aluminum are available. These are useful when anesthesia is administered in a magnetic resonance imaging (MRI) environment.
2. In recent years, cylinders with integral pressure regulators and flow-metering devices as well as handles have become available (**Fig. 1.1**). These devices are

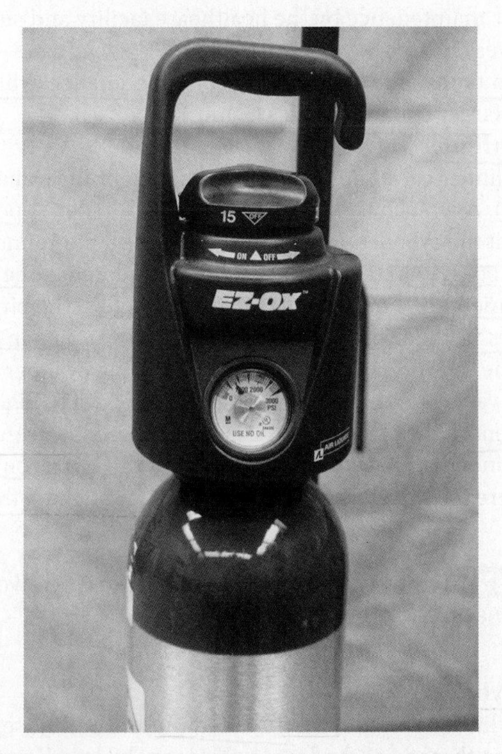

Figure 1.1 Cylinder with integral pressure regulator and flow-metering device.

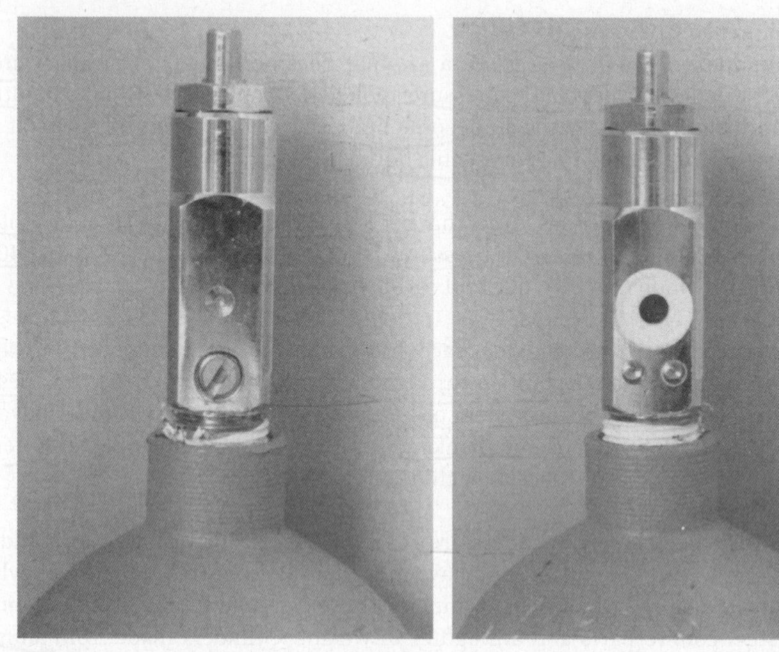

Figure 1.2 Small cylinder valves. **Left:** The conical depression is above the pressure relief device. **Right:** The port is above the Pin Index Safety System holes. A washer is over the port.

especially useful for patient transport. They eliminate the need for pressure regulator maintenance by the healthcare facility and simplify cylinder use.

B. Cylinder Valves

There are two types of cylinder valves, one for smaller cylinders (sizes A to E) and the other for larger cylinders (sizes G and H).

1. **Small Cylinder Valves**

Small cylinder valves are attached to the top of the cylinder by the manufacturer (**Fig. 1.2**). A wrench is needed to open the cylinder. A port on the side allows the gas to exit the cylinder. A washer is used to seal the connection. There is also a pin index safety system to prevent a cylinder containing one gas from being attached to equipment for a different gas (**Fig. 1.2, right**). The pin index safety system has two holes in the cylinder valve that match two pins in the receiving yoke (**Fig. 1.3**). If the pins do not align with the holes, the cylinder cannot be attached. The cylinder valve also contains a pressure relief device (**Fig. 1.2, left**) that will expel the contents if the pressure in the cylinder exceeds a preset level. It could also melt if the cylinder is subjected to a fire. Finally, there is a conical depression (**Fig. 1.2, left**) where the screw from the yoke will fit and tighten the cylinder to the yoke.

CLINICAL MOMENT If the retaining screw in the yoke is screwed into the safety relief device, it may make the cylinder unusable.

2. **Large Cylinder Valves**

Large cylinder valves have threaded outlet (bull nose) connectors (**Fig. 1.4**). When the threads of the large cylinder valve mesh with those of the nut on a regulator or the piping in a cylinder bank, the nut can be tightened, allowing

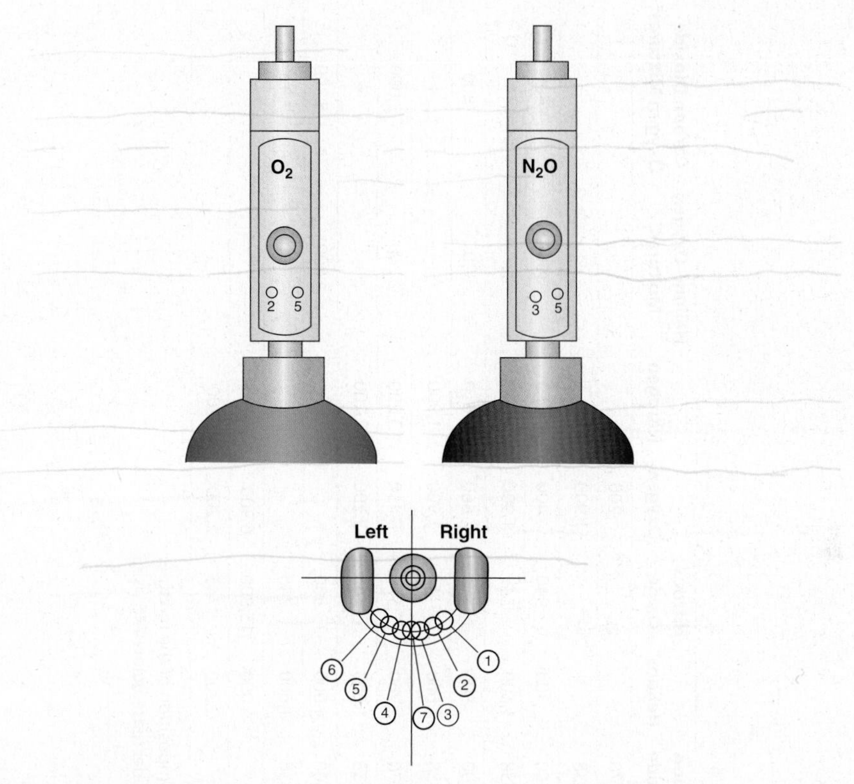

Figure 1.3 Pin Index Safety System. The bottom figure shows the six positions for pins on the yoke. The pins are 4 mm in diameter and 6 mm long, except for pin 7, which is slightly thicker. The seven-hole positions are on the circumference of a circle of 9/16-inch radius centered on the port.

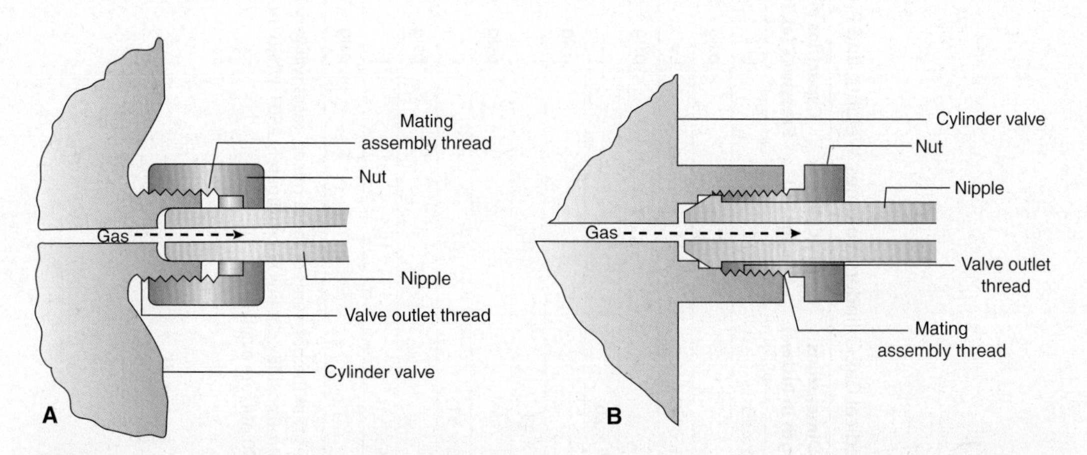

Figure 1.4 Valve outlet connections for large cylinders. **A:** The valve outlet thread is external, that is, the threads are on the outside of the cylinder valve outlet and the nut screws over the valve outlet. **B:** The valve outlet thread is internal so that the nut screws into the outlet. The specification for cylinder connections are often shown as in the following example for oxygen: 0.903-14-RH EXT. The first number is the diameter in inches of the cylinder outlet. The next number gives the number of threads per inch. The letters following this indicate whether the threads are right hand or left hand and external or internal. (Redrawn courtesy of Compressed Gas Association, 4221 Walney Road, 5th Floor Chantilly, VA 20151.)

Table 1.2 Typical Medical Gas Cylinders, Volumes, Weights, and Pressures

Cylinder Size	Cylinder Dimensions (O.D. × Length in Inches)	Empty Cylinder Weight (lb)	Capacities and Pressures (at 70°F)	Air	Carbon Dioxide	Helium	Nitrous Oxide	Oxygen	Nitrogen	Helium–Oxygen Mixtures[a]	Carbon Dioxide–Oxygen Mixtures[a]
B	3½ × 13	5	L		370			200			
			psig		838			1,900			
D	4½ × 17	11	L	375	940	300	940	400	370	300	400
			psig	1,900	838	1,600	745	1,900	1,900	+	+
E	4¼ × 26	14	L	625	1,590	500	1,590[b]	660	610	500	600
			psig	1,900	838	1,600	745[b]	1,900	1,900	+	+
M	7 × 43	63	L	2,850	7,570	2,260	7,570	3,450	3,200	2,260	3,000
			psig	1,900	838	1,600	745	2,200	2,200	+	+
G	8½ × 51	97	L	5,050	12,300	4,000	13,800			4,000	5,300
			psig	1,900	838	1,600	745			+	+
H	9¼ × 51	119	L	6,550		6,000	15,800	6,900[c]	6,400[c]		
			psig	2,200		2,200	745	2,200[c]	2,200[c]		

[a] The symbol "+" indicates that the pressures of these mixed gases will vary according to the composition of the mixture.
[b] An E-size cylinder of nitrous oxide contains approximately 250 L when the pressure begins to decrease below 745 psig.
[c] 7800-L cylinders at 2490 psig are available.

Most common

2nd common

the nipple to seat against the valve outlet and aligning the valve gas channel with the channel of the nipple. The outlets and connectors are indexed by diameter, thread size, right- and left-handed internal threading, and nipple seat design. Unfortunately, valves that are not indexed are sometimes still used (1).

C. Cylinder Contents and Pressures

Typical cylinder contents and pressures are given in **Table 1.2.** The volume of gas in a cylinder depends on whether or not the pressurized contents are partly in the liquid state (**Fig. 1.5**). Cylinder pressure will be an indication of the volume of the contents only if the contents are all in the gaseous state. If the contents are partly liquid, the pressure will remain constant until the last of the liquid has evaporated. At that point, the cylinder is nearly empty and the pressure will fall rapidly. Cylinder pressure cannot be used as a measure of the amount of the gas in the cylinder while liquid agent is present.

CLINICAL MOMENT Commit to memory the liters and pressure for a full E cylinder of oxygen (see Table 1.2).

CLINICAL MOMENT If you lose the oxygen pipeline pressure and you have a pressure of 475 psig in the oxygen cylinder, what would you do and how long can you supply oxygen from that cylinder? You know that you have a cylinder that is 25% full. This would mean that there are approximately 165 L (1/4 of 660 L) of oxygen in the cylinder. If you were running a 1 L/minute of oxygen flow, you would be able to supply oxygen for 165 minutes. If you were using a ventilator that used oxygen to compress the bellows, you would need to discontinue mechanical ventilation. This is discussed further in Chapter 6.

D. Color Coding

Cylinders are painted in various colors to indicate their contents. **Table 1.3** gives the color codes for the United States and Canada as well as the international color

Table 1.3 Medical Gases

Gas	United States	International	State in Cylinder
Oxygen	Green	White	Gas[a]
Carbon dioxide	Gray[b]	Gray	Gas + liquid (below 88°F)
Nitrous oxide	Blue	Blue	Gas + liquid (below 98°F)
Helium	Brown[c]	Brown	Gas
Nitrogen	Black	Black	Gas
Air	Yellow[d]	White and black	Gas

[a]Special containers for liquid oxygen are discussed later in this chapter.
[b]In carbon dioxide–oxygen mixtures in which the CO_2 is more than 7%, the cylinder is predominantly gray and the balance is green. If the CO_2 is less than 7%, the predominant color is green.
[c]If helium is more than 80% in a helium–oxygen mixture, the predominant color is brown and the balance is green.
[d]Air, including oxygen–nitrogen mixtures containing 19.5% to 23.5% oxygen, is color-coded yellow. Cylinders with nitrogen–oxygen mixtures other than those containing 19.5% to 23.5% oxygen are colored black and green.

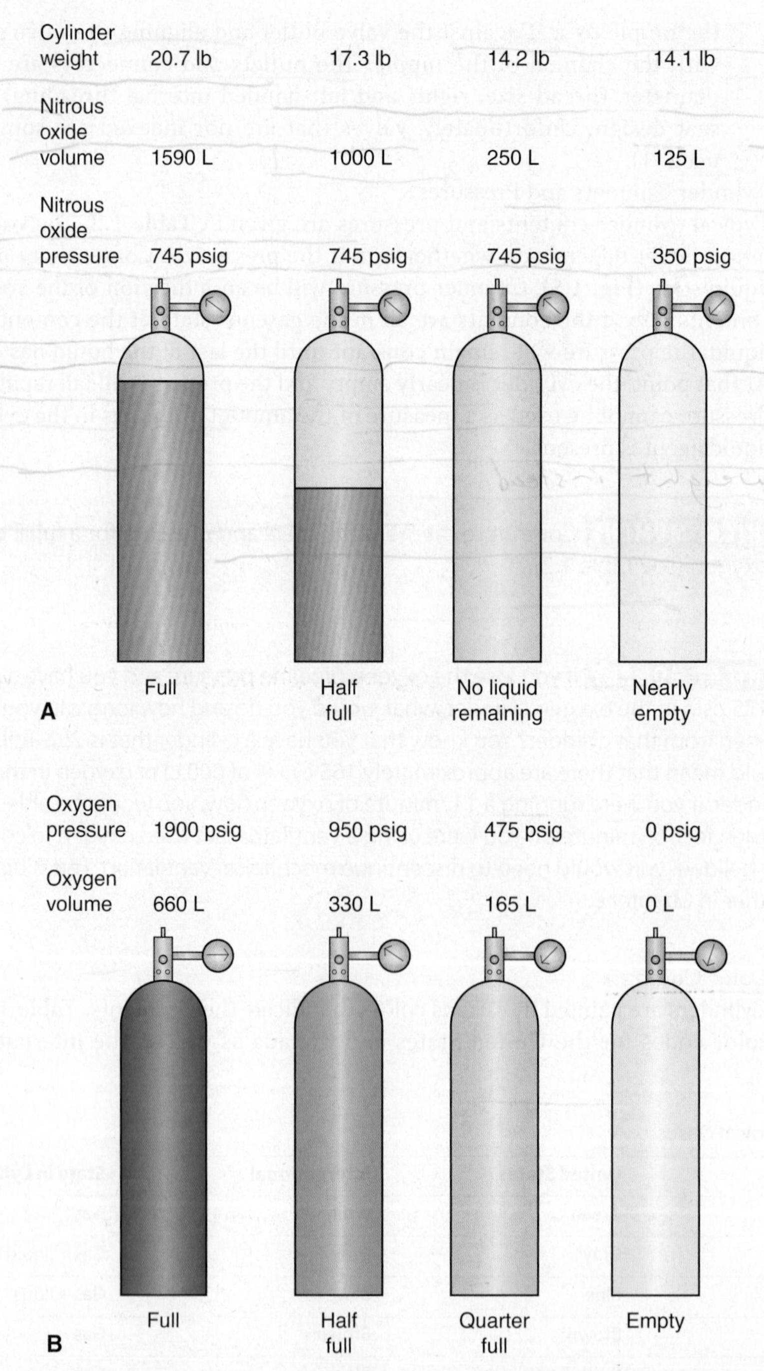

Figure 1.5 The relationship between cylinder weight, pressure, and contents. **A:** A gas stored partially in liquid form, such as nitrous oxide, will show a constant pressure (assuming constant temperature) until all liquid has evaporated, at which time the pressure will drop in direct proportion to the rate at which gas is withdrawn. **B:** A nonliquefied gas, such as oxygen, will show a steady decline in pressure until the cylinder is evacuated. Each cylinder, however, will show a steady decline in weight as gas is discharged.

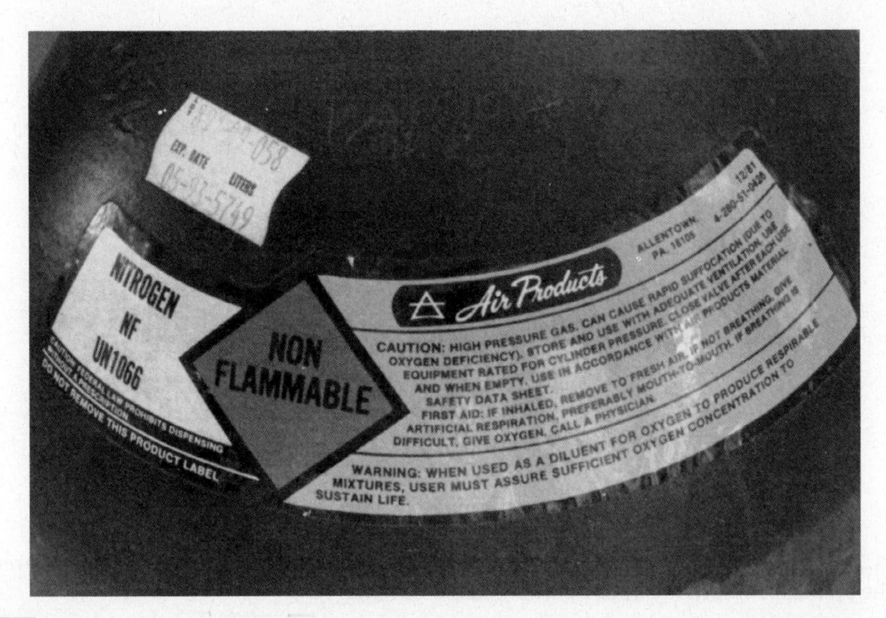

Figure 1.6 Cylinder label, showing the basic Compressed Gas Association marking system. The diamond-shaped figure denotes the hazard class of the contained gas (NONFLAMMABLE). To the left is a white panel with the name of contained gas (NITROGEN). The signal word (CAUTION) is to the right, followed by a statement of hazards and measures to be taken to avoid injury.

code. Color is not a good way of determining cylinder contents because of variations in color tones, chemical changes in paint pigments, lighting effects, and differences in color perception by personnel. Cylinders with gas mixtures may be painted the colors of both gases, which may cause confusion.

E. Cylinder Labeling

1. The label is the most reliable means of identifying the cylinder contents. **Figure 1.6** shows a typical cylinder label. It has a diamond-shaped figure denoting the hazard class of the contained gas and a white panel with the name of the contained gas to the left. The diamond indicates whether the contents contain an oxidizer, a nonflammable gas, or a flammable gas. A signal word (DANGER, WARNING, or CAUTION, depending on whether the release of gas would create an immediate, less than immediate, or no immediate hazard to health or property) is present. Following the signal word is the statement of hazard, which gives the dangers associated with reasonably anticipated handling or use of the gas. A brief precautionary statement giving measures to be taken to avoid injury or damage is usually present.
2. A label tag is shown in **Figure 1.7.** It has three sections labeled FULL, IN USE, and EMPTY, connected by perforations. When a cylinder is put into service, the FULL portion of the tag should be detached. When the cylinder is empty, the IN USE portion should be removed, leaving the EMPTY label. The tag sometimes contains a washer (seal) that fits between the small cylinder valve and the yoke or regulator. Tags normally bear the same color as the cylinder. The tag is primarily a means of denoting the amount of cylinder contents, not an identification device.

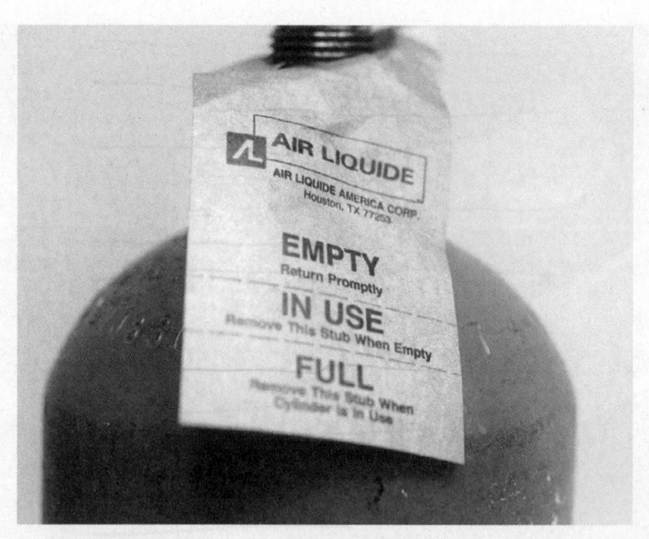
AIR LIQUIDE
AIR LIQUIDE AMERICA CORP.
Houston, TX 77253
EMPTY
Return Promptly
IN USE
Remove This Stub When Empty
FULL
Remove This Stub When
Cylinder is In Use

Figure 1.7 Cylinder tag. When the cylinder is first opened, the FULL portion of the tag should be removed. When the cylinder is empty, the IN USE portion should be removed.

F. General Rules for Safe Cylinder Handling

1. Cylinder valves, pressure regulators, gauges, or fittings should never be permitted to come into contact with oils, greases, organic lubricants, rubber, or other combustible substances. Cylinders or valves should not be handled with hands, gloves, or rags contaminated with oil or grease. Polishing or cleaning agents should not be applied to the valve, as they may contain combustible chemicals.
2. No part of any cylinder should ever be subjected to a temperature above 54°C (130°F) or below –7°C (20°F). If ice or snow accumulates on a cylinder, it should be thawed at room temperature or with water at a temperature not exceeding 54°C (130°F).
3. Connections to an anesthesia machine, piping, pressure regulators, and other equipment should always be kept tight to prevent leaks. If a hose is used, it should be in good condition.
4. The discharge port of a pressure relief device or the valve outlet should not be obstructed.
5. Pressure regulators, hoses, gauges, or other apparatus designed for use with one gas should never be used with cylinders containing other gases.
6. An adapter to change the outlet of a cylinder valve should not be used because this defeats the purpose of standardizing the outlet.
7. The valve should be kept closed at all times except when the cylinder is in use. It should be turned OFF using no more force than is necessary to prevent damage to the seat.
8. The valve is the most easily damaged part of the cylinder. Valve protection caps (metal caps that screw over the valve on large cylinders [**Fig. 1.8**]) protect the valve and should be kept in place and hand tightened, except when the cylinder is connected for use.
9. Markings, labels, decals, or tags should not be defaced, altered, or removed.
10. A cylinder should not be used as a roller or support or for any other purpose other than that for which it was intended, even if it is believed to be empty.

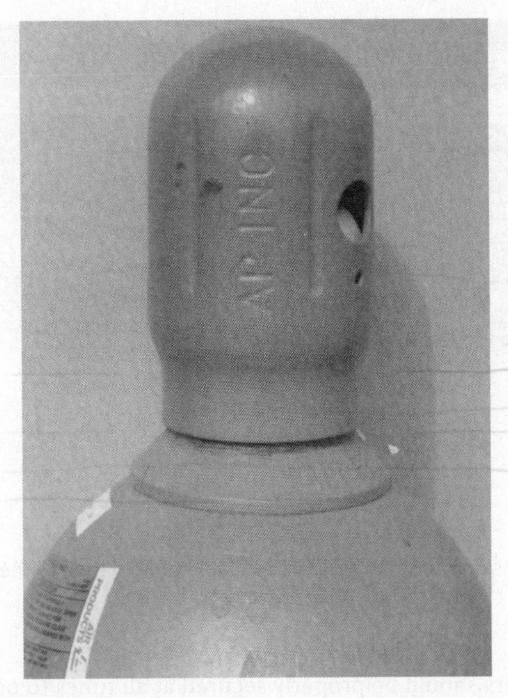

Figure 1.8 Large cylinder valve protection cap. This cap should be kept in place at all times, except when the cylinder is connected for use.

11. Care must be taken to prevent the cylinder from being damaged by an electric arc. This requires that cylinders not be placed or used in a manner in which they can become part of an electrical circuit.
12. Cylinders should not be dropped, dragged, slid, or rolled, even for short distances. Cylinders should be transported using a cart or carrier made especially for that purpose (**Figs. 1.9** and **1.10**). They should not be moved or lifted by the valve or valve protection cap.

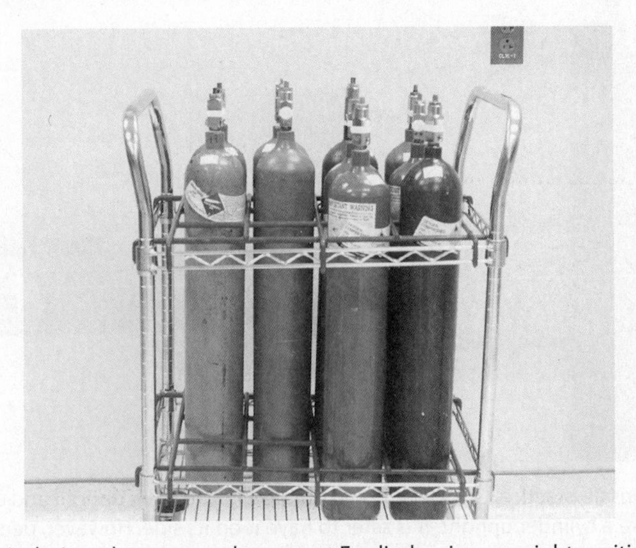

Figure 1.9 This cart is designed to store and transport E cylinders in an upright position.

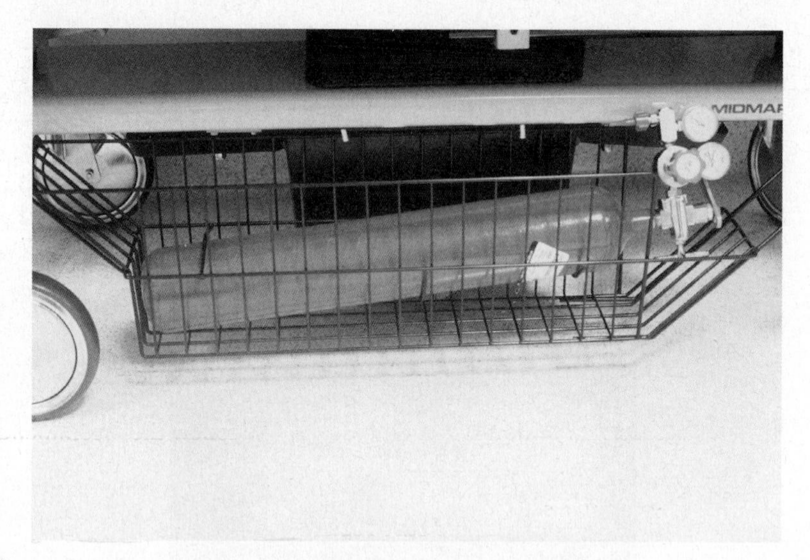

Figure 1.10 Special baskets on transport beds are available to hold the cylinder during transport.

13. Cylinders should be properly secured at all times to prevent them from falling or being knocked over (**Fig. 1.11**). They should not be dropped or permitted to violently strike each other or other surfaces. They should not be chained to movable apparatus such as a bed.

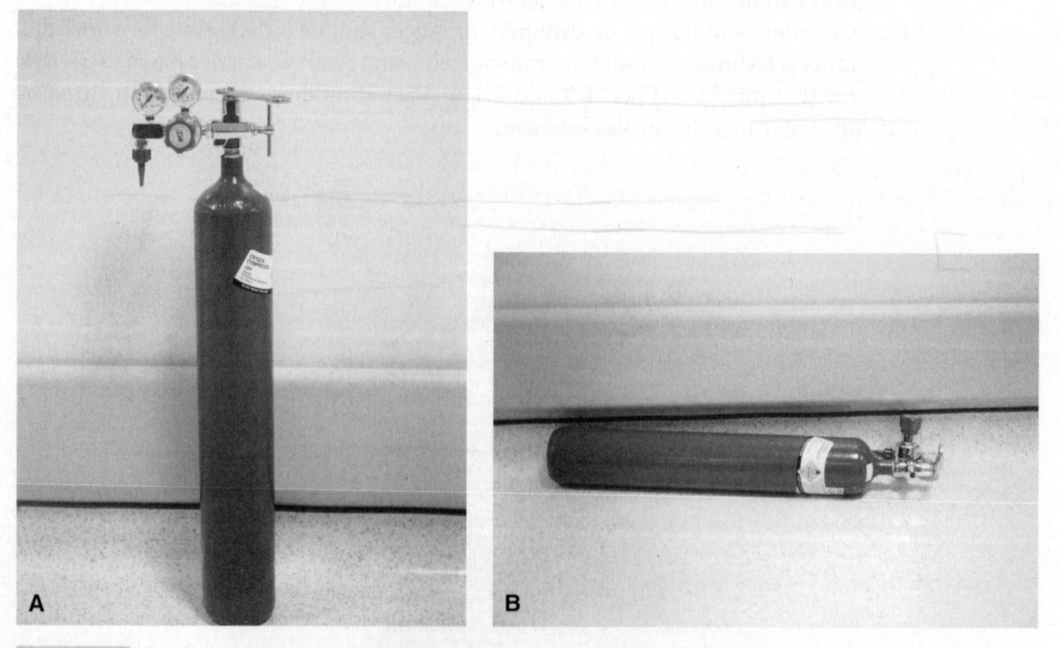

Figure 1.11 **A:** An unsafe practice. Cylinders should not be allowed to be upright and unsecured. **B:** If there is no means to secure a cylinder upright, it is safer to have it on its side. However, personnel may trip over it or damage it.

CLINICAL MOMENT Since a full oxygen cylinder has a pressure of nearly 2000 psig, if the cylinder falls and the valve is severed, the cylinder may spin rapidly or take off like a jet. This could cause serious injury to personnel in the vicinity.

14. The cylinder's owner must be notified of any damage that might impair its safety or any condition that might permit a foreign substance to enter the cylinder.

G. Rules for Safe Cylinder Use

1. Before use, the contents of the cylinder should be identified by reading the label. The cylinder color should not be relied on for identification. If the label is missing, illegible, or altered or if the cylinder color and label do not correspond, the cylinder should be returned to the manufacturer unused. The user should read the precautionary information on the label and follow the recommendations.
2. High-pressure gas released from a cylinder can be hazardous unless means for reducing the gas pressure to usable levels and for controlling the gas flow are provided. Accordingly, a pressure regulator should always be used when withdrawing cylinder contents. For cylinders attached to an anesthesia machine, the pressure regulator inside the machine performs this function. When connected to a pipeline system, the pressure regulator is part of the pipeline system.
3. Full cylinders are usually supplied with a tamper-evident seal (**Fig. 1.12**). This should be removed immediately before fitting the cylinder to the dispensing equipment.

CLINICAL MOMENT If the seal is not removed before the cylinder is fitted to the dispensing equipment, a portion of the seal may be forced into the recipient device and block the gas pathway.

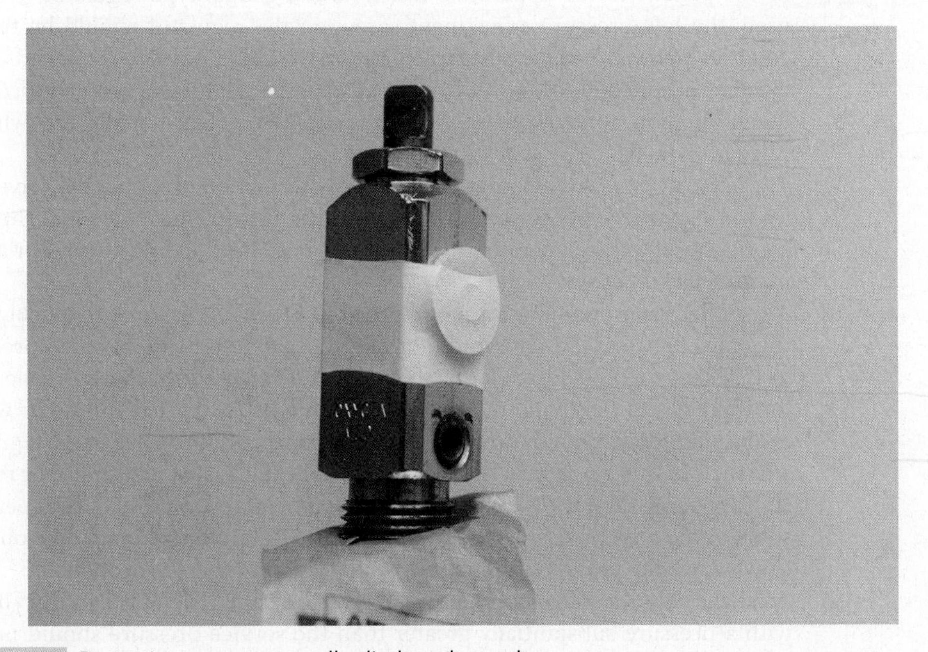

Figure 1.12 Protective cover over small cylinder valve outlet.

4. The valve protection cap on a large cylinder should be removed just before connecting the cylinder for use.
5. Before a pressure regulator is connected to a cylinder, it should be inspected for signs of damage and to make certain that it is free of foreign materials. Pressure regulators should be kept in good condition and stored in plastic bags to avoid contamination.
6. Before any fitting is applied to the cylinder valve, particles of dust, metal shavings, and other foreign matter should be cleared from the outlet by removing the protective cap or seal and then slowly and briefly opening ("cracking") the valve, with the port pointed away from the user or any other persons. This reduces the possibility of a flash fire or explosion when the valve is later opened after being attached to equipment; also, dust will not be blown into the anesthesia machine or other equipment where it could clog filters or interfere with the internal workings.
7. A sealing washer (gasket) in good condition should always be used with a small cylinder valve. It is usually supplied with a full cylinder. It fits over the port of the receiving equipment (**Fig. 1.2**). Only one washer should be used. If more than one washer is used, it may be possible to bypass the Pin Index Safety System or a leak may occur.
8. The threads on the regulator-to-cylinder valve connection and the pins on the yoke-to-cylinder valve connection should mate properly. Connectors that do not fit should never be forced.
9. Only wrenches or other tools provided or recommended by the manufacturer should be used to tighten outlets and connections. Wrenches with misaligned jaws should not be used because they may damage the equipment or slip and injure personnel. Excessive force should not be used. The handwheel should never be hammered in an attempt to open or close the valve.
10. The cylinder valve should be opened before bringing the apparatus to the patient or the patient to the apparatus. If a Bourdon gauge–type regulator is being used, the low-pressure adjustment screw on the regulator should be turned counterclockwise until it turns freely before the cylinder valve is opened. If the cylinder is attached to the yoke on an anesthesia machine or a regulator/flowmeter, the flow control valve for that gas should be closed before the cylinder valve is opened.
11. The person opening a cylinder valve should be positioned so that the valve outlet and/or the face of the pressure gauge points away from all persons. The user should stand to the side rather than in front or in back. Using goggles or a face mask is also recommended.
12. A cylinder valve should always be opened SLOWLY. If gas passes quickly into the space between the valve and the yoke or regulator, the rapid recompression in this space will generate large amounts of heat. Because there is little time for this heat to dissipate, this constitutes an adiabatic process (one in which heat is neither lost nor gained from the environment). Particles of dust, grease, and such in this space may be ignited by the heat, causing a flash fire or explosion. Opening the valve slowly prolongs the time of recompression and permits some of the heat to dissipate. The cylinder valve should continue to be opened slowly until the pressure on the gauge stabilizes and then fully opened.
13. After the cylinder valve is opened, the pressure should be checked. A cylinder with a pressure substantially greater than the service pressure should not be used but instead should be marked as defective and returned to the supplier.

A cylinder arriving with a pressure substantially below the service pressure should be checked for leaks.

14. If a cylinder valve is open but no pressure is registered on the gauge or no gas flows, the cylinder valve should be closed and the cylinder disconnected from the dispensing apparatus, marked defective, and returned to the supplier with a note indicating the problem.
15. A hissing sound when the valve is opened indicates that a large leak exists and the connection should be tightened. If the sound does not disappear, the sealing washer should be replaced (in the case of a small cylinder valve). If the hissing sound persists, soapy water, a commercial leak detection fluid, or other suitable solution should be applied to all parts. Bubbles will appear at the site(s) of the leak(s). A flame should never be used for this purpose. Should a leak be found in the cylinder valve itself, it may be possible to tighten the packing nut by turning it slightly in a clockwise direction (see special handle in **Figure 1.13**) unless the manufacturer recommends otherwise. If the leak cannot be remedied by tightening connections without using excessive force, the valve should be closed and the cylinder marked defective and returned to the supplier with a note indicating the fault.

CLINICAL MOMENT Under no circumstances should more than one washer be used.

16. Even if no hissing sound is audible when the valve is opened, a slow leak may be present and should be suspected if there is loss of pressure when no gas is being used. These leaks should be located and corrected.
17. When in use, a cylinder should be secured to a cylinder stand or to apparatus of sufficient size to render the entire assembly stable.
18. Cylinders in service or storage at user locations must be secured to prevent them from falling over.
19. The valve should always be fully open when a cylinder is in use. Marginal opening may result in failure to deliver adequate gas flow.

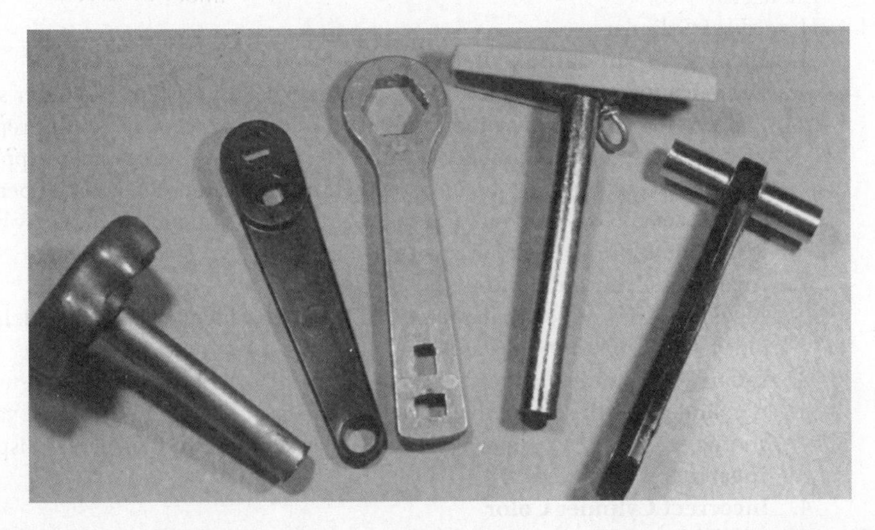

Figure 1.13 Small cylinder valve handles. The hexagonal opening at the top of the middle handle can be used to tighten the packing nut on the cylinder valve. A ratchet handle is at the right. After a cylinder has been opened, this handle must be removed, inverted, and reapplied to close the cylinder valve.

H. Rules for After Use

1. At any time an extended period of nonuse is anticipated, the cylinder valve should be closed completely and all pressure vented (bled) from the system.
2. An empty or near-empty cylinder should not be left on an anesthesia machine. A defective check valve in the yoke could result in accidental filling if the valve is left open. In addition, the presence of an empty cylinder may create a false sense of security. A yoke should not remain empty. If a full cylinder is not available, a yoke (blanking) plug (Chapter 3) should be in place.
3. Before removing a cylinder from a regulator or yoke, the valve should be closed and all downstream pressure released.
4. When a cylinder is empty, the lower part of the tag should be removed. A DOT green, yellow, or red label should be covered with an "Empty" label, or if the cylinder is provided with a combination label tag, the lower portion should be removed.
5. Valves should be completely closed on all empty cylinders. Often cylinders are not completely empty, and accidents have resulted from release of gas from a supposedly empty cylinder. If the valve remains open on an empty cylinder, debris and contaminants could be sucked into it when the temperature changes. Some gas suppliers prefer that cylinders be returned with enough pressure (e.g., 25 psig) remaining to maintain the integrity of the cylinder.

CLINICAL MOMENT When checking the pressure in a cylinder during the machine checkout, the cylinder valve should be closed after the pressure in the cylinder has been determined. If it remains open and the oxygen pipeline fails, there would be no warning that the supply had failed until the cylinder is empty.

6. Where provided, valve outlet caps or plugs should be securely affixed to the valve outlet prior to transportation.

I. Cylinder Transfilling

Transfilling contents from one cylinder to another should not be performed by the user.

J. Hazards of Cylinders

1. **Incorrect Cylinder Installed**
Despite almost universal use of the Pin Index Safety System and other systems to prevent an incorrect cylinder from being attached to an apparatus, reports of incorrect tanks being connected to yokes or regulators continue to appear (1). Yokes or regulators may be incorrectly built or altered. Pins can be bent, broken, removed, or forced into the yoke or regulator; pin index holes may become worn; and more than one washer may be used.
2. **Incorrect Cylinder Contents**
A cylinder may not contain the gas for which it is indexed and labeled. In a cylinder with a mixture, the gases may not be properly mixed.
3. **Incorrect Cylinder Valve**
A cylinder may be correctly labeled for the gas contained but have a valve for another gas. This usually will prevent its attachment to the correct dispensing apparatus.
4. **Incorrect Cylinder Color**
A cylinder may be painted other than its standard color.
5. **Incorrect Label**
A cylinder with the correct color and valve may have an incorrect label.

6. **Inoperable or Damaged Valve**
A cylinder may be delivered with an inoperable or blocked valve. If the retaining screw on the yoke is screwed into the safety relief device instead of the conical depression, the valve will be damaged. This may result in a leak. A pressure relief device may prematurely release gas from the cylinder.
7. **Asphyxia**
Sudden discharge of large quantities of gas other than oxygen from a cylinder into a closed space could displace the air from that space, creating a dangerous condition. A number of deaths due to nitrous oxide inhalation have been reported. If an oxygen-deficient atmosphere is suspected, the space should be checked with an oxygen monitor.
8. **Fires**
If an oxidizing gas is present, a fire may occur if a source of ignition and flammable material(s) are also present. Both oxygen and nitrous oxide are oxidizing gases, and their presence should be considered a source of risk. Fires are discussed in more detail in Chapter 25.
9. **Projectile Damage**
   a. If a cylinder is not properly secured and falls over, the valve may break off. Because gas in cylinders is under pressure, it will rapidly escape and cause the cylinder to shoot like a rocket or spin out of control. This could cause serious damage to equipment and personnel.
   b. Improper handling or storage of cylinders can cause them to fall over. If a valve protection cap is not present, the valve could snap off. If the packing nut rather than the stem is loosened, the stem may be ejected when the valve is opened.
   c. If a cylinder containing steel is taken into an MRI environment, it can be drawn into the magnet with such force that the magnet will be damaged or a patient or personnel in the room could be seriously injured or killed.
10. **Contaminated Cylinder Contents**
   a. Gases in cylinders may contain contaminants. Cases of poisoning due to nitrous oxide cylinders contaminated with higher oxides of nitrogen have been reported.
   b. A cylinder should not be used if the gas has an odor. The cylinder should be sequestered and the manufacturer or distributor contacted.
   c. Moisture may contaminate a cylinder and flow into the dispensing equipment. Adiabatic gas expansion as gas is released causes cooling, and the moisture could form ice and jam the regulator or yoke. In the past, this has been a significant problem with nitrous oxide cylinders.
11. **Overfilled Cylinders**
An overfilled cylinder may be delivered.
12. **Thermal Injury**
Frostbite injury from nitrous oxide has been reported in people who use the drug recreationally and in anesthesia providers and others who handle it occupationally.

CLINICAL MOMENT Some oxygen cylinders with integral flow-metering devices have fixed settings for oxygen flow. It may be possible to place the flow-selecting device between the settings. If this is done, there will be no flow. Always make sure that flow is actually occurring.

III. **Cryogenic Liquid Tanks**

A. When large amounts of oxygen are required, it is less expensive and more convenient to store it as a liquid. Oxygen is usually contained in a very large tank outside the building. The other gases may be kept in smaller portable tanks that may be stored inside the building. Liquid oxygen containers are usually refilled from supply trucks without interrupting service. Alternatively, filled liquid containers may be transported between the supplier and the facility.

B. To prevent the liquid from evaporating, it is kept in special insulated vessels. These containers vary in size and shape. They are constructed like thermos bottles, with outer and inner metal jackets separated by insulation and a layer that is near vacuum to retard heat transfer from the exterior. Gas is drawn off as required and passed through a heater to bring it up to ambient temperature and raise its pressure.

IV. **Oxygen Concentrators**

Oxygen concentrators are now being used to supply oxygen to the piping system in many facilities. This is a useful and cost-effective oxygen source, especially in areas where tanks and liquid oxygen are not readily available or where transport costs are high.

A. Technology

Most oxygen concentrators use pressure swing adsorber technology, which increases the oxygen concentration by adsorbing nitrogen onto a molecular sieve and allows oxygen and trace gases, especially argon, to pass through. Nitrogen, carbon dioxide, carbon monoxide, water vapor, and hydrocarbons are trapped. These are then desorbed (released) by venting the sieve bed to atmosphere. Regeneration of the sieve bed is then completed by purging with some product gas. The result is a gas with an oxygen concentration between 90% and 96%. The product gas from the concentrator is referred to as oxygen 93% USP (U.S. Pharmacopoeia), oxygen 90+, or oxygen-enriched air.

B. Problems with Oxygen Concentrators

1. **Fires**

Anything that generates heat such as electrical equipment or that could cause an oxygen tubing to rupture could result in a fire.

2. **Water Contamination**

Under normal circumstances, humidity is not a problem. However, very high humidity can lower the oxygen concentration in the product gas.

3. **Device Malfunction**

Device malfunction can occur from restricted air flow, clogged filters, or compressor faults.

4. **Argon Accumulation**

Argon is not trapped by the molecular sieve and is concentrated much the same as oxygen. It can reach concentrations above 5%. If oxygen 93% is added to a circle system used with low fresh gas flows, the argon may accumulate. This has not been found to be a problem if the fresh gas flow is above 0.5 L/minute. There are no known effects from long- or short-term exposure to low concentrations of argon.

V. **Air Compressors**

A. Medical air may be supplied from cylinders, a proportioning device that mixes gas from oxygen and nitrogen cylinders or motor-driven compressors. The vast majority of piped air systems employ two or more compressors that operate alternately or simultaneously, depending on demand.

B. Each compressor takes in ambient air, compressed it to above the working pressure, and supplies it to one or more receivers from which air can be withdrawn as needed. The intake location is important to ensure that the air will be as free of contaminants as possible.

C. To render the air suitable for medical use, its water content must be reduced. An aftercooler in which the air is cooled and the condensed moisture removed is usually installed downstream of each compressor. More water may condense in the receiver or may be removed by running the air through a dryer.

VI. Pipeline Systems

A pipeline system distributes oxygen, nitrous oxide, medical air, carbon dioxide, and nitrogen from their source to the areas where these gases are needed.

A. Components

1. **Supply Sources**

   The supply source for a pipeline system can include cylinders, cryogenic liquid tanks, air compressors, and/or oxygen concentrators. A typical supply system using cylinders is shown in **Figure 1.14.**

2. **Pipeline Distribution System**

   Piped system layouts vary considerably. A typical one is shown in **Figure 1.15.**

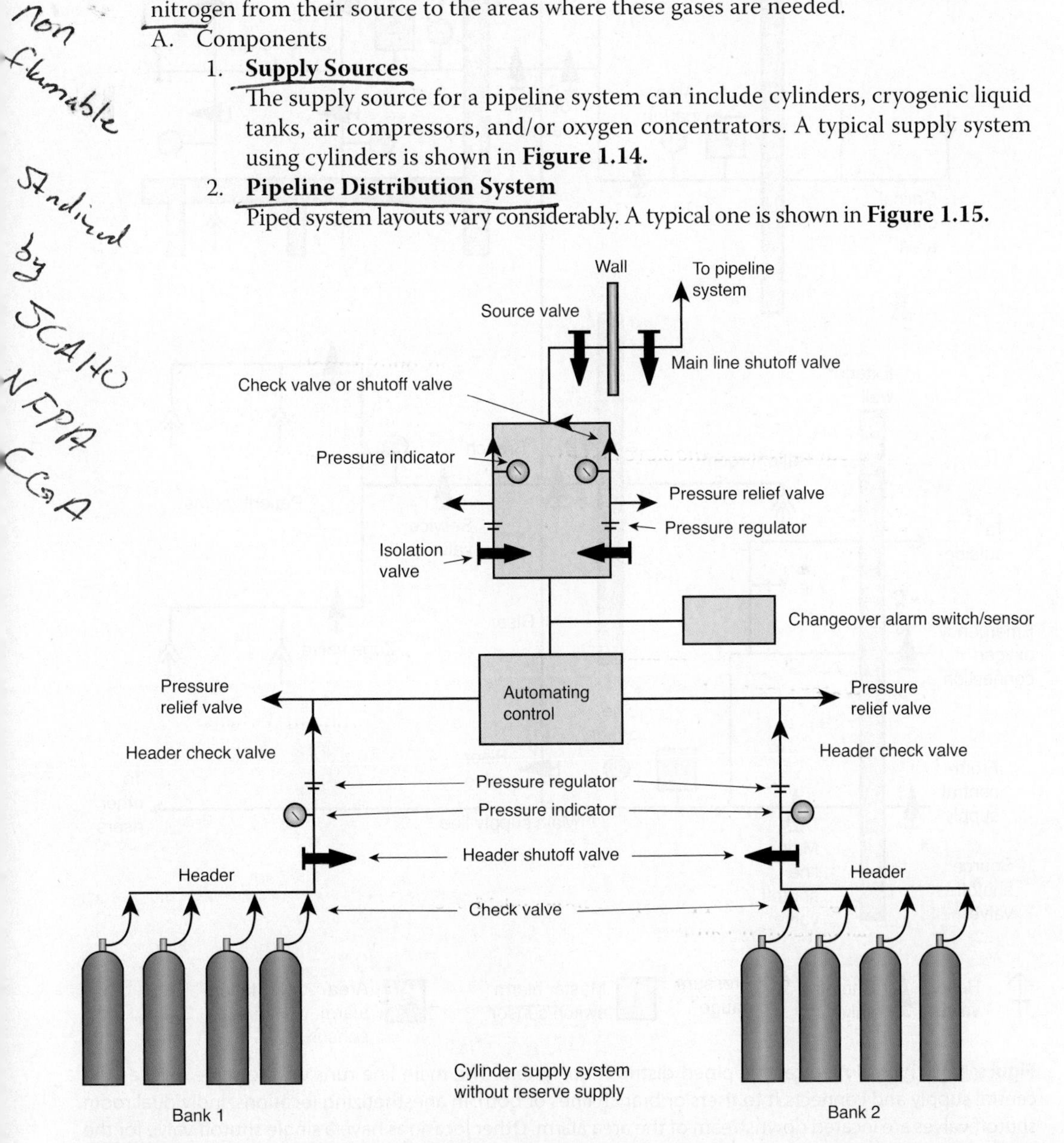

Figure 1.14 Cylinder supply system without reserve supply. This is known as an alternating supply system. The manual shutoff valves permit isolation of either bank of cylinders. Fluctuations in the distribution pressure can be decreased by reducing the pressure in two stages, so a pressure regulator is installed in the outgoing pipe. A manual shutoff valve must be located upstream of and a shutoff or check valve downstream of each pressure regulator. This makes it possible to service the regulator without shutting down the entire system. (Redrawn from a figure in National Fire Protection Association. Standard for Health Care Facilities [NFPA 99]. Quincy, MA: National Fire Protection Association, 2005.)

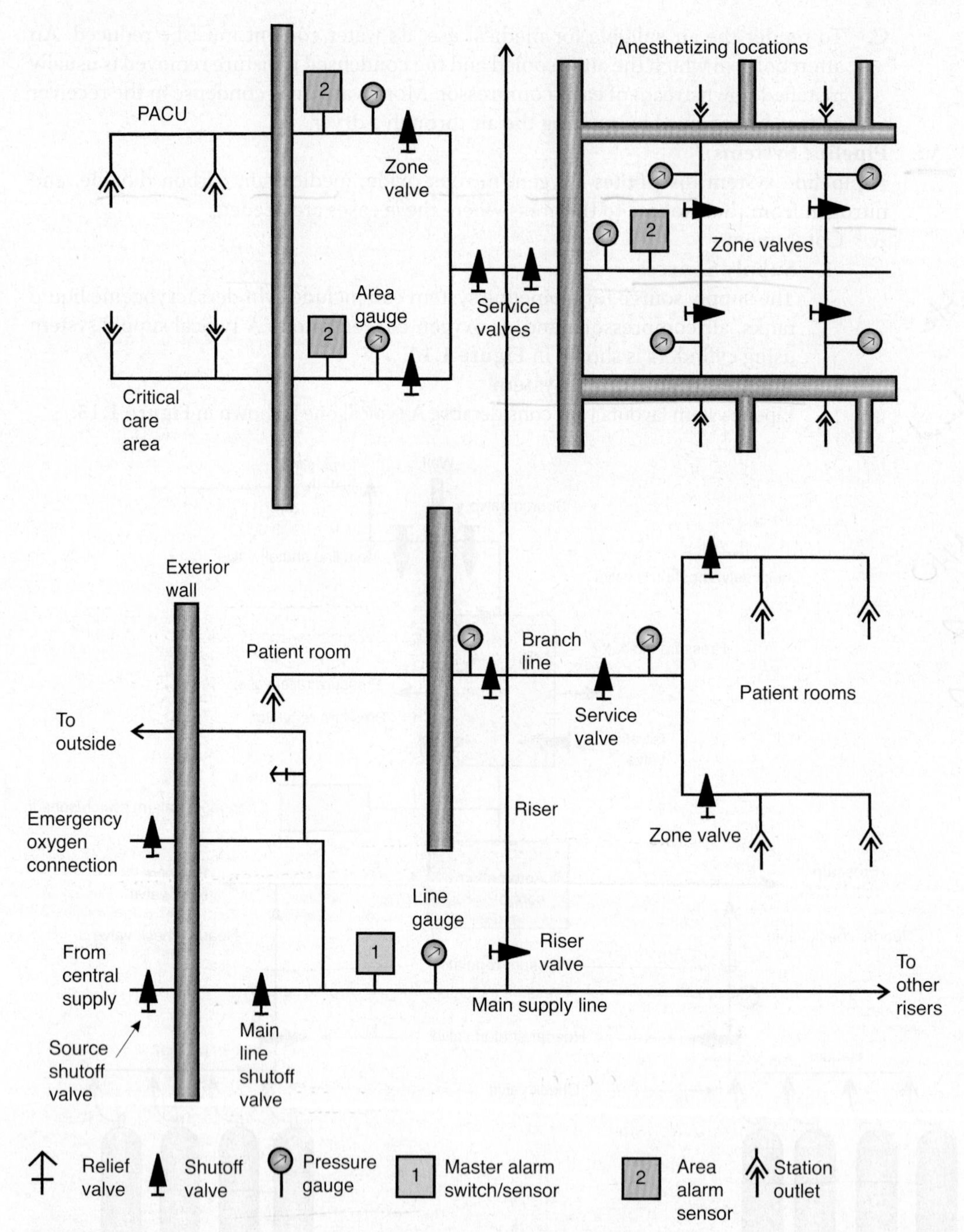

Figure 1.15 Typical medical gas piped distribution system. The main line runs on the same level as the central supply and connects it to risers or branch lines or both. In anesthetizing locations, individual room shutoff valves are located downstream of the area alarm. Other locations have a single shutoff valve for the entire area with the area alarm actuator downstream from the shutoff valve. The master alarm is activated by a 20% increase or decrease in the main line pressure. Area alarms must be installed in branch lines leading to intensive care units, postanesthesia care units (PACUs), and anesthetizing locations to signal if the pressure increases or decreases by 20% from normal operating pressure. (Redrawn from a figure in National Fire Protection Association. Standard for Health Care Facilities [NFPA 99]. Quincy, MA: National Fire Protection Association, 2005.)

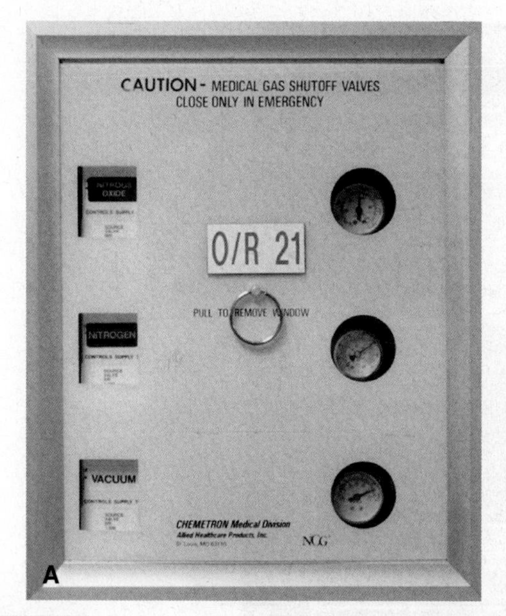

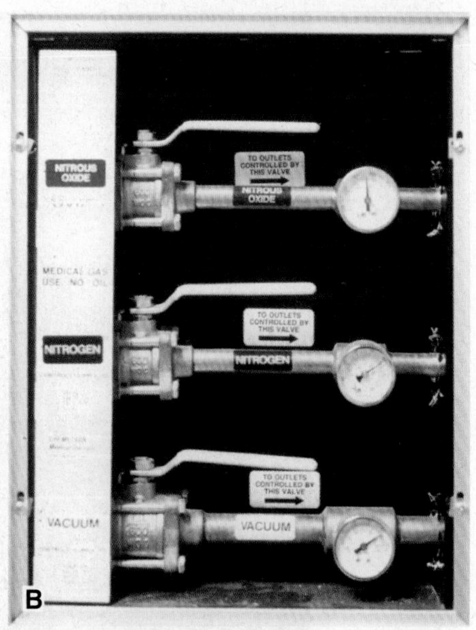

Figure 1.16 **A:** Box with shutoff valves. The window can be easily removed by pulling the ring in the center. Note that the operating room controlled by the shutoff valves is identified. **B:** Box with cover removed. To close a valve, the handle is pulled a quarter turn. Note that the pipes are labeled to show the gases contained. The front cover cannot be installed if a valve is closed.

3. **Shutoff Valves**

   There are various shutoff valves that allow the system to be maintained, added onto, or shut off in the event of an emergency. Shutoff valves for each operating room are usually located just outside the rooms that they control. They are usually in a box with a plastic cover that can be easily removed (see **Fig. 1.16**).

4. **Alarms**

   Area alarms that warn of pipeline failure or decreased pipeline pressure are situated in critical areas throughout the facility (**Fig. 1.17**).

5. **Pressure gauges**

   Pressure gauges are located downstream of shutoff valves and on all anesthesia machines. Those on the anesthesia machines should be periodically checked for adequate pipeline pressure.

CLINICAL MOMENT Anesthesia providers need to know the location and functioning of all shutoff valves, alarm panels, and pressure gauges. Your knowledge may be checked by facility credentialing agencies.

6. **Terminal Units**

   Terminal units are the points in the operating room where anesthesia machines and other equipment are connected to the pipeline system. There are two types of gas-specific terminal units: the Diameter Index Safety System (DISS) and quick connectors.

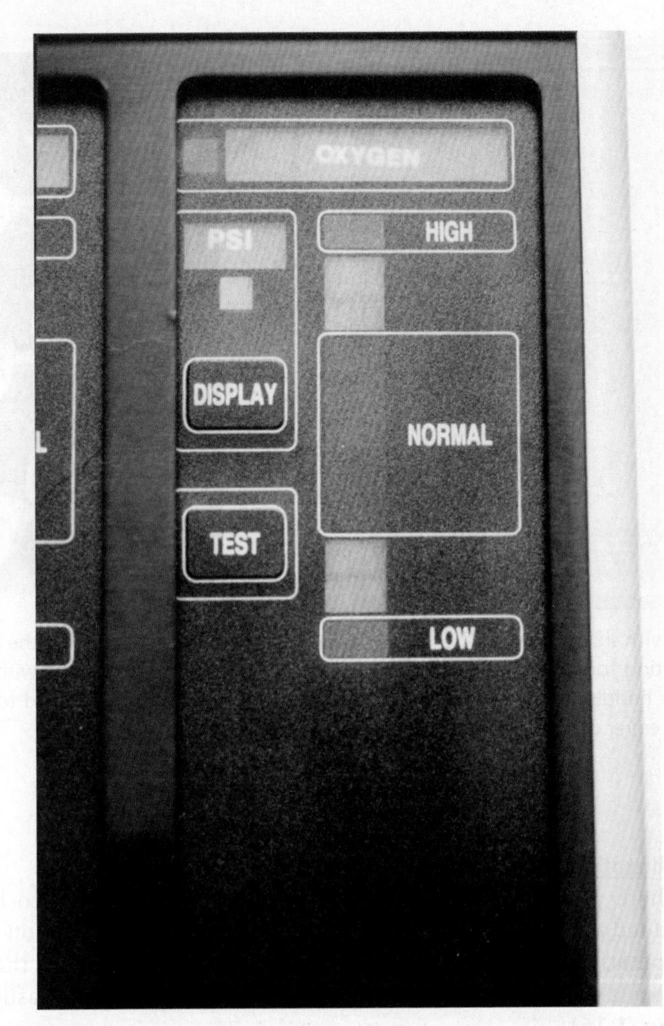

Figure 1.17 Part of area (local) alarm panel. The gas pressure is monitored and a warning is provided if the pressure increases or decreases from the normal operating pressure. A button for testing the alarm is provided. Area alarm systems are provided for anesthetizing locations and other vital life-support areas such as the postanesthesia care, intensive care, and coronary care units.

a. Diameter Index Safety System DISS

The Diameter Index Safety System was developed to provide noninterchangeable connections for medical gas lines at pressures of 1380 kPa (200 psi) or less. As shown in **Figure 1.18,** each DISS connector consists of a body, nipple, and nut combination. There are two concentric and specific bores in the body and two concentric and specific shoulders on the nipple. To achieve noninterchangeability between different connectors, the two diameters on each part vary in opposite directions so that as one diameter increases, the other diameter decreases. Only properly mated parts will fit together and allow the threads to engage. This system is used to connect gas hoses to each anesthesia machine. It may also be used to connect the hoses to the pipeline system.

b. Quick Connectors

Quick connectors (**Fig. 1.19**) allow apparatus (hoses, flowmeters, etc.) to be connected or disconnected by a single action using one or both hands without the use of tools or undue force. The style and method of ensuring

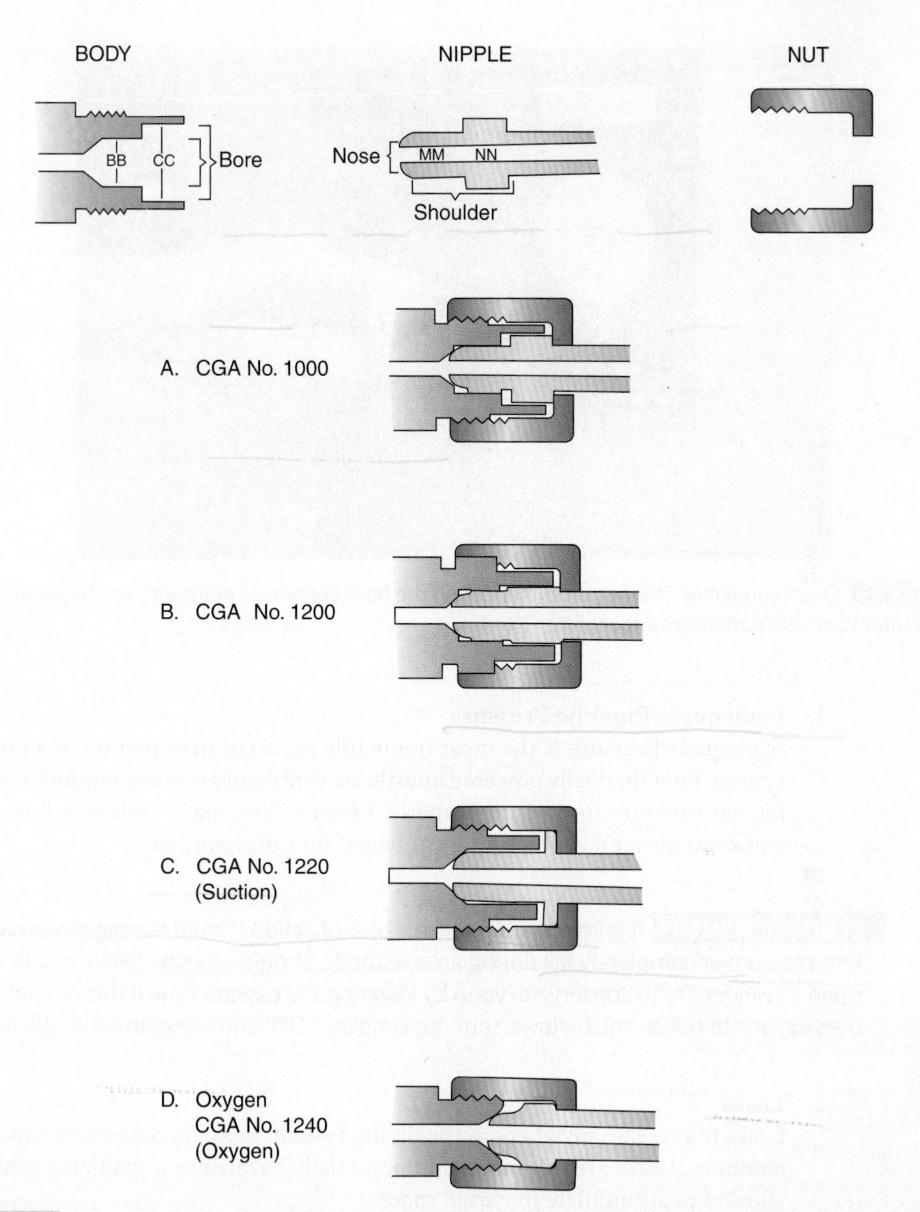

Figure 1.18 Diameter Index Safety System. With increasing Compressed Gas Association (CGA) number, the small shoulder (MM) of the nipple becomes larger and the large diameter becomes smaller. If assembly of a nonmating body and nipple is attempted, either MM will be too large for small bore (BB) or large shoulder (NN) will be too large for large bore (CC). (Redrawn courtesy of the Compressed Gas Association.)

noninterchangeability between gases vary with the manufacturer. Quick connectors are more convenient than DISS fittings but tend to leak more.

c. Face Plate

The face plate holds the female DISS or quick-connect component of the noninterchangeable connection. It should be permanently marked with the name and/or symbol of the gas that it conveys. The identifying color may also be present.

B. Problems with Piping Systems

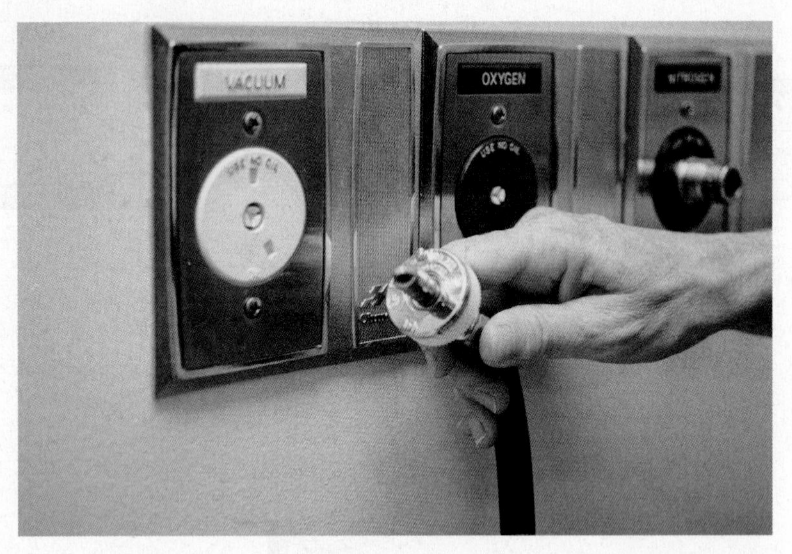

Figure 1.19 Quick connector. The two prominences on the hose connector mate with the two slots on the wall outlet to ensure noninterchangeability.

1. **Inadequate Pipeline Pressure**
   Inadequate pressure is the most frequently reported malfunction of a pipeline system. Pneumatically powered anesthesia ventilators require a minimum driving gas pressure to operate properly. Pressure loss may result in a flow inadequate to power a ventilator but sufficient for other purposes.

CLINICAL MOMENT It is important to have a plan of action should the pipeline system lose pressure or completely fail during an anesthetic. Should pipeline failure occur, open a cylinder. Try to conserve oxygen by lowering the oxygen flow. If the ventilator uses oxygen to power the bellows, turn the ventilator OFF and use manual ventilation.

2. **Leaks**
   Leaks may occur anywhere in the piping system. Leaks in outlets are especially common. Leaks are expensive and potentially hazardous if oxidizing gases are allowed to accumulate in closed spaces.
3. **Excessive Pressure**
   Excessive pressure can cause damage to equipment and barotrauma to patients. Some ventilators will not operate properly if the line pressure is too high.

CLINICAL MOMENT When excessive pipeline pressure occurs, it is best to disconnect apparatus from the pipeline system and use cylinders until the problem is corrected.

4. **Alarm Problems**
   Failure, absence, or disconnection of an alarm is common. The alarm may not be heard or the person who hears it may not know the proper course of action or fail to respond. The anesthesia machine will annunciate an alarm if

the pipeline or cylinder pressure fails. Repeated false alarms can cause complacency among personnel, which may have serious consequences if a real emergency occurs.

5. **Gas Cross Connection**

   Although an uncommon event, accidental substitution of one gas for another can have devastating consequences. The most frequent crossovers are associated with alterations to the piping system. Most crossovers have been between nitrous oxide and oxygen, but various other combinations have been reported. Crossovers could occur if the hoses to the anesthesia machine have incorrect connections on either end. Face plates or terminal units may be incorrect. Pipeline alarms indicate only pressure faults and give no signal that an incorrect gas is present. The oxygen monitor on the anesthesia machine should be used to detect cross connections. Oxygen monitors should be used in other areas where oxygen is administrated such as obstetrics, the nursery, and intensive care units.

CLINICAL MOMENT If the oxygen monitor is not showing the expected oxygen concentration as judged from the flows on the flowmeters, what would you do? (A) Turn OFF the nitrous oxide. (B) Assume that the oxygen monitor is incorrect. (C) Disconnect the central gas supply and open the oxygen tank.

Turning OFF the nitrous oxide flowmeter would allow pure nitrous oxide to flow through the oxygen flowmeter if the lines were crossed. A well-serviced oxygen analyzer is rarely incorrect. The best course is to go to cylinder supply until the nature of the problem is determined. If the problem is a crossover in the anesthesia machine, it is best to ventilate the patient using a separate cylinder and a resuscitation bag until the machine can be replaced.

6. **Gas Contamination**

   a. Various types of contaminants can be found in the pipeline system, including particulate matter remaining after construction, cleaning solvents and other volatile liquids, bacteria, and water. Currently, no available monitor can detect the entire spectrum of potential contaminants.

CLINICAL MOMENT If contamination of piped gases is suspected, a switch to cylinder supply should be made and the anesthesia machine disconnected from the pipeline. If the pipeline is not disconnected, the machine will continue to use gas from the pipeline, even though the cylinder valve is open.

   b. Filters can be used in equipment to prevent contaminants such as particles, bacteria, and liquid water from entering the apparatus and harming attached medical devices and patients (**Fig. 1.20**). These filters are usually too coarse to contain small contaminants and are not useful for volatile liquids or gases.

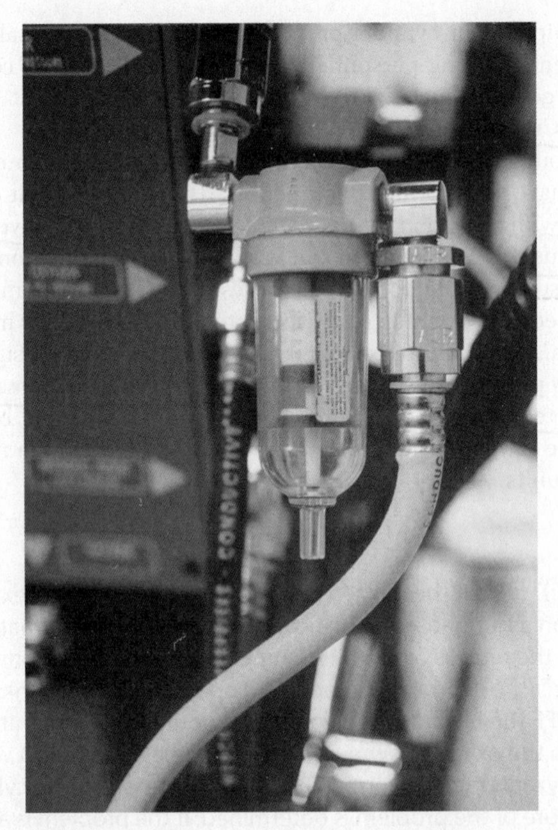

Figure 1.20 Water trap with drain and filter in the air hose leading to the anesthesia machine.

REFERENCE

1. McLachlan JK, Campkin N. Medical gas misconnection. Anaesthesia 2006;61:1228.

SUGGESTED READINGS

Anderson WR, Brock-Utne JG. Oxygen pipeline supply failure: a coping strategy. J Clin Monit 1991;7:39–41.

Anonymous. Medical gas safety; Read the labels! They're the only sure identifier of gas cylinder contents. Health Devices. 2001;30(3):87–89.

Dorsch J, Dorsch S. Medical gas cylinders and containers. In: Understanding Anesthesia Equipment. Fifth edition. Philadelphia: Wolters Kluwer/Lippincott Williams & Wilkins, 2008:1–24.

Dorsch J, Dorsch S. Medical gas pipeline systems. In: Understanding Anesthesia Equipment. Fifth edition. Philadelphia: Wolters Kluwer/Lippincott Williams & Wilkins, 2008:25–50.

Dorsch J, Dorsch S. Oxygen concentrators. In: Understanding Anesthesia Equipment. Fifth edition. Philadelphia: Wolters Kluwer/Lippincott Williams & Wilkins, 2008:76–81.

Friesen RM. Oxygen concentrators and the practice of anaesthesia. Can J Anaesth 1992;39:R80–R84.

Friesen RM, Raber MB, Reimer DH. Oxygen concentrators; a primary oxygen supply source. Can J Anesth 1999;46:1185–1190.

Klemenzson G, Perouansky M. Contemporary anesthesia ventilators incur a significant "oxygen cost." Can J Anesth 2004; 51:616–620.

Lorraway PG, Savoldelli GL, Joo HS, et al. Management of simulated oxygen supply failure: is there a gap in the curriculum? Anesth Analg 2006;102:865–867.

Peterson TG, Evans F. Shutdown of gas supply system need not be danger. APSF Newslett 1994;9(3):32–34.

Petty WC. Medical gases, hospital pipelines and medical gas cylinders: how safe are they? AANA J 1995;63:307–312.

Weller J, Merry A, Warman G, Robinson B. Anaesthetists' management of oxygen pipeline failure: room for improvement. Anaesthesia 2007;62:122–126.

2 Suction Equipment

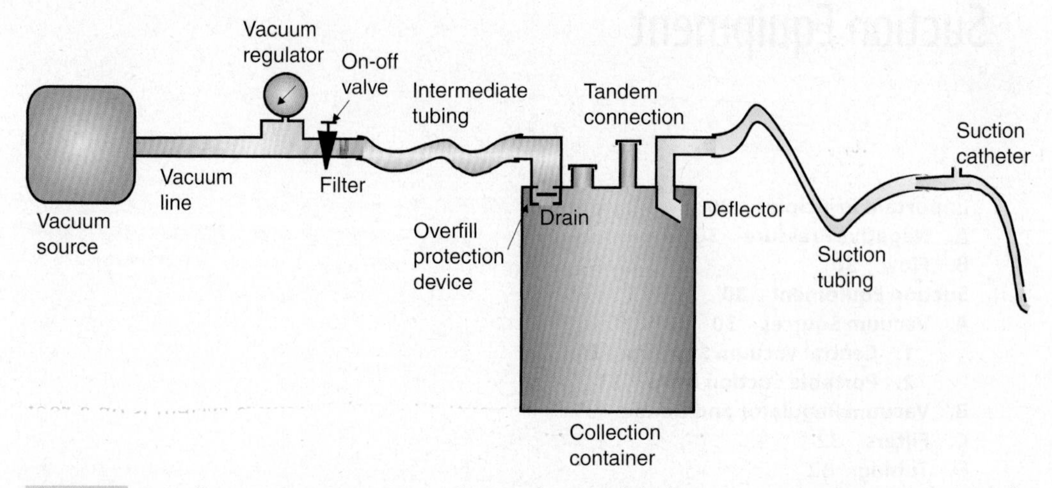

Figure 2.1 Complete suction system. Normally, liquids and solids do not move any farther than the collection container. Note the deflector on the collection container.

SUCTION SYSTEMS ARE USED TO remove and/or collect solids, gases, and liquids from the patient, the breathing system, and the environment. A complete suction apparatus is shown in **Figure 2.1.**

I. Important Principles

A. Negative Pressure

1. "Vacuum" will be used in this chapter to denote a pressure less than atmospheric (negative pressure). "Suction" (mechanical aspiration) is the movement of gases, liquids, or solids caused by vacuum.
2. Vacuum is usually stated in gauge pressure, the difference between the measured pressure and ambient atmospheric pressure (which is zero on the gauge). Pressure is the amount of force acting on a given area. **Table 2.1** gives some commonly used pressure units.

B. Flow

1. All suction equipment from the source to the patient connection can be thought of as a tube of varying diameter. When a vacuum source is attached and turned ON, flow through the equipment will occur. The rate of flow will depend on the pressure difference between the ends of the tube and the resistance to flow. To ensure good flow, the maximum vacuum and the shortest possible length of tubing should be used, the internal diameter of tubings, connectors, and the suction catheter should be as large as possible, and the vacuum system should

Table 2.1 Pressure Equivalents

Unit	kPa	Inches Hg	mm Hg	cm H_2O
1 kPa	1	0.295	7.501	111.5
1 inch Hg	3.386	1	25.4	330
1 mm Hg	0.1333	0.004	1	0.77
1 cm H_2O	1.73	0.052	13	1

not leak. Increasing the number of intakes will result in a decrease in vacuum and flow at each intake.

2. Flow through suction apparatus is also affected by the physical characteristics (elasticity, viscosity, adhesion, and cohesion) of the material being suctioned. Water or saline drawn through a suction catheter before use may act as a lubricant and improve flow. After material enters the collection container, it no longer causes resistance to flow.

II. Suction Equipment

A. Vacuum Sources

1. **Central Vacuum Systems**

   Healthcare facilities usually have a central vacuum system. This consists of vacuum pumps that supply a piping system that extends into patient care areas where suction will be needed. The outlet from the vacuum system is on a roof or other area where it is not likely to come in contact with personnel.

2. **Portable Suction Units**

   Portable suction units are used in places where a central system is not available. These are electrically or manually powered and contain all the parts necessary to perform suction.

B. Vacuum Regulator and Gauge

To regulate the amount and type of suction required, a vacuum regulator, a gauge, and ON and OFF controls are needed (**Fig. 2.2**). An ON/OFF switch may be located on the anesthesia machine.

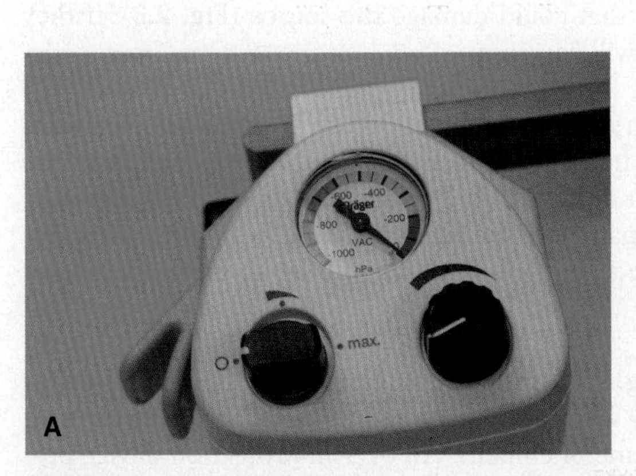

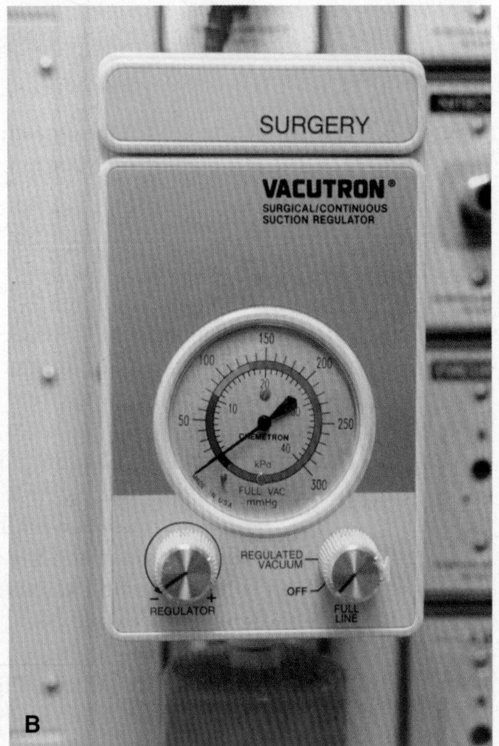

Figure 2.2 Vacuum regulators and gauges. Note that the indicator on the gauge may move counterclockwise **(A)** or clockwise **(B)**.

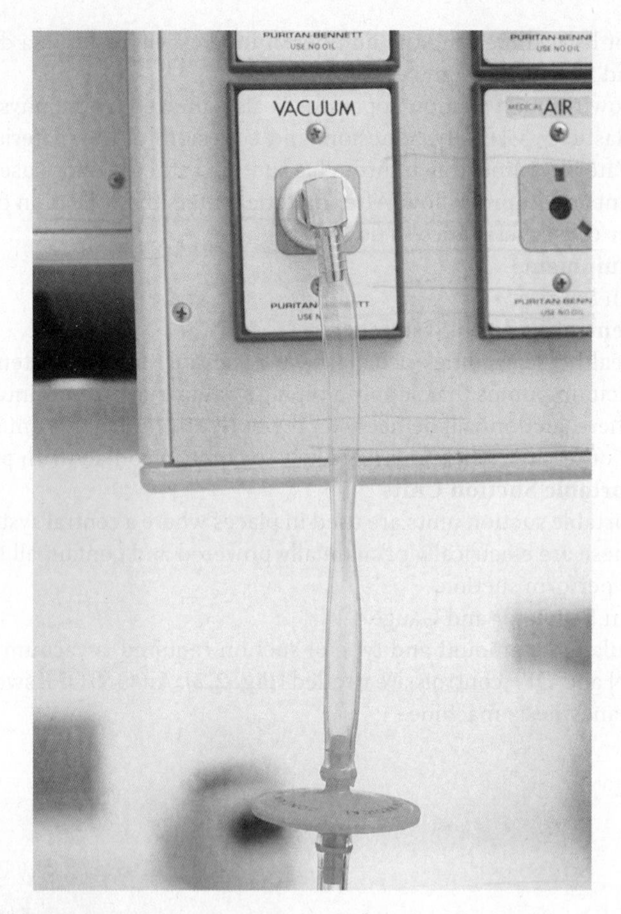

Figure 2.3 A filter will help to protect the vacuum source from liquids or solids.

C. Filters

Filters are used between the collection container and the vacuum source to remove any liquids or particulate matter that could damage the source (**Fig. 2.3**). If they become wet or dirty, the vacuum will decrease.

D. Tubing

There are two pieces of tubing in a suction system unless the collection bottle is directly attached to the pipeline inlet. The intermediate tubing extends from the wall to the collection container. It does not transfer any liquids or solids. Between the collection container and the patient is the suction tubing, which transfers liquids and solids. It is best to have a long intermediate tubing and a short suction tubing whenever possible.

E. Collection Container

1. The collection container (**Fig. 2.4**) is the repository for the liquids and solids that are removed. It is usually wholly or partially disposable. There is a scale on the side to measure the volume of effluent. An overfill protection device prevents effluent from entering the intermediate tubing (**Fig. 2.5**).

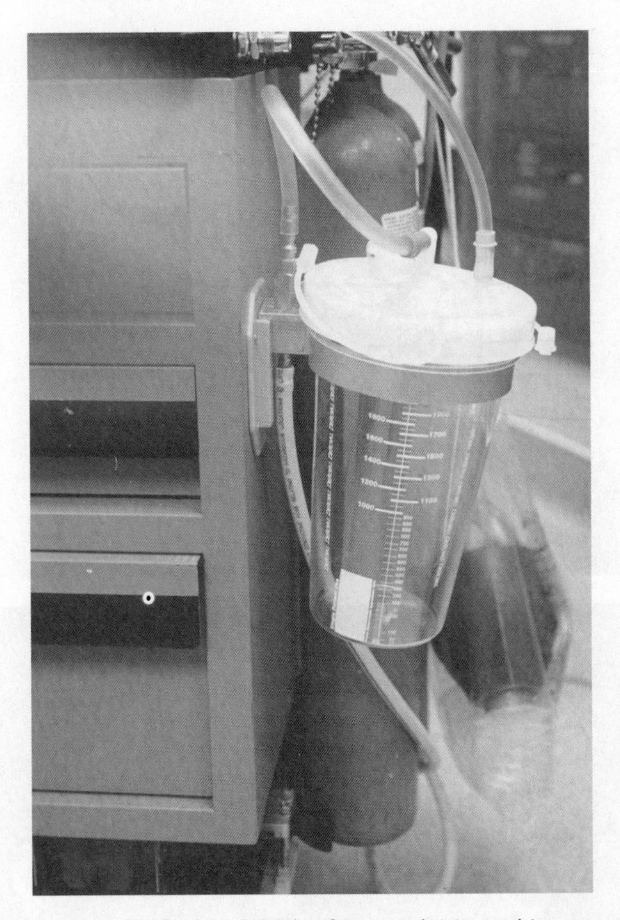

Figure 2.4 Collection container attached to the side of an anesthesia machine.

2. The location of the collection container is important. It should be close to the point of use and placed where it is unlikely to be tipped or cause tripping. An advantage of having it lower than the patient is that gravity helps to remove liquids and solids. If it is located higher than the patient, it may be easier to observe but more negative pressure will be required to lift materials into the container. An additional problem with a higher location is that if the vacuum is interrupted, fluid in the suction tubing could return to the patient.
3. There are no firm guidelines as to when the collection container should be changed. In busy operating rooms, the container is usually changed between cases if it was used. In outpatient and office surgical procedures, the canister is often changed when full or at the end of the day.

F. Suction Catheters

1. **Catheter Types**

   There are two general types of suction catheters: flexible and rigid.

   a. Flexible Catheters

   A flexible catheter is especially useful for suctioning through a tube. There is usually an opening to atmosphere that can be controlled by the user to alter or release the suction. There are a number of different style tips on

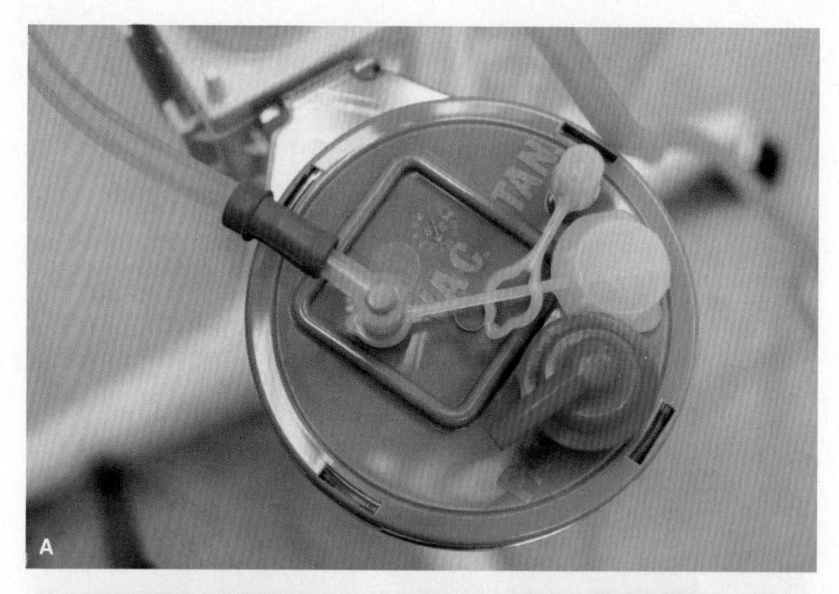

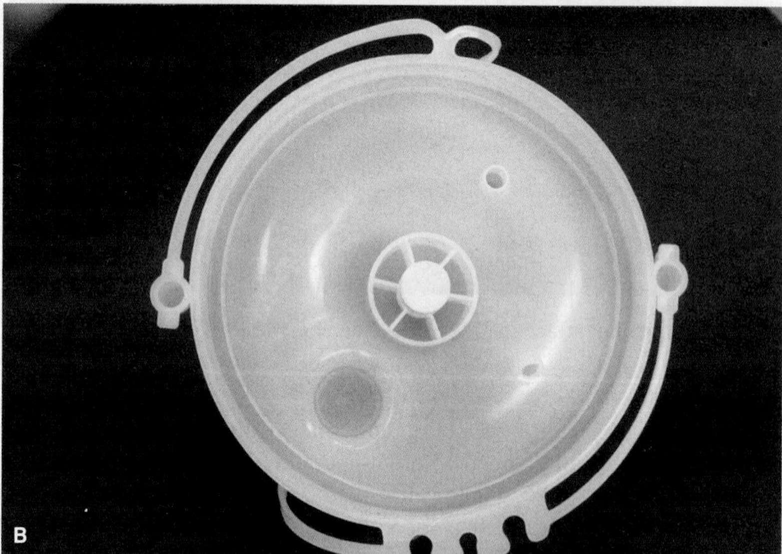

Figure 2.5 Lid for collection container. **A:** There are two ports the red one is to receive suction from the patient and the other is for connecting the suction bottle to another in tandem. The large port between the suction ports is for emptying the container. **B:** The underside of the lid. The overfill protection device is in the center.

these catheters (**Fig. 2.6**). Curved tips are useful to direct the catheter into a specific orifice.

b. Rigid Suction Catheters

The rigid (Yankauer) suction catheter (**Fig. 2.7**) is useful for removing solids and liquids from the mouth or other open space. Its rigidity allows good tip control. There is a guard over the patient end to prevent it being closed by tissue.

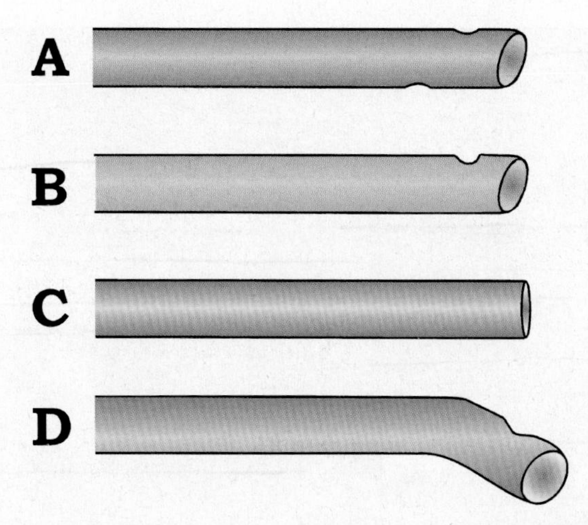

Figure 2.6 Flexible suction catheter tips. **A:** The whistle tip catheter has two side holes, usually perpendicular to each other. **B:** Tip with a single side hole. **C:** Tip with a single end hold and no side holes. **D:** A curved (Coude) tip is often used for bronchial suctioning.

c. Closed Suction Catheters
Closed suction catheters are used primarily in critical care areas where suctioning may need to be performed frequently. The catheter (**Fig. 2.8**) is flexible and can be retracted into a plastic sheath to prevent contamination between uses.

2. **Catheter Sizes**
Suction catheters are sized by the external diameter and shaft length, both in millimeters. For closed-system catheters, the marked length is the length that can be inserted into the patient's airway. The outside diameter may also be expressed in French gauge (Charriere) size, which is three times the external diameter in millimeters.

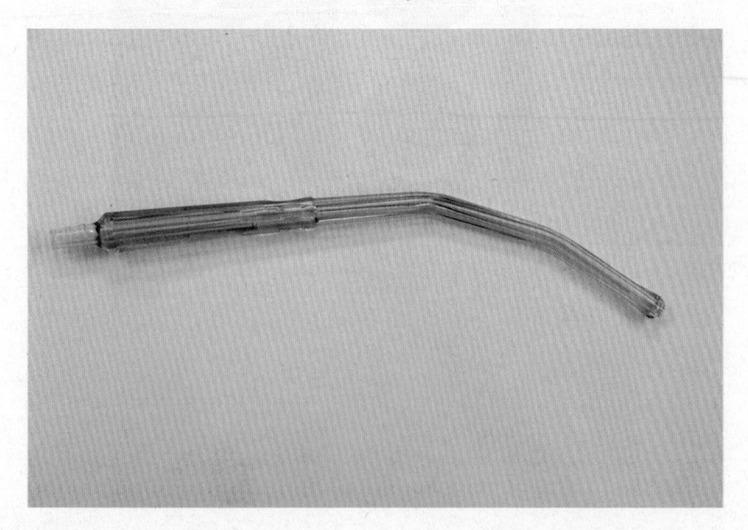

Figure 2.7 Yankauer suction catheter. Most Yankauer suction catheters have a single hole and several eyes near the tip. Some have finger vents.

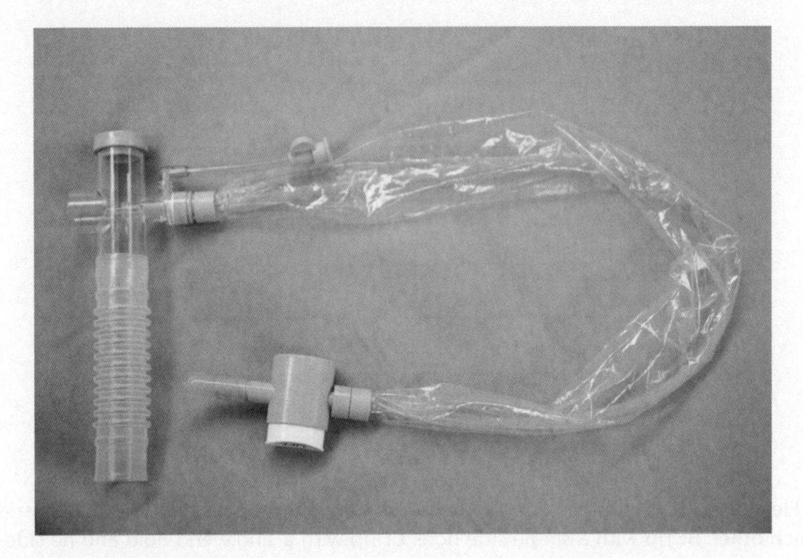

Figure 2.8 Closed suction catheter.

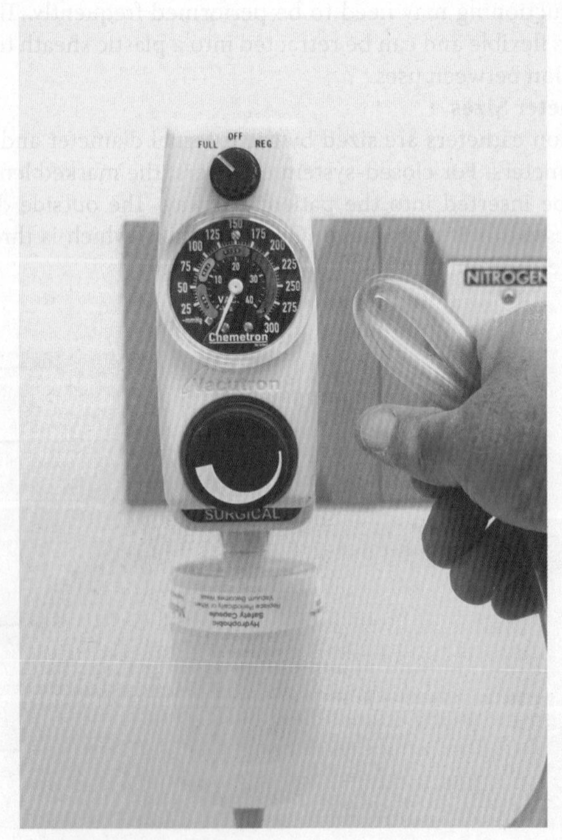

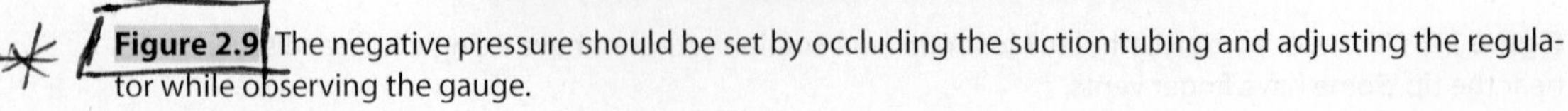

Figure 2.9 The negative pressure should be set by occluding the suction tubing and adjusting the regulator while observing the gauge.

III. Suctioning Techniques

The catheter should be large enough to remove secretions rapidly but not block the airway. Catheter size is especially important if the catheter is placed inside a tracheal or tracheostomy tube. Smaller catheters allow more air to be entrained around the catheter, limiting the negative pressure that is applied to the lungs. Thin, copious secretions can usually be removed with a relatively small catheter, whereas thick, tenacious secretions require a larger one.

The first step is to set the maximum negative pressure. Before adjusting this pressure, the regulator outlet must be occluded. This can be done either by placing a finger over the collection container intake or by crimping the suction tubing (**Fig 2.9**). The gauge will then register the maximum vacuum that can be generated at that setting.

CLINICAL MOMENT When not in use, the vacuum source should be turned OFF or the suction tubing kinked (**Fig. 2.10**) to reduce the load on the system and improve the pressure and flow available at other inlets. It also prevents dust and debris from being suctioned into the regulator and other equipment. Kinking the suction tubing allows maximum vacuum to be quickly restored.

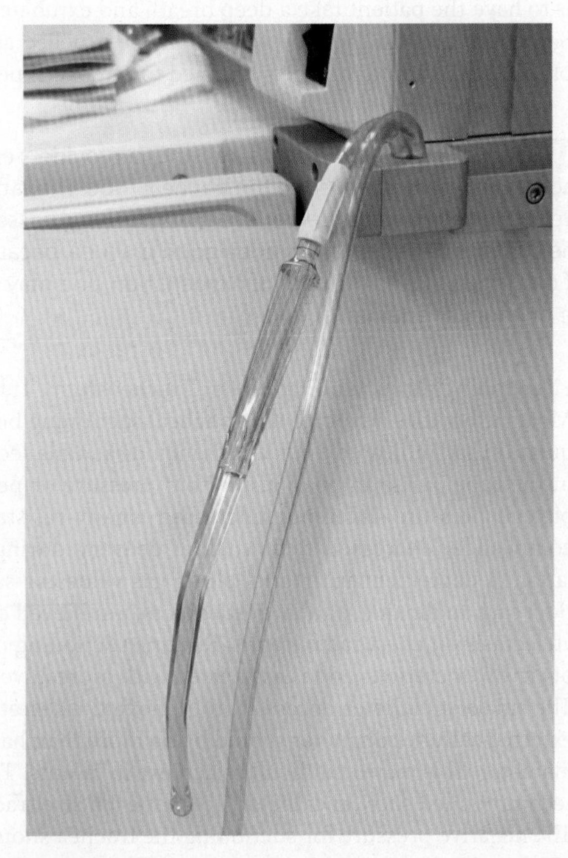

Figure 2.10 Keeping the suction tubing kinked when not in use will allow maximum vacuum to be restored quickly. It also reduces the strain on the vacuum system.

A. Mouth and Pharyngeal Suctioning
1. Either a rigid or flexible catheter may be used. A 14 to 18 size is usually used for adults.
2. A flexible catheter can be inserted through a nasopharyngeal or oropharyngeal airway. The external surface of the catheter should first be thoroughly lubricated.
3. If the teeth are clenched, it may be possible to insert the catheter laterally behind the last molar or where teeth are missing.
4. While most fluids in the mouth and pharynx are easily removed, water may need to be instilled to remove a large amount of blood or vomitus.
5. Suctioning through the nasal cavity without a nasal airway in place may result in epistaxis.
6. The vacuum control on the catheter should be open while inserting the catheter. The catheter should be withdrawn slowly with a twisting motion while intermittently occluding the vacuum control.

B. Suctioning Associated with Extubation
1. Prior to extubation, secretions in the mouth and pharynx should be removed. This can be accomplished with the same catheter that was used for tracheal tube suctioning.
2. After oropharyngeal suctioning, the tracheal tube cuff should be deflated and the tube removed while applying continuous positive pressure. An alternative is to have the patient take a deep breath and extubate at the end of inspiration. Secretions around the tube will usually be expelled as the patient exhales. The oropharynx should then be suctioned to remove expelled secretions.

CLINICAL MOMENT In the past, some anesthesia providers extubated the patient while suction was being applied to the tracheal tube. The rationale behind this maneuver was to remove any secretions that may have passed into the trachea when the cuff was deflated. This is not a good practice, because it depletes the lungs of oxygen, removes the path of oxygenation, and may result in negative pressure pulmonary edema.

C. Open Suctioning through a Tracheal or Tracheostomy Tube
1. Most authorities advocate that tracheal suctioning be performed no more frequently than indicated. Indications include audible secretions, secretions visible in the tube, a rise in peak inspiratory pressure or peak inspiratory pressure–plateau pressure difference, increased airway resistance, decreased dynamic compliance, decreased tidal volume delivery during pressure-limited ventilation, a decrement in arterial blood gas values or saturation, increased end-tidal carbon dioxide, patient restlessness, unrelieved coughing, and evidence of atelectasis on chest radiographs. Routine suctioning may stimulate production of airway secretions and is associated with more adverse effects.
2. The smallest catheter necessary to remove the secretions should be used. The external catheter diameter should be no more than half the inside tracheal tube diameter. This may be difficult to achieve in infants. Table 2.2 shows the largest recommended suction catheter sizes for each size tracheal tube.
3. The negative pressure for suctioning the trachea should be no more than 70 to 150 mm Hg (9.3 to 20 kPa, 50 to 115 cm H_2O) in adults. For infants, the negative pressure should be no more than 60 to 80 mm Hg (8.0 to 10.7 kPa). When

Table 2.2 Maximum Recommended Suction Catheters

Tracheal Tube Size	Suction Catheter Size (French)
5.0	8
6.0	8
7.0	10
8.0	12
9.0	14

copious or viscous secretions are present, it may be necessary to increase the vacuum to allow more effective removal.

4. Normal saline, water, or water-soluble jelly may be used to lubricate the outside of the catheter prior to insertion. Drawing water or saline through a catheter before use may improve flow and checks catheter patency.
5. Hyperoxygenation, hyperventilation, and hyperinflation prior to and following suctioning will help prevent hypoxemia, as will oxygen insufflation during the procedure.
6. Instilling saline into the tracheal tube before suctioning to dilute secretions or generate a cough is controversial. It should have little effect on clearing secretions, because mucus and water are immiscible. An exception may be postoperative head and neck surgery patients who often have bloody secretions.

CLINICAL MOMENT The saline used to flush intravenous lines or intravenous normal saline solutions should not be instilled into the trachea because the preservative may burn lung tissue.

7. There are a number of possible negative consequences to instilling saline into the trachea. It can dislodge bacteria or secretions from the tracheal tube wall and wash them into the lower airways. Vials are frequently contaminated during opening. Irrigation fluid may pool in the swivel and ventilator connectors, causing saline to mix with bacteria in this area. Subsequent procedures such as turning the patient or lowering the head may cause contaminated fluid to enter the patient's lower airways. Instilling saline may cause hypoxemia and have an adverse effect on patient comfort. Another concern is more environmental contamination due to increased splashing.
8. A suction catheter used for tracheal suctioning can also be used for oral and pharyngeal suctioning. A catheter that has been used for suctioning in the upper airway should be discarded and a new, sterile catheter touched only with a sterile glove used if tracheal suctioning is needed.
9. The catheter should be inserted with a smooth, gentle motion, without force and without applying negative pressure. The tracheal tube should be handled carefully to avoid coughing and straining.
10. If deep suctioning (entering a mainstem bronchus) is not needed, the catheter should be passed just beyond the end of the tracheal tube (**Fig. 2.11**). If the catheter is inserted too far, mucosal trauma is more likely. If insertion is too shallow, secretions in the tube may not be cleared. The best way to determine how far to insert the catheter is to place the suction catheter next to another

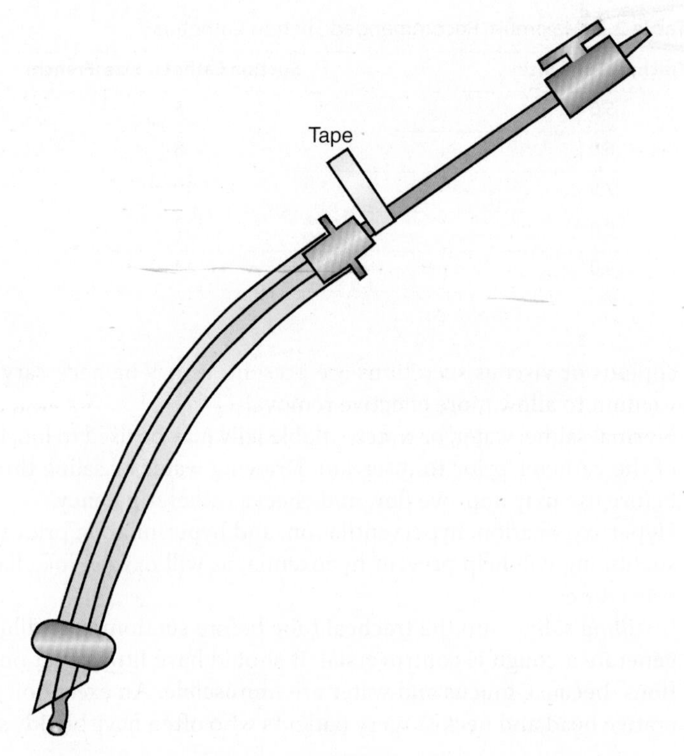

Figure 2.11 Unless deep suctioning is needed, the suction catheter should extend only just beyond the end of the tracheal tube. Placing a piece of tape on the suction catheter will prevent deep insertion.

tracheal tube of the same size. If the length from the patient end is marked on the catheter, this scale can be used to determine the correct depth to insert the catheter. If resistance is met during catheter insertion, the catheter should be withdrawn 0.5 cm before suction is applied to avoid invaginating the mucosa into the catheter.

11. After the catheter is inserted, suctioning should begin immediately. Most authors recommend that the vacuum control be closed intermittently while the catheter is withdrawn, although some recommend continuous suctioning. The catheter may be rotated gently during withdrawal. It should not be jabbed up and down. If the operator feels resistance during withdrawal, the vacuum control should be opened immediately.
12. The catheter should be in the tube no longer than necessary and never more than 10 to 15 seconds in adults. Shorter times should be used for pediatric patients.

CLINICAL MOMENT A convenient way to dispose of the catheter is to coil it, pull off the glove with the catheter inside, and dispose of both as a unit.

CLINICAL MOMENT If hyperoxygenation is used to avoid hypoxia during suctioning, it is important to turn the oxygen down to the previous level at the conclusion of suctioning.

IV. Hazards Associated with Suctioning

A. Hypoxemia

Arterial oxygen saturation decreases during tracheal suctioning and for some time afterward. Children desaturate more quickly than adults. The amount of desaturation depends on the suctioning duration and whether ventilation is continued during suctioning. The size of the catheter in relation to the size of the tracheal tube and the amount of negative pressure are also factors. The drop in oxygen saturation is more severe and persistent with pressure-controlled ventilation than with volume-controlled ventilation.

A number of maneuvers have been recommended to prevent hypoxemia associated with suctioning. These may be used separately or in combination.

1. **Maintaining Ventilation**

   If suctioning is performed during artificial ventilation, the drop in oxygenation is less. This can be accomplished by using special adaptors, closed-system suctioning, or high-frequency jet ventilation through a channel in the tracheal tube wall.

2. **Hyperoxygenation**

   a. Hypoxemia can be avoided or attenuated by administering oxygen at an FIO_2 greater than the patient was receiving. In adults, this is usually with an FIO_2 close to 100%, although 20% above maintenance is adequate in most cases. In newborns, an FIO_2 10% to 20% above baseline is recommended.

   b. Insufflation can be accomplished by using a suction catheter or a tracheal tube with an extra lumen that allows continuous oxygen delivery. This can be an effective method of avoiding or minimizing hypoxemia. A high oxygen flow should be used.

3. **Hyperinflation**

   a. Hyperinflation (inflation of the lungs with a volume greater than baseline tidal volume) before or after suctioning when used in conjunction with hyperoxygenation may be effective in maintaining PaO_2. Hyperinflation without hyperoxygenation does not consistently prevent hypoxemia. There is a progressive improvement in oxygenation with increasing volume. Up to 1.5 times the baseline tidal volume has been recommended. Another recommendation is a peak pressure that is 10% to 20% above baseline tidal volume, triggering preset sighs on a ventilator equipped with this feature, or manually hyperinflating with a resuscitation bag. The use of a ventilator is usually superior to the resuscitation bag. It is also more efficient, as it requires only one person and no additional equipment. Most manual resuscitation bags are not attached to a spirometer, so there is no way to accurately measure volumes.

   b. Hyperinflation can result in patient discomfort, cardiovascular disturbances, and barotrauma. It could propel secretions farther into the airway. For these reasons, each patient should be assessed individually to determine the need for hyperinflation and the appropriate volume. If saturation drops despite hyperoxygenation, hyperinflation should be added and the changes in SpO_2 and other parameters assessed. Hyperinflation should be avoided when intracranial pressure is a concern and used with caution in unstable cardiac patients.

4. **Hyperventilation**

   Hyperventilation, an increase in ventilation above baseline, is often performed before or after suctioning. Because of inconsistent tidal volume delivery with a manual resuscitation bag, it is recommended that a ventilator be used. Hyperventilation is often used in conjunction with hyperoxygenation. It should be used with caution in head-injured patients.

5. **Limiting the Duration of Suctioning**
The longer the suction is applied to the tracheobronchial tree, the greater the magnitude of the hypoxemia. Suctioning should be limited to less than 10 to 15 seconds in adults. Adequate rest periods should be taken between suctioning procedures to allow correction of hypoxia and hypercarbia.
6. **Avoiding Laryngeal Spasm**
Laryngeal spasm may be avoided by inserting the catheter during inspiration and using topical or intravenous lidocaine. If laryngeal spasm occurs, the operator should immediately cease suctioning, open the vent to air, and insufflate oxygen through the catheter.
7. **Proper Technique**
   a. Negative pressure should be applied only while the catheter is being withdrawn. Excessive negative pressure should not be used. Finally, the outside diameter of the catheter should be no greater than one half of the inside diameter of the tracheal or tracheostomy tube.
   b. Closed suctioning techniques cause less hypoxia than open suctioning ones.

B. Adverse Effects on Respiratory Mechanics
Tracheal suctioning increases respiratory resistance. A loss of end-expiratory lung volume and a fall in compliance are commonly seen. Right upper lobe collapse in children has been associated with deep suctioning.

C. Trauma
1. Whenever suctioning is performed, there is the possibility that there will be damage to the airway. Reported problems include irritation, edema, inflammation, decreased mucociliary function, ulceration, necrosis, perforation, granulation tissue formation, and lobar emphysema. Suctioning through the nose may result in epistaxis.
2. Trauma is related to the frequency of suctioning, the technique used, and the magnitude of the negative pressure. The suction catheter has a minor role in determining the amount of mucosal damage.
3. To minimize trauma, unnecessary suctioning should be avoided. The catheter should be inserted only slightly more than the length of the tracheal tube unless deep suctioning is required. Poking or prodding should be avoided. If blood-stained secretions are observed in the absence of obvious reasons (lung contusion, recent tracheostomy), the entire suctioning technique should be examined.
4. Suctioning via the nasopharynx often causes trauma to the nasal mucosa. If the catheter tip is directed gently along an inferior and medial path with rotation, it will tend to follow the nasal cavity floor and trauma to the turbinates will be minimized. Prior nasal airway insertion will usually result in less trauma and more consistent catheter positioning.

D. Cross Infection
1. Many aspirated fluids contain high concentrations of microorganisms or blood, so cross contamination between patients or staff is a hazard. Caution should be used in handling all suction equipment.
2. Cross infection can occur either by direct contact with contaminated equipment or fluid or from aerosols. Microorganisms are aerosolized into the collection container during suctioning. When the container is opened, the microorganisms may be released into the environment. During open suctioning, condensate spray and tracheal secretions expelled during exhalation or coughing may contaminate the operator and atmosphere.

3. Personnel should be encouraged to regard all suction waste as potentially infectious and to handle and dispose of it properly. Hands should be washed after touching suction equipment, even if gloves were worn.

E. Bacteremia

Transient bacteremia can occur during suctioning through a tracheal tube or nasotracheal suctioning. Minimizing trauma and using aseptic technique can reduce this risk.

F. Cardiovascular Disturbances

Cardiac dysrhythmias, tachycardia, bradycardia, hypotension, hypertension, or even cardiac arrest can occur during suctioning. These problems are often related to hypoxemia. Another possible cause is coughing. In the unintubated patient, vocal cord stimulation may cause cardiac dysrhythmias. Cardiovascular disturbances are less with closed suctioning using a ventilator rather than a manual resuscitation bag for hyperinflation/hyperoxygenation and using insufflation rather than preoxygenation. Limiting the depth that the catheter is inserted should reduce the risk of vagal stimulation.

G. Increased Intracranial Pressure

Intracranial pressure may increase during suctioning. Measures to limit the increase include preoxygenation; hyperventilation prior to and following suctioning; limiting the duration of suctioning; not rotating the head; limiting the depth of catheter insertion; allowing adequate recovery time following suctioning; and administering drugs such as lidocaine, sedatives, or paralyzing agents. For severely head-injured patients in whom intracranial pressure is a concern, hyperinflation during and/or after suctioning should not be used in conjunction with hyperoxygenation.

H. Negative Pressure Pulmonary Edema

Pulmonary edema can occur if negative pressure is applied to a catheter that is inserted through the vocal cords closed because of laryngeal spasm. If this happens, suctioning should be discontinued and oxygen insufflated through the suction catheter.

I. Inadequately Removed Material

Consequences of inadequately removing material such as secretions or vomitus include hypoxia, atelectasis, infection, increased airway pressures (with increased risk of barotrauma), patient discomfort and anxiety and excessive coughing. Tracheal tube narrowing from secretion buildup may occur, especially with prolonged intubation.

J. Inadequate Suction

1. Inadequate suction may result from using one or more Y connectors to increase the number of vacuum inlets (**Fig. 2.12**).
2. Misassembling a suction system so that no collection jar is incorporated in the system can result in loss of suction. The system will appear to function during testing, but once fluid reaches the suction controller, the filter will be occluded and vacuum will be lost.
3. The suction tubing may become obstructed by viscous or particulate material.
4. It is possible for the overfill protection mechanism to interrupt the flow if it is bumped or jarred. Restoring suction requires disconnection of the vacuum source and reopening of this valve. This problem can be avoided by mounting the container securely and not allowing the container to become too full.

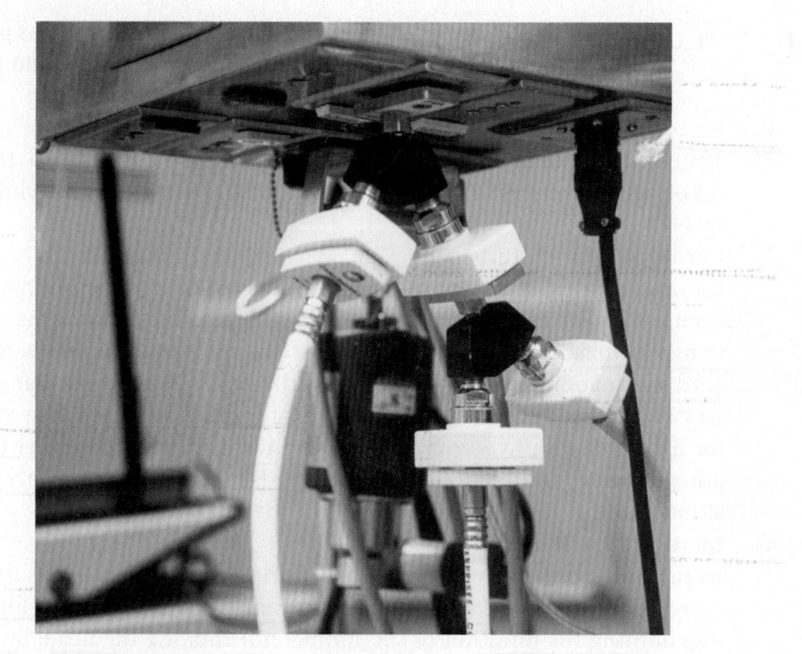

Figure 2.12 Use of multiple Y connectors will result in reduced vacuum and flow.

5. If the filter becomes wet or clogged, the flow will be interrupted. This can be caused by liquid, foam, or aerosol products from lasers or electrosurgery.
6. The vacuum control on a suction catheter may be a source of obstruction if the glove on the finger occluding it is sucked into the catheter.

K. Impacted Suction Catheter

A suction catheter can become impacted in a tracheal tube if the suction catheter exits through the Murphy eye. The patient may need to be reintubated. An alternative is to cut the machine end of the tracheal tube and try to remove the catheter from the shortened tube.

CLINICAL MOMENT If the catheter cannot be pulled out of a tracheal tube with a Murphy eye, there is a possibility that it is caught in the eye. The tube may need to be removed to free it from the suction catheter.

L. Inability to Pass Suction Catheter through a Tracheal Tube

There are a number of reasons why a suction catheter may not pass through a tracheal tube. The catheter may be too large. The tracheal tube may have a special configuration that makes passage difficult. The inner surface of the tracheal tube may be sticky, causing the catheter to hang up as it is inserted. There may be an obstruction or narrowing within the tracheal tube lumen.

M. Dental Damage

Dental damage can occur when rigid suction catheters are used, especially if the patient bites down on the catheter while being suctioned.

N. Broken Catheter

Part of a catheter can break off and lodge in the airway.

SUGGESTED READINGS

Baun MM, Stone KS, Rogge JA. Endotracheal suctioning: open versus closed with and without positive end-expiratory pressure. Crit Care Nurs Q 2002;25:13–26.

Brooks D, Anderson CM, Carier MA, et al. Clinical practice guidelines for suctioning the airway of the intubated and nonintubated patient. Can Respir J 2001;8:163–181.

Dean B. Evidence-based suction management in accident and emergency: a vital component of airway care. Accid Emerg Nurs 1997;5:92–97.

Dorsch J, Dorsch S. Suction equipment. In: Understanding Anesthesia Equipment. Fifth edition. Philadelphia: Wolters Kluwer/Lippincott Williams & Wilkins, 2008:51–75.

Glass CA, Grap MJ. Ten tips for safer suctioning. Am J Nurs 1995;95:51–53.

Lasocki S, Lu Q, Sartorius A, et al. Open and closed-circuit endotracheal suctioning in acute lung injury. Efficiency and effects on gas exchange. Anesthesiology 2006;104:39–47.

Lindgren S, Almgren B, Hogman M, et al. Effectiveness and side effects of closed and open suctioning: an experimental evaluation. Intensive Care Med 2004;30:1630–1637.

Morrow BM, Futter MJ, Argent AC. Endotracheal suctioning: from principles to practice. Intensive Care Med 2004;30: 1167–1174.

Royer K. Fluid management products. Outpatient Surg Magazine 2003;4:24–30.

Simmons CL. How frequently should endotracheal suctioning be undertaken? Am J Crit Care 1997;6:4–6.

Wainwright SP, Gould D. Endotracheal suctioning in adults with severe head injury: literature review. Intensive Crit Care Nurs 1996;12:303–308.

Wood CJ. Endotracheal suctioning: a literature review. Intensive Crit Care Nurs 1998;14:124–136.

SUGGESTED READINGS

Anesthesia Machines and Breathing Systems

3 The Anesthesia Machine

I. Introduction

A. The anesthesia machine is a complex piece of equipment consisting of many components. It is usually part of the anesthesia workstation which also includes devices such as vaporizers, a ventilator, breathing and scavenging systems, and monitors. These will be discussed in other chapters.

B. There are two general systems comprising the anesthesia machine: the electrical system and the pneumatic system.

C. There is a trend toward computer-driven electronic anesthesia machines. These are extremely complex and differ between manufacturers and even between models from the same manufacturer. Familiarity with one machine does not imply that a person can use another machine correctly. It is not possible in a text such as this to give all the information necessary to correctly use these machines. The user manual is the final authority as to their proper use.

CLINICAL MOMENT When being introduced to a new machine, especially one of the electronically controlled models, the user manual must be studied carefully.

II. Electrical System

A. Master Switch

1. A master (main power) switch (**Fig. 3.1**) activates both the pneumatic and electrical functions. On most machines, when the master switch is in the OFF position, the only electrical components that are active are the backup battery charger and the electrical outlets. On some machines, electrical components

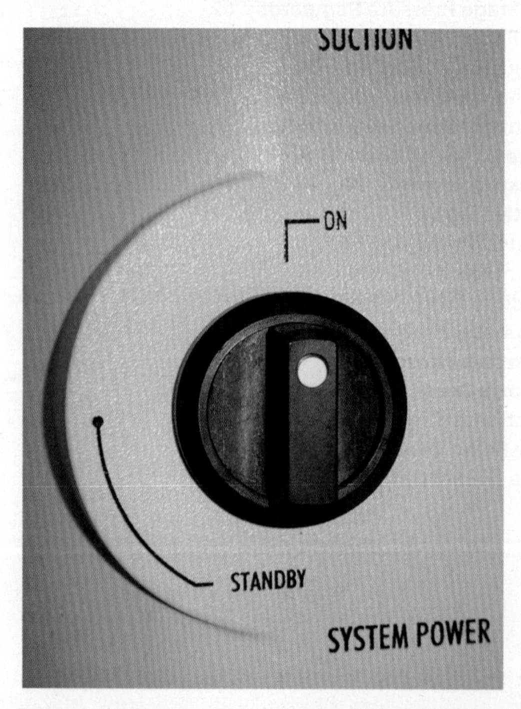

Figure 3.1 Master switch. Turning the master switch to the ON position activates both pneumatic and electrical functions of the machine as well as certain alarms and safety features.

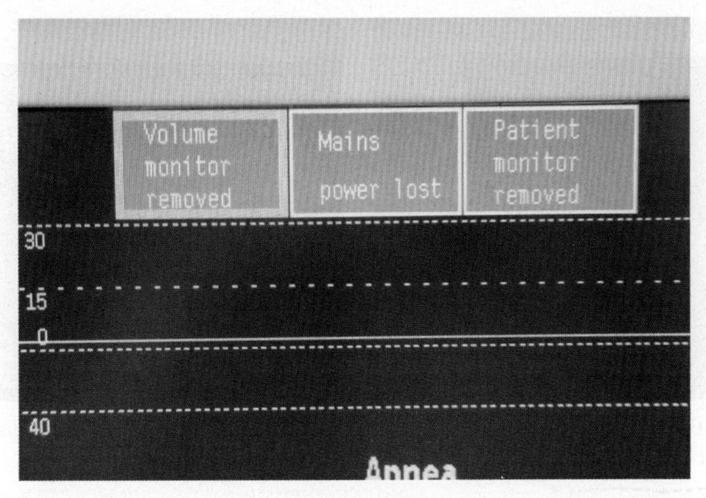

Figure 3.2 The machine will usually give an indication when mains power is lost.

can be activated without pneumatic power. A standby position may be present to allow the machine to be quickly powered up.

2. Electronic machines utilize a complicated power-up procedure that includes a system checkout. In addition to an electronic checkout, the computer gathers data that are necessary for proper function.

CLINICAL MOMENT In most cases, a machine must be turned OFF and the computer rebooted at least every 24 hours to clear previously stored start-up data. Failure to do this could cause the computer to malfunction. Check the user manual for the recommendations for your particular machine.

B. Power Failure Indicator

Most machines are equipped with a visual and/or audible indicator to alert the anesthesia provider to the loss of mains electrical power (**Fig. 3.2**).

CLINICAL MOMENT If the power indicator shows loss of mains electrical power or that the battery is in use, first check that the power line has not become loose or disconnected. Do what you can to conserve electrical energy until the problem is fixed.

C. Reserve Power

1. Since electricity is crucial for most anesthesia machines, a backup source is provided. Generally, this will provide power for 30 minutes, depending on usage. A noninterruptible power source may be added to the anesthesia machine to extend the backup period.
2. Most electronic anesthesia machines have a way for the user to determine the charge in the battery and whether the battery is in use (**Fig. 3.3**). The anesthesia provider should check the battery status during the preuse checkout procedure.

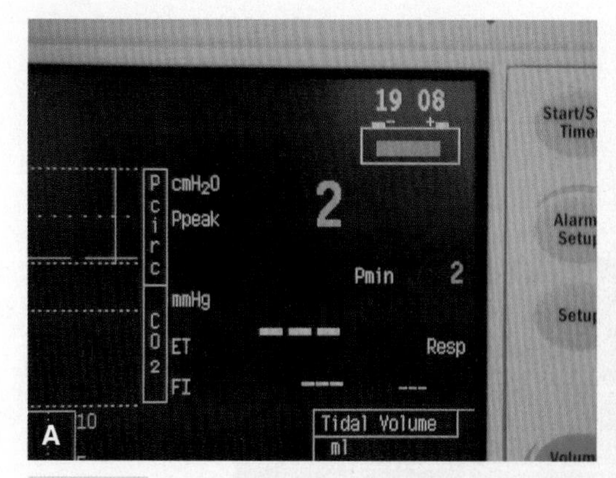

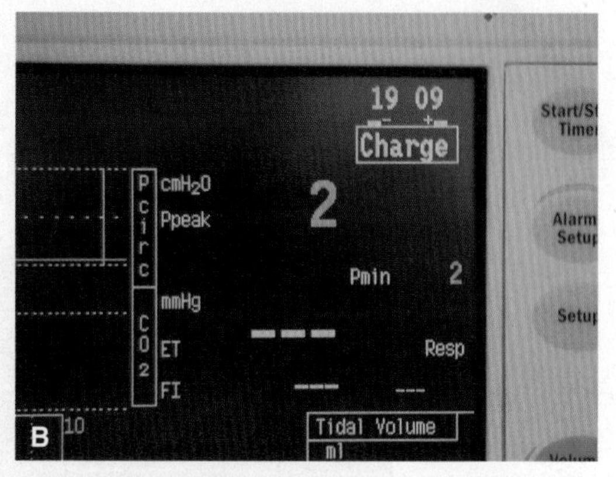

Figure 3.3 **A:** In the right corner of the screen, the amount of energy in the battery is displayed. **B:** If the battery does not carry a full charge, it can be charged by using mains power.

CLINICAL MOMENT Since many or all machine functions can cease if the electrical power fails, the user must know which functions are still available. This varies with the particular machine. The user manual will give this information. A plan to utilize the features available if electrical power is lost should be in place.

D. Electrical Outlets

Most modern anesthesia machines have electrical outlets at the back of the machine (**Fig. 3.4**). These are intended to power monitors and other anesthesia devices. They usually cannot supply electricity if there is a power failure.

CLINICAL MOMENT These outlets should not be used to power anything other than anesthesia devices and must not be used to power other devices such as operating room tables, floor vacuums, or electrosurgical units.

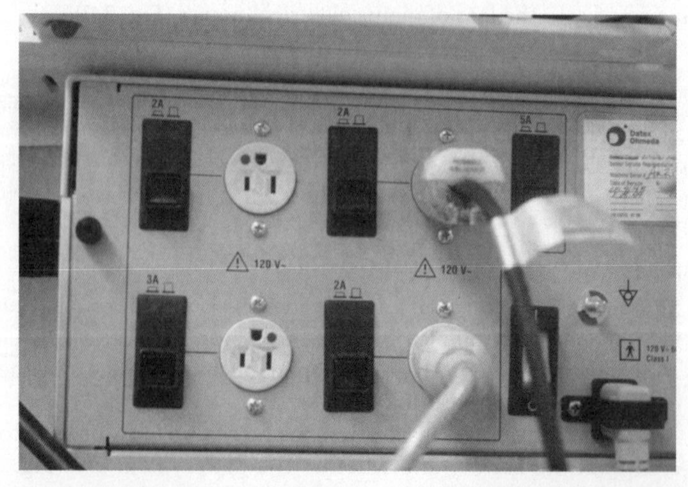

Figure 3.4 Convenience electrical outlets at the back of the anesthesia machine. These should be used only for anesthesia monitors and not for general operating room use. Note the cautions regarding the total electrical load. Next to each outlet is a circuit breaker.

E. Circuit Breakers

There are circuit breakers for both the anesthesia machine and the electrical outlets (**Fig. 3.4**). When a circuit breaker is activated, the electrical load should be reduced and the circuit breaker reset.

CLINICAL MOMENT The location of the circuit breakers varies with the specific anesthesia machine. Know where they are so that you can reset them quickly.

F. Data Communication Ports

Most modern anesthesia machines have data communication ports. These are used to transfer information among the anesthesia machine, monitors, and a data management system.

III. Pneumatic System

As shown in **Figure 3.5**, the pneumatic part of the machine can be conveniently divided into three parts: high-, intermediate-, and low-pressure systems.

A. The High-Pressure System

The high-pressure system receives gases from cylinders at high, variable pressures and reduces those pressures to a lower, more constant pressure suitable for use in the machine.

1. **Hanger Yoke**

The hanger yoke (**Fig. 3.6**) orients and supports the cylinder, provides a gas-tight seal, and ensures a unidirectional gas flow. It is composed of several parts: the body, which is the principal framework and supporting structure; the retaining screw, which tightens the cylinder in the yoke; the nipple, through which gas enters the machine; the Pin Index Safety System pins (see Chapter 1), which prevent an incorrect cylinder from being attached; the washer, which helps to form a seal between the cylinder and the yoke; and a filter to remove particulate matter that could come from the cylinder.

2. **Check Valve**

a. The check valve allows gas from a cylinder to enter the machine but prevents gas from exiting the machine when there is no cylinder in the yoke. It allows an empty cylinder to be replaced with a full one without losing gas from other cylinders of the same gas that are open or from the intermediate pressure system. The check valve also prevents gas from being transferred from a cylinder with a higher pressure to another one with a lower pressure when both are connected to a double yoke and opened at the same time.

CLINICAL MOMENT A yoke should not be left vacant. As soon as a cylinder is exhausted, it should be replaced by a full one. If a full cylinder is not available, a yoke plug (dummy cylinder block or plug, blanking cap or plug) (**Fig. 3.7**) should be placed in the empty yoke. The yoke plug is a solid piece of metal or other material that has a conical depression on one side to fit the tip of the retaining screw and a hollowed area on the other side to fit over the nipple. When in place, the plug forms a seal to prevent the gas from escaping from the machine. Manufacturers often chain yoke plugs to the machine.

b. To prevent transfilling between paired cylinders as a result of a defective check valve, only one cylinder of a gas should be open at a time.

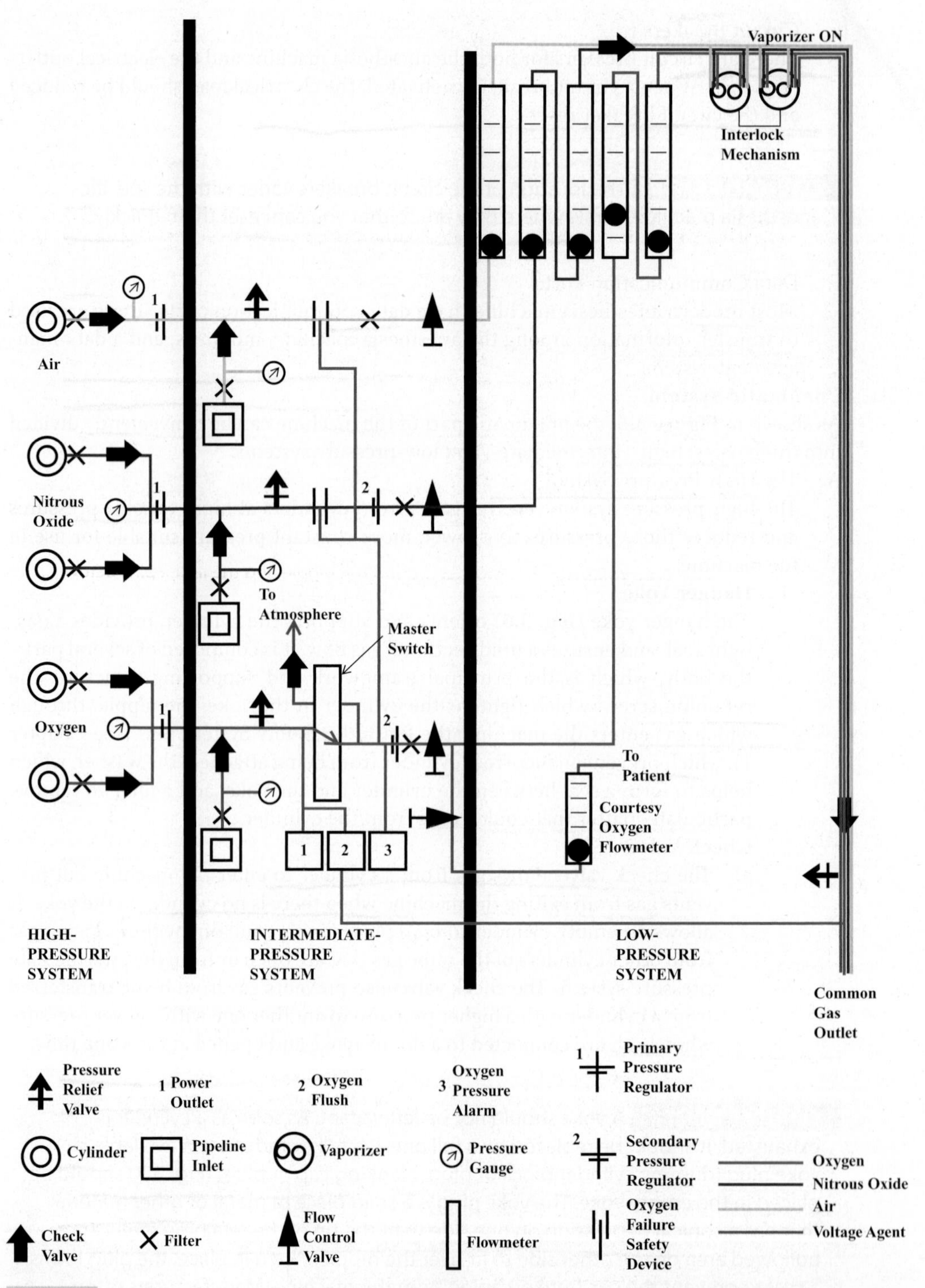

Figure 3.5 Diagram of a generic three-gas anesthesia machine. The components and their arrangement may differ somewhat with machines from different manufacturers.

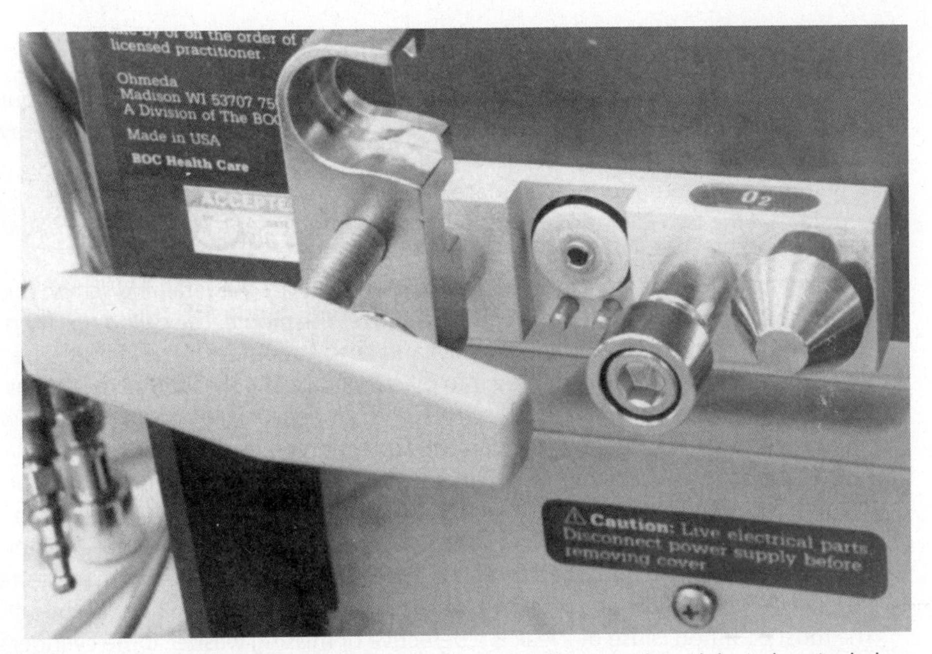

Figure 3.6 Swinging gate-type yoke. Note the washer around the nipple and the index pins below.

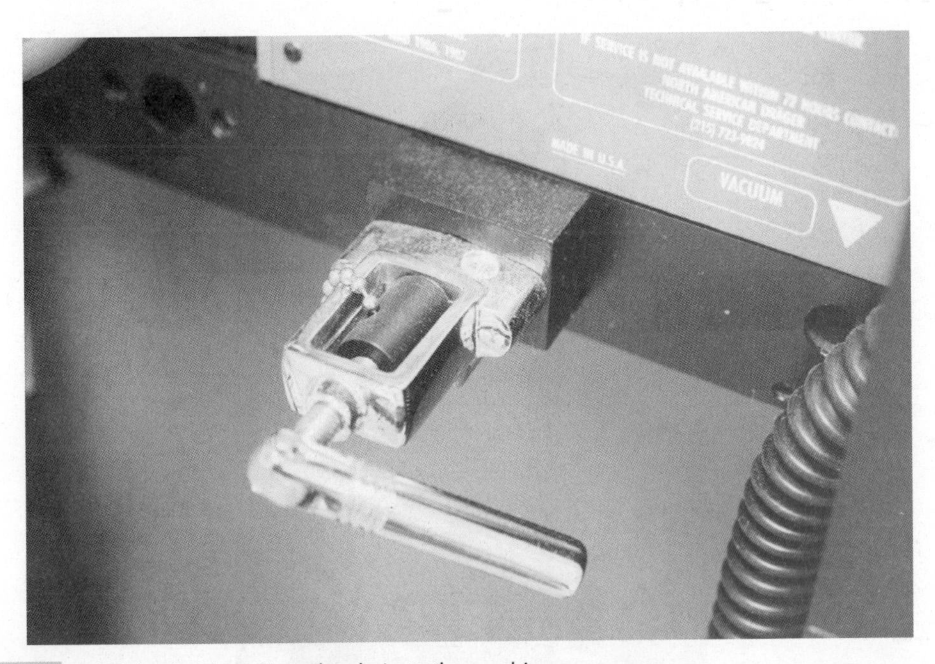

Figure 3.7 Yoke plug in place. Note the chain to the machine.

CLINICAL MOMENT When placing a cylinder in a yoke, it is important that the cylinder valve and yoke not be contaminated with oil or grease, because this could cause a fire (see Chapter 24). The person placing a cylinder in a yoke should always wash his/her hands first.

Before a cylinder is mounted in place, the yoke should be checked to make certain that the two Pin Index Safety System pins are present. A missing pin could allow the safety system to be bypassed.

The first step in placing a cylinder in a yoke is to retract the retaining screw. The gate is swung open and the washer is placed over the nipple. The cylinder is then supported with the foot (E cylinders only) and raised into the yoke (**Fig. 3.8**). The port on the cylinder valve is steered into place over the nipple and the index pins are engaged in the appropriate holes. The gate is then closed. The retaining screw is tightened so that it contacts the conical depression on the cylinder valve and pushes the valve over the nipple and index pins. It is important to ensure that the cylinder is correctly placed before tightening the retaining screw. Otherwise, the retaining screw may be inserted into the safety relief device on the cylinder. After the cylinder has been tightened onto the yoke, it should be opened to make certain that the cylinder is full and that there is no leak (as evidenced by a hissing sound). The most common cause of a leak is a defective or missing washer. If the cylinder valve leaks or is difficult to operate, the cylinder should be returned to the supplier.

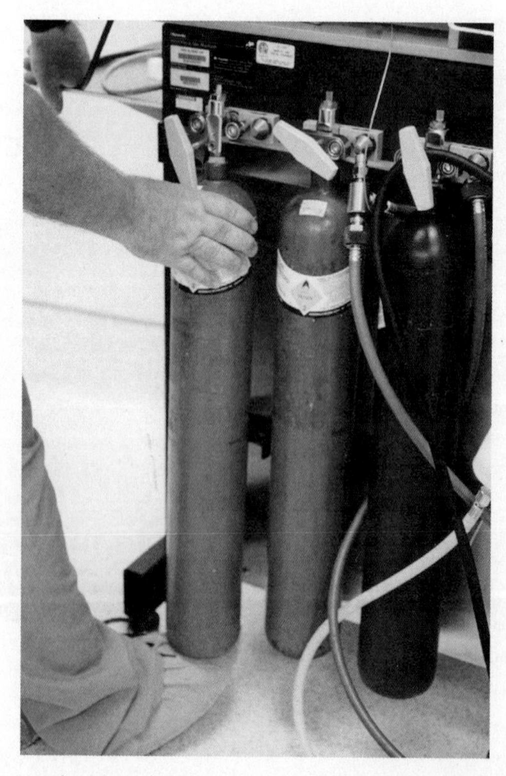

Figure 3.8 Placing cylinder in yoke. The cylinder is supported by the foot and guided into place manually.

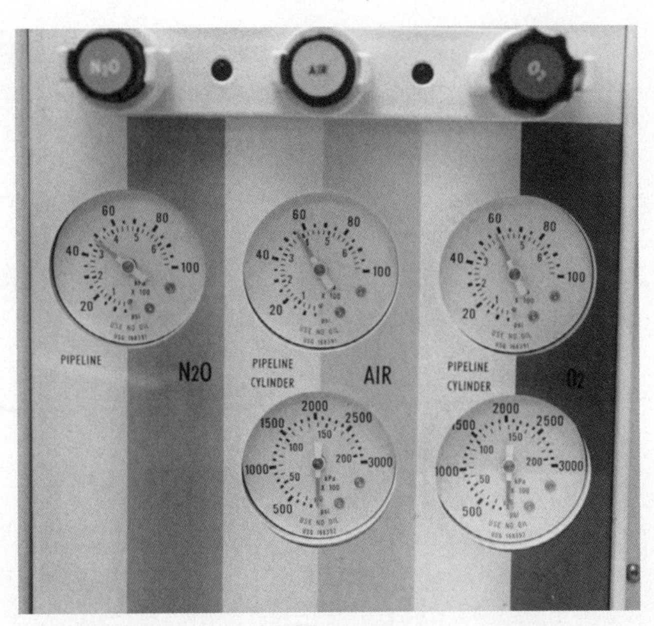

Figure 3.9 Cylinder and pipeline pressure indicators. Kilopascals × 100 are indicated in the inside of the dial, whereas pounds per square inch gauge are indicated on the outside.

CLINICAL MOMENT After the cylinder has been attached to the yoke, the valve should be closed unless it is to be the primary gas supply for the machine. If the pipeline is the primary supply and the valve remains open, fluctuations in the gas pressure in the machine could allow some or all of the gas to exit the cylinder. In the event that pipeline pressure is lost, gas could be used from the cylinder without the user being aware of the change. The first time that the user becomes aware of the lost pipeline pressure could be when the cylinder becomes empty. If only one gas cylinder is present, there would be no gas available.

3. **Cylinder Pressure Gauge (Indicator)**
   a. Many cylinder pressure gauges (indicators) (**Fig. 3.9**) are the Bourdon tube (Bourdon spring, elastic element) type. A hollow metal tube is bent into a curve and then sealed and linked to a clocklike mechanism. The other end is connected to the gas source. An increase in gas pressure inside the tube causes it to straighten. As the pressure falls, the tube resumes its curved shape. Because the open end is fixed, the sealed end moves. These motions are transmitted to the indicator, which moves over a calibrated scale. A drawback of these mechanical pressure gauges is that their readings cannot be transferred to a data management system.
   b. Most new anesthesia machines indicate cylinder pressure digitally (**Fig. 3.10**). Light-emitting diodes may also be used to indicate adequate pressure in the cylinder.
4. **Pressure Regulator**
   a. A pressure regulator reduces the high and variable pressure delivered from a cylinder to a lower, more constant pressure suitable for use in an anesthesia machine. Without a regulator, it would be necessary for the anesthesia

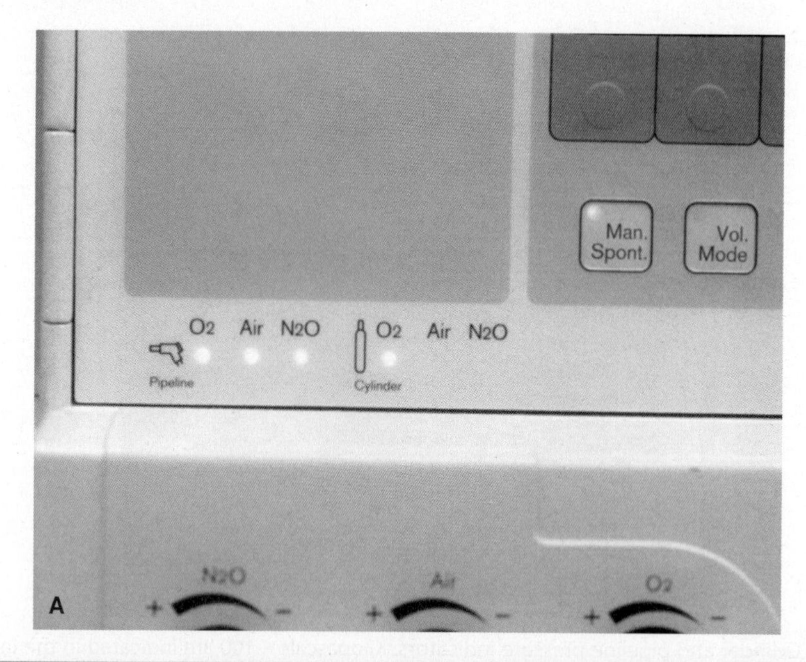

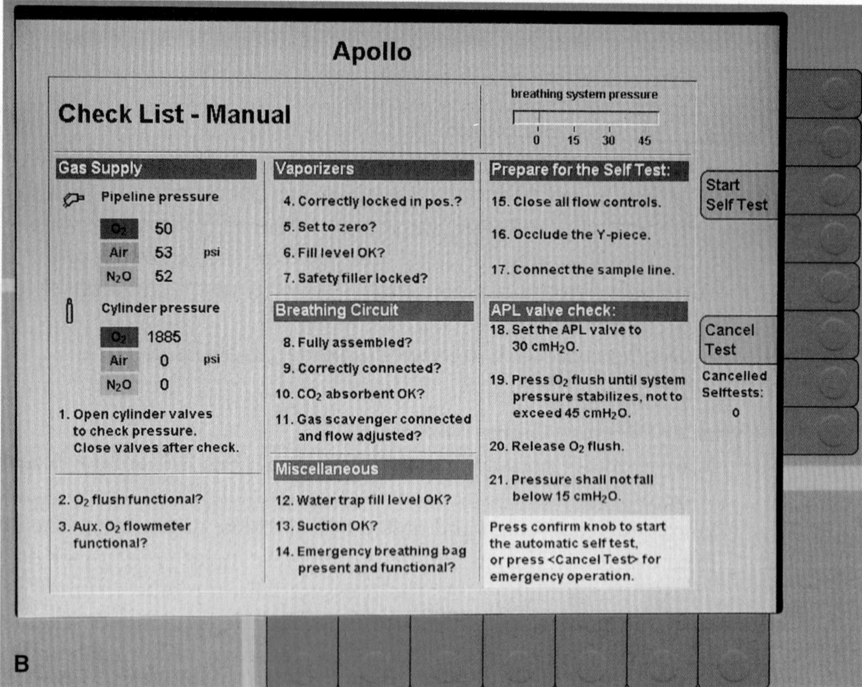

Figure 3.10 **A:** Light-emitting diodes (LEDs) indicate cylinder pressure. If the cylinder valve is open and the pressure is adequate, the LED will be green. If the valve is open but the pressure is inadequate, the LED will flash red. It will be dark if the cylinder valve is not open. **B:** Cylinder pressure can shown digitally on the checkout screen during the checkout phase or on the main screen during the case.

provider to constantly alter the flow control valve to maintain a constant flow through the flowmeter as the pressure in the cylinder decreases.

b. Pressure regulators used in anesthesia machines are preset at the factory. The pressure at the regulator outlet is set lower than the pipeline pressure. This ensures that pipeline gas is used preferentially to the cylinder supply if the cylinder valve is open while oxygen from the piping system is being used. This differential pressure may not always prevent the cylinder from becoming exhausted since pressure fluctuations in the pipeline may cause the pressure in the machine to drop below the pressure from the pressure regulator.

B. Intermediate-Pressure System

The intermediate-pressure system (**Fig. 3.5**) receives gases from the pressure regulator or the pipeline inlet. Components in this system include the pneumatic part of the master switch, pipeline inlet connections, pipeline pressure indicators, piping, the gas power outlet, oxygen pressure failure devices, the oxygen flush, additional pressure regulators (if so equipped), the alternate oxygen control (if so equipped), and the flow control valves.

1. **Master Switch (Pneumatic Component)**

The pneumatic portion of the master switch is located in the intermediate-pressure system downstream of the inlets for the cylinder and pipeline supplies. The oxygen flush is usually independent of this switch. When the master switch is turned OFF, the pressure in the intermediate-pressure system will drop to zero.

2. **Pipeline Inlet Connections**

a. The pipeline inlet connections are the entry points for gases from the pipelines. There are usually connections for air, oxygen, and nitrous oxide.

b. The pipeline inlets are fitted with threaded noninterchangeable Diameter Index Safety System (DISS) connectors (Chapter 1) (**Fig. 3.11**).

c. Each inlet contains a unidirectional (check) valve to prevent reverse gas flow from the machine into the piping system (or to atmosphere if no hose

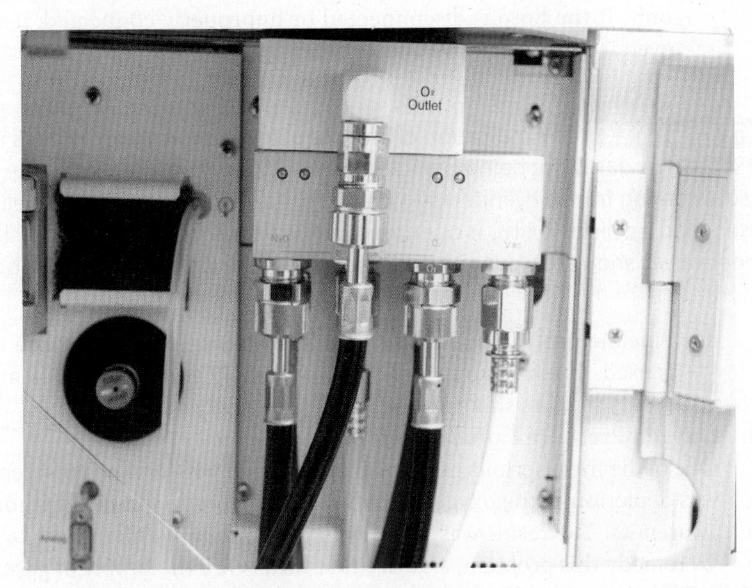

Figure 3.11 Gas pipeline connections for oxygen, air, nitrous oxide and vacuum. There is also an oxygen outlet that could drive a ventilator or an accessory flowmeter. The connections to the anesthesia machine have DISS fittings.

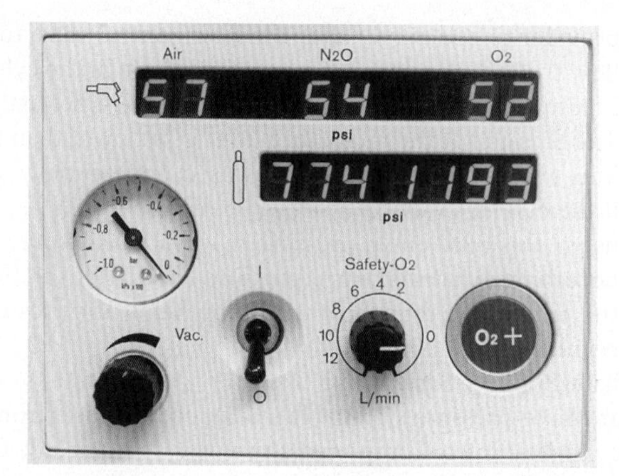

Figure 3.12 Digital pressure indicators. Pipeline pressures are at the top. Cylinder pressures are below. At the left below is the vacuum regulator and gauge and ON–OFF control for suction. To the right of this is the alternative oxygen source, which can be used if there is total loss of electrical power. To the right is the recessed oxygen flush control.

is connected) and a filter to prevent debris from the pipeline entering the anesthesia machine.

3. **Pipeline Pressure Gauges**
   a. Gauges are present to monitor the pipeline pressure of each gas (**Figs. 3.9** and **3.12**). They are usually on a panel on the front of the machine (or the information screen, if present) and color coded for the gases they monitor.
   b. Some machines have digital pressure gauges (**Fig. 3.12**) that display pressure either continuously or on demand. Some use light-emitting diodes (LEDs) to indicate adequate pipeline pressure.
   c. The sensing point for the pipeline pressure gauge is located on the pipeline side of the check valve. In this location it will monitor pipeline pressure only. If the hose is disconnected or improperly connected, it will read "0" even if a cylinder valve is open.

CLINICAL MOMENT The indication of an adequate pipeline pressure does not guarantee that gas is not being drawn from a cylinder. If for any reason the gas pressure coming from a cylinder via a pressure regulator exceeds the pipeline pressure and a cylinder valve is open, gas will be drawn from the cylinder. Therefore, cylinder valves should always remain closed when the pipeline supply is in use.

   d. Pipeline pressure indicators should always be checked before the machine is used. The pressure should be between 50 and 55 psig (345 and 380 kPa). The indicators should be scanned repeatedly during use.

4. **Oxygen Pressure Failure Devices**
   One of the most serious mishaps that occurred with earlier anesthesia machines was depletion of the oxygen supply (usually from a cylinder) without the user's awareness. The result was delivery of gas containing no oxygen to the patient. To remedy this problem, a device that turns OFF the supply of gases other than oxygen (oxygen failure safety device) is used. In addition, an alarm to warn when oxygen pressure has fallen to a dangerous level is used.

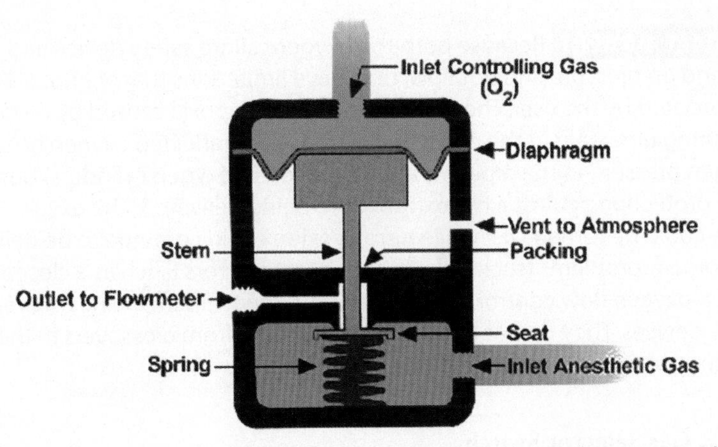

Figure 3.13 Oxygen failure safety valve. When oxygen pressure in the machine is normal, it will push the diaphragm and stem downward, opening the valve. The anesthetic gas flows in at the inlet around the stem and through the outlet to the flowmeter. When the oxygen pressure falls, the stem moves upward, closing the valve. The middle chamber is vented to atmosphere to prevent mixing of anesthetic gas and oxygen in the event that the diaphragm ruptures or the packing leaks. (Redrawn from a drawing furnished by Ohmeda, a division of BOC, Inc., Madison, Wisconsin.)

a. Oxygen Pressure Failure Safety Device
   1) The oxygen failure safety valve (fail safe) placed in the piping system for nitrous oxide (and on some machines air) shuts off or proportionally decreases and ultimately interrupts the supply of the other gas if the oxygen supply pressure decreases.
   2) When the pneumatic system is activated, oxygen pressure opens the oxygen pressure failure safety device, allowing other gases to flow. A decrease in oxygen pressure causes it to interrupt the flow of other gases to their flow control valves.
   3) One such device is shown diagrammatically in **Figure 3.13.** When oxygen pressure is normal, the plunger and the seal assembly are depressed so that anesthetic gas can flow through the valve. When the oxygen pressure decreases, the spring forces the plunger and the seal assembly upward, narrowing the valve opening in proportion to oxygen supply pressure loss. If the oxygen supply pressure fails completely, the valve closes.

CLINICAL MOMENT To determine whether a machine has a properly functioning oxygen failure safety device, the flows of oxygen and the other gas (usually nitrous oxide) are turned ON. The source of oxygen pressure (cylinder or pipeline) is then removed. If the oxygen failure safety device is functioning properly, the flow indicator for the other gas will fall to the bottom of the tube just before the oxygen indicator falls to the bottom of its tube. Restoring oxygen pressure should restore the other gas in the previous proportion.

b. Oxygen Supply Failure Alarm
   An oxygen supply pressure alarm will sound within 5 seconds of the oxygen pressure falling below 30 psig.

CLINICAL MOMENT Because both the oxygen failure safety device and the alarm depend on pressure and not flow, they have limitations that are not always fully appreciated by the user. They aid in preventing hypoxia caused by problems occurring upstream in the machine circuitry (disconnected oxygen hose, low oxygen pressure in the pipeline, and depletion of oxygen cylinders) but do not offer total protection against a hypoxic mixture being delivered. The oxygen flow control valve could be turned OFF while nitrous oxide could continue to be delivered. Equipment problems (such as leaks) or operator errors (such as a closed or partially closed oxygen flow control valve) that occur downstream are not prevented by these devices. They do not guard against hypoxia from crossovers in the pipeline system or a cylinder containing the wrong gas.

5. **Gas Selector Switch**
   Many machines have a gas selector switch that prevents air and nitrous oxide from being used together. Two types of switches are shown in **Figures 3.14** and **3.15.**
6. **Second-Stage Pressure Regulator**
   Some machines have additional pressure regulators in the intermediate pressure system just upstream of the flow adjustment controls. The second-stage regulator receives gas from either the pipeline or the cylinder pressure regulator and reduces it further to around 26 psi (177 kPa) for nitrous oxide and 14 psi (95 kPa) for oxygen. Reducing the pressures below the normal fluctuation range causes the flow from the flowmeters to remain more constant. Not all anesthesia machines incorporate this device.
7. **Oxygen Flush**
   a. The oxygen flush (oxygen bypass, emergency oxygen bypass) (**Fig. 3.16**) receives oxygen from the pipeline inlet or cylinder pressure regulator and directs a high (35 to 75 L/minute) unmetered flow directly to the common gas outlet. It is commonly labeled "O_{2+}." On most anesthesia machines, the

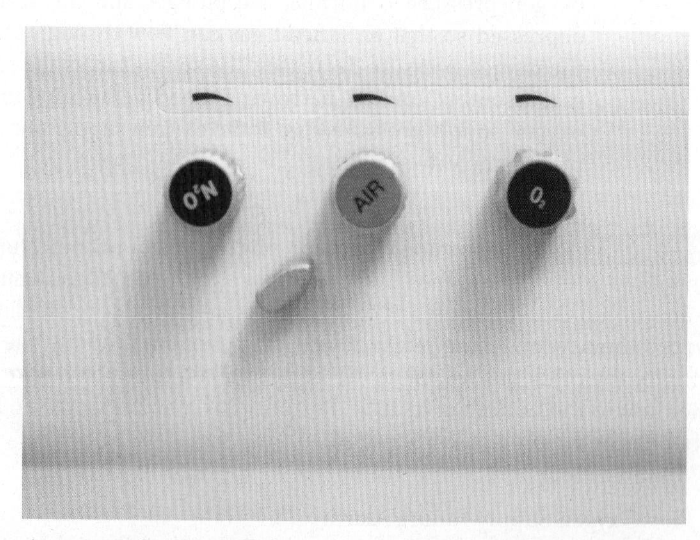

Figure 3.14 Gas selector switch. In the N_2O position, only oxygen and nitrous oxide can be used. In the air position, only oxygen and air can be administered.

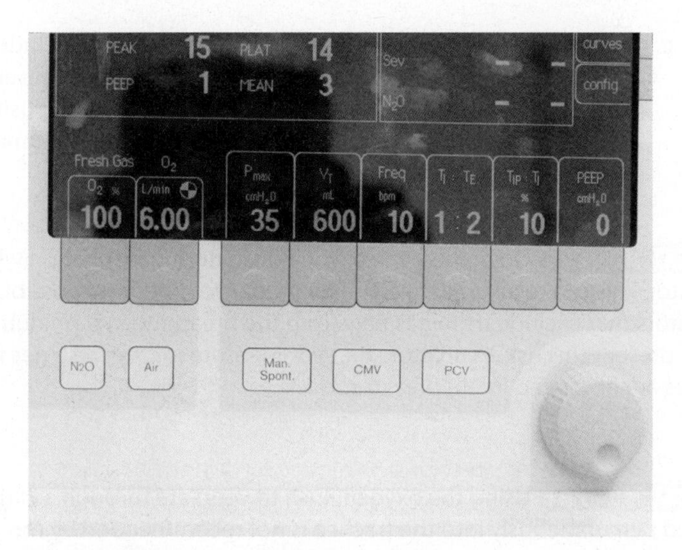

Figure 3.15 Electronic gas selector switch. Either nitrous oxide or air can be selected by pushing the appropriate button (lower left). Total gas flow and oxygen percentage are set by pushing the hard keys and rotating the wheel at the lower right. The balance of the fresh gas flow will be the other gas chosen (nitrous oxide or air).

oxygen flush can be activated regardless of whether the master switch is turned ON or OFF.

b. Oxygen flush activation may or may not result in other gas flows being shut OFF and may result in either a positive or negative pressure in the machine circuitry, depending on the design of the inlet and the flush line into the common gas line. This pressure may be transmitted backward on other structures in the machine, such as flow indicators and vaporizers, and may change the vaporizer output and the flow indicator readings. The effect will depend on the pressure generated, the presence or absence of check valves in the machine, and the relationship of the oxygen flush valve to other components.

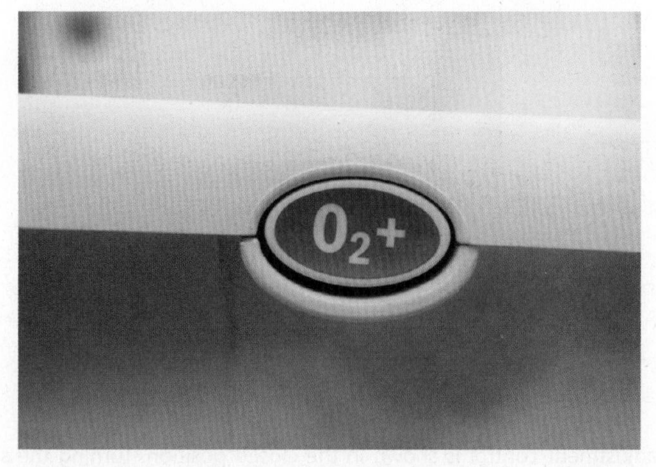

Figure 3.16 Oxygen flush valve. Note the protective ring to prevent accidental activation. O_2+ is a symbol for the oxygen flush valve.

c. Reported hazards associated with the oxygen flush include accidental activation and internal leakage, which result in an oxygen-enriched mixture being delivered. The flush valve may stick in the ON position. It may also stick and obstruct flow from the flowmeters. Barotrauma and awareness during anesthesia have resulted from its activation.

CLINICAL MOMENT Do not use the oxygen flush during inspiration when using a ventilator. This can result in delivery of high tidal volumes and possible barotrauma. Ventilators that exclude fresh gas flow from the breathing system during inspiration do not present this risk. Ventilators that compensate for the fresh gas flow do. These features are discussed in Chapters 6 and 10.

CLINICAL MOMENT Using the oxygen flush to ventilate through a catheter inserted percutaneously into the trachea is not recommended by most anesthesia machine manufacturers. Some machines provide sufficient pressure for effective jet ventilation, but others do not.

8. **Flow Adjustment Control**

The flow adjustment control (**Fig. 3.17**) regulates the flow of oxygen, air, and other gases to the flowmeters. There is one flow adjustment control per gas and

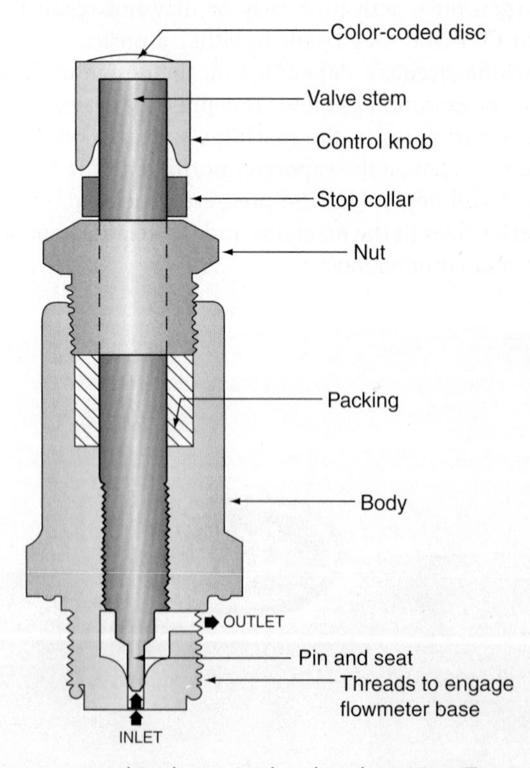

Figure 3.17 Flow adjustment control is shown in the closed position. Turning the stem creates a leak between the pin and the seat so that gas flows to the outlet. The stop collar prevents overtightening of the pin in the seat. (Redrawn from a drawing furnished by Foregger Co., a division of Puritan Bennett Co., Inc.)

it must be adjacent to or identifiable with its associated flowmeter. There are two types of flow adjustment controls: mechanical and electronic.

a. Mechanical Flow Control Valves

1) The mechanical flow control valve utilizes a stem with fine threads that when turned clockwise will move inward to decrease or stop gas flow. When turned counterclockwise, the stem will move outward to increase the gas flow. When the valve is closed, the pin at the end of the stem fits into a seat, occluding the orifice so that no gas can pass through the valve.

2) It is advantageous to have stops for the OFF and MAXIMUM flow positions. A stop for the OFF position avoids damage to the valve seat by overtightening the valve. A stop for the MAXIMUM flow position prevents the stem from becoming disengaged from the valve body.

3) The control knob is joined to the stem. If it is a rotary-style knob, the oxygen flow control knob has a fluted profile (**Figs. 3.9, 3.14, 3.18,** and **3.19**) and is larger than that for any other gas. All other flow control knobs are round. If other types of flow control valves are present, the oxygen control must look and feel different from the other controls.

4) Accidental changes in position can be minimized by a shield, bar, or other protective mechanism (**Figs. 3.18** and **3.19**) and by placing the control knob high enough above the working surface to lessen the likelihood of contact with objects on that surface.

5) Flow control valves should be closed when not in use. If there is no yoke plug or cylinder in the yoke or the one-way valve in the pipeline inlet does not work well, gas from an unused gas system could flow retrograde through a flowmeter with an open flow control valve and leak to atmosphere.

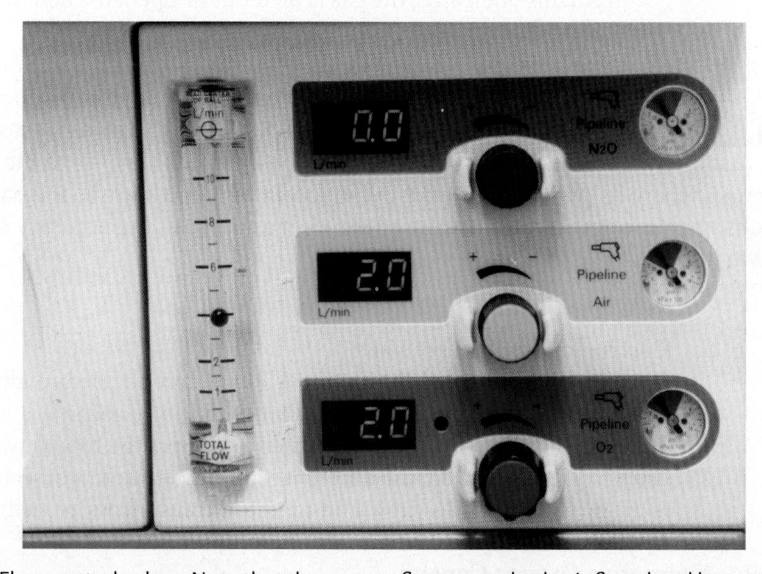

Figure 3.18 Flow control valves. Note that the oxygen flow control valve is fluted and larger than the other flow control valve. Also note the guard around each flow control valve. To the left of each valve is the flow. At the left is a flowmeter for total flow.

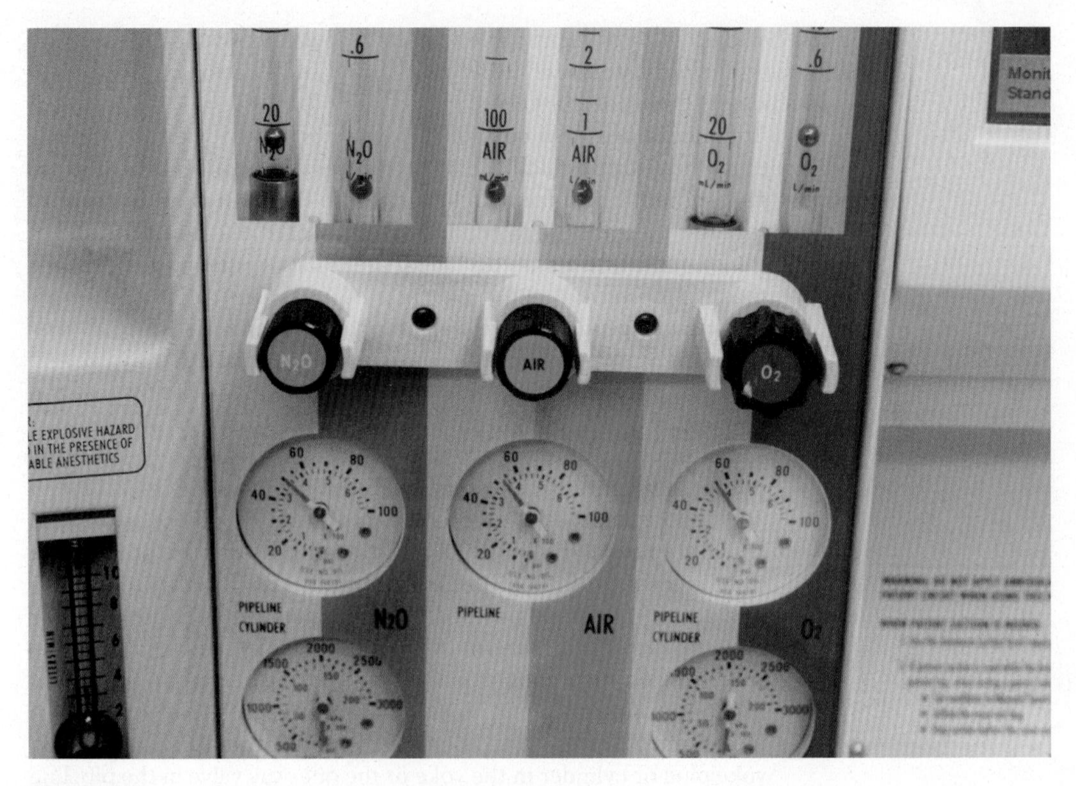

Figure 3.19 Flow control valves below conventional flowmeters.

6) Before a machine is used, the flow control valves should be checked to make certain that they are closed. Sometimes, a flow control valve remains open after the gas is bled out or opened when the machine is cleaned or moved.

CLINICAL MOMENT If the gas supply to an open flow control valve is restored and the associated flow indicator is not observed, the indicator may rise to the top of the tube where its presence may not be noticed. Even if no harm to the patient results, the sudden indicator rise may damage it and impair the accuracy of the flowmeter.

b. Electronic Flow Control Valves

Electronically activated flow control valves can be used to alter gas flows (**Fig. 3.15**). A common configuration is that one control is used to alter the oxygen concentration and another to control the total flow. If less than 100% oxygen is desired, the difference is made up from the second gas such as air or nitrous oxide. Flow and pressure transducers as well as temperature sensors are used to maintain accuracy.

9. **Alternative Oxygen Control**

When using a computer-controlled anesthesia machine, there is always the possibility that the electronics will fail. Different machines deal with this problem

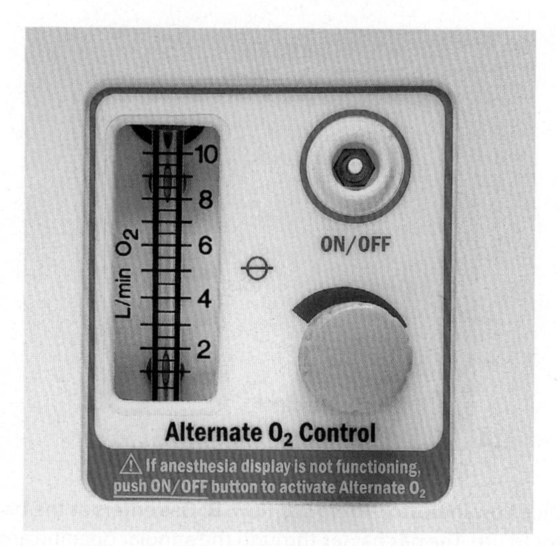

Figure 3.20 Alternative oxygen source. This can be used to supply oxygen in case of total loss of electrical power.

in different ways. As shown in **Figures 3.12** and **3.20,** this is usually accomplished by a means to administer oxygen. This is separate from the auxiliary (courtesy) flowmeter. If there is a mechanical total flow flowmeter (**Fig. 3.18**), it can be used to measure the delivered oxygen.

CLINICAL MOMENT Different anesthesia machines handle computer control loss differently. Check the user manual to determine how to handle this problem. Have a plan to handle electronic failure in place.

C. The Low-Pressure System

The low-pressure system (**Fig. 3.5**) is located between the flow control devices and the machine outlet. Pressure in this section is only slightly above atmospheric, and variable rather than constant. Pressure fluctuations depend on the flow from the flow control valves, the presence of back-pressure devices (check valves), and back pressure from the breathing system. Components found in this section include flowmeters, hypoxia prevention safety devices, unidirectional valves, pressure relief devices, and the common gas outlet. Vaporizers and their mounting devices are found in the low-pressure system but will be considered in Chapter 4.

1. **Flowmeters**

Flowmeters may be mechanical or electronic. Electronic flowmeters that are on many new machines use sensors to measure gas flow. There may be a representation of a mechanical flowmeter on a screen. Even with electronic flowmeters, there may be a mechanical flowmeter for total fresh gas flow at the common gas outlet to provide a sense of security for clinicians who do not fully trust electronic flowmeters.

a. Physical Principles

1) Traditional mechanical flow indicators used in anesthesia machines are the variable orifice (variable area, Thorpe tube) type. A vertical glass

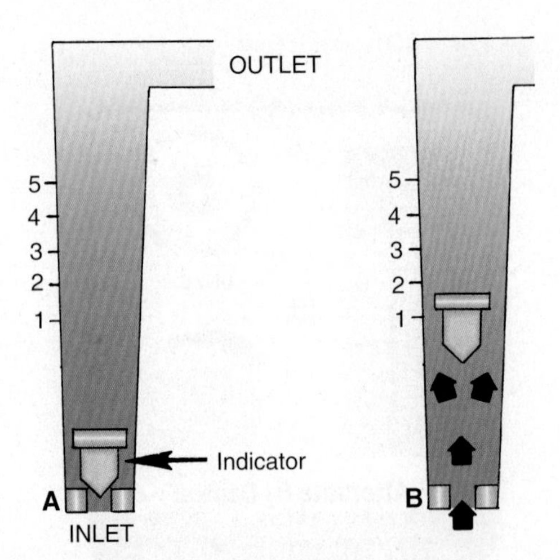

Figure 3.21 Variable orifice flow indicator. **A:** No gas flow. **B:** Gas enters at the base and flows through the tube, causing the indicator to rise. The gas passes through the annular opening around the float. The area of this annular space increases with the height of the indicator. Thus, the height of the indicator is a measure of gas flow.

tube (**Fig. 3.21**) has an internal taper with its smallest diameter at the bottom. It contains an indicator that is free to move up and down inside the tube. When there is no gas flow, the indicator rests at the bottom of the tube. As shown in **Figure 3.21 B,** when the flow control valve is opened, gas enters at the bottom and flows up the tube, elevating the indicator. The gas passes through the annular opening between the indicator and the tube wall and on to the outlet at the top of the tube. The indicator floats freely in the tube at a position where the downward force caused by gravity equals the upward force caused by the gas pressure on the bottom of the indicator. As gas flow increases, the number of gas molecules hitting the indicator bottom increases, and it rises. Because the tube is tapered, the size of the annular opening around the indicator increases with height and allows more gas flow. When the flow is decreased, gravity causes the indicator to settle to a lower level. A scale on or beside the tube indicates the gas flow rate.

2) The flow rate through the tube will depend on three factors: the pressure drop across the constriction, the size of the annular opening, and the physical properties of the gas.
3) As gas flows around the indicator, it encounters frictional resistance between the indicator and the tube wall. There is a resultant loss of energy, so the pressure drops. This pressure drop is constant for all positions in the tube and is equal to the weight of the float divided by its cross-sectional area. For this reason, these flowmeters are often called constant-pressure flowmeters. Increasing the flow does not increase the pressure drop but causes the indicator to rise to a higher position in the tube, thereby providing greater flow area for the gas.
4) The physical characteristics of the gas affect the gas flow through the flowmeter tube. When a low gas flow passes through the tube, the annular opening between the float and the tube wall will be narrow. As flow increases, the annular opening becomes larger. The physical property that relates gas flow to the pressure difference across the

constriction varies with the form of the constriction. With a longer and narrower constriction (low flows), flow is laminar and is mainly a function of the viscosity of the gas (Hagen–Poiseuille equation). When the constriction is shorter and wider (high flows), flow is more turbulent and depends more on the gas density (Graham's law).

5) Flowmeters are calibrated at atmospheric pressure (760 torr) and room temperature (20°C). Temperature and pressure changes will affect the gas viscosity and density and so influence the indicated flow rate accuracy. Variations in temperature as a rule are slight and do not produce significant changes.

CLINICAL MOMENT In a hyperbaric chamber, a flowmeter will deliver less gas than indicated. With decreased barometric pressure (increased altitude), the actual flow rate will be greater than that indicated.

b. Flowmeter Assembly

1) The flowmeter assembly consists of the tube through which the gas flows, the indicator inside the tube, a stop at the top of the tube, and the scale that indicates the flow. Lights are available on most anesthesia machines to allow the flowmeters to be observed in a dark room. Each assembly is marked with the appropriate color and name or chemical symbol of the gas measured. Flowmeters are usually protected by a plastic shield. The flowmeter assembly empties into a common manifold that delivers the measured amount of gases into the low-pressure system.

2) Flowmeter tubes are usually made of glass. Glass tubes intended for a ball indicator have rib guides, thickened bars that run the length of the tube and keep the ball indicator in the center of the tube (**Fig. 3.22**). As the tube widens, the space between the indicator and the inside of the tube increases.

3) The flowmeter tube can have a single or double taper (**Fig. 3.23**). Single-taper tubes have a gradual increase in diameter from the bottom to the top. They are usually used where there are different tubes for low and high flows. Dual-taper flowmeter tubes have two different tapers on the inside of the same tube. The lower taper is more gradual and is used when fine flows are in use. The less gradual taper is used for higher flows. These tubes are used when only one tube is used for a gas.

CLINICAL MOMENT Flowmeter tubes are most accurate in the middle half of the tube. Accuracy decreases at the bottom and top. This is why separate tubes are often used for low flows.

4) The indicator (float, ball, rotameter or bobbin) is a free-moving device within the tube. It is important to observe the indicator frequently and especially when the flow is altered. If the indicator moves erratically, the readings may be inaccurate. The widest diameter of the indicator is the point where the flow should be read (**Fig. 3.24**).

5) The stop at the top of the flowmeter tube (**Fig. 3.25**) prevents the indicator from plugging the outlet, which could lead to tube damage.

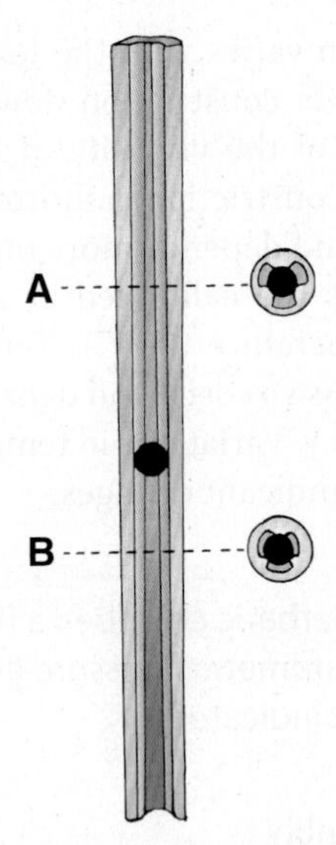

Figure 3.22 Flow indicator tube with rib guides. This is used with ball indicators. The triangular thickening of the inside of the tube keeps the ball centered. The area through which the gas flows increases with increasing height in the tube. (Redrawn courtesy of Fraser Harlake, Inc.)

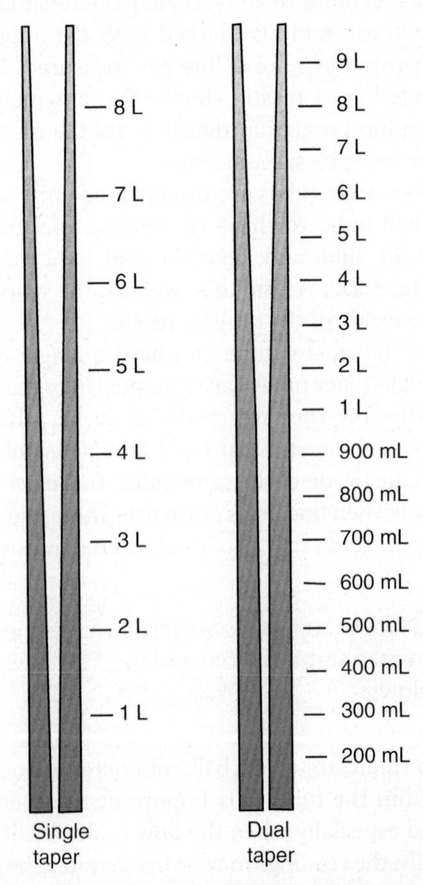

Figure 3.23 Dual- and single-taper flow indicator tubes. With the single-taper tube, the opening gradually increases from the bottom to the top of the tube. With the dual-taper tube, the opening size increases more rapidly above 1 L/minute.

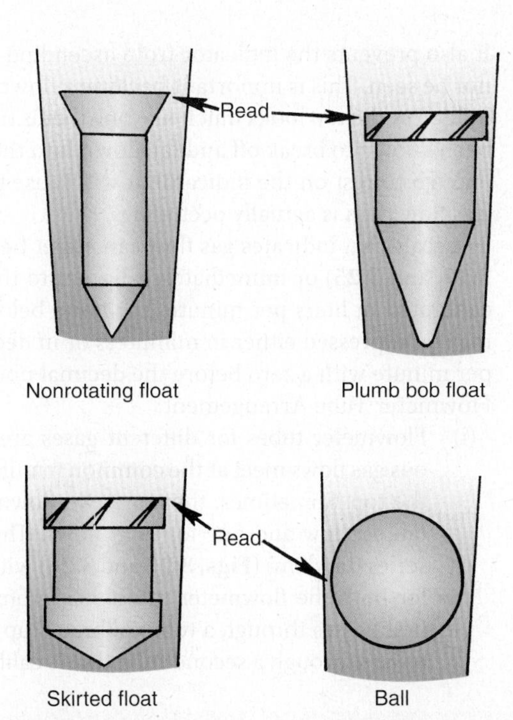

Figure 3.24 Flow indicators. The plumb bob and skirted floats are kept centered in the tube by constant rotation. The reading is taken at the top. The ball indicator is kept centered by rib guides. The reading is taken at the center. The nonrotating float does not rotate and is kept centered by gas flow. (Adapted from Binning R, Hodges EA. Flowmeters. Can they be improved? Anaesthesia 1967;22:643–646.)

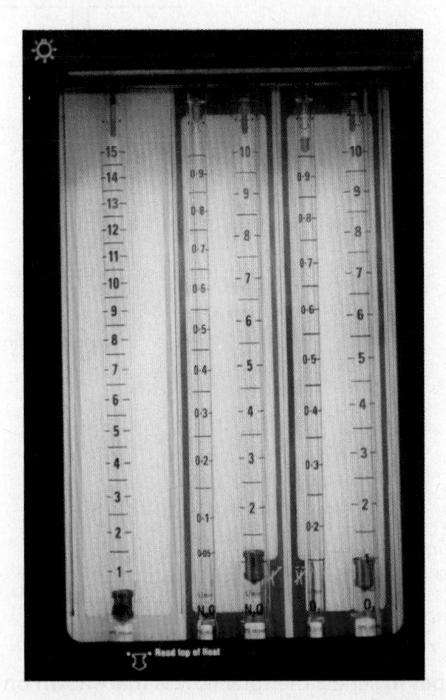

Figure 3.25 Skirted float indicators. Note the stops at the top of the flow indicator tubes. The flow indicator tubes are in series. The total flow is that shown on the higher flow tube, not the sum of the two tubes.

It also prevents the indicator from ascending to a point where it cannot be seen. This is important because a flowmeter with the indicator hidden at the top looks much like one that is turned OFF. The stop has been known to break off and fall down into the tube. If it descends far enough to rest on the indicator, it will cause the indicator to register less flow than is actually occurring.

6) The scale that indicates gas flow can either be marked on (**Figs. 3.18, 3.19,** and **3.25**) or immediately adjacent to the tube. Flowmeters are calibrated in liters per minute. For flows below 1 L/minute, the flow may be expressed either in milliliters or in decimal fractions of a liter per minute with a zero before the decimal point.
7) Flowmeter Tube Arrangement:
   (i) Flowmeter tubes for different gases are side by side. The various gas flows meet at the common manifold (mixing chamber) at the top. Sometimes, there are two flowmeters for the same gas: one for low and one for high flows. The tubes are arranged in series (tandem) (**Figs. 3.25** and **3.26**) with one flow control valve for both the flowmeter tubes. Gas from the flow control valve first passes through a tube calibrated up to 1 L/minute and then passes through a second tube that is calibrated for higher flows.

CLINICAL MOMENT The total flow through two-series flowmeters is not the sum of the two tubes but that shown on the higher flow tube.

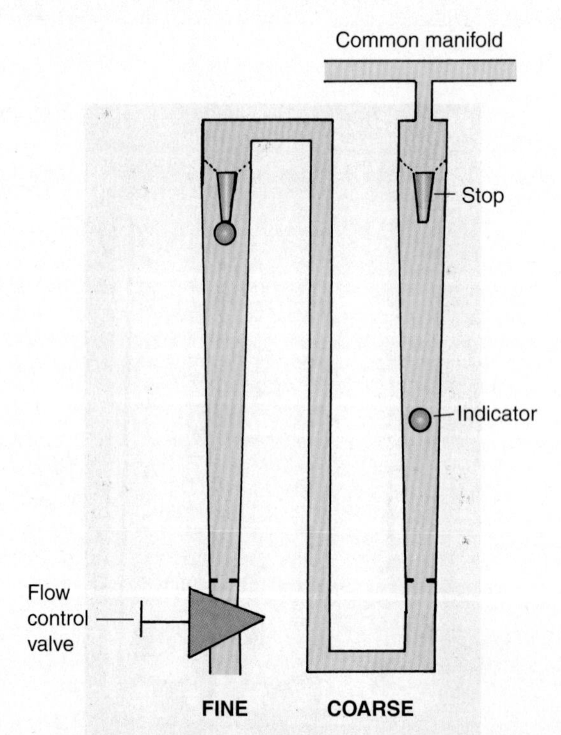

Figure 3.26 Flow indicator tubes in series. The total flow is that shown on the higher flow tube, not the sum of the two tubes.

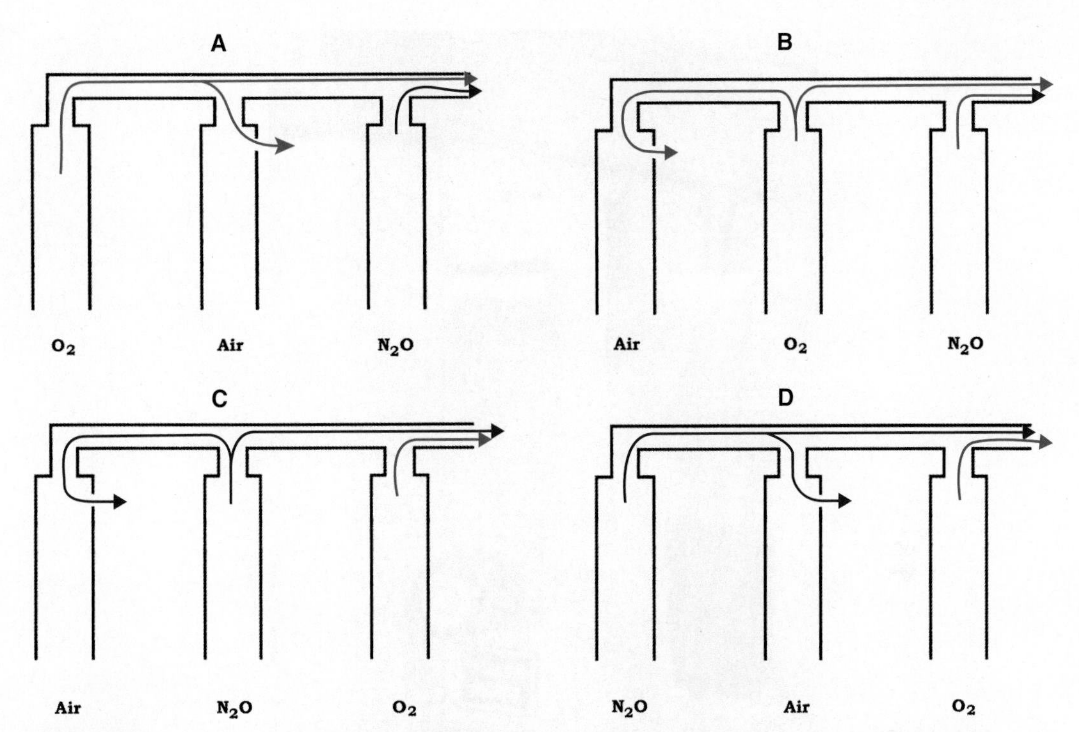

Figure 3.27 Flow indicator sequence. **A,B:** Potentially dangerous arrangements, with the oxygen flow indicator upstream. If a leak occurs, oxygen will be selectively lost. **C,D:** Oxygen is downstream from other gases, which is a safer situation because anesthetic gas rather than oxygen will be lost. Arrows represent flows of gases. (Redrawn from Eger EI, Hylton RR, Irwin RH, et al. Anesthetic flowmeter sequence—a case for hypoxia. Anesthesiology 1963;24:396–397.)

(ii) Flowmeter tube sequence is important to prevent hypoxia. **Figure 3.27** shows four different arrangements for oxygen, nitrous oxide, and air flowmeters. Normal gas flow is from bottom to top in each tube and then from left to right at the top. In **Figure 3.27 A/B,** a leak is shown in the unused air flowmeter, showing potentially dangerous arrangements because the nitrous oxide flowmeter is located in the downstream position. A substantial portion of oxygen flow passes through the leak while all the nitrous oxide is directed to the common gas outlet. Safer configurations are shown in **Figure 3.27 C/D.** By placing the oxygen flowmeter nearest the manifold outlet, a leak upstream from the oxygen results in loss of nitrous oxide rather than oxygen.

(iii) Before discovering that flowmeter sequence was important in preventing hypoxia, there was no consensus on where the oxygen flowmeter should be in relation to the flowmeters for other gases. To avoid confusion, the American workstation standard requires that the oxygen flowmeter be placed on the right side of the flowmeter group as viewed from the front. In many countries, the oxygen flowmeter is on the left side with the manifold outlet also on the left. This sets the stage for potential operator error if a user administers anesthesia in a country other than where he or she was trained. There is no consensus on the

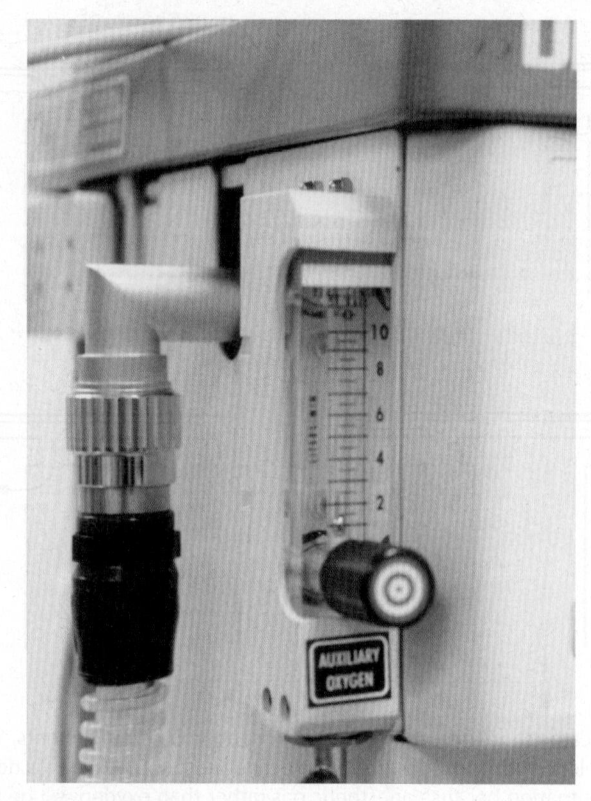

Figure 3.28 Courtesy (auxiliary) oxygen flowmeter.

location of the air or nitrous oxide flowmeters as long as they do not occupy the location next to the manifold outlet.

c. Auxiliary Oxygen Flowmeter

An auxiliary (courtesy) oxygen flowmeter (**Fig. 3.28**) is a self-contained flowmeter with its own flow control valve, flow indicator, and outlet. It is not affected by computer control. It usually has a short tube with a maximum flow of 10 L/minute and a barbed fitting on the outlet for connection to a face mask or nasal cannula. It is used to supply oxygen to the patient without turning ON the anesthesia machine.

CLINICAL MOMENT On some older machines, this flowmeter will work only on pipeline gas. On newer machines, it will work on either cylinder or pipeline supplies. Check your machine by disconnecting the pipeline and opening the oxygen cylinder. If oxygen flows, either the pipeline or the cylinder may be the gas source.

d. Flowmeter Problems

1) The flowmeter scale, tube, and indicator must be regarded as an inseparable unit. The tube assembly calibrated for one gas cannot be used for a different gas. If a tube, indicator, and scale calibrated for one gas are used for another gas, they will deliver an incorrect gas flow.

CLINICAL MOMENT If any part of the flowmeter is damaged, the flowmeter, scale, and indicator all need to be replaced with a new set. Flowmeter components are calibrated as a set and if only one component is changed there will be inaccuracy.

2) Damage to the flow indicator can result if it is suddenly propelled to the top of the tube when a cylinder is opened or a pipeline hose is connected while the flow control valve is open. Flow indicators can become worn or distorted with use. The stop at the top of the flowmeter tube can become dislodged and rest on top of the indicator.

CLINICAL MOMENT Mechanical flowmeters should be protected by turning each flow control valve OFF at the end of the day or when a cylinder valve is opened or a pipeline hose is connected to the machine. This prevents the indicator from suddenly rising to the top of the tube, which might damage the indicator or allow it to go unnoticed.

3) A leak in a flowmeter downstream of the indicator but upstream of the common manifold will result in a lower-than-expected concentration of that gas in the fresh gas. A leak may occur if a flow control valve is left open and there is no cylinder or yoke plug in the yoke. The indicator at the bottom of the tube will not prevent gas backflow.
4) Anesthesia providers are accustomed to a certain flowmeter sequence. When this sequence is altered, there may be mistakes that result in an unintended gas being administered. This problem is most likely to occur between air and nitrous oxide because the position of oxygen is fixed by national custom or standards.

e. Electronic Flowmeters

Most of the electronic anesthesia machines available at this time use a conventional flow control valve and an electronic flow sensor. Different technologies are used to measure gas flow. They are discussed in Chapter 18. The flow measured by the sensor is then represented digitally and/or by a simulated flowmeter on the anesthesia machine screen (**Fig. 3.29**). An advantage of electronic flow measurement is that this information is available in a form that can be sent to a data management system.

f. Hypoxia Prevention Safety Devices

1) One of the hazards associated with flowmeters is the possibility that the operator will set the flows that could deliver a hypoxic mixture. Various devices have been developed to prevent this problem.

CLINICAL MOMENT The hypoxia prevention devices discussed here should not be confused with the oxygen pressure failure device discussed earlier. The oxygen pressure failure device prevents hypoxia due to a loss of oxygen pressure in the machine, whereas hypoxia prevention devices prevent the operator from accidentally setting a hypoxic gas mixture.

2) Some older anesthesia machines required a minimum mandatory oxygen flow of 50 to 250 mL/minute. This does not in itself prevent a hypoxic gas concentration from being delivered. It is not usually found on electronic anesthesia machines.

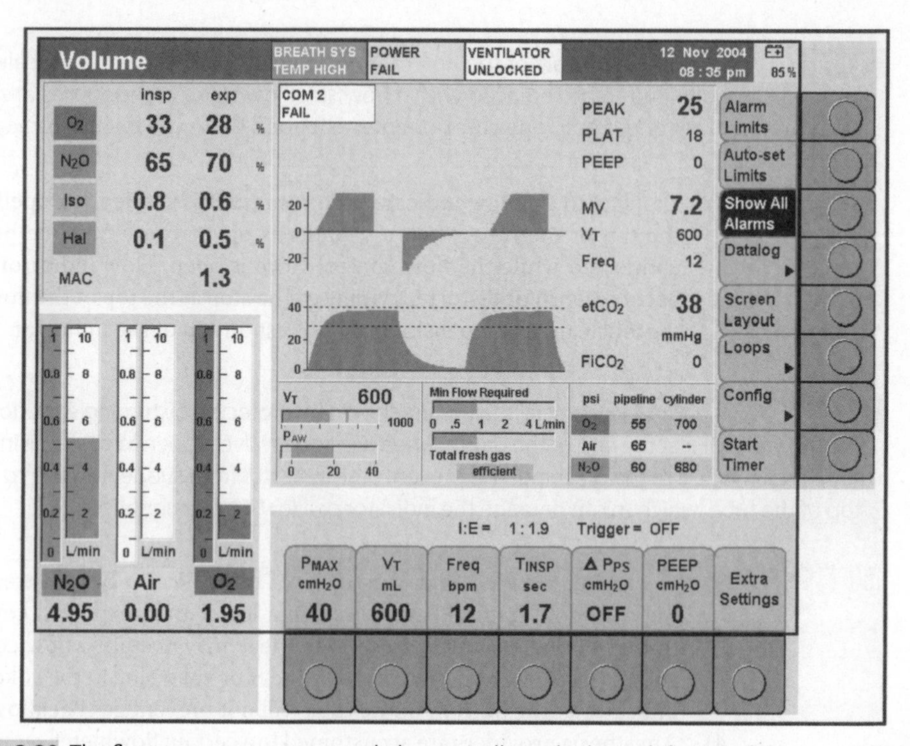

Figure 3.29 The flowmeters are represented electronically at the lower left part of the screen. The flows are set by using conventional flow control valves and then the flows are measured electronically. Note that the simulated flowmeter tubes are in series. At the top are a series of messages, including ones showing that there is no mains power and the battery has 85% of its charge. This screen also shows the pipeline and cylinder pressures. (Courtesy of Drager Medical, Lubeck, Germany.)

CLINICAL MOMENT The minimum mandatory oxygen flow makes it difficult to use a closed system anesthesia technique because the flow can be higher than the metabolic oxygen uptake. This means that excess gas must be periodically released from the system.

3) To protect against an operator-selected delivery of a mixture of oxygen and nitrous oxide having an oxygen concentration below 21% oxygen (V/V), a minimum oxygen ratio device is used. If the oxygen flow is decreased to a point where the oxygen concentration would be less than 25%, the device will lower the nitrous oxide flow to maintain an oxygen concentration of at least 25%. In some cases, if the nitrous oxide is increased, the oxygen flow will also increase by the necessary amount. Alarms are available on some machines to alert the operator that the oxygen:nitrous oxide flow ratio has fallen below the minimum.

2. **Unidirectional (Check) Valve**

When ventilation is controlled or assisted, positive pressure from the breathing system can be transmitted back into the machine. Using the oxygen flush valve may also create a positive back pressure. This pressure can affect flowmeter readings and the concentration of volatile anesthetic agents delivered from the vaporizers on the machine. Some machines have a unidirectional (check) valve to minimize these effects. This valve is located between the vaporizers and the common gas outlet, upstream of where the oxygen flush flow joins the fresh gas flow. This valve will lessen the pressure increase but not prevent it, because gas will be continually flowing from the flowmeters toward a blocked valve. These valves are not present on all machines. If present, they will interfere with checking for leaks upstream of the machine outlet. This is discussed in Chapter 25.

3. **Pressure Relief Device**
   a. Some machines have a pressure relief device near the common gas outlet to protect the machine from high pressures. This valve opens to atmosphere and vents gas if a preset pressure is exceeded.
   b. A pressure relief device may limit the ability of an anesthesia machine to provide adequate pressure for jet ventilation through a catheter inserted through the cricothyroid membrane.

CLINICAL MOMENT Anesthesia machine manufacturers do *not* recommend that the common gas outlet and oxygen flush be used to provide jet ventilation. Some machines offer a connection from the pipeline or intermediate pressure system for a jet ventilation device.

4. **Common (Fresh) Gas Outlet**
   a. The common (fresh) gas outlet receives all of the gases and vapors from the machine and delivers the mixture to the breathing system. Some outlets have a 15-mm female slip-joint fitting (that will accept a tracheal tube connector). They may also have a manufacturer-specific fitting. There is a mechanism to prevent a disconnection between the machine and the hose to the breathing system.
   b. Many new anesthesia machines have internal connections to the breathing system. These machines may not have the conventional common gas outlet described.
   c. The common gas outlet should not be used to administer supplemental oxygen to a patient. This will delay conversion to the breathing system if an emergency arises. Another potential problem is that a vaporizer on the back bar may be accidentally left ON, leading to undesired administration of the inhalation agent.

CLINICAL MOMENT Do not use the common gas outlet to administer supplemental oxygen to a patient. Use the auxiliary oxygen flowmeter or a separate flowmeter.

SUGGESTED READINGS

Brockwell RC. Understanding Your Anesthesia Machine (ASA Refresher Course #506). Atlanta, GA: ASA, 2005.

Dorsch J, Dorsch S. The Anesthesia Machine in Understanding Anesthesia Equipment. Fifth edition. Philadelphia: Wolters Kluwer/Lippincott Williams & Wilkins, 2008:83–120.

Stone AGH, Howell PR. Use of the common gas outlet for the administration of supplemental oxygen during Caesarean section under regional anaesthesia. Anaesthesia 2002;57:690–692.

4 Vaporizers

I. Introduction

A vaporizer (anesthetic agent or vapor delivery device) changes a liquid anesthetic agent into its vapor and adds a controlled amount of that vapor to the fresh gas flow to the breathing system. Up to three vaporizers are commonly attached to an anesthesia machine, but only one can be used at a time.

II. Physics

A. Vapor Pressure

1. **Figure 4.1A** shows a volatile liquid inside a container that is closed to atmosphere. Molecules of liquid break away from the surface and enter the space above, forming a vapor. If the container is kept at a constant temperature, a dynamic equilibrium is established between the liquid and vapor phases so that the number of molecules in the vapor phase remains constant. These molecules bombard the walls of the container, creating a pressure. This is called the *saturated vapor pressure* and is represented by the density of dots above the liquid.
2. If heat is supplied to the container (**Fig. 4.1B**), the equilibrium will be shifted so that more molecules enter the vapor phase and the vapor pressure will rise. If the liquid temperature is lowered (**Fig. 4.1C**) or is lowered because a carrier gas flows through the vaporizer and the agent is vaporized (**Fig. 4.1D**), more molecules will remain in the liquid state, causing the vapor pressure to be lower. It is meaningless, therefore, to talk about vapor pressure without specifying the temperature. Vapor pressures of some anesthetic agents at 20°C are shown in **Table 4.1.** Vapor pressure depends only on the liquid and the temperature. It is not affected by ambient pressure within the range of barometric pressures encountered in anesthesia.

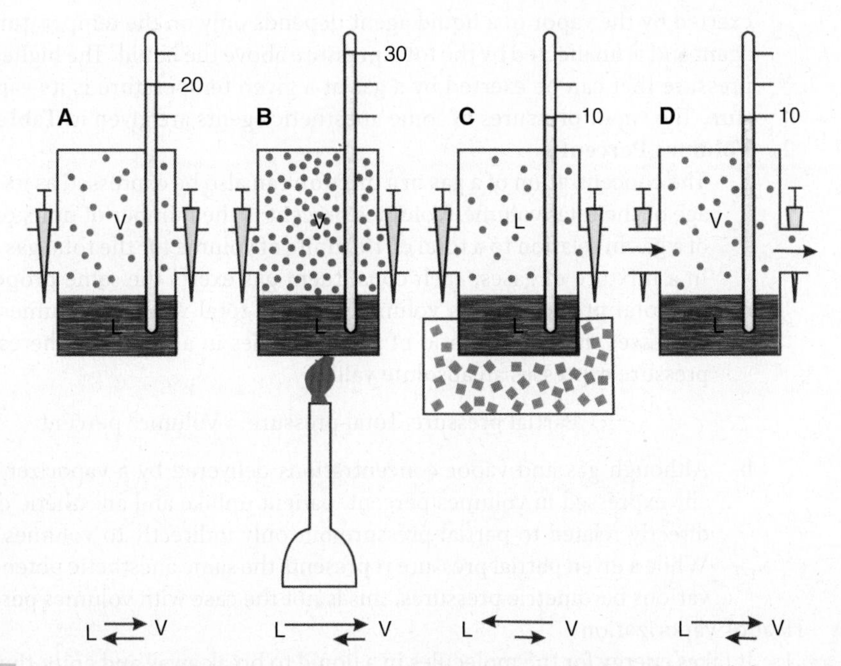

Figure 4.1 Vapor pressure changes with varying temperature. **A:** The liquid (L) and the vapor (V) are in equilibrium. **B:** The application of heat causes the equilibrium to shift so that more molecules enter the vapor phase, as illustrated by the increased density of dots above the liquid. **C:** Lowering the temperature causes a shift toward the liquid phase and a decrease in vapor pressure. **D:** Passing a carrier gas over the liquid shifts the equilibrium toward the vapor phase. The heat of vaporization is supplied from the remaining liquid. This causes a drop in temperature.

Table 4.1 Properties of Common Anesthetic Agents

Agent	Boiling Point (°C, 760 mm Hg)	Vapor Pressure (torr, 20°C)	Density of Liquid (g/mL)	MAC[a] in O_2 (%)
Halothane	50.2	243	1.86 (20°C)	0.75
Isoflurane	48.5	238	1.496 (25°C)	1.15
Desflurane	22.8	669	1.45 (20°C)	6.4
Sevoflurane	58.6	157		2.0

[a]Minimum anesthetic concentration.

B. Boiling Point

A liquid's boiling point is the temperature at which its vapor pressure is equal to the atmospheric pressure. The boiling point will be lower with lower atmospheric pressure. The boiling points for some anesthetic agents are shown in **Table 4.1.**

C. Gas Concentration

Two methods are commonly used to express the concentration of a gas or vapor: partial pressure and volumes percent (vol %).

1. **Partial Pressure**

   A mixture of gases in a closed container will exert a pressure on the walls of the container. The part of the total pressure due to any one gas in the mixture is called the partial pressure of that gas. The total pressure of the mixture is the sum of the partial pressures of the constituent gases. The partial pressure exerted by the vapor of a liquid agent depends only on the temperature of that agent and is unaffected by the total pressure above the liquid. The highest partial pressure that can be exerted by a gas at a given temperature is its vapor pressure. The vapor pressures of some anesthetic agents are given in **Table 4.1.**

2. **Volumes Percent**

   a. The concentration of a gas in a mixture can also be expressed as its percentage of the total volume. Volumes percent is the number of units of volume of a gas in relation to a total of 100 units of volume for the total gas mixture. In a mixture of gases, each constituent gas exerts the same proportion of the total pressure as its volume is of the total volume. Volumes percent expresses the relative ratio of gas molecules in a mixture, whereas partial pressure expresses an absolute value.

   Partial pressure/Total pressure = Volumes percent

   b. Although gas and vapor concentrations delivered by a vaporizer are usually expressed in volumes percent, patient uptake and anesthetic depth are directly related to partial pressure but only indirectly to volumes percent. While a given partial pressure represents the same anesthetic potency under various barometric pressures, this is not the case with volumes percent.

D. Heat of Vaporization

1. It takes energy for the molecules in a liquid to break away and enter the gaseous phase. A liquid's heat of vaporization is the number of calories necessary to convert 1 g of liquid into vapor. Heat of vaporization can also be expressed as the number of calories necessary to convert 1 mL of liquid into vapor.
2. Liquid temperature decreases as vaporization proceeds. As the temperature falls, a gradient is created so that heat flows from the surroundings into the liquid. The lower the liquid temperature, the greater the gradient and the greater

the flow of heat from the surroundings. Eventually, equilibrium is established so that the heat lost to vaporization is matched by the heat supplied from the surroundings. At this point, the temperature ceases to drop.

3. In **Figure 4.1D,** a gas (carrier gas) is passed through the container and carries away molecules of vapor. This causes the equilibrium to shift so that more molecules enter the vapor phase. Unless some means of supplying heat is available, the liquid will cool. As the temperature drops, so does the vapor pressure of the liquid and fewer molecules will be picked up by the carrier gas so that there is a decrease in partial pressure in the gas flowing out of the container.

E. Specific Heat

1. A substance's specific heat is the quantity of heat required to raise the temperature of 1 g of the substance by 1°C. The higher the specific heat, the more heat is required to raise the temperature of a given quantity of that substance. A slightly different definition of specific heat is the amount of heat required to raise the temperature of 1 mL of the substance by 1°C. Water is the standard with a specific heat value of 1 cal/g/°C or 1 cal/mL/°C.
2. Specific heat is important when considering the amount of heat that must be supplied to a liquid anesthetic to maintain a stable temperature when heat is lost during vaporization.
3. Specific heat is also important for choosing the material to construct a vaporizer. Temperature changes more gradually for materials with a high specific heat than for those with a low specific heat.

F. Thermal Conductivity

1. Another consideration in choosing material from which to construct a vaporizer is thermal conductivity. This is a measure of the speed with which heat flows through a substance. The higher the thermal conductivity, the better the substance conducts heat.
2. Thermostabilization is achieved by constructing a vaporizer of a metal with high thermal conductivity (copper, bronze) to minimize temperature changes when the vaporizer is in use. In a vaporizer containing a wick, it is important that the wick be in contact with a metal part so that heat lost as a result of vaporization can be quickly replaced.

III. Vaporizer Design

A. Concentration Calibration

Nearly all the vaporizers in use today in the United States are calibrated by agent concentration as expressed in percentage of vapor output. They are known as *concentrated-calibrated vaporizers*. Vaporizer output is controlled by a single dial that is calibrated in volumes percent.

CLINICAL MOMENT Concentration-calibrated vaporizers are designed to be located between the flowmeters and the common gas outlet on the anesthesia machine (**Fig. 4.2**). They are not designed to be used between the common gas outlet and the breathing system or in the breathing system.

1. **Variable Bypass Vaporizers**

a. The vapor pressures of most anesthetic agents at room temperature are much greater than the partial pressure required to produce anesthesia. To produce clinically useful concentrations, a vaporizer dilutes saturated vapor. This can be accomplished by splitting the fresh gas flow that passes through the vaporizer (**Fig. 4.3**). Some of the gas flows through the vaporizing

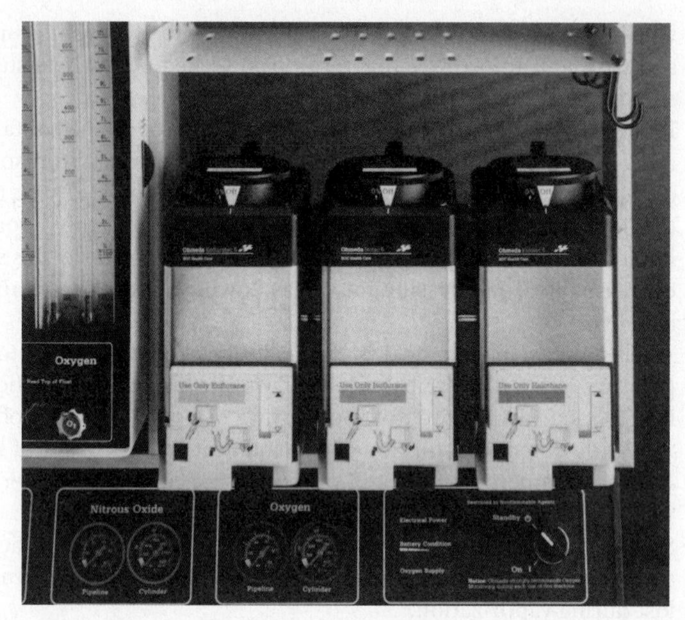

Figure 4.2 Tec 5 vaporizers. The locking lever for the filling device is on the lower left side of each vaporizer. The lever for filling/draining is at the base, below the sight glass. To fill, the bottle adaptor is inserted into the rectangular port and clamped in place by pulling the locking lever down. The bottle is then lifted up and the filling/draining lever pulled forward. When filling is complete, the filling/draining lever is returned to the closed position, the bottle is lowered, the clamping lever is pushed upward, and the bottle and adaptor are removed. Draining the vaporizer is accomplished by using the same levers but by lowering the bottle rather than lifting it up. Behind each control dial is a locking lever in the locked position. The lever must be in the locked position before the vaporizer can be turned ON. There is a mechanism to prevent more than one vaporizer from being turned ON. (Courtesy of Ohmeda, now a part of General Electric.)

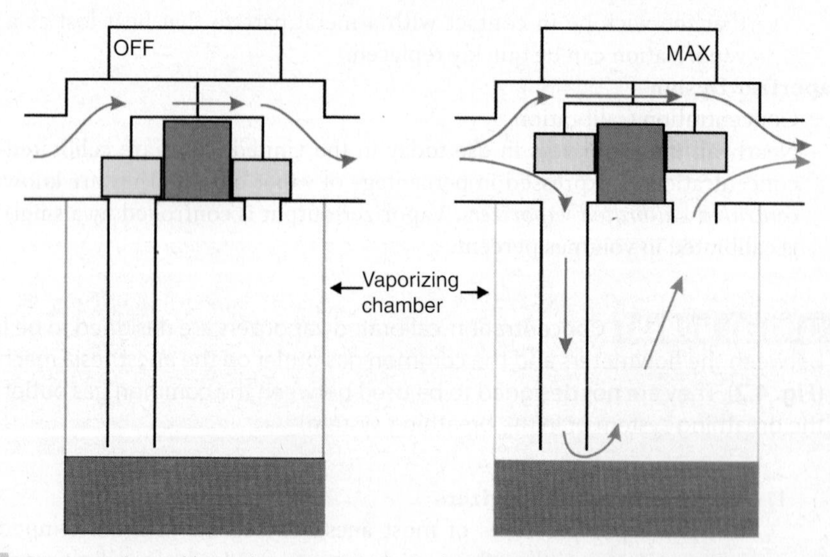

Figure 4.3 Concentration-calibrated vaporizer. **Left:** In the OFF position, all of the inflowing gas is directed through the bypass. **Right:** In the ON position, gas flow is divided between the bypass and the vaporizing chamber. In the MAX position, all of the gas flow allowed by the vaporizer goes to the vaporizing chamber.

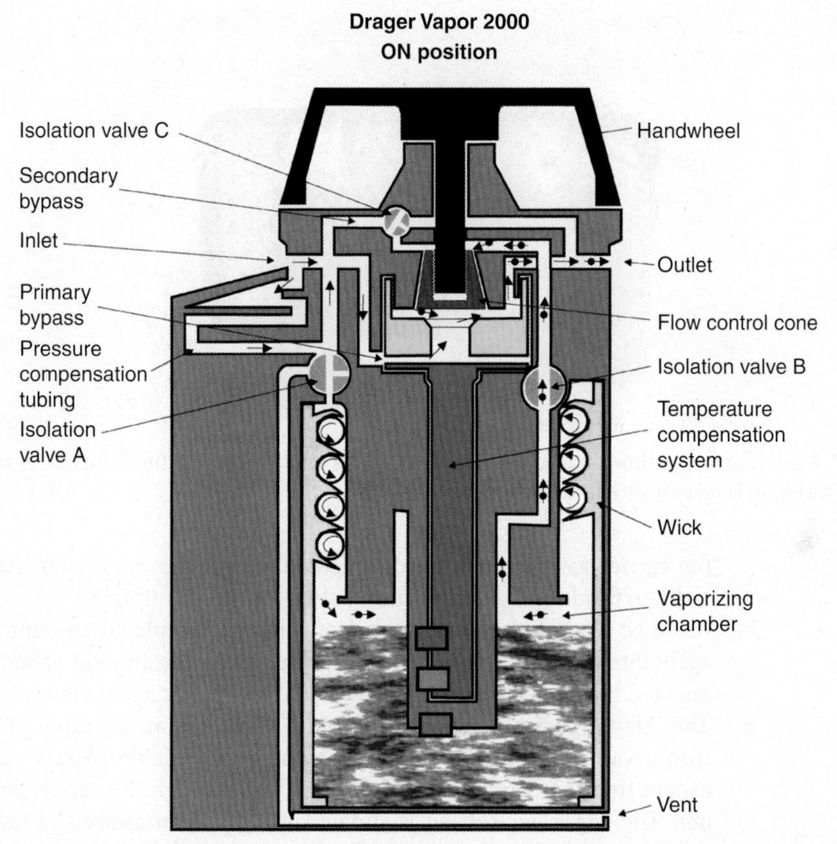

Figure 4.4 Vapor 2000 vaporizer in ON position. (Redrawn courtesy of Drager Medical, Telford, PA.)

chamber (the part containing the liquid anesthetic agent), and the remainder goes through a bypass to the vaporizer outlet. Both gas flows join downstream of the vaporizing chamber, where gas at the desired concentration exits the vaporizer.

b. The ratio of bypass gas to gas going to the vaporizing chamber is called the splitting ratio and depends on the resistances in the two pathways. This, in turn, depends on the variable (adjustable) orifice, which is controlled by the concentration dial. This orifice may be in the inlet to the vaporizing chamber but is in the outlet in most modern vaporizers.

c. **Figure 4.4** shows the internal construction of a typical concentration-calibrated vaporizer. Gas enters at the left and is split into the bypass and vaporizing chamber flows. In the center of the vaporizer is a thermostat that alters flow in the bypass. The vaporizing chamber gas flow passes through a spiral channel to enter the vaporizing chamber where it then passes through a spiral of wicks. The vapor-laden gas then exits the vaporizing changer through a channel controlled by the control dial and joins the bypass gas. The gas then exits the vaporizer.

2. **Electronic Vaporizers**

a. In an electronic vaporizer, the volume of carrier gas necessary to produce the desired agent concentration may be determined by a computer that calculates

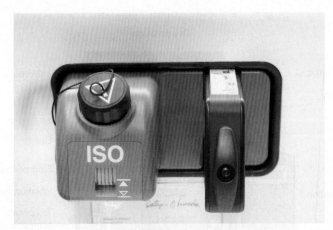

Figure 4.5 Aladin cassette vaporizer in place. The cassette fits into a recess on the front of the anesthesia machine. The liquid level indicator is below the filling device.

the carrier gas flow that needs to pass through the vaporizing chamber in order to produce the desired anesthetic agent concentration.

b. Another type of electronic vaporizer injects a calculated amount of liquid agent into the breathing system or fresh gas flow. The amount of liquid that is injected is adjusted to achieve the desired anesthetic agent concentration.

c. The Aladin cassette vaporizer (**Figs. 4.5–4.7**) is an example of an electronic vaporizer. It is similar to mechanical variable bypass vaporizers except that the computer controls the flow through the vaporizing chamber. The vaporizer setting is shown on the screen above the handwheel that is used to alter the setting. The plastic cassette holds the liquid agent.

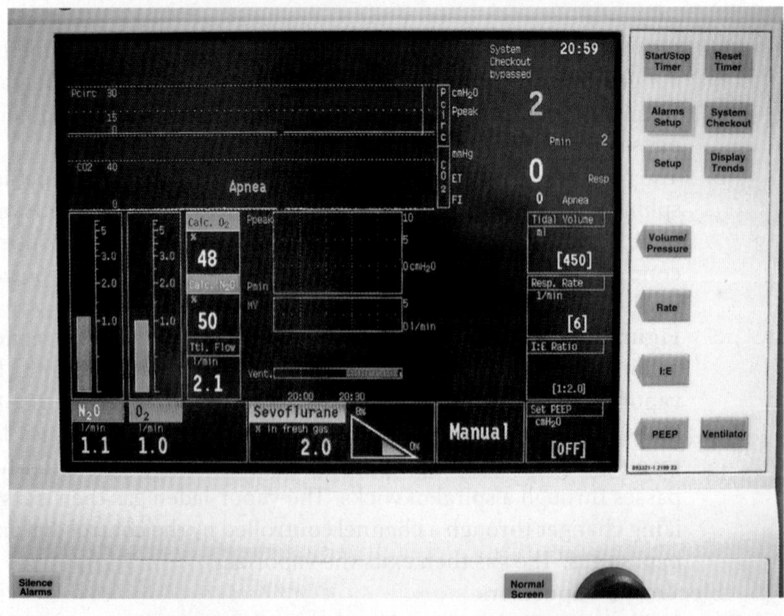

Figure 4.6 Display screen showing the agent and the setting at the bottom in the center. The agent is identified in the text and is color coded. The setting is in numerals and represented by a triangular graph.

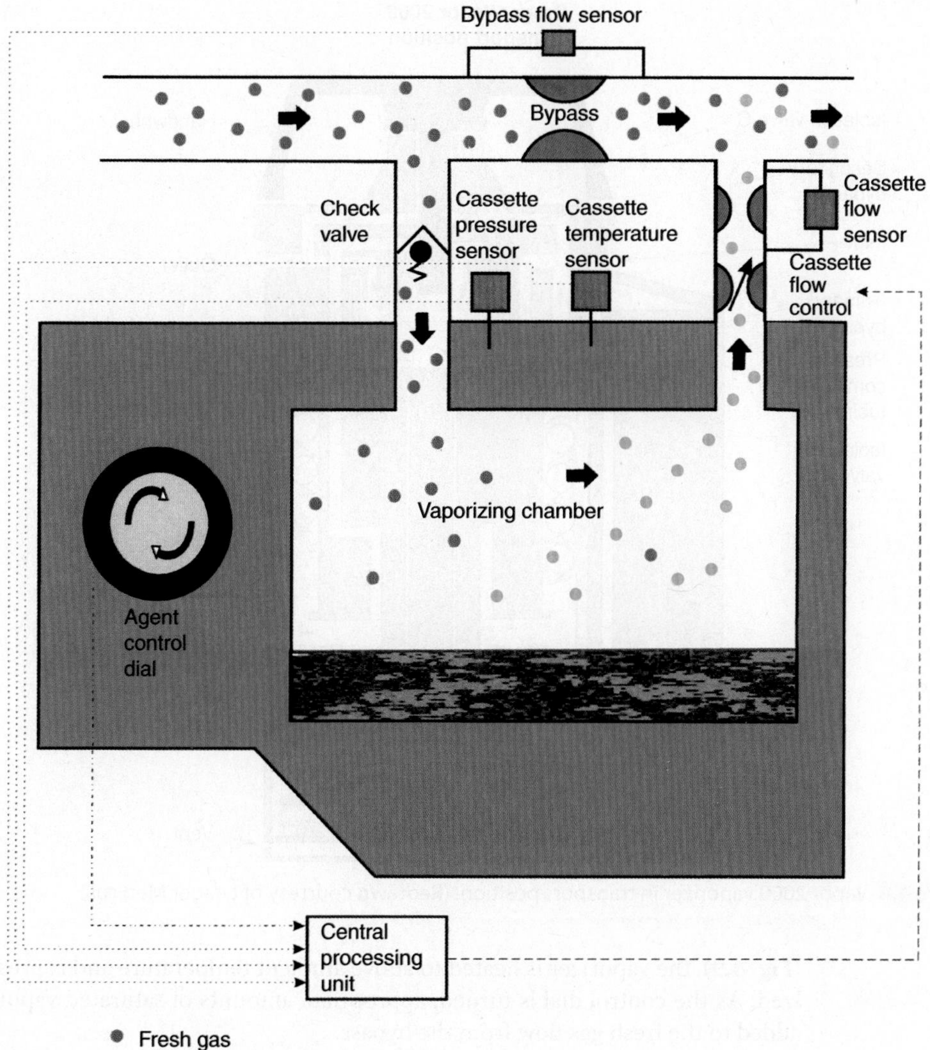

Figure 4.7 Diagram of Aladin cassette vaporizer.

Temperature variations are compensated for by increasing or decreasing the flow through the vaporizing chamber.

B. Vaporization Methods

1. **Flow-over**

In a flow-over vaporizer, a stream of carrier gas passes over the surface of the liquid. Increasing the area of the carrier gas–liquid interface enhances vaporization efficiency. This can be done by using baffles or spiral tracks to lengthen the gas pathway over the liquid or employing wicks that have their bases in the liquid. The liquid moves up the wicks by capillary action. The vaporizers in **Figures 4.4** and **4.8** are examples of flow-over vaporizers.

2. **Injection**

Certain vaporizers control the vapor concentration by injecting a known amount of liquid anesthetic into a known volume of gas. In desflurane vaporizers

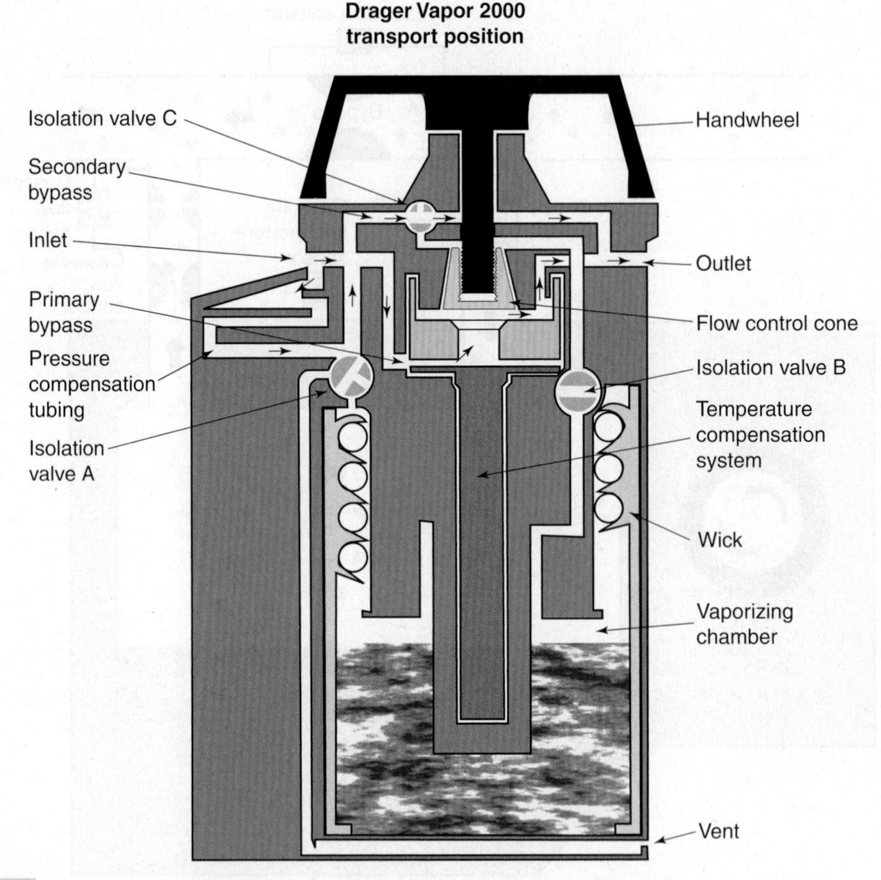

Figure 4.8 Vapor 2000 vaporizer in transport position. (Redrawn courtesy of Drager Medical.)

(**Fig. 4.9**), the vaporizer is heated to above ambient temperature and is pressurized. As the control dial is turned, appropriate amounts of saturated vapor are added to the fresh gas flow from the bypass.

3. **Temperature Compensation**

As a liquid is vaporized, heat is lost. As the liquid temperature decreases, so does the vapor pressure. Most concentration-calibrated vaporizers compensate for temperature changes by altering the splitting ratio so that the percentage of carrier gas directed through the vaporizing chamber is increased or decreased (**Fig. 4.4**). An electric heater can be used to supply heat to a vaporizer and maintain it at a constant temperature (see **Fig. 4.9**).

IV. **Effects of Altered Barometric Pressure**

Most vaporizers are calibrated at sea level. Because they are sometimes used in hyperbaric chambers or at high altitudes where atmospheric pressure is low, it is important to know how they will perform when the barometric pressure is changed. The documents accompanying each vaporizer should be consulted.

V. **Effects of Intermittent Back Pressure**

When assisted or controlled ventilation is used, the positive pressure generated during inspiration is transmitted from the breathing system back to the machine and the vaporizers. Back pressure also occurs when the oxygen flush is activated. Back pressure may either increase (pumping effect) or decrease (pressurizing effect) the vaporizer output.

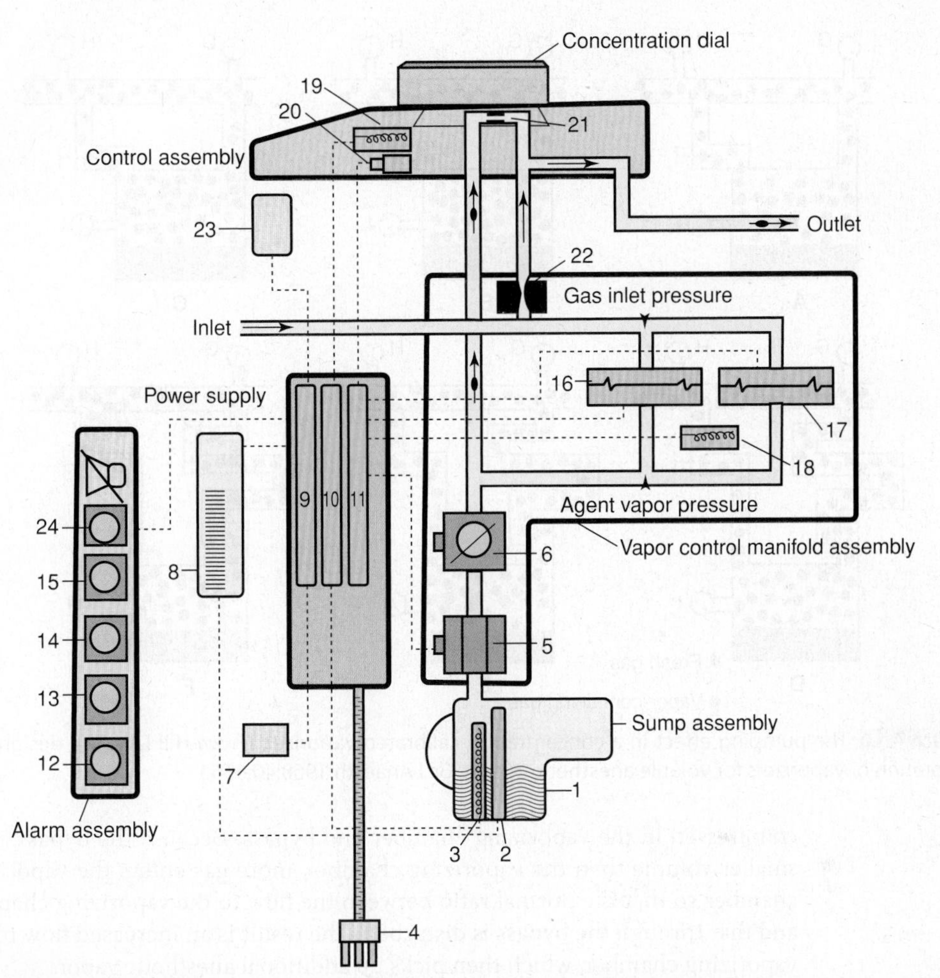

Figure 4.9 Diagram of Tec 6 vaporizer: (*1*) agent, (*2*) level sensor, (*3*) sump heaters, (*4*) electrical mains, (*5*) shutoff valve, (*6*) agent pressure-regulating valve, (*7*) battery for alarms, (*8*) LCD level display, (*9*) alarm electronics, (*10*) heater electronics, (*11*) control electronics, (*12*) alarm battery low LED, (*13*) warm-up LED, (*14*) low agent LED, (*15*) no output LED, (*16*) pressure transducer, (*17*) pressure monitor, (*18*) heater in vapor manifold, (*19*) heater in valve plate, (*20*) solenoid interlock, (*21*) variable resistor (controlled by rotary valve), (*22*) fixed restrictor, (*23*) tilt switch, and (*24*) operational LED. (See text for details.) (Redrawn from a diagram furnished by Ohmeda, a division of BOC Health Care, Inc., Madison, WI.)

A. Pumping Effect

1. Studies have shown that concentrations delivered by some vaporizers are higher during controlled or assisted ventilation than when the vaporizer is used with free flow to atmosphere. This change is most pronounced when there is less liquid agent in the vaporizing chamber, when carrier gas flow is low, when the pressure fluctuations are high and frequent, and when the dial setting is low.
2. A proposed mechanism for the pumping effect in concentration-calibrated variable bypass vaporizers is shown in **Figure 4.10. Figure 4.10A** shows the vaporizer during exhalation. The relative resistances of the outlets from the bypass and vaporizing chamber determine the flows to each.
3. **Figure 4.10B** shows inspiration. Positive pressure at point H prevents gas and vapor outflow. Pressure is transmitted to points G and I. This results in gas being

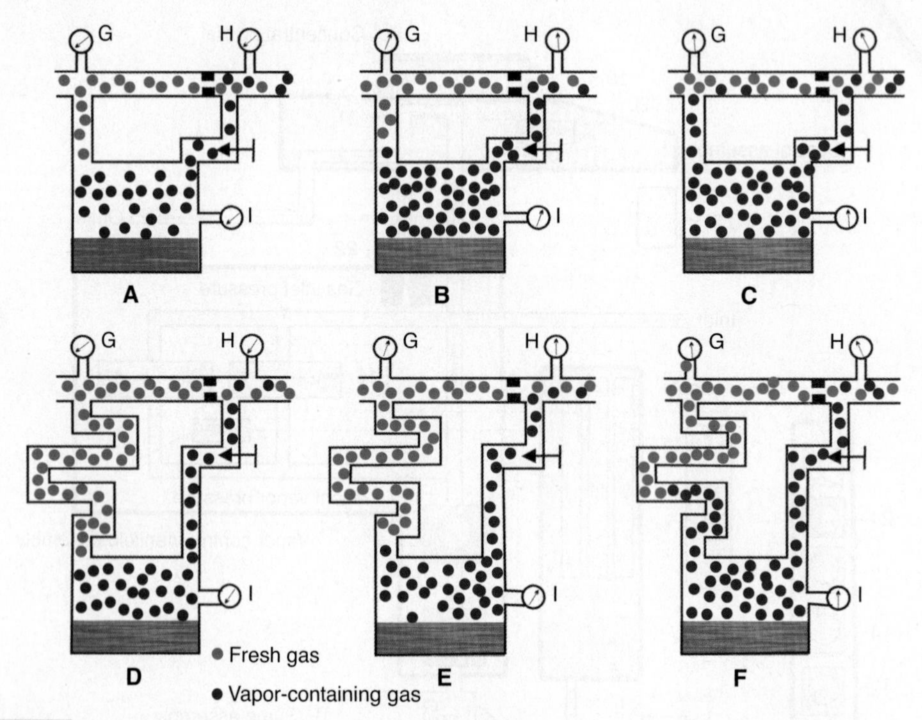

Figure 4.10 The pumping effect in a concentration-calibrated vaporizer. (From Hill DW. The design and calibration of vaporizers for volatile anesthetic agents. Br J Anaesth 1968;40:656.)

compressed in the vaporizing chamber and bypass. Because the bypass has a smaller volume than the vaporizing chamber, more gas enters the vaporizing chamber so that the normal ratio between the flow to the vaporizing chamber and that through the bypass is disturbed. The result is an increased flow to the vaporizing chamber, which then picks up additional anesthetic vapor.

4. **Figure 4.10C** shows the situation after the beginning of exhalation. The pressure at point H falls rapidly and gas flows from the vaporizing chamber and the bypass to the outlet. Because the bypass has less resistance than the vaporizing chamber outlet, the pressure in the bypass falls more quickly than that in the vaporizing chamber and gas containing vapor flows from the vaporizing chamber into the bypass. Because the gas in the bypass (which dilutes the gas from the vaporizing chamber) now carries vapor and the gas flowing from the vaporizing chamber is still saturated, the concentration in the vaporizer output is increased.
5. To decrease the pumping effect, the vaporizer can be kept relatively full, decreasing the space above the liquid. The tubing that the gas passes through before entering the vaporizing chamber can be elongated in a spiral as shown in **Figures 4.10D–F** and **4.4.** Check valves in the machine or at the vaporizer outlet may be used to reduce pressure fluctuations.

B. Pressurizing Effect

1. The output of some vaporizers used in conjunction with automatic ventilators has been found to be lower than during free flow to atmosphere. The effect is greater with high flows, large pressure fluctuations, and low vaporizer settings.
2. **Figure 4.11A** shows a vaporizer flowing free to atmosphere. The pressure in the vaporizing chamber and the bypass is *P*. As gas flows to the outlet, the pressure is reduced to *R*. The number of molecules of anesthetic agent picked up by each

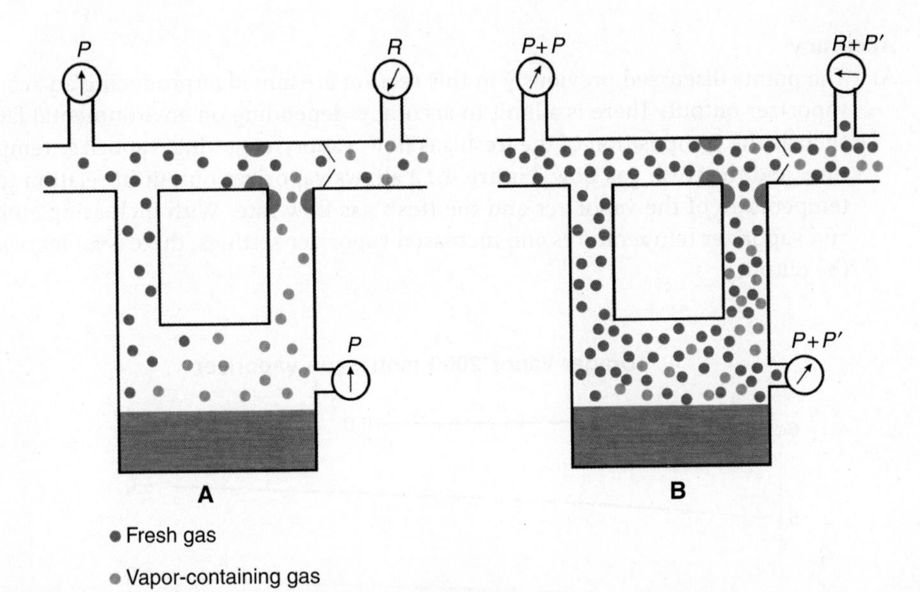

Figure 4.11 The pressurizing effect. An increase in pressure (*P′*) causes an increase in pressure (*P*) inside the vaporizer. The vapor pressure of the volatile anesthetic is unaffected by changes in the total pressure of the gas mixture above it. As a result, the concentration is reduced.

milliliter of carrier gas depends on the density of the anesthetic vapor molecules in the vaporizing chamber. This, in turn, depends on the agent's vapor pressure.

3. **Figure 4.11B** shows the situation when an increased pressure is applied to the vaporizer outlet and transmitted to the vaporizing chamber. The increased pressure will compress the carrier gas so that there will be more molecules per milliliter. The number of anesthetic vapor molecules in the vaporizing chamber will not be increased, however, because this depends on the saturated vapor pressure of the anesthetic and not on the pressure in the container. The net result is a decrease in the concentration of anesthetic in the vaporizing chamber and the vaporizer outlet.

VI. Effects of Rebreathing

The vaporizer dial setting reflects the concentration of inhalational agent delivered to the breathing system. When the fresh gas flow is high, there may be little, if any, exhaled gas rebreathed and the inspired concentration should be close to the vaporizer setting. As the fresh gas flow is lowered, exhaled gases contribute a more significant portion of anesthetic agent to the inspired gases. Rebreathing causes a difference between the vaporizer setting and the inspired concentration. If minute volume is increased, there will be more rebreathing and a greater effect. With significant rebreathing, only an agent analyzer can provide an accurate value for the inspired agent concentration.

CLINICAL MOMENT Some anesthesia providers think that the vaporizer output is low because the concentration in the breathing system is lower than the dial setting at the beginning of an anesthetic. This difference is caused by the relatively large volume of the breathing system and low fresh gas flow to the breathing system. Agent uptake by the patient is also important, especially in the early stages of the anesthetic. The difference will decrease with time.

VII. Accuracy

A. The points discussed previously in this section are aimed at producing an accurate vaporizer output. There is a limit to accuracy, depending on environmental factors such as the composition of the fresh gas flow, vaporizer setting, vaporizer temperature, and the fresh gas flow. **Figure 4.12** shows vaporizer output in relation to the temperature of the vaporizer and the fresh gas flow rate. With increasing ambient and vaporizer temperatures and increased vaporizer settings, there is an increase in the output.

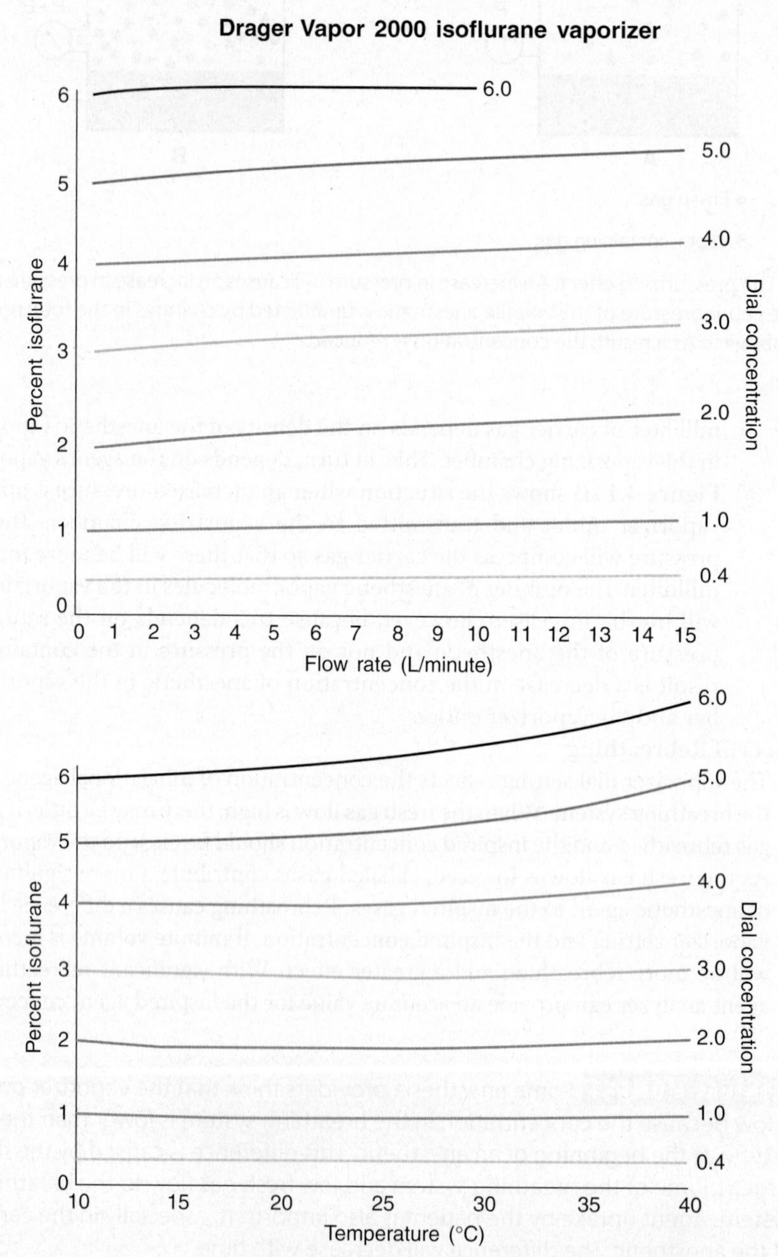

Figure 4.12 Performance of isoflurane Vapor 2000 vaporizer. (Redrawn from graphs furnished by Drager Medical.)

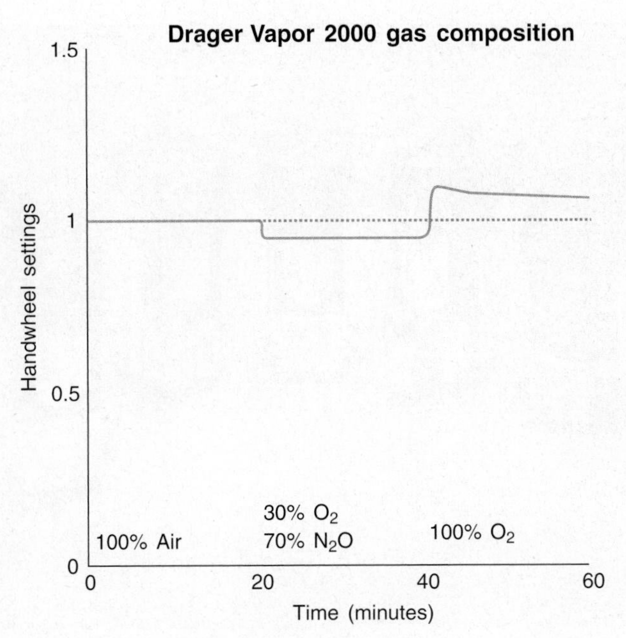

Figure 4.13 Effect of carrier gas composition on the output of the halothane Vapor 2000 vaporizer. (Redrawn from graphs furnished by Drager Medical.)

CLINICAL MOMENT When in doubt about vaporizer accuracy, check the accuracy with an anesthetic agent monitor by placing the sample line inside the fresh gas outlet while gas is flowing.

B. The fresh gas composition can have an effect on vaporizer output. **Figure 4.13** illustrates the change in vapor output with air, followed by a combination of 30% oxygen and 70% nitrous oxide and finally 100% oxygen. If this occurs with a particular vaporizer, it should be noted in the user manual.

C. Fortunately, at temperatures normally encountered in the operating room and the fresh gas flows and vaporizer settings usually used in clinical practice, nearly all vaporizers deliver outputs close to the dial settings.

D. Some electronic vaporizers maintain their accuracy by a feedback loop. This system compensates for differences in fresh gas flow and temperature. The concentration in the breathing system determines the vaporizer output necessary to produce the desired concentration. The computer alters the fresh gas flow through the vaporizing chamber.

VIII. Filling Systems

There are a number of different filling systems available at this time (**Fig. 4.14**). Some are designed to allow a vaporizer to be filled only with a specific agent. Some systems are specific to one vaporizer manufacturer or anesthetic agent, whereas some can be used with vaporizers from different manufacturers.

CLINICAL MOMENT Vaporizers should always be filled in the vertical position.

A. Bottle Keyed System

1. Several filling systems have a means to prevent the filler from being attached to a bottle that has an incorrect agent. This system consists of a bottle collar with

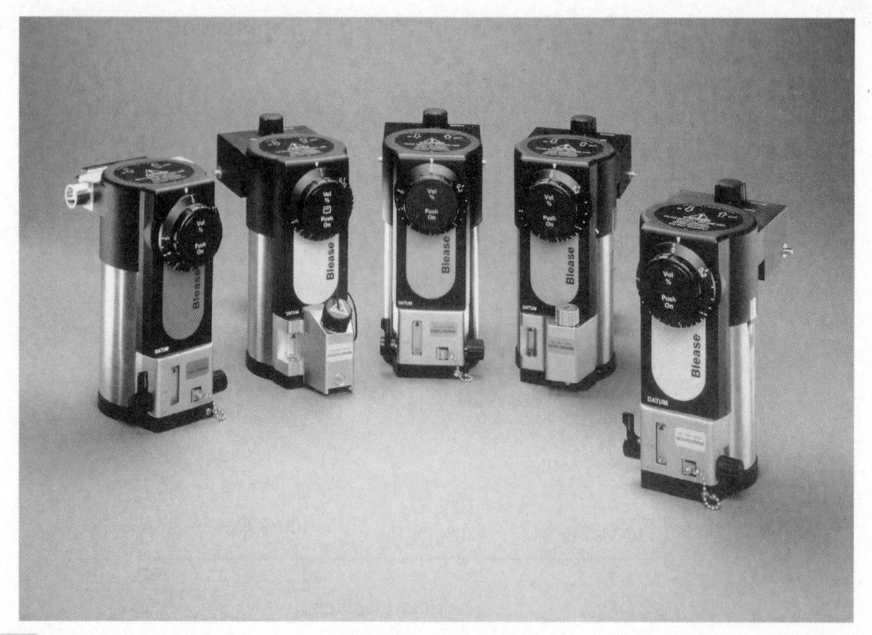

Figure 4.14 Various filling systems for vaporizers. **Left to right:** Keyed fill, Quick-Fill, keyed filled, funnel fill, and keyed filled.

two projections that differ in size (**Fig. 4.15**). The filler can be screwed only onto the bottle if the grooves on the filler fit the protrusions on the collar.

2. There are potential problems with the design. The projections for the isoflurane and sevoflurane bottles have the collar protrusions at the same place but in mirror image. If the bottle collar is placed on the bottle upside down, an incorrect filler could be placed on the bottle. It may be possible to enlarge the smaller groove on the filling adapter so that it fits on the incorrect bottle.

B. Funnel Fill System

The funnel fill system (**Fig. 4.14**) employs a funnel on the front of the vaporizer with a screw-in plug. To fill the vaporizer, the plug is removed and the liquid is poured into the funnel. When the vaporizer is full, liquid will remain in the funnel or possibly spill out. There is a drain that can allow the liquid to be removed into a container.

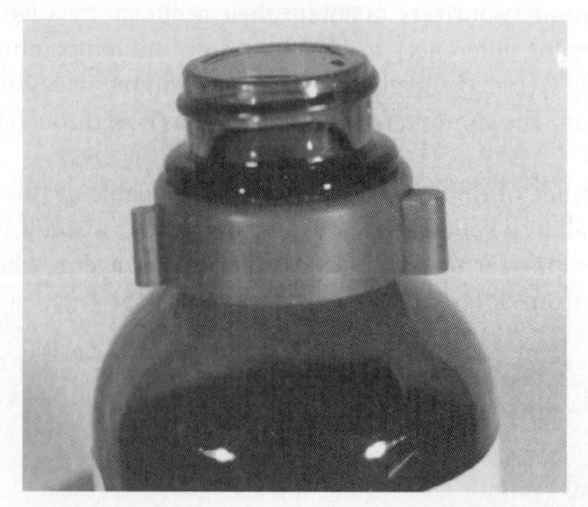

Figure 4.15 Bottle collar. The collar is color coded according to the bottle contents. It has two projections, one thicker than the other, which are designed to mate with corresponding grooves on the bottle adaptor.

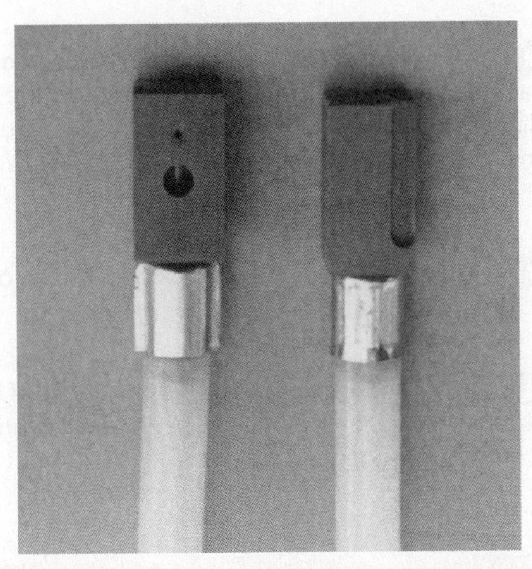

Figure 4.16 Male adaptor. The groove corresponds to a projection on the vaporizer filler receptacle. The larger hole is for anesthetic agent, and the smaller hole is for air.

This system can be converted to an agent-specific system with a screw-in adaptor keyed to the agent bottle collar.

C. Keyed Filling System

Keyed filling systems have been used by many manufacturers for a variety of vaporizers.

1. The filling device attaches to the bottle, using the collar with protrusions (**Fig. 4.15**). At the other end of the filling device is a rectangular plastic piece with a groove specific to each agent (**Fig. 4.16**). When fitted into the correct vaporizer filling block, a pin in the block lines up with the groove. Without this alignment, the filling device cannot be placed in the filler block.
2. There are two holes in the vaporizer end of the filling device (**Fig. 4.16**). One is to allow the liquid in the bottle to enter the vaporizer and the other is to allow air in the vaporizer to pass through a separate channel into the bottle.
3. The vaporizer has a mechanism to seal the filling piece into the filling block. There might also be a vent on the vaporizer filling block. The bottle is held above the filling point to allow the vaporizer to fill. After filling, the filling block must be closed. This may involve inserting a metal block.
4. To drain the vaporizer, the filler is attached to the bottle and the vaporizer in the same way but the bottle is held lower than the vaporizer.

CLINICAL MOMENT Failure to tighten the adaptor on the bottle or the keyed component, a blocked fluid path inside the vaporizer, or leakage in the valve or adapter can result in liquid anesthetic agent leaking during filling.

CLINICAL MOMENT Filling systems that use a metal block to seal the vaporizer also have a vent that must be opened to fill the device. If the metal block is not replaced and tightened, gas will leak from the filler port when the vaporizer is turned ON. No liquid will be expelled. Vapor can leak out if the fill or drain valve is not closed.

CLINICAL MOMENT A filling system that has a single opening for filling and emptying has a means to open and close the vaporizer. If the opening device is not closed after filling, there will be a leak to atmosphere and liquid anesthetic may spew out when the vaporizer is turned ON.

CLINICAL MOMENT If the filler tube is lost, it is not possible to fill the vaporizer.

CLINICAL MOMENT With some filling devices, up to 27 mL of liquid agent may be left in the bottle after the vaporizer is filled. The residual liquid can be poured into another bottle of the same agent.

CLINICAL MOMENT Some anesthesia providers try to speed filling a vaporizer by turning ON the concentration dial and/or loosening the bottle end of the adaptor. These practices should be discouraged because overfilling may result.

D. Quick-Fill System

1. The Quick-Fill system is used only for sevoflurane. It is seen in **Figures 4.14** and **4.17.**
2. The vaporizer filler on the vaporizer has a screw-on cap. The filler neck has three grooves that can accept only a special filler device. The bottle has a permanently attached, agent-specific filling device that has three ridges that fit into slots in the filler. A valve prevents liquid from draining when the bottle is inverted, before it is inserted into the vaporizer.

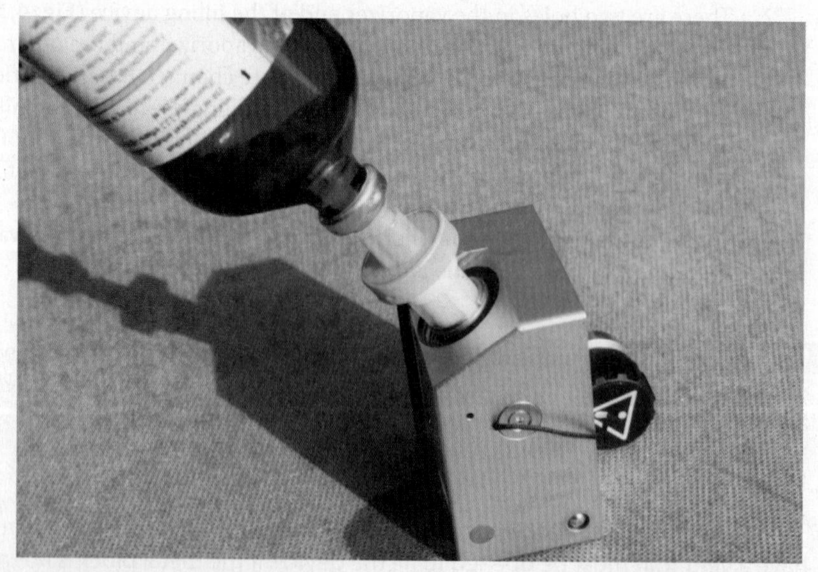

Figure 4.17 The Quick-Fil System. Bottle inserted into the filler block. Note the projections on the bottle that fit into the indentations on the filler block.

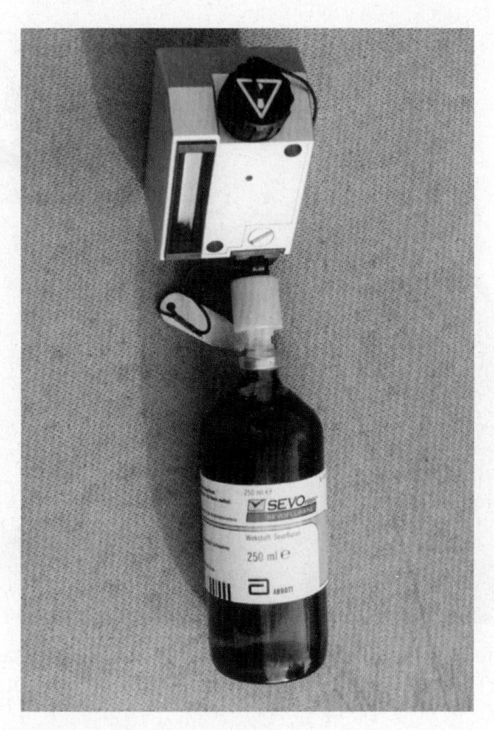

Figure 4.18 The Quick-Fil System. Draining the vaporizer.

3. To fill the vaporizer, the filler and bottle caps are removed. The bottle is inserted so that the projections fit the corresponding grooves in the filler neck (**Fig. 4.17**). The bottle is pushed into the vaporizer as far as it will go and held firmly in place. This will open a valve and allow liquid agent to flow into the vaporizer. After filling, the bottle is removed and the filler and bottle caps are replaced.
4. To empty the vaporizer, the filler cap is removed from the vaporizer. The drain attachment is fitted to the bottom of the block. The bottle is then inserted into the drain attachment (**Fig. 4.18**). The drain plug is unscrewed using the tool attached to the filler cap. Fluid will flow from the vaporizer. After draining, the drain plug is tightened and the filler cap is replaced and tightened.

E. Easy-Fill System

1. The Easy-Fill system is used for all Tec 7 vaporizers. The vaporizer component (block) (**Figs. 4.5** and **4.19B**) has a cap with a tool that is used to open and close the drain on the end that is inserted into the vaporizer. Inside the filler channel are two keys (ridges) that fit grooves on the bottle adapter.
2. The bottle adaptor (**Figs. 4.19A** and **4.20**) attaches to the bottle by aligning the notches with the projections on the bottle collar. The adaptor has grooves that must be aligned with the projections on the vaporizer.
3. To fill the vaporizer, the bottle adaptor is attached securely to the bottle and the filler cap on the vaporizer is removed. The bottle nozzle is inserted into the filler block, aligning the adaptor grooves with projections in the filler block. When the bottle is fully inserted, liquid will flow into the vaporizer. When the vaporizer is full or the bottle is empty, the bottle is released and then removed from the vaporizer filler. The filler cap is replaced and the cap is put back on the agent bottle. The filler cap is tightened in place.

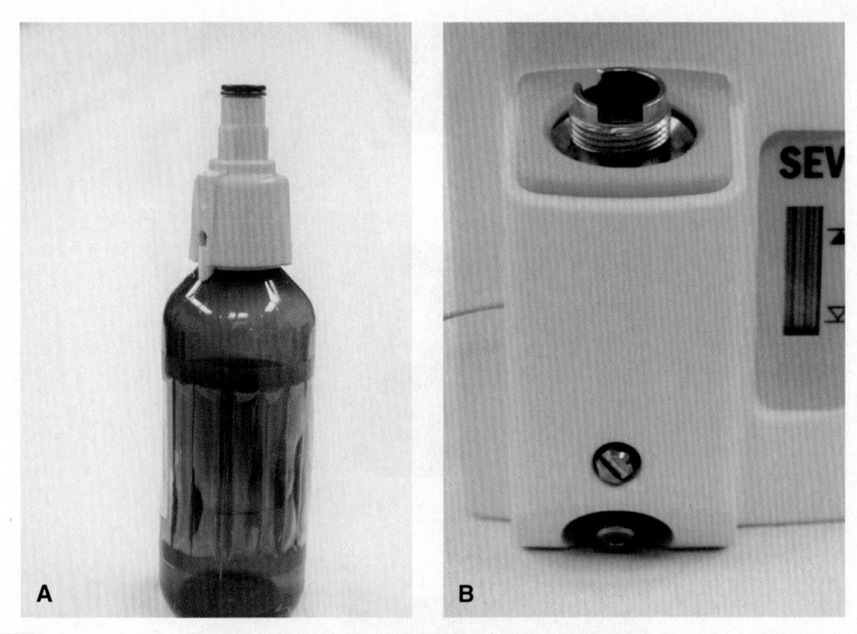

Figure 4.19 **A:** Easy-Fil System. The bottle adaptor fits over the bottle and has two ridges that fit into the grooves on the vaporizer. **B:** The grooves fit over the ridges on the bottle adaptor. Note the drain screw near the bottom of the vaporizer.

4. To drain the vaporizer, the cap is removed from the filler. A suitable container is placed under the drain nozzle. The drain plug (**Fig. 4.19B**) is unscrewed using the tool attached to the filler cap. Liquid should then flow into the container. After draining, the drain plug is tightened and the filler cap is replaced and tightened.
5. While this system appears similar to the Quick-Fill system, they are not compatible and so the Quick-Fill bottle adaptor cannot be inserted into the Easy-Fill vaporizer.

F. Desflurane Filling Systems

1. Filling systems for vaporizers used with desflurane are different from other filling systems. All use the same bottle to fill the vaporizer. This bottle has a crimped-on adaptor (**Fig. 4.21**). The bottle adaptor has a spring-loaded valve that opens when the bottle is pushed into the filling port on the vaporizer.

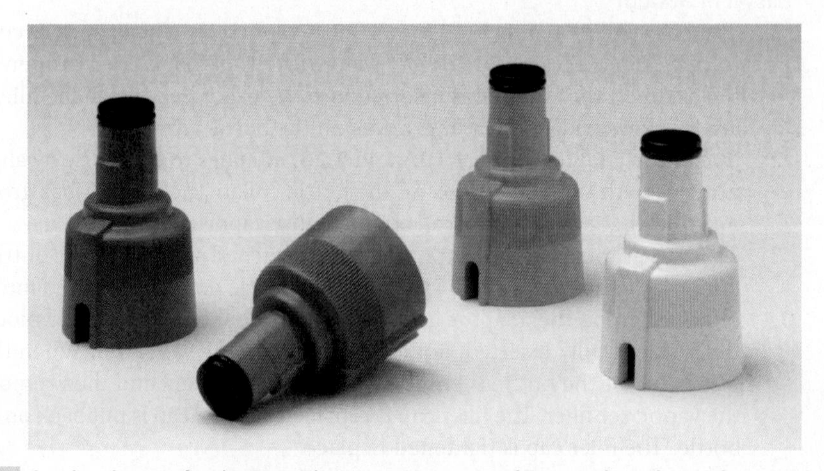

Figure 4.20 Bottle adaptors for the East-Fil system. (Courtesy of Datex-Ohmeda, Madison, WI.)

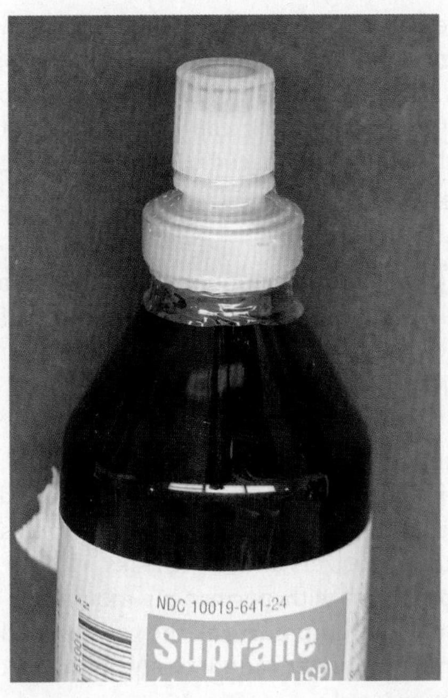

Figure 4.21 Bottle for desflurane. The protection cap has been removed and is at the right. (Courtesy of Ohmeda, a division of BOC Health Care, Inc.)

2. To fill the Tec 6 vaporizer, the bottle protection cap is removed and the bottle is fitted to the filler port and pushed up against the spring (**Fig. 4.22**). After the bottle is fully engaged in the port, it is rotated upward. The bottle is held in this position while filling.
3. When the liquid level gauge indicates that the sump is full or when the bottle is empty, the bottle is rotated downward and removed from the vaporizer. The

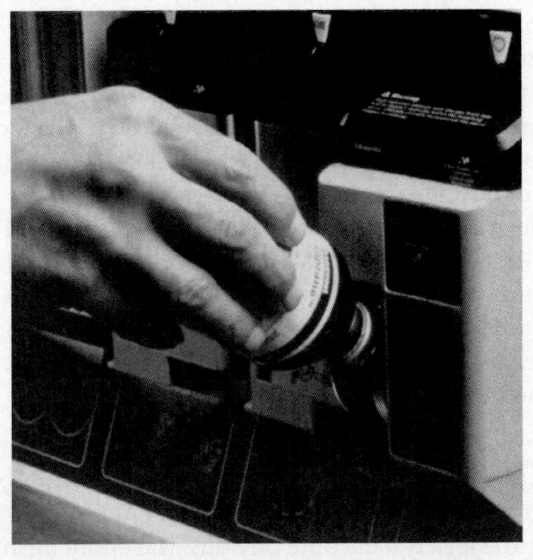

Figure 4.22 Filling Tec 6 vaporizer. The bottle is fitted to the filler port. After it is engaged in the filler port, it is rotated upward. When it reaches the upper stop, the agent will enter the vaporizer. (Courtesy of Ohmeda, a division of BOC Health Care, Inc.)

valve on the bottle closes automatically to prevent agent spill. The filling port has a spring valve to prevent the agent from escaping.

4. Problems with these filling systems have been reported. Bottles containing desflurane that do not have the cap properly in place can leak the agent. If the O-ring on the bottle is damaged or missing, the agent may leak during filling.

IX. Vaporizer Mounting Systems

CLINICAL MOMENT The order of vaporizers on anesthesia machines should be the same throughout a department to reduce errors. The desflurane vaporizer should always be on the right because the electric cord may interfere with mounting a vaporizer to the right of it.

A. Permanent Mounting

1. Permanent mounting means that tools are required to remove or install a vaporizer on the anesthesia machine. Advantages of this system include less physical damage to the vaporizers and fewer leaks.
2. There are problems with permanent mounting. The machine may not have enough room to accommodate all the vaporizers that are likely to be needed. A malfunctioning vaporizer cannot easily be changed, especially while anesthesia is being administered.

B. Detachable Mounting

1. Detachable mounting systems are standard on most new anesthesia machines. They allow the vaporizer to be mounted and removed without using tools. Vaporizers cannot be exchanged between different manufacturers' systems, although they may appear similar. If a vaporizer from one manufacturer is to be mounted on a different manufacturer's machine, it must be fitted with the proper mounting system for that machine.
2. The Select-a-Tec system is shown in **Figures 4.23** and **4.24.** It consists of a pair of port valves for each vaporizer position. Each vaporizer has a special mounting bracket containing two plungers (spindles), which fits over the port valves. The vaporizer's weight and an O-ring around each port valve create a seal between the mounting system and the vaporizer. On the back of each vaporizer is a locking lever.
3. Before mounting a vaporizer, the control dial must be in the OFF position. Adjacent vaporizers must also be turned OFF. The locking lever on the vaporizer should be unlocked. The vaporizer is fitted onto the mounting system and locked in position.
4. To remove a vaporizer, the control dial is turned OFF and the locking lever is moved to the unlock position. The vaporizer can then be lifted off the manifold.
5. When the vaporizer is turned ON (**Fig. 4.24, right**), the two plungers move downward, opening the valve ports and connecting the vaporizer into the fresh gas stream. When the vaporizer is turned OFF (**Fig. 4.24, left**), it is isolated from the fresh gas flow.

CLINICAL MOMENT If the vaporizer is not correctly mounted or if the O-ring is absent or broken, a leak will not be present when the vaporizer is turned OFF. When it is turned ON, the leak will become obvious. The entire fresh gas flow may be lost through the leak.

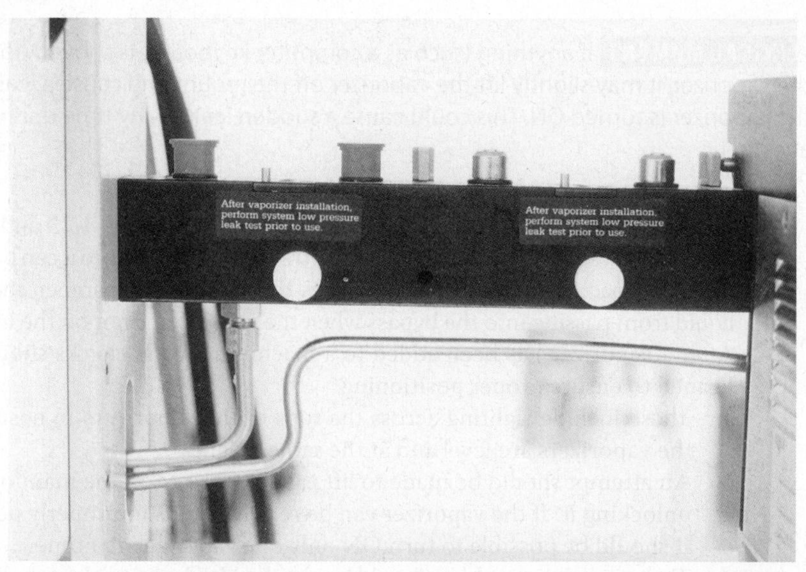

Figure 4.23 Select-a-Tec mounting system. A vaporizer is mounted on the right. In the center position, the nipples and O-rings are in place, ready to accept a vaporizer. Caps are over the nipples and O-rings on the left to protect them. The projections between the sets of nipples are to prevent two vaporizers from being turned ON at the same time (vaporizer exclusion or interlock system). The plastic projections are interconnected so that they move from side to side. The rod shown on the vaporizer to the right contacts the right projection. When that vaporizer is turned ON, the rod moves to the left, causing that projection to move to the left. The left projection also moves to the left. If there were vaporizers in these positions, their rods would also be moved in a such way that their dials could not be turned ON. The inlet and outlet pipes are below the mounting system. They enter at opposite ends so that they cannot be interchanged.

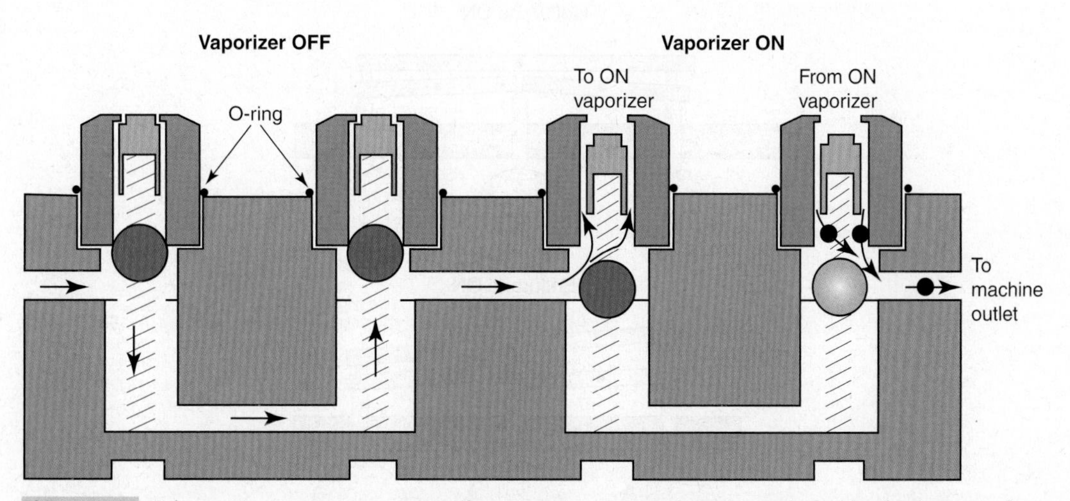

Figure 4.24 Select-a-Tec mounting system. The mounting system has channels for the fresh gas to flow from the flowmeters toward the machine outlet. When a vaporizer is mounted and turned ON, two plungers push the valves down so that gas passes through the vaporizer. If the mounting position is empty or the vaporizer is turned OFF, the gas passes directly through the mounting system. (Reproduced from a drawing furnished by Datex-Ohmeda.)

CLINICAL MOMENT If anything (such as a computer keyboard) is shoved up under the vaporizer, it may slightly lift the vaporizer off the mount and cause a leak when the vaporizer is turned ON. This could cause a sudden leak at any time during an anesthetic.

6. The Drager Medical mounting system is shown in **Figures 4.25** and **4.26.** The Vapor 2000 vaporizer must be in the "T" (travel) position before it can be unlocked from the machine. This position isolates the vaporizing chamber and prevents liquid from passing into the bypass when the vaporizer is not on the machine.
7. After a vaporizer has been added to a machine, several checks should be performed to ensure proper positioning.
   a. These include sighting across the tops of the vaporizers to ensure that all the vaporizers are level and at the same height.
   b. An attempt should be made to lift each vaporizer off the manifold without unlocking it. If the vaporizer can be removed, it is improperly positioned.
   c. It should be possible to turn ON only one vaporizer at a time.
   d. The anesthesia machine should be checked for leaks, with each vaporizer in both the ON and OFF position as described in Chapter 25.

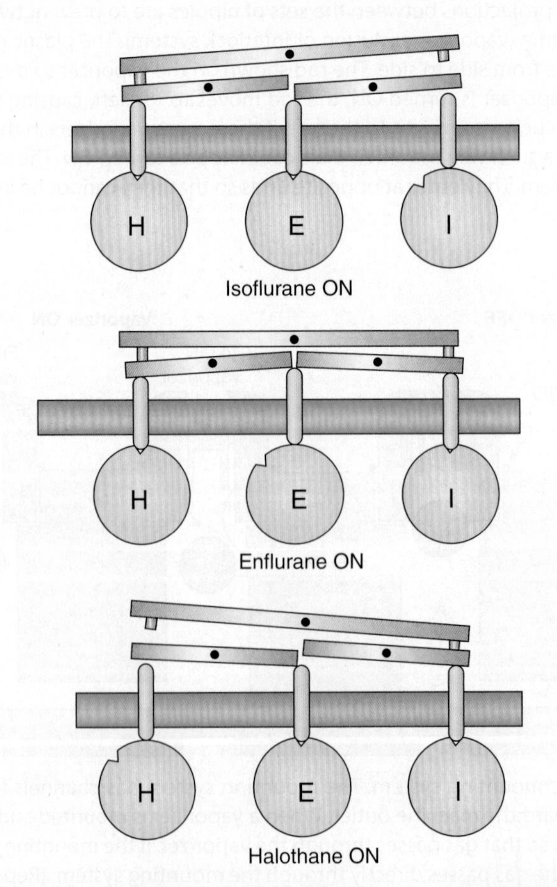

Figure 4.25 North American Drager interlock system. When the vaporizer of choice is turned ON, a pin is forced into a notch on the concentration control knob of each of the other vaporizers. These vaporizers are then locked in the OFF position. (Reproduced from a drawing furnished by North American Drager, Inc., Telford, PA.)

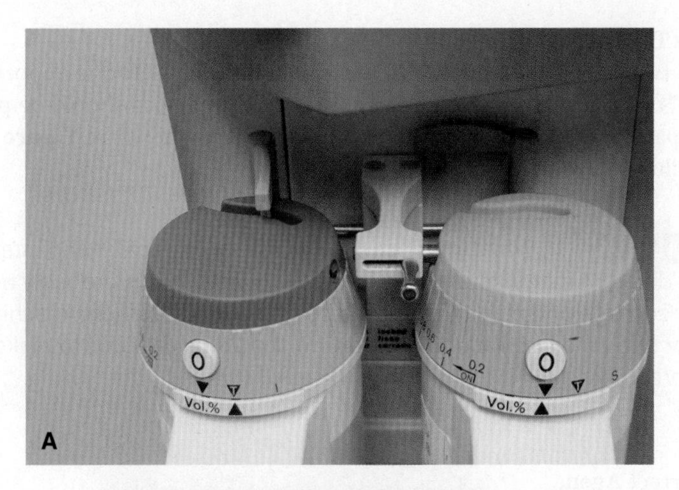

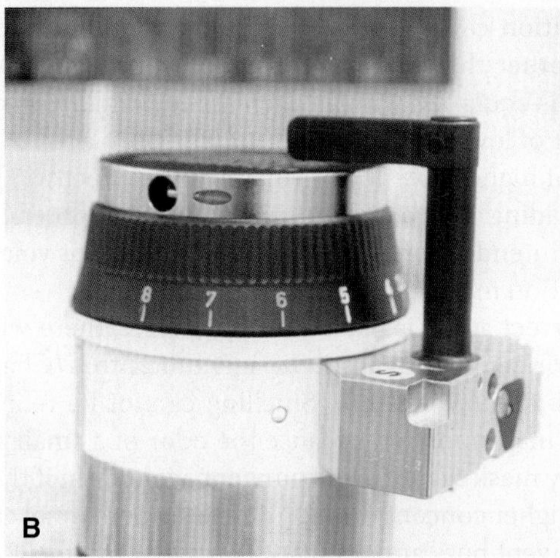

Figure 4.26 Mounting system for Vapor 2000 vaporizer. **A:** View of Vapor 2000 vaporizers from the top. The "0" button on the handwheel (above the control dial) must be depressed to turn the vaporizer ON or to put it into the transport position. To the right of this is the "T" (transport) mark. When the handwheel is turned to this position (left vaporizer), the lever at the back of the vaporizer fits into the groove on the top so that the dial cannot be removed. The vaporizer can then be removed. A slidebar between the vaporizers prevents two vaporizers from being turned ON at the same time. The slidebar fits into a hole in the control dial, preventing that vaporizer from being turned ON. **B:** Side view showing the locking lever. Below the lever is the mounting system. The hole for the slidebar is seen near the top of the dial.

8. Detachable mounting systems have a number of advantages. An anesthesia machine with fewer mounting locations can be used. Vaporizers can be easily removed and replaced, even during a case. This may be especially useful if the patient has a history of malignant hyperthermia or if it occurs during the anesthetic.
9. There are a number of disadvantages of these mounting systems. Partial or complete obstruction to gas flow as a result of problems associated with the mounting system has been reported. Leaks may occur. A common leak source is an absent or damaged O-ring. Another cause is leaving the locking lever in the unlocked position. Differences among vaporizers and interlocks from different manufacturers can pose problems of compatibility. Several cases have been reported, in which failure to deliver anesthetic agent was associated with problems with mounting systems.

X. Interlock Devices

Interlock (vaporizer exclusion) systems prevent more than one vaporizer from being turned ON at the same time. Checking the interlock device should be part of the anesthesia apparatus checkout procedure. One system is shown in **Figure 4.25.** Interlock system failures have been reported.

CLINICAL MOMENT While interlock devices may seem similar and interchangeable among different manufacturers and their vaporizers, this is probably not the case. If a vaporizer from one manufacturer is attached to an anesthesia machine of another manufacturer, the interlocking mechanism should be checked to make sure that it works properly.

XI. Hazards

A. Incorrect Agent

1. Concentration-calibrated vaporizers are agent-specific. Filling a vaporizer with an agent other than the one for which it was designed is less of a risk if the vaporizer is equipped with an agent-specific filling system.
2. If an agent of low potency or low volatility is placed in a vaporizer designed for an agent of higher potency or volatility, the effect will be an output of less than the dial reading. Conversely, if an agent of high potency or volatility is used in a vaporizer intended for an agent of low potency or volatility, a dangerously high concentration may be delivered.
3. If an incorrect agent is placed in a vaporizer, there will be a mixture of agents in the vaporizer. Some anesthetic agent monitors (Chapter 17) will detect agent mixtures but some will not. Smelling cannot be relied on to tell which agent is present in a vaporizer, because the odor of a small amount of one agent can completely mask that of a less pungent agent even if the second agent is present in much higher concentration. Anesthesia personnel can detect the presence of a volatile agent but cannot identify an agent by smell.

CLINICAL MOMENT If a vaporizer is filled with the wrong agent, it must be completely drained and all liquid discarded. Gas should be allowed to flow through it with the concentration dial fully ON until no agent can be detected in the outflow. Draining cannot be relied on to completely empty a vaporizer and remove the agent from the wicks.

B. Tipping

1. If some vaporizers are tipped more than 30 degrees, liquid from the vaporizing chamber may get into the bypass or outlet. If this occurs, a high concentration will be delivered when the vaporizer is first used.
2. Tipping can be prevented by mounting vaporizers securely and handling them with care when they are removed. Vaporizers should be turned OFF or placed in a travel (T) setting if they are being moved.

CLINICAL MOMENT Should tipping occur, a high flow of gas should be run through the vaporizer with the concentration dial set at a low concentration until the output shows no excessive concentration.

3. Many new vaporizers have a mechanism that blocks the entrance and exit from the vaporizing chamber. This prevents the problems associated with tipping the vaporizer when it is transported. Consult the user manual to determine whether your particular vaporizer is susceptible to problems from tipping.

C. Overfilling

1. If a vaporizer is overfilled, liquid agent may enter the fresh gas line and lethal concentrations may be delivered. Another result of overfilling may be complete vaporizer failure so that it produces no output.
2. Most vaporizers have the filling port situated so that overfilling cannot occur. Liquid will pour over the edge of the funnel before the level inside the vaporizer rises to a dangerous level. If an agent-specific filling system is used, filling will cease when the vaporizer is full.
3. If a vaporizer is tipped during the filling process, it is possible that it could be overfilled. The vaporizer should be securely attached to the anesthesia machine and vertical when it is filled.
4. Agent-specific filling devices prevent overfilling by connecting the air intake in the bottle to the inside of the vaporizer chamber.

CLINICAL MOMENT Many users who have the keyed filling system have found that slightly unscrewing the bottle adaptor or turning the vaporizer concentration dial ON during filling can speed the filling process. Such practices should be avoided because they can result in overfilling.

D. Reversed Flow

1. Although the anesthesia machine standard requires that the vaporizer inlet be male and the outlet female, the direction of gas flow be marked, and the inlet and outlet labeled, it may be possible to connect the fresh gas delivery line from the anesthesia machine to the outlet and the delivery tube to the breathing system to the inlet. Reversed flow through a vaporizer has also been reported after improper connection or repairs to the selector valve.
2. In most cases, reversed flow through a vaporizer will result in an increased output.

CLINICAL MOMENT None of the concentration-calibrated vaporizers are designed to be placed in the fresh gas hose between the anesthesia machine and the breathing system. They offer too much resistance to gas flow, especially when the oxygen flush is activated. Back pressure compensation may be disabled.

E. Control Dial in Wrong Position

After previous vaporizer use or servicing, the vaporizer control dial may be left ON. For this reason, the dial should be inspected as part of the preuse checking procedure. The control dial may be changed during a case without the operator's knowledge.

CLINICAL MOMENT Whenever an anesthesia machine is moved with assistance of others, check the vaporizers because someone may have grasped a control dial and altered the concentration or inadvertently turned a vaporizer ON.

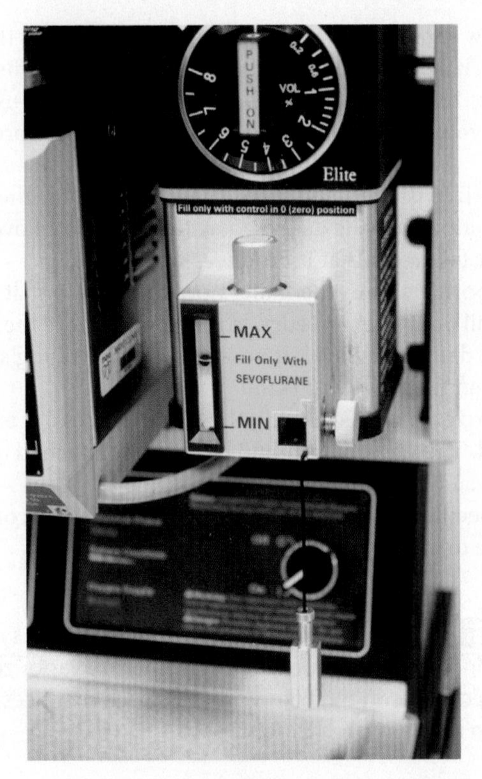

Figure 4.27 Failure to replace the filler plug will result in a leak when the vaporizer is turned ON.

F. Leaks

1. The effects of a leak on a vaporizer will depend on the size and location of the leak and whether or not there is a check valve at the vaporizer outlet. In addition to affecting fresh gas composition and flow, leaks pollute the operating room air, especially if the leak is downstream of the vaporizing chamber.
2. A common cause of leaks is failure to replace or adequately tighten the filler cap. If the fill valve or vent on a keyed filling system is not closed or the plug is not replaced and tightened in place, a leak will occur when the vaporizer is turned ON (**Fig. 4.27**).
3. If an incorrect cap is used on the filler device, a leak may result. The fitting between a vaporizer and its inlet or outlet connection may become loose or broken. A vaporizer may not be properly mounted.
4. With a leak in a vaporizer or its mount, the machine will often function normally until the vaporizer is turned ON. At that point, the fresh gas flow from the machine will be lost through the leak and the total flow to the breathing system will be reduced or nonexistent.
5. The leak may contain little or no vapor, especially if it is in the mounting mechanism.
6. A leak should be suspected if a vaporizer requires filling with unusual frequency, if an odor can be detected, or if there is a loss or reduction in the fresh gas flow to the breathing system after the vaporizer is turned ON.

7. A loose or missing filler cap may be detected by liquid being forced out under pressure when the vaporizer is turned ON. If the liquid level is low or below the filler, liquid may not be splattered.
8. A leak can sometimes be located by using the sampling tube from an anesthetic agent monitor to "sniff" around the vaporizer.

CLINICAL MOMENT Personnel who fill vaporizers should be instructed to always close filler caps and vents tightly. A leak in a vaporizer can be detected when the anesthesia machine is tested before use if the vaporizer is turned ON (Chapter 25). Even after a proper preuse check, if anything is pushed under the vaporizer and the vaporizer is lifted even slightly from its mount, a leak may occur.

G. Vapor Leak into the Fresh Gas Line

Some vaporizers leak small amounts of vapor into the bypass when turned OFF. Interlock devices or selectors will not prevent this problem if there is still a diffusion pathway via the selector valve. The amount of such a leak depends on the ambient temperature as well as the size and configuration of the internal ports. Although the amounts delivered are usually too small to produce a clinical effect, it might cause a "sensitized" individual to react to a halogenated agent or trigger an episode of malignant hyperthermia. These leaks can be reduced by not turning a vaporizer from the OFF to the "0" setting unless it is to be used.

CLINICAL MOMENT If it is important that a "sensitized" patient not receive any volatile agent, it is best to use a dedicated agent-free machine. If this is not possible, all vaporizers should be removed from the machine to be used and the machine flushed well with oxygen before beginning the anesthetic.

H. Contaminants in the Vaporizing Chamber

1. It is possible for various substances to be poured into a bottle that contains anesthetic agent and that combination used to fill a vaporizer.
2. Cleaning agents may collect in the funnel filler and be washed into the vaporizing chamber when it is filled with a liquid agent.
3. Water and other foreign substances can cause corrosion (**Fig. 4.28**).

CLINICAL MOMENT If foreign substances are known to have entered the vaporizer, the manufacturer should be contacted to determine what measures need to be taken.

I. Physical Damage

Shock, excessive vibration, or mistreatment may lead to malfunction. Damage to vaporizers that are permanently mounted on a machine is significantly less than in those that are frequently moved. A sufficient number of vaporizers should be purchased so that they do not need to be moved during routine use. If a vaporizer must be removed, care should be taken to protect it from physical damage.

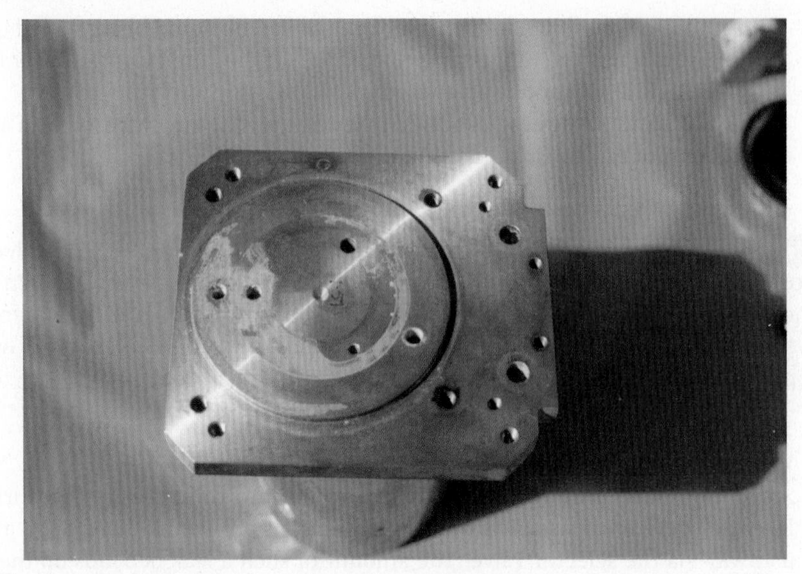

Figure 4.28 Corrosion in vaporizer caused by water and other foreign substances.

> **CLINICAL MOMENT** If a vaporizer has been dropped or otherwise tempered with, it should be sent back to the manufacturer to be checked or serviced. If an agent monitor indicates that there is a disparity between the dialed output and the delivered output, it should also be sent to the manufacturer.

J. No Vapor Output
   1. The most common cause of no vapor output is an empty vaporizer.
   2. Incorrect vaporizer mounting can result in little or no vapor output. In most cases, this can be detected by checking for leaks with the vaporizer ON (Chapter 25).
   3. An overfilled vaporizer may deliver no vapor.
   4. Blood entering the vaporizer can cause vaporizer failure.
   5. If an anesthesia machine is turned OFF and then ON again, electronic vaporizer settings may default to zero.
   6. Failure to deliver adequate vapor can be detected by an anesthetic gas monitor (Chapter 17).

K. Projectile

   A case has been reported in which a portable vaporizer carried into the magnetic resonance imaging (MRI) suite was rapidly attracted to the magnet.

> **CLINICAL MOMENT** Some vaporizers that are MRI safe only when they are attached to a rack on the wall or the anesthesia machine may need to be attached to the wall. Consult the user manual for information on your particular vaporizer.

XII. **Disposing of Liquid Anesthetics**

After a vaporizer has been drained, the question of what do with the liquid agent arises. Some of these agents will react with plastic. A simple solution is to place the agent in a bottle or tray and set it outside, where personnel will not be exposed to the vapor. An evaporator has been described. It consists of a glass flask with a stopper that has two holes. A glass tubing open to room air is inserted through one hole. The glass tubing that is inserted through the other hole is connected to the vacuum system. The liquid is allowed to evaporate, and the vapor is removed by the vacuum system.

SUGGESTED READINGS

Abel M, Eisenkraft JB. Performance of erroneously filled sevoflurane, enflurane and other agent-specific vaporizers. J Clin Monit 1996;12:119–125.

Block FE, Schulte GT. Observations on use of wrong agent in an anesthesia agent vaporizer. J Clin Monit 2000;15: 57–61.

Dorsch J, Dorsch S. Vaporizers in Understanding Anesthesia Equipment. Fifth edition. Philadelphia: Wolters Kluwer/ Lippincott Williams & Wilkins, 2008:121–190.

Hendrickx JFA, De Cooman S, Deloof TM, Vandeput D, et al. The ADU vaporizing unit: a new vaporizer. Anesth Analg 2001;93:391–395.

Keresztury MF, Newman AG, Kode A, Wendling WW. A surprising twist: an unusual failure of a keyed filling device specific for a volatile inhaled anesthetic. Anesth Analg 2006;103:124–125.

Weiskopf RB, Sampson D, Moore MA. The desflurane (Tec 6) vaporizer: design, design considerations and performance evaluation. Br J Anaesth 1994;72:474–479.

5 Breathing Systems

I. Physics

A. Resistance

When gas passes through a tube, the pressure at the outlet will be lower than that at the inlet. The drop in pressure is a measure of the resistance that must be overcome. Resistance varies with the volume of gas passing per unit of time. Therefore, flow rate must be stated when a specific resistance is stated.

The nature of the flow is important in determining resistance. There are two types of flow: laminar and turbulent. In clinical practice, flow is usually a mixture of both.

1. **Laminar Flow**
   a. **Figure 5.1A** illustrates laminar gas flow. The flow is smooth and orderly, and particles move parallel to the walls of the tube. Flow is fastest in the center of the tube, where there is less friction.

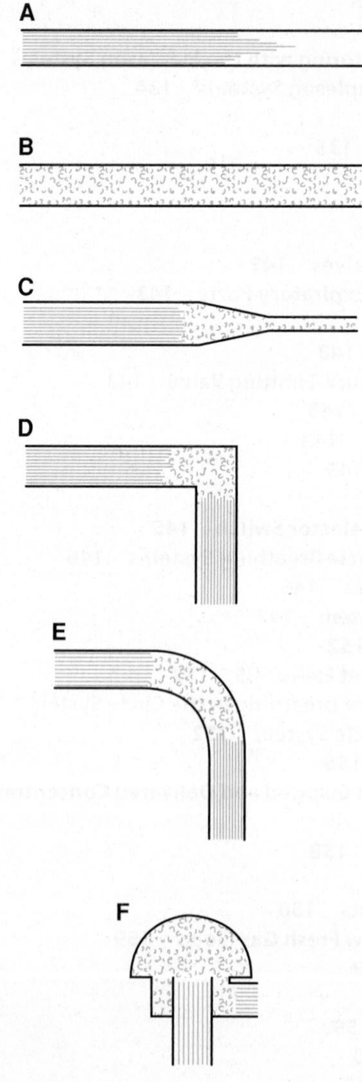

Figure 5.1 Laminar and turbulent flows. **A:** Laminar flow; the lines of flow are parallel and flow is slower near the sides of the tube because of friction. **B:** Generalized turbulent flow, which occurs when the critical flow rate is exceeded. Eddies move across or opposite the general direction of flow. **C–F:** Localized turbulence, which occurs when there is change in direction or the gas passes through a constriction.

b. When flow is laminar, the Hagen–Poiseuille law applies. This law states that

$$\Delta P = \frac{(L \times \nu \times V)}{r^4}$$

where r is the radius of the tube, ΔP is the pressure gradient across the tube, ν is the viscosity of the gas, L is length, and V is the flow rate. Resistance is directly proportional to flow rate during laminar flow.

2. **Turbulent Flow**
   a. **Figure 5.1B** illustrates turbulent gas flow. The flow lines are no longer parallel. Eddies, composed of particles moving across or opposite the general direction of flow, are present. The flow rate is the same across the tube. During turbulent flow, the factors responsible for the pressure drop include those described for laminar flow, but gas density becomes more important than viscosity.
   b. Turbulent flow can be generalized or localized. When the gas flow through a tube exceeds a certain value, called the *critical flow rate*, generalized turbulent flow results. As seen in **Figure 5.1C–F,** when gas flow is below the critical flow rate but encounters constrictions, curves, valves, or other irregularities, an area of localized turbulence results. The increase in resistance will depend on the type and number of obstructions encountered.
   c. To minimize resistance, gas-conducting pathways should have minimal length and maximal internal diameter and be without sharp curves or sudden changes in diameter.

B. Significance of Resistance
   1. Resistance imposes a strain on the patient with ventilatory modes in which the patient must do part or all of the respiratory work (e.g., spontaneous respiration, intermittent mandatory ventilation, or pressure support ventilation). Changes in resistance tend to parallel changes in the work of breathing. Flow-volume loops (Chapter 18) can show changes in resistance to flow in a breathing system.

CLINICAL MOMENT The tracheal tube is usually the source of more resistance and a more important factor in determining the work of breathing than the breathing system.

   2. There is a lack of agreement about what level of resistance is excessive. Anesthesia providers should be aware of how much resistance components of breathing systems offer and to employ, wherever possible, those offering the least resistance. For some patients, increased expiratory resistance may be desirable. This should be achieved by using devices designed for that purpose.

C. Compliance
Compliance is the ratio of a change in volume to a change in pressure. It is a measure of distensibility and is usually expressed in milliliters per centimeter of water (mL/cm H_2O). The most distensible breathing system components are the reservoir bag and the breathing tubes. Compliance will help determine the tidal volume. Compliance can be illustrated graphically with a pressure–volume loop (Chapter 18).

II. Rebreathing

Rebreathing means to inhale previously respired gases from which carbon dioxide may or may not have been removed. There is a tendency to associate the word *rebreathing* with carbon dioxide accumulation. This is unfortunate because although it is true that rebreathing can result in higher inspired carbon dioxide concentrations than normal, it is possible to have partial or total rebreathing without an increase in carbon dioxide concentration when carbon dioxide is removed by an absorbent. Rebreathing carbon dioxide, depending on the amount, is not necessarily bad for the patient.

A. Factors Influencing Rebreathing

1. **Fresh Gas Flow**

The amount of rebreathing varies inversely with the total fresh gas flow. If the volume of fresh gas supplied per minute is equal to or greater than the patient's minute volume, there will be no rebreathing, as long as provision is made for unimpeded exhaust to a scavenging system or atmosphere at a point close to the patient's respiratory tract. If the total volume of gas supplied per minute is less than the minute volume, some exhaled gases must be rebreathed to make up the required volume (assuming no air dilution).

2. **Mechanical Dead Space**

a. Mechanical (apparatus) dead space is the volume in a breathing system occupied by gases that are rebreathed without any change in composition. It can be minimized by separating the inspiratory and expiratory gas streams as close to the patient as possible. Apparatus such as connectors added between the patient and the breathing system will increase the dead space.

CLINICAL MOMENT Adding dead space between the breathing system and the patient is not usually a problem with adult patients but can result in serious rebreathing with pediatric patients.

b. The mechanical dead space should be distinguished from the physiological dead space, which includes anatomical dead space, consisting of the patient's conducting airway down to the alveoli, and alveolar dead space, which is the volume of alveoli ventilated but not perfused.

c. The gas composition in the mechanical dead space will vary according to whether it is occupied by anatomical dead space gas, alveolar gas, or mixed exhaled gas. Gas exhaled from the anatomical dead space has a composition similar to inspired gas but is saturated with water vapor and is warmer. Alveolar gas is saturated with water vapor at body temperature and has less oxygen and more carbon dioxide than inspired gas. The anesthetic agent concentration in alveolar gas will differ from that in the inspired gas. Mixed expired gas will have a composition intermediate between that of anatomical dead space and alveolar gas.

3. **Breathing System Design**

In addition to these factors, breathing system components may be arranged so that there is more or less rebreathing.

B. Effects of Rebreathing

With no rebreathing, the inspired gas composition is identical to that of the fresh gas delivered from the anesthesia machine. With rebreathing, the inspired gas is composed partly of fresh gas and partly of rebreathed gas.

1. **Heat and Moisture Retention**

Fresh gas from the anesthesia machine is dry and at room temperature. Exhaled gases are warm and saturated with moisture. Rebreathing reduces the patient's heat and moisture loss. In most breathing systems, heat is rapidly lost to atmosphere, and gas that is reinhaled has a lower temperature and moisture content than exhaled gas.

2. **Altered Inspired Gas Tensions**
   The effects of rebreathing on inspired gas tensions will depend on how much exhaled gases are rebreathed and whether these gases pass to the alveoli (and so influence gas exchange) or only to the anatomical dead space.
   a. Oxygen
      Rebreathing alveolar gas will cause a reduction in the inspired oxygen tension.
   b. Inhaled Anesthetic Agents
      Rebreathing alveolar gas exerts a "cushioning" effect on changes in inspired gas composition with alterations in fresh gas composition. During induction, when alveolar tensions are lower than those in the fresh gas, rebreathed alveolar gas will reduce the inspired concentration and prolong induction. During recovery, the alveolar concentration exceeds that of the inspired gases and rebreathing slows agent elimination.
   c. Carbon Dioxide
      1) Rebreathing alveolar gas will cause an increased inspired carbon dioxide tension unless the gas passes through an absorbent before being rebreathed. Because carbon dioxide is concentrated in the alveolar portion of expired gases, the efficiency with which it is eliminated from a breathing system varies. If the system is designed so that alveolar gas is preferentially eliminated through the adjustable pressure-limiting (APL) valve or the ventilator spill valve, carbon dioxide retention will be minimal, even with a low fresh gas flow.
      2) During spontaneous respiration, carbon dioxide in the inspired gas is generally considered undesirable. Although the patient can compensate by increasing minute volume, a price is paid in terms of increased work of breathing Compensation may or may not be adequate.
      3) During controlled ventilation, some carbon dioxide in the inhaled gases may be advantageous. Rebreathing allows normocarbia and heat and moisture retention during hyperventilation.

III. Discrepancy between Inspired and Delivered Volumes

A. The volume of gas discharged by a ventilator or reservoir bag usually differs from that which enters the patient.

B. When a ventilator is used and the fresh gas flow rate is greater than the rate at which it is absorbed by the patient or lost through leaks, the fresh gas flow delivered during inspiration may be added to the tidal volume delivered by the ventilator. The added fresh gas increases with higher fresh gas flows and inspiratory to expiratory (I:E) ratios and lower respiratory rates. Modern anesthesia ventilators have been designed to eliminate or compensate for the additional tidal volume caused by fresh gas flow (see Chapter 6).

C. A reduction in the tidal volume delivered to the patient will result from gas compression and breathing system component distention during inspiration. This is referred to as *wasted ventilation*. Wasted ventilation increases with increases in airway pressure, tidal volume, breathing system volume, and component distensibility. Proportionally, more of the set tidal volume is lost with small patients.

D. Tidal volume is decreased by leaks in the breathing system. The amount lost will depend on the size and location of the leaks and the pressure in the breathing system.

E. Tidal volumes are best measured between the patient and the breathing tubes (Chapter 18). Measuring tidal volume at the end of the expiratory limb will reflect increases caused by fresh gas flow and decreases resulting from leaks in the breathing system but will miss decreases from wasted ventilation. Leaks between the volume sensor located at the patient port and the patient can be detected by comparing the inspired and exhaled tidal volumes. If there is a significant leak, the exhaled volume will be less than the inspired volume.

IV. **Discrepancy between Inspired and Delivered Oxygen and Anesthetic Gas Concentrations**

The composition of the gas mixture that exits the machine may be modified by the breathing system so that the mixture the patient inspires differs considerably from that delivered to the system. There are several contributing factors.

A. Rebreathing

The effect of rebreathing will depend on the volume of the rebreathed gas and its composition. This will depend on the factors discussed previously.

B. Air Dilution

1. If the fresh gas supplied per respiration is less than the tidal volume, negative pressure in the breathing system may cause air dilution.
2. Air dilution makes it difficult to maintain a stable anesthetic state. It causes the anesthetic concentration in the inspired mixture to fall. This results in a lighter level of anesthesia with stimulated spontaneous ventilation. The increased ventilation causes more air dilution. The opposite is also true. Deepening anesthesia depresses ventilation. Respiratory depression decreases air dilution, which causes an increase in the inspired anesthetic agent concentration. This, in turn, leads to further depressed spontaneous respiration.

C. Leaks

With a leak, positive pressure in the breathing system will force gas out of the system. The composition and amount of the gas lost will depend on the location and size of the leak, the pressure in the system, and the compliance and resistance of the breathing system and the patient.

D. Anesthetic Agent Uptake by Breathing System Components

Anesthetic agents may be taken up or adhere to rubber, plastics, metal, and carbon dioxide absorbent. This will lower the inspired concentration.

E. Anesthetic Agent Released from the System

Anesthetic agent elimination from the breathing system will depend on the same factors as those of uptake. The system may function as a low-output vaporizer for many hours after a vaporizer has been turned OFF even if the rubber goods and absorbent are changed. This can result in a patient being inadvertently exposed to the agent.

V. **Common components**

Some components are found in only one type of breathing system. These will be discussed with the individual systems. The following components are found in more than one type of breathing system.

A. Bushings

A bushing (mount) serves to modify the component's internal diameter. Most often, it has a cylindrical form and is inserted into, and becomes part of, a pliable component such as a reservoir bag or breathing tube.

B. Sleeves

A sleeve alters the external diameter of a component.

C. Connectors and Adaptors

1. A connector is a fitting intended to join together two or more similar components. An adaptor establishes functional continuity between otherwise disparate or incompatible components.
2. A variety of connectors and adaptors are available (**Fig. 5.2**). An adaptor or connector may be distinguished by (a) shape (e.g., straight, right angle [elbow], T, or Y); (b) component(s) to which it is attached; (c) added features (e.g., with nipple); and (d) size and type of fitting at either end (e.g., 15-mm male, 22-mm female).

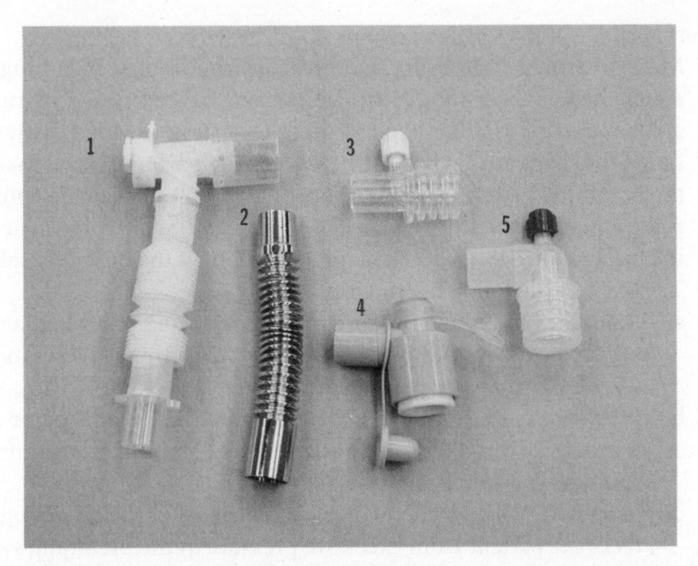

Figure 5.2 Various connectors. **1:** A swivel connector that can be used to insert a flexible fiberscope. It has a flexible accordion-type side arm. **2:** A flexible metal connector that can be used between the tracheal tube and the breathing system. It cannot be used with a mask. **3:** Straight connector with a side gas sampling port. **4:** Right angle connector for insertion of a flexible fiberscope. It can accommodate different sized fiberscopes by changing the diaphragm. The large cap is used if no diaphragm is present. **5:** Right angle connector with gas sampling port.

3. All anesthesia breathing systems terminate at the patient connection port. This is the point where the breathing system connects to a device (face mask, tracheal tube, or supraglottic airway device) that establishes continuity with the patient's respiratory system.
4. All face masks have a 22-mm female opening, whereas other devices (supraglottic devices and tracheal tubes) have a 15-mm male fitting. To facilitate the change from mask to tracheal tube or supraglottic device, a component having a 22-mm male fitting with a concentric 15-mm female fitting is used at the patient connection port. Usually, this component is a right angle connector (**Fig. 5.2**), also known as an elbow adaptor, elbow joint, elbow connector, mask angle piece, mask adaptor, or mask elbow.
5. Connectors and adaptors can be used to:
   a. Extend the distance between the patient and the breathing system. This is especially important in head and neck surgery when the presence of the breathing system near the head may make it inaccessible to the anesthesia personnel and/or interfere with the surgical field.
   b. Change the angle of connection between the patient and the breathing system.
   c. Allow a more flexible and/or less kinkable connection between the patient and the breathing system.
   d. Increase the dead space.

CLINICAL MOMENT Using a connector or adaptor between the breathing system and the patient will increase the dead space. In adults, some added dead space will be of little importance. In pediatric patients, added dead space is more significant.

D. Reservoir Bag

1. Most breathing systems have a reservoir (respiratory, breathing, or sometimes erroneously, rebreathing) bag. Most bags are composed of rubber or plastic and have an ellipsoidal shape so that they can be grasped easily with one hand. Latex-free bags are available. The neck is the part of the bag that connects with the breathing system. The neck must have a 22-mm female connector. The tail is the end opposite from the neck. A loop may be provided near the tail to hold the bag upside down, which facilitates drying if the bag is reusable.
2. The bag has the following functions:
   a. It allows gas to accumulate during exhalation, providing a reservoir of gas for the next inspiration. This permits rebreathing, allows more economical use of gases, and prevents air dilution.
   b. It provides a means whereby ventilation may be assisted or controlled.
   c. It can serve through visual and tactile perceptions as a monitor of a patient's spontaneous respiration.
   d. Because the bag is the most distensible part of the breathing system, it protects the patient from excessive pressure in the breathing system.
3. The pressure–volume characteristics of bags become important if there is no way for gases to escape from the system while inflow continues. Adding volume to a bag normally causes a negligible rise in pressure until the nominal capacity is reached. As more volume continues to be added, the pressure rises rapidly to a peak and then reaches a plateau. As the bag distends further, the pressure falls slightly. The peak pressure is of particular interest, because this represents the maximal pressure that can develop in a breathing system.

CLINICAL MOMENT Since new bags develop greater pressures when first used, it is a good idea to stretch the bag by overinflating it before use. This can be done while testing the breathing system for leaks as part of the preuse procedure.

4. Bags are available in a variety of sizes. The size that should be used will depend on the patient, the breathing system, and the user's preference. A 3-L bag is traditionally used with adults. A larger bag may be difficult to squeeze and will make monitoring the patient's spontaneous respiration more difficult because the excursions will be smaller. A small bag, on the other hand, provides less safety with respect to pressure limitation and may not provide a large enough reservoir or tidal volume.

CLINICAL MOMENT A spare reservoir bag should always be kept immediately available in case the bag develops a leak or becomes lost.

E. Breathing Tubes

1. A large-bore (approximately 22-mm diameter) corrugated breathing (conducting) tube (hose) provides a flexible, low-resistance, lightweight connection from one part of the breathing system to another. Corrugations increase flexibility and help to prevent kinking. Breathing tubes have some distensibility, but not enough to prevent excessive pressures from developing. Smaller diameter breathing tubings are available for circle systems used for pediatric patients. If it is necessary to have the anesthesia machine at some distance from the patient's head, several breathing tubes may be connected in a series or extra-long tubings

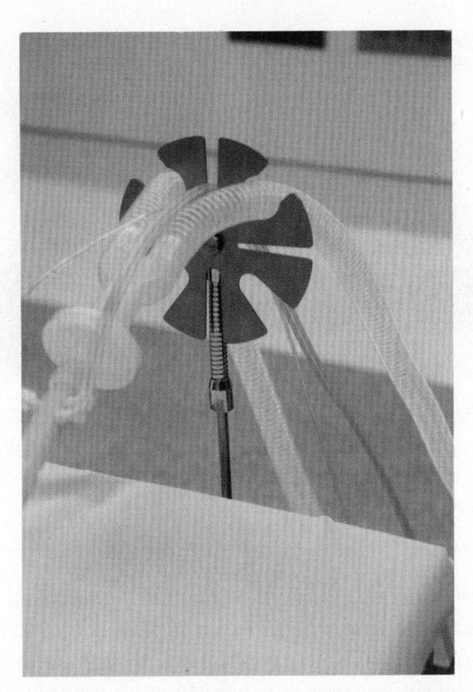

Figure 5.3 A tube retainer (tube tree) is useful to hold the breathing tubes and other tubes in place.

can be used. Special tubings that can be elongated are available. A tube holder (tree) (**Fig. 5.3**) can be used to support breathing tubes and prevent them from exerting a pull on the airway device.

F. Adjustable Pressure-Limiting Valve

1. The APL valve (**Figs. 5.4** and **5.5**) is the only gas exit from a breathing system unless a ventilator is being used. It is used to control the pressure in the breathing system

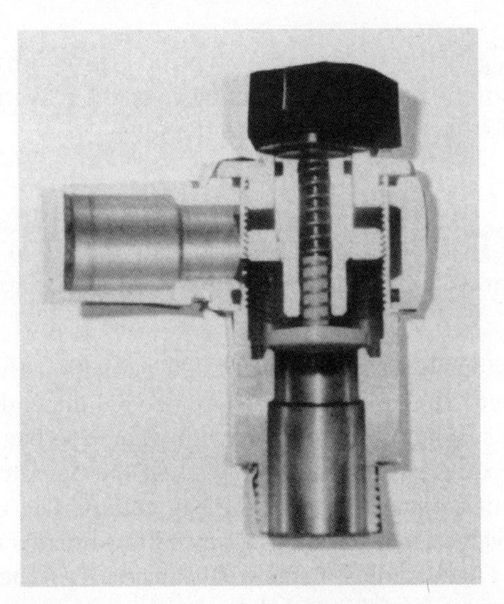

Figure 5.4 Adjustable pressure-limiting valve with spring-loaded disc. Gas from the breathing system enters at the base and passes into the gas collecting assembly at the left. Turning the control knob varies the tension in the spring and the pressure necessary to lift the disc off its seat. When the cap is fully tightened, the spring is compressed enough to prevent the valve leaflet from lifting at any airway pressure.

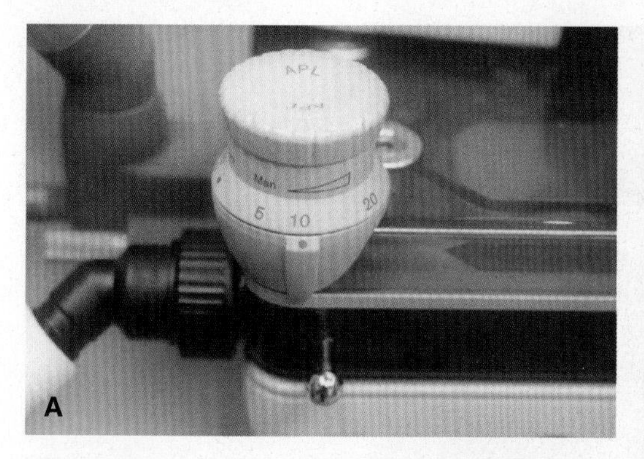

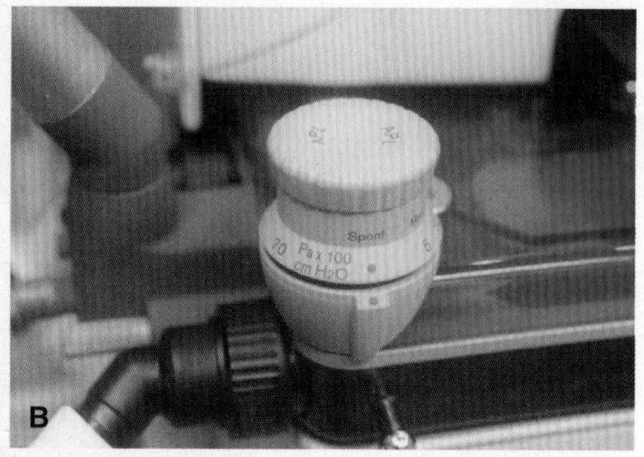

Figure 5.5 Another type of adjustable pressure-limiting valve. The control knob is rotated counterclockwise to increase the opening pressure. **A:** The valve is set for manual ventilation. The valve can be fully opened by pulling up on the control knob. **B:** The valve is set for spontaneous ventilation. Note that the control knob is slightly elevated.

during spontaneous, assisted, or manually controlled respiration. It employs an adjustment knob that when rotated increases or decreases the gas outlet size to adjust amount of gas that leaves the breathing system. There may also be a means to quickly release the pressure in the breathing system should it rise to a dangerous level (**Fig. 5.5**). There is also a collecting device to capture the gases that leave the breathing system and allow them to flow to the scavenging system.

2. During spontaneous ventilation, the APL valve should be fully open. There is a slight amount of positive pressure to be overcome when the valve is fully open to prevent negative pressure in the scavenging system from pulling gas from the breathing system. This pressure also allows the bag to fill and keeps it from deflating during spontaneous ventilation.

CLINICAL MOMENT If there is not enough positive pressure in the APL valve, gas can be pulled from the breathing system by an active scavenging system. To prevent this, the APL valve may need to be closed slightly.

CLINICAL MOMENT If the APL valve is less than fully open, the spontaneously breathing patient will be breathing against continuous airway pressure.

3. During manually assisted or controlled ventilation, the APL valve should be partially closed. The amount of closure needed depends on the gas flow into the breathing system, the frequency with which the bag is squeezed, and the tidal volume. Excess gas is vented only when the operator squeezes the bag. If the valve is not sufficiently open, the bag volume will increase with each breath. The APL valve should be adjusted every few breaths until the correct balance is achieved. Further adjustments will be necessary if the fresh gas flow, respiratory frequency, or tidal volume is altered.
4. When a ventilator is used, there is a spill valve that replaces the APL valve in the breathing system to vent excess respiratory gas (see Chapter 6). When the selector switch is turned to "ventilator," the APL valve will be isolated from the breathing system.

CLINICAL MOMENT Some older anesthesia machine breathing systems did not isolate the APL valve when the selector switch was turned to "ventilator". If the APL valve is not isolated when the ventilator is turned ON, the APL valve must be fully closed. If the valve is isolated, it need not be closed when the ventilator is in use.

G. Positive End-Expiratory Pressure Valves

1. Positive end-expiratory pressure (PEEP) and continuous positive airway pressure (CPAP) are used to improve oxygenation. PEEP may be used with spontaneous or controlled ventilation, whereas CPAP is used both during spontaneous ventilation and during one-lung ventilation (Chapter 16).
2. Some older anesthesia machines have manually controlled PEEP valves that are a component of the breathing system. On newer anesthesia machines, the PEEP valve is controlled electronically with the ventilator. For a machine not equipped with a PEEP valve, a disposable PEEP valve can be placed in the exhalation limb.

CLINICAL MOMENT If it is necessary to use a disposable PEEP valve, make certain that it is attached on the expiratory side. If the PEEP valve is unidirectional, it must be installed so that gas flows in the proper direction. If installed backward, it can obstruct exhalation.

H. Filters

1. **Use**
   a. Filters are used both to protect the patient from microorganisms and airborne particulate matter and to protect anesthesia equipment and the environment from exhaled contaminants. When placed between the patient and the breathing system, a filter may help to increase the inspired humidity (see Chapter 9). Another benefit of filters is preventing exposure to latex allergens.
   b. Using filters is controversial. Convincing evidence that their use is of benefit in preventing postoperative infections is lacking. Problems with filters (see the following text) have resulted in serious complications.
   c. The Centers for Disease Control and Prevention and the American Society of Anesthesiologists make no recommendation for placing a filter in the breathing system unless there is suspicion that the patient has an infectious pulmonary disease. The Association of Anaesthetists of Great Britain and Ireland (AAGBI) and others recommend that either a new filter be placed between the patient and the breathing system for each adult patient or a new breathing system be used for each patient. For pediatric patients, the increased resistance and relative inefficiency of pediatric filters may make other means of humidification and infection control more attractive. The AAGBI recommends that a filter not be used for pediatric patients but the breathing system be replaced between cases.
   d. Pediatric filters are available. Considerations when using filters in pediatrics include increased work of breathing and increased dead space versus increased humidification and bacterial and particulate filtration.
2. **Types**
   a. There are two types of filters: mechanical and electrostatic. Both are manufactured with and without additional heat- and moisture-exchange elements.

b. Mechanical filters utilize a compact fiber matrix. They are pleated to increase surface area. They have very small pores and act by physically preventing microorganisms and particles from passing. Electrostatic filters use a felt-like material that is polarized in an electromagnetic field. They rely on electrostatic forces to hold organisms within a loosely woven charged filter element. The fibers are less dense than those present in mechanical filters; hence, the pore size is larger. Most studies show that the filtration performance of these filters is less satisfactory than that of mechanical filters, especially with extreme challenges. However, studies show that they are effective in preventing breathing system contamination.

3. **Filtration Efficiency**
Filter efficiency varies. It depends on the experimental test conditions. To evaluate filter efficiency, the size of the challenge particle or organism must be disclosed. A high-efficiency particulate aerosol (HEPA) device is defined as one capable of trapping at least 99.97% of particles having a diameter of 0.3 μm. The approximate size of the human immunodeficiency virus (HIV) particle is 0.08 μm, hepatitis C virus 0.06 μm, *Mycobacterium tuberculosis* 0.3 μm, *Pseudomonas aeruginosa* 0.5 μm, and *Staphylococcus aureus*, 1.0 μm.

4. **Filter Location in the Breathing System**
A filter can be attached to a disposable breathing tube for connection to the absorber, attached to a ventilator hose, or placed between the breathing system and the patient. A filter placed at the patient port may permit disposable breathing systems to be reused.

CLINICAL MOMENT A filter should not be placed downstream of a humidifier or nebulizer because it may become less efficient when wet. An increase in resistance, sometimes to a hazardous level, may also be seen.

5. **Problems Associated with Filters**

a. Increased Resistance and Dead Space

1) A filter increases the resistance to gas flow. Resistance increases with condensation. While increased resistance is usually not a problem during controlled ventilation, it may be problematic with spontaneous respiration.

2) Adding a filter between the patient and the breathing system increases the dead space. Unless ventilation is increased, significant rebreathing can occur. Spontaneously breathing patients who derive a major portion of their minute volume from shallow breaths may find the increase in dead space excessive. A large filter should not be used in this location with pediatric patients.

b. Obstruction
A filter may become obstructed by blood, edema, or regurgitant fluid, a manufacturing defect, sterilization of a disposable filter, nebulized drugs, or insertion of a unidirectional filter backward. A filter should not be used with a patient who produces copious secretions or downstream of a humidifier or nebulizer. An increase in peak inspiratory pressure may indicate the need to replace a filter.

c. Leaks
A defect in a filter can cause a leak.

d. Liquid Penetration

Since filters located between the breathing system and the patient are sometimes exposed to liquids, the ability to contain that liquid is important. Microbes can pass through a filter by way of a liquid that passes through the filter. There is a great variability among filters with regard to the pressure that will cause liquid to penetrate the filter material. In general, pleated mechanical filters are more resistant to liquid passage than electrostatic filters.

I. Equipment to Administer Bronchodilators

Intraoperative bronchospasm can be a very serious problem. Studies show that medications administered by the inhalational route are just as effective as parenteral therapy with fewer adverse effects.

1. **Apparatus**

   a. Manufacturers have adapted metered-dose inhalers (MDIs) for use with anesthesia breathing circuits. Numerous commercial adapters and homemade devices have been described in the literature. Most adapters are T-shaped with the injection port on the side (**Fig. 5.6**). The gas sampling port in the breathing system or the sampling lumen of a specialized tracheal tube (Chapter 15) may be used to deliver medications. Medication may be delivered by a catheter that extends to the tracheal tube tip.

   b. The aerosol adapter should be placed close to the patient port. There should not be a filter or heat and moisture exchanger (HME) between the adapter and the patient.

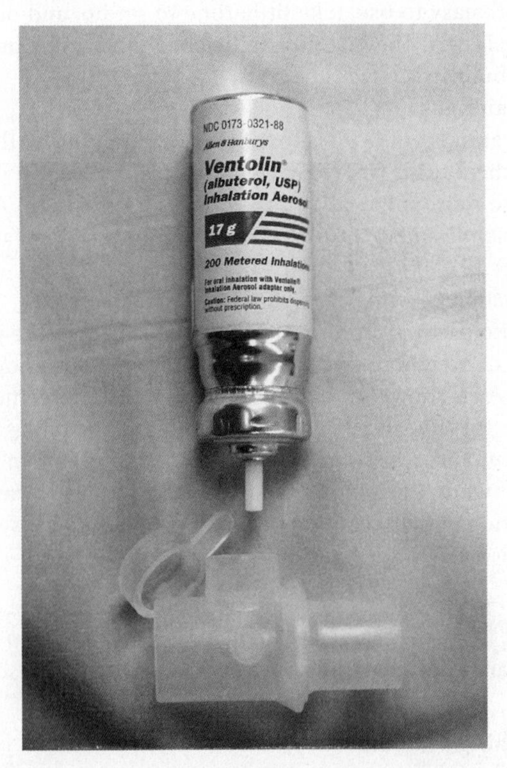

Figure 5.6 Adaptor for administering bronchodilators by using a multidose inhaler. Note the cap that can be fitted over the port when it is not in use. The hole in the inhaler should point toward the patient unless an upstream spacer is used.

c. A spacer (aerosol-holding chamber, reservoir chamber, or auxiliary or accessory device [extension or reservoir]) may be placed downstream or upstream of the MDI to slow the flow of aerosol and increase impaction and sedimentation of large particles. Rigid spacers result in more efficient medication delivery than collapsible ones.

2. **Use**

a. The inhaler should be shaken well prior to use. Bronchodilator discharge is maximal when the canister is upright. The hole in the adapter should point toward the patient, unless an upstream spacer is used. Actuating the inhaler just after inspiration begins will maximize delivery to the airways. If a spacer is used, the MDI should be actuated 1 to 2 seconds before inspiration or near the end of exhalation.

b. A slow, deep inspiration, followed by a pause of 2 to 3 seconds before exhalation will enhance the amount of medication deposited in the airway. There should be at least a 30- to 60-second pause between puffs.

c. If possible, humidification should be discontinued when an MDI is used. High humidification causes the aerosol droplets to increase in size, which causes them to rain out.

d. Using a spacer will increase bronchodilator delivery and reduce the number of puffs required. When a spacer is used, as many as 10 to 15 puffs may be required to achieve the desired results. The patient should be monitored for the appearance of beneficial and adverse side effects.

3. **Advantages**

MDIs are easy to use, take little time to set up, and occupy little space on the anesthesia cart. They are more efficient at delivering medications and less costly than nebulizers.

4. **Disadvantages**

A large amount of drug is lost because of rainout in the breathing system and the tracheal tube. Improper technique is one factor. The smaller the tracheal tube, the more medication is deposited in the tube. Another problem is that the carrier gas may cause erroneous readings with an anesthetic agent analyzer (Chapter 17).

J. Breathing System Classification

1. A favorite pastime among anesthesia providers in the past has been the classification of breathing systems. The result has been a hopelessly confused terminology. As is shown in **Table 5.1,** there is little agreement on terminology.

2. Because this hopelessly confused jumble of meanings for terms such as *open, semiopen,* and *semiclosed* makes it impossible for individuals to understand what is meant, the authors recommend that these terms should not be used. A description of the breathing system (e.g. Mapleson D system, circle system) and the fresh gas flow gives all the information needed.

CLINICAL MOMENT The terms *open, semiopen,* and *semiclosed* are obsolete and do not convey meaningful information. An equipment-based description is preferred.

VI. Mapleson Breathing Systems

A. Operating Principles

1. The Mapleson systems are characterized by the absence of unidirectional valves to direct gases to or from the patient. Because there is no means for absorbing

Table 5.1 Terminology for Classification of Breathing Systems

Author	Open	Semiopen	Semiclosed	Closed	Insufflation
Dripps RD, Echenhoff JE, Vandam LD. Introduction to Anesthesia. 3rd edition. Philadelphia: WB Saunders, 1968.	Pt inhales only gas delivered from machine ± bag. No CO_2 absorption	Exhaled gas to be rebreathed. No CO_2 absorption. Bag and directional valve optional	Some exhaled gases go to scavenging system and part +fresh gas are rebreathed. CO_2 absorption, directional valves, and bag present	Complete rebreathing expired gas	No valves, reservoir bag, or CO_2 absorption
Moyers JA. Nomenclature for methods of inhalation anesthesia. Anesthesiology 1953;14:609–611.	No reservoir bag or rebreathing	Reservoir bag with no rebreathing	Reservoir bag with partial rebreathing	Complete rebreathing	
Collins VJ. Principles of Anesthesiology. Philadelphia: Lea & Febiger, 1966.	Pt breathes anesthetic and air. No reservoir or rebreathing	Reservoir bag open to atmosphere with no rebreathing. Air dilutes anesthetic agent.	System closed on inspiration but open on exhalation. Reservoir bag closed to atmosphere	No access to atmosphere. Complete rebreathing	
Adriani J. The Chemistry and Physics of Anesthesia. Springfield, IL: Charles C Thomas, 1962.	Open drop mask		Closed system with no air dilution	Complete rebreathing	Gas flow over nasopharynx mouth or trachea
Conway CM. Anaesthetic circuits. In: Scurr C, Feldman S, eds. Foundations of Anaesthesia. Philadelphia: FA Davis, 1970:399–405.	No boundaries to fresh gas flow	Partial boundaries. Some restriction of fresh gas flow	Excess gas overflow with or without CO_2 absorption	No excess gas overflow. Complete rebreathing	
Hall J. Wright's veterinary Anaesthesia. 6th edition. London: Bailliere Tindall & Cox, 1966.	No reservoir or rebreathing	No reservoir bag with partial rebreathing	Reservoir bag with partial rebreathing	Complete breathing and reservoir bag	
McMahon J. Rebreathing as a basis for classification of inhalation techniques. J Am Assoc Nurse Anesth 1951;19:133–158.	No rebreathing Fresh gas flow rate equal to or more than minute volume		Some rebreathing	Complete rebreathing	
Baraka A. Functional classification of anaesthesia circuits. Anaesth Intensive Care 1977;5:172–178.	CO_2 eliminated by washout No reservoir bag	CO_2 washout with reservoir bag	Some rebreathing Reservoir bag and CO_2 absorption	CO_2 absorption. Fresh gas flow equals uptake	
Marini JJ, Culver BH, Kirk W. Flow resistance of exhalation valves and positive end-expiratory pressure devices used in mechanical ventilation. Am Rev Respir Dis 1984;131:850–854.	No reservoir bag. Open drop. Insufflation	Reservoir bag present. The Magill and Mapleson systems			

CO_2, the fresh gas flow must wash CO_2 out of the circuit. For this reason, these systems are sometimes called *carbon dioxide washout circuits* or *flow-controlled breathing systems.*

2. Because there is no clear separation of inspired and exhaled gases, rebreathing can occur when the patient's inspiratory flow exceeds the fresh gas flow. The composition of the inspired mixture will depend on how much rebreathing takes place. A number of studies designed to determine the fresh gas flow needed to prevent rebreathing with these systems have been performed, often with widely differing results. This is partly because different criteria have been used to define the onset of rebreathing and because variables such as minute ventilation, respiratory waveform, CO_2 production, patient responsiveness, stimulation, and physiological dead space may be unpredictable in anesthetized patients. Monitoring end-tidal CO_2 is the best method to determine the optimal fresh gas flow. It should be noted that with rebreathing, the arterial CO_2 to end-tidal CO_2 gradient decreases.
3. As shown in **Figure 5.7,** these systems are classified into five basic types: A through F. The B and C configurations will not be discussed because they are little used.

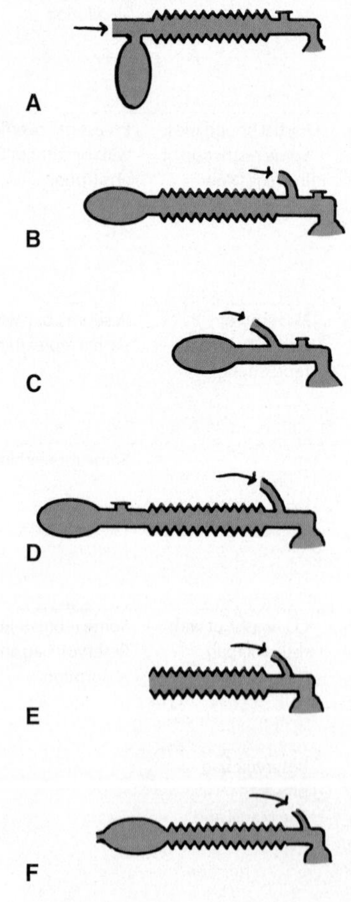

Figure 5.7 The Mapleson systems. Components include a reservoir bag, corrugated tubing, the adjustable pressure-limiting valve, fresh gas inlet, and patient connection. They lack CO_2 absorbers, unidirectional valves, and separate inspiratory and expiratory limbs. (Redrawn from Mapleson WW. The elimination of rebreathing in various semiclosed anesthetic systems. Br J Anaesth 1954;26:323–332.)

B. Mapleson A System

1. **Description**

a. The Mapleson A system (Magill attachment or system) is shown in **Figure 5.7A**. It differs from the other Mapleson systems in that fresh gas does not enter the system near the patient connection but at the other end of the system near the reservoir bag. A tube connects the bag to the APL valve at the patient end of the system.

b. The sensing site for a respiratory gas monitor (Chapter 17) may be located between the APL valve and the corrugated tubing. In adults, it may be placed between the APL valve and the patient. In small patients, this location could result in excessive dead space.

2. **Use**

a. Spontaneous Respiration

1) The sequence of events during the respiratory cycle using the Mapleson A system with spontaneous ventilation is shown in **Figure 5.8.** As the patient exhales (**Fig. 5.8C**), first dead space and then alveolar gases flow into the tube toward the bag. At the same time, fresh gas flows into the bag. When the bag is full, the pressure in the system rises until the APL valve opens. The first gas vented will be alveolar gas. During the remainder of exhalation, only alveolar gas is vented

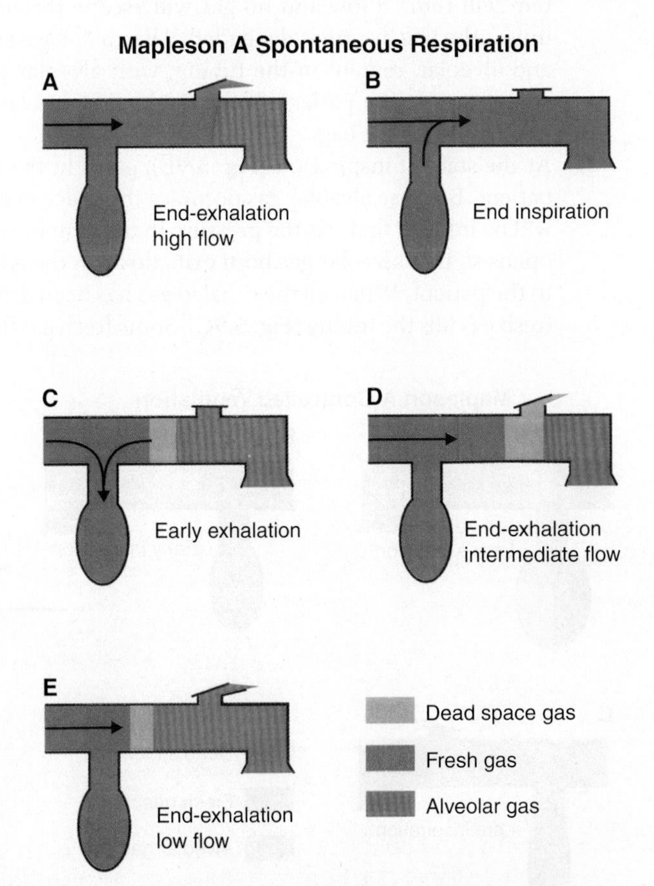

Figure 5.8 The Magill system with spontaneous ventilation. (Redrawn from Kain ML, Nunn JF. Fresh gas economies of the Magill circuit. Anesthesiology 1968;29:964–974.)

through the open APL valve. The continuing fresh gas inflow reverses the exhaled gas flow in the tube. Some alveolar gas that bypassed the APL valve now returns and exits through it. If the fresh gas flow is high (**Fig. 5.8A**), it will also force the dead space gas out. If the fresh gas flow is intermediate (**Fig. 5.8D**), some dead space gas will be retained in the system. If the fresh gas flow is low (**Fig. 5.8E**), more alveolar gas will be retained.

2) At the start of inspiration, the first gas inhaled will be from the dead space between the patient and the APL valve. The next gas will be either alveolar gas (if the fresh gas flow is low), dead space gas (if the fresh gas flow is intermediate), or fresh gas (if the fresh gas flow is high) (**Fig. 5.8B**). Changes in the respiratory pattern have little effect on rebreathing.

3) With the Mapleson A system, investigators have found that rebreathing begins when the fresh gas flow is reduced to 56 to 82 mL/kg/minute, or 58% to 83% of minute volume. Fresh gas flows of 51 to 85 mL/kg/minute and 42% to 88% of minute volume have been recommended to avoid rebreathing.

b. Controlled or Assisted Ventilation

1) During controlled or assisted ventilation (**Fig. 5.9**), the gas flow pattern changes. During exhalation (**Fig. 5.9A**), the pressure in the system will remain low and no gas will escape through the APL valve, unless the bag becomes distended. All exhaled gases, both dead space and alveolar, remain in the tubing, with alveolar gas occupying the space nearest the patient. If the tidal volume is large, some alveolar gas may enter the bag.

2) At the start of inspiration (**Fig. 5.9B**), gases in the tubing flow to the patient. Because alveolar gas occupies the space nearest the patient, it will be inhaled first. As the pressure in the system rises, the APL valve opens so that alveolar gas both exits through the APL valve and flows to the patient. When all the exhaled gas has been driven from the tube, fresh gas fills the tubing (**Fig. 5.9C**). Some fresh gas flows to the patient,

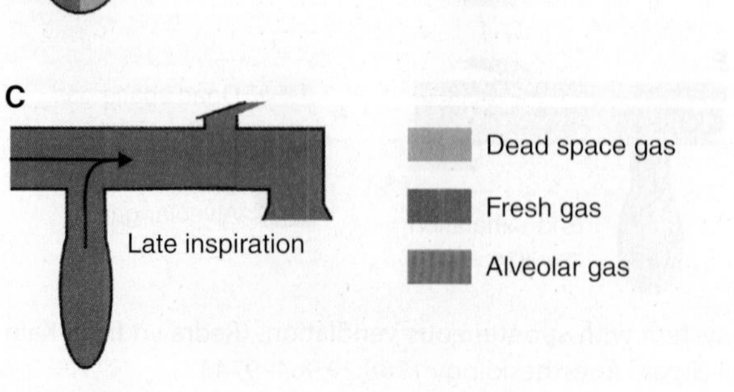

Figure 5.9 The Magill system with controlled ventilation.

and some is vented through the valve. Thus, during controlled ventilation, there is considerable rebreathing of alveolar gases and fresh gas is vented. The composition of the inspired gas mixture depends on the respiratory pattern. The system becomes more efficient as the expiratory phase is prolonged. Most investigators believe that it is illogical to use the Mapleson A system for controlled ventilation.

3) During assisted ventilation, the Mapleson A system is somewhat less efficient than with spontaneous ventilation but more efficient than with controlled ventilation.

3. **Hazards**

A mechanical ventilator that vents excess gases should not be used with this system, because the entire system then becomes dead space. The ventilators found on most anesthesia machines in the United States are unsuitable for use with the Mapleson A system.

4. **Preuse Checks**

The Mapleson A system is tested for leaks by occluding the patient end of the system, closing the APL valve, and pressurizing the system. Opening the APL valve will confirm that it is properly functioning. In addition, the user or a patient should breathe through the system.

CLINICAL MOMENT A frequently asked question on examinations is "Which Mapleson system is most efficient for the spontaneously breathing patient?" The answer is the Mapleson A system.

C. Mapleson D System

The Mapleson D, E, and F systems (**Fig. 5.7**) all have a T-piece near the patient and function similarly. The T-piece is a three-way tubular connector with a patient connection port, a fresh gas port, and a port for connection to corrugated tubing.

1. **Description**

a. Classic Form

1) The Mapleson D system is shown in **Figures 5.7D** and **5.10.** A tubing connects the T-piece at the patient end to the APL valve and the reservoir bag adjacent to it. The tubing length determines the distance the user can be from the patient but has minimal effects on ventilation.

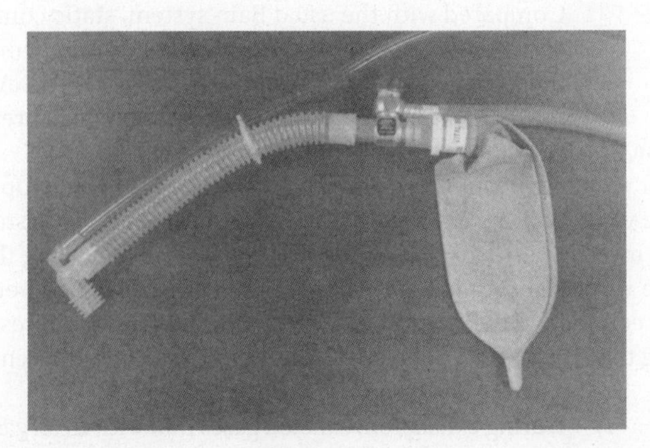

Figure 5.10 The Mapleson D system. A tube leading to the scavenging system is attached to the adjustable pressure-limiting valve.

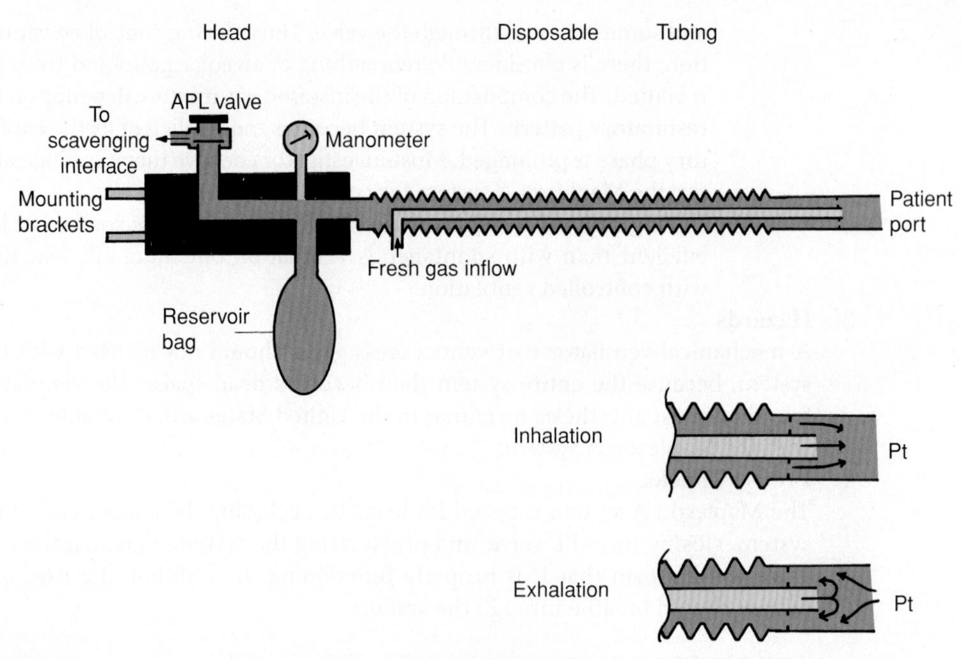

Figure 5.11 The Bain modification of the Mapleson D system. The fresh gas supply tube is inside the corrugated tubing. APL, adjustable pressure limiting; Pt, patient.

2) The sensor or sampling site for a respiratory gas monitor may be located at the T-piece, or between the corrugated tubing and the APL valve. In adults, it may be placed between the T-piece and the patient. Carbon dioxide monitoring may be inaccurate because exhaled carbon dioxide will be contaminated with fresh gas.

b. Bain Modification

1) In the Bain modification (**Fig. 5.11**), the fresh gas supply tube runs coaxially inside the corrugated tubing and ends at the point where the fresh gas would enter if the classic Mapleson D system were used. The outer tube is attached to a mount that includes a pressure gauge, a reservoir bag, and the APL valve.

2) A longer version of the Bain system may be used for anesthesia delivery in locations such as the magnetic resonance imaging (MRI) unit. Compared with the usual Bain system, static compliance is increased with a reduction in peak inspiratory pressure and tidal volume with the same ventilator settings. PEEP is increased. A longer Bain system presents increased resistance to spontaneous breathing.

2. **Use**

For spontaneous respiration, the APL valve is left fully open and excess gases are vented during expiration. Manually controlled or assisted ventilation is performed by partially closing the APL valve and squeezing the bag. Excess gases are vented during inspiration. Mechanically controlled ventilation is achieved by connecting the hose from a ventilator in place of the reservoir bag and closing the APL valve. Excess gases are vented through the ventilator spill valve.

a. Spontaneous Respiration

1) During exhalation, exhaled gases mix with fresh gases and flow through the corrugated tube toward the bag. After the bag has filled, gas exits via the APL valve. During the expiratory pause, fresh gas pushes exhaled gases down the corrugated tubing.

2) During inspiration, the patient inhales gas from the fresh gas inlet and the corrugated tubing. If the fresh gas flow is high, all the gas drawn from the corrugated tube will be fresh gas. If the fresh gas flow is low, some exhaled gas containing CO_2 will be inhaled. The ventilatory pattern will help to determine the amount of rebreathing. Factors that tend to decrease rebreathing include a high I:E time ratio, a slow rise in the inspiratory flow rate, a low flow rate during the last part of exhalation, and a long expiratory pause.
3) As gas containing CO_2 is inhaled, the end-tidal CO_2 will rise. Provided rebreathing is not extreme, a normal end-tidal CO_2 can be achieved but only at the cost of increased work of breathing by the patient. The end-tidal CO_2 tends to reach a plateau. At that point, no matter how hard the patient works, the end-tidal CO_2 cannot be lowered. If the patient's respiration is depressed, end-tidal CO_2 will rise.
4) End-tidal CO_2 depends on both the ratio of minute volume to fresh gas flow and their absolute values. If the expired volume is greater than the fresh gas flow, end-tidal CO_2 will be determined mainly by fresh gas flow. If fresh gas flow is greater than minute volume, end-tidal CO_2 will be determined mainly by minute volume. Recommendations for fresh gas flows based on body weight vary from 100 to 300 mL/kg/minute. Most studies have recommended that the fresh gas flow be 1.5 to 3.0 times the minute volume, whereas others have held that a fresh gas flow approximately equal to minute ventilation is adequate.

b. Controlled Ventilation

1) During exhalation (**Fig. 5.12**), gases flow from the patient down the corrugated tubing. At the same time, fresh gas enters the tubing. During the expiratory pause, the fresh gas flow continues and pushes exhaled gases down the tubing.
2) During inspiration, fresh gas and gas from the corrugated tubing enter the patient. If the fresh gas flow is low, some exhaled gases may be inhaled. Prolonging the inspiratory time, increasing the respiratory rate, or adding an inspiratory plateau will increase rebreathing. Rebreathing can be decreased by allowing a long expiratory pause so that fresh gas can flush exhaled gases from the tubing.
3) When the fresh gas flow is high, there is little rebreathing and the end-tidal CO_2 is determined mainly by minute ventilation. Tidal volume, the volume of the expiratory limb, and expiratory resistance also affect rebreathing. When minute volume substantially exceeds fresh gas flow, the fresh gas flow is the main factor controlling CO_2 elimination. The higher the fresh gas flow, the lower the end-tidal CO_2.
4) Combining fresh gas flow, minute volume, and arterial CO_2 levels, a series of curves can be constructed (**Fig. 5.13**). An infinite number of combinations of fresh gas flow and minute volume can be used to produce a given $PetCO_2$. High fresh gas flows and low minute volumes or high minute volumes and low fresh gas flows or combinations in between can be used. In **Figure 5.13,** at the left, with a high fresh gas flow, the circuit is nonrebreathing and end-tidal CO_2 depends only on ventilation. Such high flows are uneconomical and associated with lost heat and humidity. End-tidal CO_2 depends on minute volume, which is difficult to accurately adjust, especially in small patients. On the right is the region of hyperventilation and partial rebreathing.

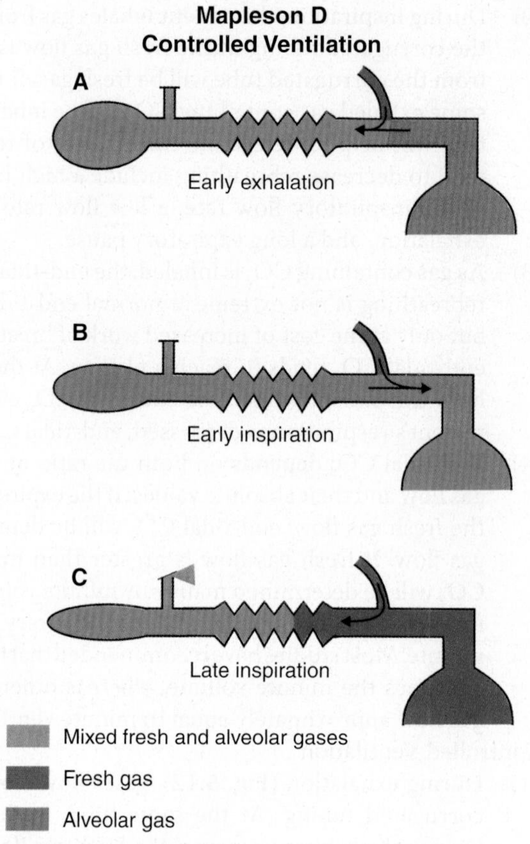

Figure 5.12 Functioning of the Mapleson D system.

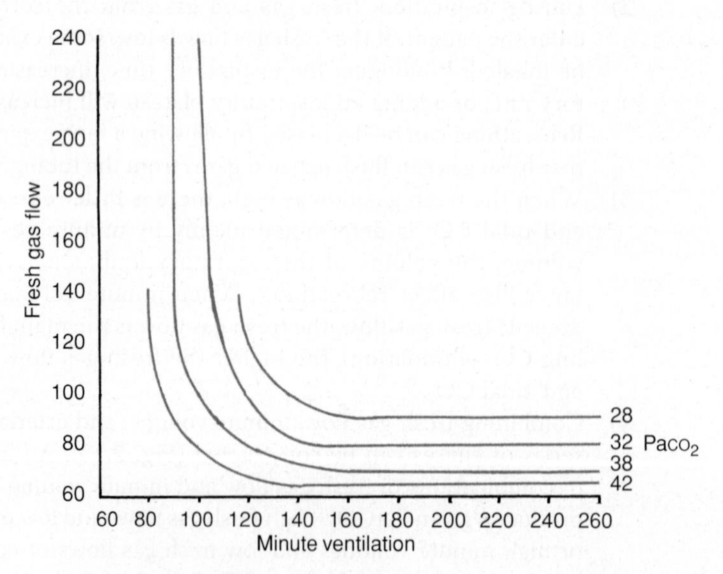

Figure 5.13 The Mapleson D system used with controlled ventilation. Each isopleth represents a constant level of $Paco_2$. Note that essentially the same $Paco_2$ can be achieved for fresh gas flows from 100 to 240 mL/kg/minute. (Redrawn from Froese AB. Anesthesia Circuits for Children [ASA Refresher Course]. Park Ridge, IL: American Society of Anesthesiologists, 1978.)

End-tidal CO_2 is regulated by adjusting the fresh gas flow. Lower fresh gas flows (and increased rebreathing) are associated with higher humidity, less heat loss, and greater fresh gas economy. Hyperventilation can be used without inducing hypocarbia. Individual differences in the ratio of dead space to tidal volume are minimized at high minute volumes. For these reasons, in most cases, it is advantageous to aim for the right side of the graph. In patients with stiff lungs, poor cardiac performance, or hypovolemia, using the left side of the graph with relatively low ventilation and a high fresh gas flow may be beneficial.

CLINICAL MOMENT Another frequently asked examination question is "Which Mapleson system is most efficient for controlled ventilation?" The answer is the Mapleson D system.

CLINICAL MOMENT With assisted ventilation, Mapleson D system efficiency is intermediate between that for spontaneous and controlled ventilation.

3. **Hazards**
   If the inner tube of the Bain system becomes detached from its connections at either end or develops a leak at the machine end, the fresh gas supply tube becomes kinked or twisted, the system is incorrectly assembled (such as using standard corrugated tubing), or there is a defect in the metal head so that fresh gas and exhaled gas mix, the dead space will be increased.
4. **Preuse Checks**
   a. The Mapleson D system is tested for leaks by occluding the patient end, closing the APL valve, and pressurizing the system. The APL valve is then opened. The bag should deflate easily if the valve and the scavenging system are working properly. Either the user or the patient should breathe through the system to detect obstructions.
   b. The Bain modification of the Mapleson D system requires special testing to confirm the integrity of the inner tubing. This can be performed by setting a low flow on the oxygen flowmeter and occluding the inner tube (with a finger or the plunger from a small syringe) at the patient end while observing the flowmeter indicator. If the inner tube is intact and correctly connected, the indicator will fall. The inner tube integrity can also be confirmed by activating the oxygen flush and observing the bag. A Venturi effect caused by the high flow at the patient end will create a negative pressure in the outer tubing, which will cause the bag to deflate. If the inner tube is not intact, this maneuver will cause the bag to inflate slightly. This test will not detect a system in which the inner tube is omitted or does not extend to the patient port or one that has holes at the patient end of the inner tube.
5. **Continuous Positive Airway Pressure and Patient Transport**
   a. During one-lung ventilation with a double-lumen tube (Chapter 16), a modified Mapleson D system attached to the lumen leading to the nondependent lung is often used to apply CPAP to that lung. A number of configurations have been described. One is shown in **Figure 5.14.** An oxygen source is connected to the system. The APL valve is set to maintain the desired pressure. A PEEP valve may be added to function as a high-pressure relief device.

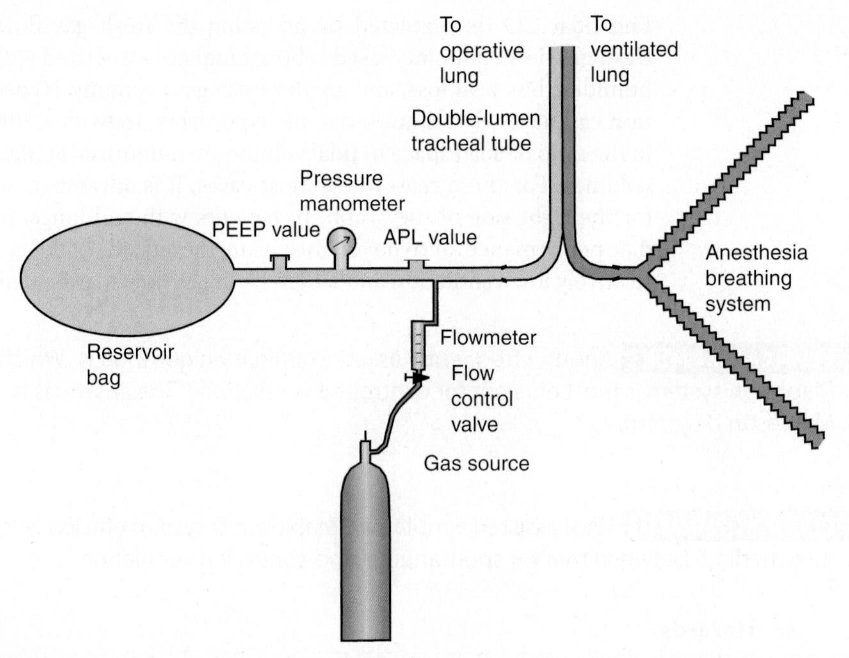

Figure 5.14 System for continuous positive airway pressure. (See text for details.) PEEP, positive end-expiratory pressure; APL, adjustable pressure limiting.

b. The Mapleson D system is frequently used for patient transport requiring controlled ventilation.

CLINICAL MOMENT Never try to provide CPAP to a tracheal tube by connecting the oxygen source directly to the tube. The Mapleson D system can be used safely because the amount of pressure can be controlled by adjusting the APL valve, which furnishes an exit for excess gas.

D. Mapleson E System

1. **Description**

a. The Mapleson E (T-piece) system is shown in **Figure 5.7E.** It does not have a bag. A tubing may be attached to the T-piece to form a reservoir. The expiratory port may be enclosed in a chamber from which excess gases are evacuated.

b. The sensor or sampling site for the respiratory gas monitor may be placed between the expiratory port and the expiratory tubing. In larger patients, it may be placed between the T-piece and the patient, but this location should be avoided in small patients because it increases dead space.

c. Numerous modifications to the original T-piece have been made. Many have the fresh gas inlet extending inside the body of the T-piece toward the patient connection to minimize dead space. A pressure-limiting device may be added to the system.

2. **Use**

a. Using the Mapleson E system for anesthesia administration has decreased because of the difficulty in scavenging excess gases, but it is commonly used to administer oxygen or humidified gas to spontaneously breathing patients.

b. For spontaneous ventilation, the expiratory limb is open to atmosphere. Controlled ventilation can be performed by intermittently occluding the expiratory limb and allowing the fresh gas flow to inflate the lungs. Assisted respiration is difficult to perform.

c. The sequence of events during the respiratory cycle is similar to that of the Mapleson D system shown in **Figure 5.12.** The presence or absence and the amount of rebreathing or air dilution will depend on the fresh gas flow, the patient's minute volume, the volume of the exhalation limb, the type of ventilation (spontaneous or controlled), and the respiratory pattern.

d. With spontaneous ventilation, no rebreathing can occur if there is no exhalation limb. If there is an expiratory limb, the fresh gas flow needed to prevent rebreathing will be the same as that for the Mapleson D system. During controlled ventilation, there can be no rebreathing because only fresh gas will inflate the lungs.

e. No air dilution can occur during controlled ventilation. During spontaneous ventilation, air dilution cannot occur if the exhalation tube volume is greater than the patient's tidal volume. If there is no expiratory limb or if the volume of the limb is less than the patient's tidal volume, air dilution can be prevented by providing a fresh gas flow that exceeds the peak inspiratory flow rate, normally three to five times the minute volume. A fresh gas flow of twice the minute volume and a reservoir volume one third of the tidal volume will prevent air dilution.

3. **Hazards**

Controlling ventilation by intermittently occluding the expiratory limb may lead to overinflation and barotrauma. This is a danger associated with this system in particular because the anesthesia provider does not have the "feel of the bag" during inflation that he or she has with other systems. The pressure-buffering effect of the bag is absent, and there is no APL valve to moderate the pressure in the lungs. To overcome this potential hazard, it has been recommended that a pressure-limiting device be placed in the system.

E. Mapleson F System

1. **Description**

The Mapleson F (Jackson-Rees, Rees, or Jackson-Rees modification of the T-piece) system has a bag with a mechanism for venting excess gases (**Fig. 5.7F**). The mechanism can be a hole in the tail or side of the bag that is occluded by using a finger to provide pressure. It may be fitted with a device to prevent the bag from collapsing while allowing excess gases to escape. An anesthesia ventilator may be used in place of the bag. An APL valve may be placed near the patient connection to provide protection from high pressure. Scavenging can be performed either by enclosing the bag in a chamber from which waste gases are suctioned or by attaching various devices to the relief mechanism in the bag.

2. **Use**

a. For spontaneous respiration, the relief mechanism is left fully open. For assisted or controlled respiration, the relief mechanism is occluded sufficiently to distend the bag. Respiration can then be controlled or assisted by squeezing the bag. Alternately, the hole in the bag can be occluded by the user's finger during inspiration. For mechanical ventilation, the bag is replaced by the hose from a ventilator.

b. The Mapleson F system functions much like the Mapleson D system. The flows required to prevent rebreathing during spontaneous and controlled respiration are the same as those required with the Mapleson D system. This system offers slightly less work of breathing than a pediatric circle system.

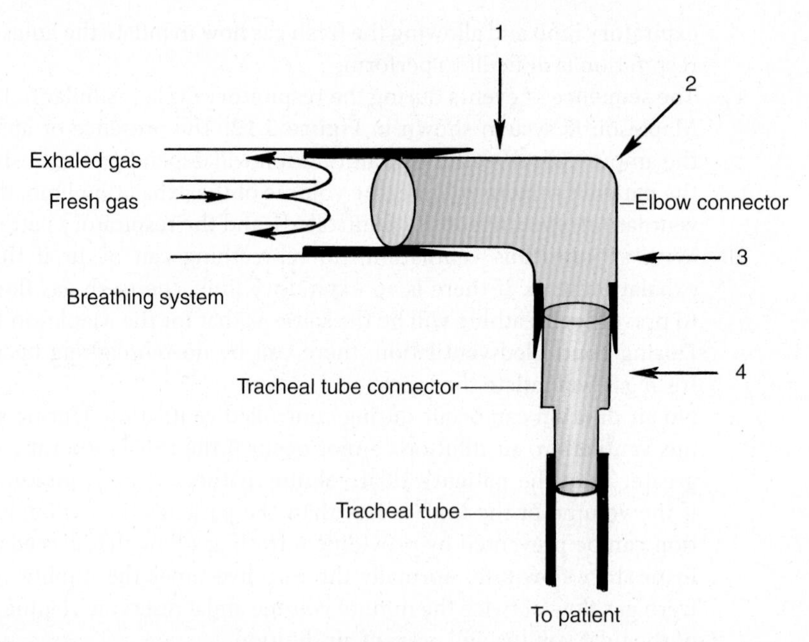

Figure 5.15 Respiratory gas sampling with a Mapleson system. Accurate values for expiratory concentrations can be obtained by sampling at sites 3 and 4. Sampling at site 2 will yield accurate values only if the fresh gas flow is not high. Sampling at site 1 will yield inaccurate values even at low fresh gas flows. (Redrawn from Gravenstein N, Lampotang S, Beneken JEW. Factors influencing capnography in the Bain circuit. J Clin Monit 1985;1:6–10.)

F. Respiratory Gas Monitoring with the Mapleson Systems

All of the Mapleson systems except the A system have the fresh gas inlet near the patient connection port. This may make it difficult to obtain a reliable sample of exhaled gases. One study examined four sampling sites (**Fig. 5.15**): at the junction of the breathing system and elbow connector, at the corner of the elbow connector, 2 cm distal in the elbow connector, and in the tracheal tube connector. If sampling were carried out at the two sites closest to the patient, values would be accurate. Significant errors were noted when samples were taken from the corner of the elbow connector, but only if a high fresh gas flow was used. Significant errors were noted when sampling was performed at the junction of the breathing system and elbow connector even if low fresh gas flows were used. A cannula that projects into the airway can be used to improve sampling.

G. Advantages of the Mapleson Systems

Mapleson systems are made from simple equipment and have no moving parts. They are easy to disinfect and sterilize. Resistance to breathing is low during spontaneous breathing. Since there is no CO2 absorbent, the problems with carbon monoxide and compound A, which are discussed later in this chapter, are not present. They can be used in remote situations such as in the MRI unit if the metal parts do not contain ferrous material.

H. Disadvantages

These systems require high gas flows. This results in higher costs, increased atmospheric pollution, and difficulty assessing spontaneous ventilation. The optimal fresh gas flow is difficult to determine and differs between spontaneous and controlled ventilation. High flows tend to lower heat and humidity.

CLINICAL MOMENT If a patient develops malignant hyperthermia, use the circle system rather than a Mapleson system.

VII. Circle Breathing System

The circle system is so named because gases flow in a circular pathway through separate inspiratory and expiratory channels. Carbon dioxide exhaled by the patient is removed by an absorbent.

A. Components

1. **Absorber**

The absorber is usually attached to the anesthesia machine but may be separate. An absorber assembly consists of an absorber, two ports for connection to breathing tubes, and a fresh gas inlet. Other components that may be mounted on the absorber assembly include inspiratory and expiratory unidirectional valves, an APL valve, and a bag mount. Modern anesthesia machines often incorporate components of the anesthesia ventilator into the absorber assembly. Disposable absorbers and absorber assemblies are available.

a. Construction

1) The absorbent is held in canisters (carbon dioxide absorbent containers, chambers, units, or cartridges). The side walls are transparent so that absorbent color can be monitored. A screen at the bottom of each canister holds the absorbent in place.

2) Some absorbers use two canisters in a series (**Fig. 5.16**). Many newer machines use a single, small, disposable canister that can be quickly changed during anesthesia without interrupting breathing system continuity (**Fig. 5.17**).

3) Prepackaged absorbent containers are available and may be used alone or placed inside a canister. These eliminate the need to pour absorbent into the canister.

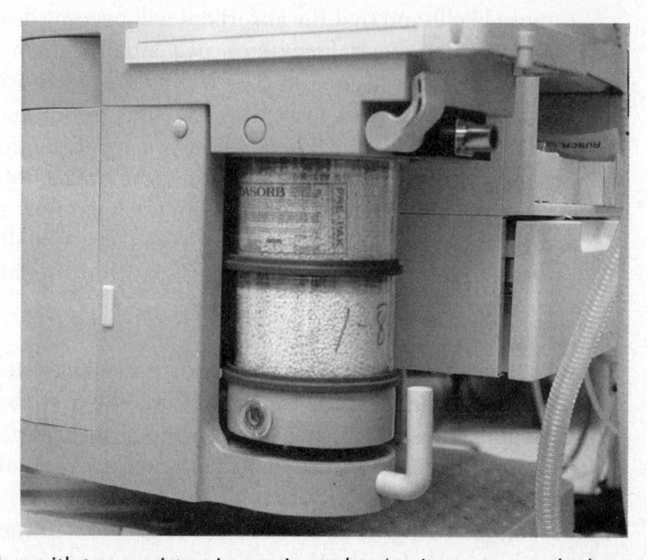

Figure 5.16 Absorber with two canisters in a series, a dust/moisture trap at the bottom and a drain at the side. The lever at the right is used to tighten and loosen the canisters. Note that the date the absorbent was last changed is marked on the lower canister.

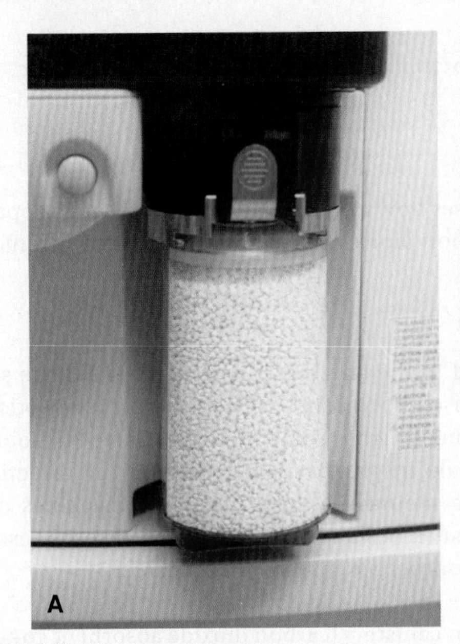

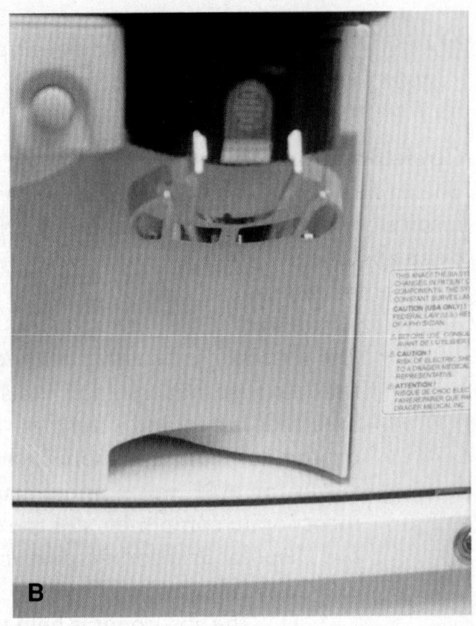

Figure 5.17 Absorber with a single disposable canister. **A:** With canister in place. **B:** With canister removed. The canister fits into grooves in the bracket and is pushed up to lock it in place. Note the release button.

CLINICAL MOMENT Prepackaged absorbent containers frequently come with a plastic covering to seal the absorbent and prevent drying. If this is not removed, there will be complete breathing system obstruction.

4) Canisters of varying capacity have been used. An advantage of large canisters is longer intervals between absorbent changes, but there is more likelihood that the absorbent will become desiccated.
5) Newer anesthesia machines use small canisters that must be changed more frequently, providing fresh absorbent with proper water content and lessening the likelihood that toxic products will be produced or anesthetic agents will be adsorbed. Another advantage of small absorbers is that the breathing system volume is reduced. This will allow changes in fresh gas flow composition to be reflected more quickly in the inspired gas. Usually, these canisters can be changed during anesthesia without opening the breathing system.

b. Absorption Pattern

The absorption pattern within a properly packed canister is shown in **Figure 5.18.** Gases enter at the top or bottom. The first absorption occurs at the inlet and along the canister sides. As this absorbent becomes exhausted, carbon dioxide will be absorbed farther downstream in the canister.

c. Baffles

Baffles, annular rings that serve to direct gas flow toward the central part of the canister, are frequently used to increase the travel path for gases that pass along the sides of the canister and compensate for the reduced flow resistance along the walls of the canister.

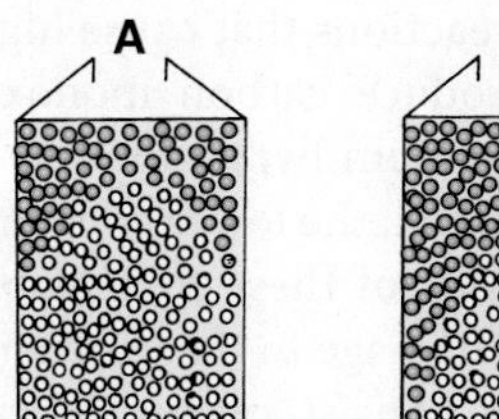

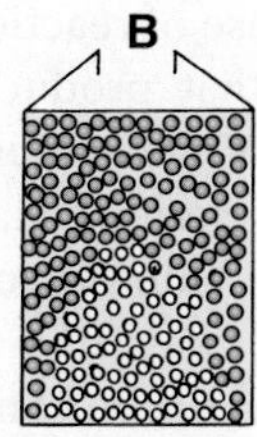

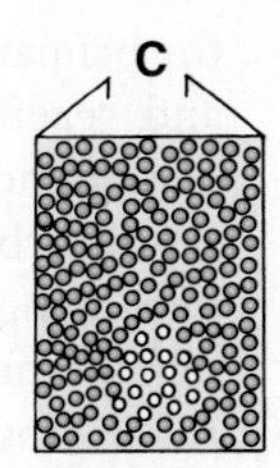

Figure 5.18 Pattern of carbon dioxide absorption in a canister. *Darkened circles* represent exhausted absorbent. **A:** After limited use; absorption has occurred primarily at the inlet and to a lesser extent along the sides. **B:** After extensive use; the granules at the inlet and along the sides are exhausted. **C:** Carbon dioxide is filtering through the canister; in the distal third of the canister, a spot remains where the granules are still capable of absorbing carbon dioxide. (Redrawn from Adriani J, Rovenstein EA. Experimental studies on carbon dioxide absorbers for anesthesia. Anesthesiology 1941;2:10.)

d. Side or Center Tube

There must be a way to conduct gases to or from the bottom of the canister. Some absorbers have a side tube external to the canister(s). The tube may also be in the center of the absorber (**Fig. 5.19**).

2. **Absorbents**

a. Composition

1) Carbon dioxide absorption employs the general principle of a base neutralizing an acid. The acid is carbonic acid formed by the reaction of carbon dioxide with water. The end products are water and a carbonate. Heat is liberated in the reaction.

2) Some absorbents, including such traditional ones as soda lime, at one time contained relatively high amounts of potassium and/or sodium hydroxide. When these absorbents become desiccated, they react with volatile anesthetics to form carbon monoxide. Compound A, formaldehyde, and methanol can be formed with sevoflurane. These absorbents do not change color when dry. Their capacity to absorb carbon dioxide is decreased by decreased moisture, and they adsorb anesthetic agents more when dry. These absorbents have a longer life than those that have no potassium or sodium hydroxide.

3) Absorbents no longer contain potassium hydroxide and contain reduced concentrations of sodium hydroxide. Potassium hydroxide is

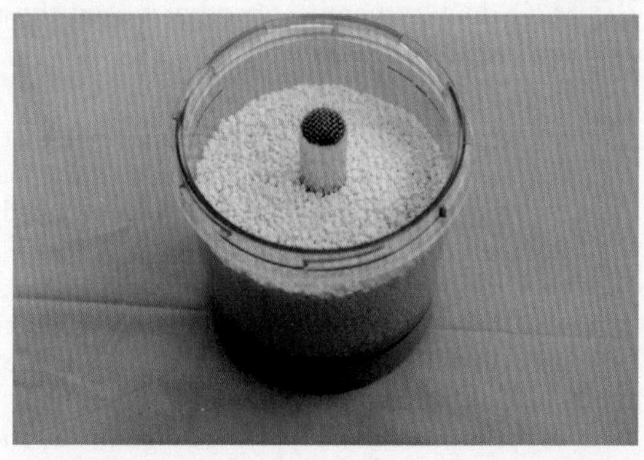

Figure 5.19 Center tube in canister. Note the grooves around the edge that allow the canister to be screwed tightly in place.

the primary cause of reactions that cause high internal temperatures and reactions that produce carbon monoxide, formaldehyde, and compound A. While sodium hydroxide will react with agents when the absorbent is desiccated, the lower concentrations should not produce dangerous amounts of these toxic substances or high enough temperatures to cause damage to the canister.

4) Alkali-free absorbents consist mainly of calcium hydroxide, with small amounts of other agents added to accelerate carbon dioxide absorption and bind water. With these absorbents, there is no evidence of carbon monoxide formation with any anesthetic agent, even if the absorbent becomes desiccated. There is little or no compound A or formaldehyde formation with sevoflurane even with low fresh gas flows and desiccated absorbent. The indicator in these absorbents changes color on drying. Once exhausted, these absorbents do not revert to their original color. The carbon dioxide absorption capacity of these absorbents is less than that of absorbents containing strong alkali but does not deteriorate when moisture is lost.

5) The Anesthesia Patient Safety Foundation has provided a number of recommendations that an anesthesia department should take to prevent absorbent desiccation if the department continues to use strong alkaline absorbents with volatile anesthetic agents. These, and a few more from the literature, are as follows:
   (i) All gas flows should be turned OFF after use with each patient. This is probably the most important measure. When the daily schedule is finished, the anesthesia machine should be disconnected from the medical gas pipeline system at the pipeline outlet.
   (ii) Vaporizers should be turned OFF when not in use. At the end of each case, the breathing system should be flushed with gas that is free of volatile anesthetic.
   (iii) The absorbent should be changed routinely, at least once a week, preferably on a Monday morning, and whenever fresh gas has been flowing for an extensive or indeterminate period of time. The canister should be labeled with the filling date (**Fig. 5.16**). Checking this date should be part of the daily checkout procedure.

CLINICAL MOMENT If a double-chamber absorber is used, the absorbent in both canisters should be changed at the same time.

   (iv) Canisters on an anesthesia machine that is not commonly used for a long period of time should not be filled with absorbent that contains alkali or should be filled with fresh absorbent before each use.
   (v) The integrity of the absorbent packaging should be verified prior to use. Opened containers that contain absorbent should be carefully closed after use, and the rest of the absorbent should be used as soon as possible.
   (vi) The practice of supplying oxygen for a patient who is not receiving general anesthesia through the circle system should be strongly discouraged. This is associated with other hazards, including

accidental administration of nitrous oxide and volatile anesthetics. Supplemental oxygen should be obtained from a flowmeter that is connected directly to the oxygen pipeline system or the auxiliary oxygen flowmeter on the anesthesia machine (Chapter 3).

(vii) Using fresh gas to dry breathing system components should be strongly discouraged.

(viii) The negative pressure relief valve on a closed scavenging system (Chapter 8) should be checked regularly. Failure of this valve to pull in room air may result in fresh gas from the machine being drawn through the absorbent if the APL valve is open.

(ix) The temperature in the canister should be monitored and the absorbent changed if excessive heat is detected. A simple patient temperature monitor may be used for this purpose. If the temperature approaches 50°C, excessive heating from anesthetic breakdown should be suspected. If the probe is not in the area where the temperature increase occurs, the rise in temperature may be missed.

(x) Consideration should be given to removing absorbent from canisters in induction rooms and using high fresh gas flows to eliminate rebreathing.

CLINICAL MOMENT Flushing the breathing system with fresh gas before use will not prevent carbon monoxide exposure.

b. Indicators

1) An indicator is an acid or base whose color depends on pH. It is added to the absorbent to show when the absorbent's ability to absorb carbon dioxide is exhausted. Some of the commonly used indicators and their colors are shown in **Table 5.2.**

2) Some alkali-free absorbents change color when desiccated. The user should always know which indicator is being used and what color change is expected when the absorption capacity is exhausted or the absorbent is desiccated. During certain flow conditions, water may accumulate on the granules and block CO_2 absorption.

CLINICAL MOMENT The presence of inspired CO_2 is the best indication of absorbent exhaustion. Color change of the absorbent is less reliable.

Table 5.2 Indicators for Absorbents

Indicator	Color When Fresh	Color When Exhausted
Phenolphthalein	White	Pink
Ethyl violet	White	Purple
Clayton yellow	Red	Yellow
Ethyl orange	Orange	Yellow
Mimosa Z	Red	White

c. Shape and Size
Absorbents are supplied as pellets or granules. Pellets and small granules provide larger surface area and decrease gas channeling along low-resistance pathways. However, they may cause more resistance and caking.

d. Hardness
Some absorbent granules fragment easily, producing dust (fines). To prevent this, small amounts of a hardening agent are added. There are variations in the dust content of different absorbents. Excessive powder produces channeling, resistance to flow, and caking. Dust may be blown through the system to the patient or may cause system components to malfunction.

e. Excessive Heat and Fires
1) The interaction of desiccated barium hydroxide absorbent and sevoflurane can produce temperatures of several hundred degrees centigrade. Cases of fires and/or melted components in the absorber have been reported. Barium hydroxide lime is no longer available for use.

CLINICAL MOMENT Fires have occurred primarily with barium hydroxide lime, which is now off the market, although fires involving desiccated soda lime have also been reported. Damage to absorber parts from excessive heat can occur.

2) It is possible that damage from excessive heat is not reported more often because absorption of the toxic products by the patient reduces their concentrations below the lower limit of flammability. Cases of melted or burned absorber parts should be reported to the Food and Drug Administration (FDA), suppliers, and the Emergency Care Research Institute.

f. Absorbent Storage and Handling
Loose absorbent containers are sealed prior to use. They should be resealed after absorbent has been removed to prevent reaction with ambient carbon dioxide, indicator deactivation, and moisture loss. They need to be handled gently to avoid fragmentation and exposure to absorbent dust, which can irritate the eyes, skin, and respiratory tract.

g. Changing the Absorbent
1) There are a number of criteria that indicate that the absorbent should be changed. If small canisters that can be changed without opening the breathing system are used, the absorbent can be changed when inspired carbon dioxide is detected. In large absorbers, color change can be used as a criterion. Desiccation may occur before the color changes.
2) The following considerations should be kept in mind when using an indicator:
   (i) A phenomenon known as *peaking* or *regeneration* is seen with absorbents that contain strong bases. The absorbent appears to be reactivated with rest. After a number of such periods of efficient absorption with intervening periods of rest, terminal exhaustion occurs.

CLINICAL MOMENT Color change when the canister is not in use can give a false impression that the absorbent has regenerated. The color can change quickly upon use.

(ii) When the exhausted color shows strongly, the absorbent is at or near the point of exhaustion. When little or no color change shows, active absorbent may be present, but the amount is indeterminate and may be quite small.
(iii) Alkali-free absorbents may change color when dried.
(iv) If channeling occurs, the absorbent along the channels will become exhausted and carbon dioxide will pass through the canister. If channeling occurs at sites other than the sides of the canister, the color change may not be visible.
(v) The absorbent may not contain an indicator. Some companies make an industrial absorbent that does not contain an indicator, and this product may be supplied as the result of an administrative error.
(vi) Ethyl violet undergoes deactivation even if it is stored in the dark. Deactivation is accelerated in the presence of light, especially high-intensity or ultraviolet light.

CLINICAL MOMENT If an absorbent containing sodium hydroxide is used, it should be changed at least once a week, regardless of the color. Monday morning is recommended in the event that a continuous fresh gas flow that could desiccate the absorbent occurred over the weekend. If a dual-chamber absorber is being used, both the canisters must be changed at the same time.

3. **Unidirectional Valves**
   a. Two unidirectional (flutter, one-way, check, directional, dome, flap, nonreturn, inspiratory, and expiratory) valves are used in each circle system to ensure that gases flow toward the patient in one breathing tube and away in the other. They are usually part of the absorber assembly. The valves are either marked with a directional arrow or the words *inspiration* or *expiration.*
   b. A typical horizontal unidirectional valve is shown diagrammatically in **Figure 5.20.** A light, thin disc (leaflet) seats horizontally on an annular seat. The disc has a slightly larger diameter than the circular edge on which it

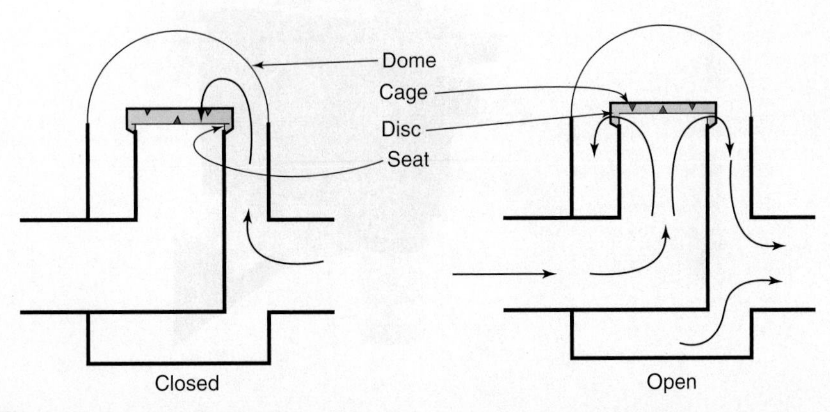

Figure 5.20 Unidirectional valve. **Left:** Reversing the gas flow causes the disc to contact its seat, stopping further retrograde flow. **Right:** Gas flowing into the valve raises the disc from its seat and then passes through the valve. The guide (cage) prevents lateral or vertical displacement of the disc. The transparent dome allows observation of disc movement.

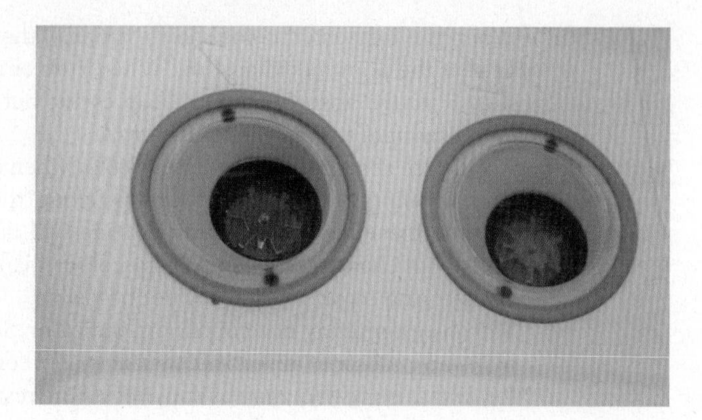

Figure 5.21 Horizontal unidirectional valves. Note the cages that prevent the discs from being displaced.

sits. A cage or guide mechanism (retainer) (such as projections from the seat and the dome) may be present to prevent the disc from becoming dislodged (**Fig. 5.21**). The disc is hydrophobic so that condensate does not cause it to stick and increase resistance to opening. The valve top is covered by a clear plastic dome so that the disc can be observed. Gas enters at the bottom, raising the disc from its seat, and then passes under the dome and on through the breathing system. Reversing the gas flow will cause the disc to contact the seat, preventing retrograde flow. A unidirectional valve may be vertical rather than horizontal (**Fig. 5.22**). The disc is hinged at the top.

c. One or both unidirectional valves may become incompetent. Disc movement does not guarantee valve competence. Because an incompetent valve offers less resistance to flow than one that must open, the gas flow will be primarily through the incompetent valve, resulting in rebreathing. The valve on the exhalation side is most prone to this problem because it is exposed to more moisture. A unidirectional valve leak produces a characteristic waveform on the capnograph (Chapter 17). A unidirectional valve may jam, obstructing gas flow.

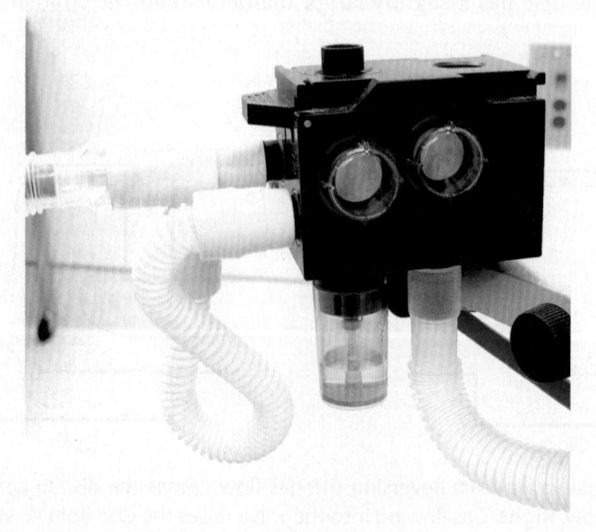

Figure 5.22 Vertical unidirectional valves.

CLINICAL MOMENT Disc movement in a unidirectional valve does not mean that there is no retrograde flow through it.

CLINICAL MOMENT The function of a unidirectional valve is to ensure that gas flows in only one direction. When checking the valve for proper action, it should be subjected to back pressure to make certain that gas does not flow in the wrong direction. Methods to check unidirectional valves for proper functioning are discussed in Chapter 26.

4. **Inspiratory and Expiratory Ports**
   The inspiratory port is just downstream from the inspiratory unidirectional valve and has a 22-mm male connector through which gases flow toward the patient during inspiration. The expiratory port is just upstream of the unidirectional valve and has a 22-mm male connector through which gases flow during exhalation. These ports are usually mounted on the absorber assembly.
5. **Y-piece**
   a. The Y-piece (Y-piece connector, Y-adaptor) is a three-way tubular connector with two 22-mm male ports for connection to the breathing tubes and a 15-mm female patient connector for a tracheal tube or supraglottic airway device. The patient connection port usually has a coaxial 22-mm male fitting to allow connection to a face mask. In most disposable systems, the Y-piece and breathing tubes are permanently attached. A septum may be placed in the Y-piece to decrease the dead space.
   b. Coaxial circle systems (**Fig. 5.23**) have a component that replaces but serves the same function as the Y-piece. The inner (inspiratory) tube ends just before the connection to the patient. The exhalation channel though the outer tube begins just downstream of the end of the inspiratory tubing.
6. **Fresh Gas Inlet**
   The fresh gas inlet may be connected to the common gas outlet on the anesthesia machine by flexible tubing. On most new anesthesia machines, there is a direct connection between the machine outlet and the breathing system so that the user does not see a fresh gas hose.
7. **Adjustable Pressure-Limiting Valve**
   The APL valve was discussed earlier in this chapter.
8. **Pressure Gauge**
   Many circle systems have an analog pressure gauge (manometer) attached to the exhalation pathway. On newer machines, breathing system pressure is monitored electronically and displayed on a screen. The analog pressure gauge may not be present. A virtual pressure gauge may be displayed on the screen (**Fig. 5.24**).
9. **Breathing Tubes**
   a. Two breathing tubes carry gases to and from the patient. Each tube connects to a port on the absorber at one end and the Y-piece at the other. The dead space in the system extends from the Y-piece to the patient. The length of the tubes does not affect the amount of dead space or rebreathing because the gas flow is unidirectional. Longer tubes allow the anesthesia

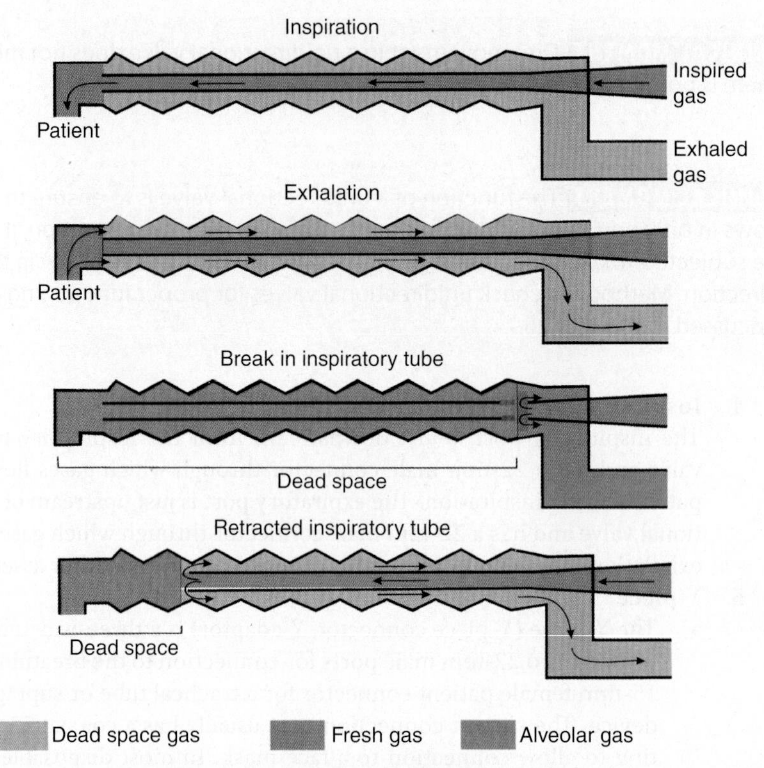

Figure 5.23 Coaxial circle breathing system. If there is a break in the inspiratory tube or the inspiratory tube becomes retracted, there will be an increase in dead space.

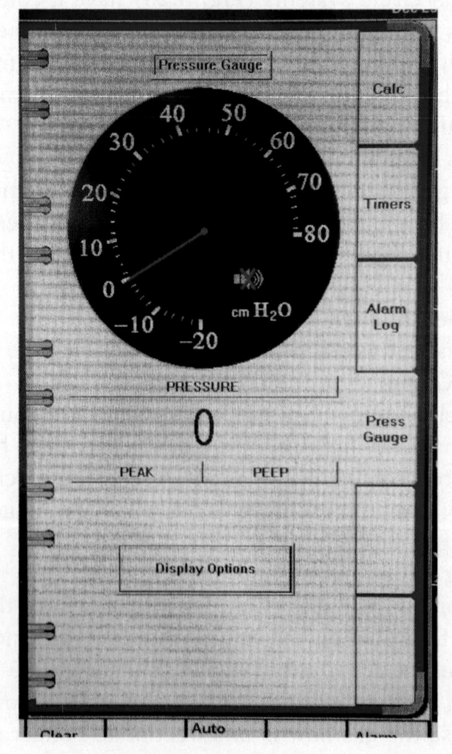

Figure 5.24 Virtual pressure gauge on anesthesia machine display. This can be displayed on demand.

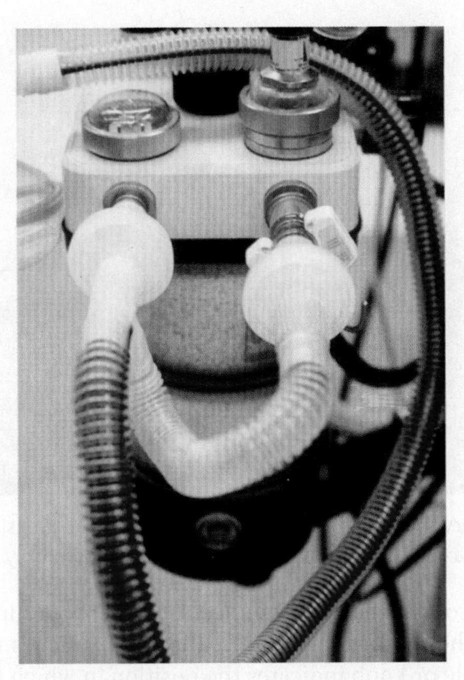

Figure 5.25 Coaxial system attached to the absorber.

machine and other equipment to be located farther from the patient's head. Expandable tubes are available.

b. Coaxial circle systems are available. The breathing tubes may be concentric or placed side by side. As shown in **Figure 5.25,** the tubings attach to a conventional absorber assembly. Gases flow through the inner tube to the patient, and exhaled gases flow to the absorber assembly via the outer tube (**Fig. 5.23**). Advantages of this system include compactness and modestly increased inspired heat and humidity. A disadvantage is the increased resistance. If the inner tube has a leak or becomes retracted at the patient end (**Fig. 5.23**), the dead space will be increased. This problem may not be easily detected and may result in hypercapnea. If the gas flow is reversed, entering the breathing system through the outer tube and returning through the smaller inner tubing, the resistance during exhalation will be increased.

10. **Reservoir Bag**

    Bags were discussed earlier in this chapter. The bag is usually attached to a 22-mm male bag port (bag mount or extension). It may also be placed at the end of a length of corrugated tubing or a metal tube leading from the bag mount (**Fig. 5.26**), giving the anesthesia provider more freedom of movement.

11. **Ventilator**

    In the past, the ventilator was considered a replacement for the reservoir bag and was attached at the bag mount. As machines and ventilators have evolved, the ventilator has become an integral part of the circle system. Ventilators are discussed in Chapter 6.

12. **Bag/Ventilator Selector Switch**

    a. A bag/ventilator selector switch (**Fig. 5.27**) provides a convenient means to rapidly shift between manual or spontaneous respiration and automatic ventilation without removing the bag or ventilator hose from its mount. As shown in **Figure 5.28,** the selector switch is essentially a three-way

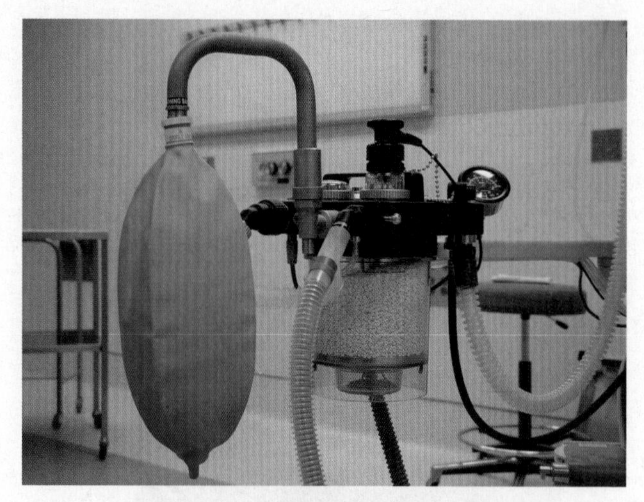

Figure 5.26 Having the reservoir bag on an extended arm may make it easier for the anesthesia provider to move around. Note the coaxial system attached to the absorber assembly.

stopcock. One port connects to the breathing system. The second is attached to the bag mount. The third attaches to the ventilator hose. The handle or knob indicates the position in which the switch is set.

b. When the selector switch is in the ventilator position, the APL valve is isolated from the circuit so that it does not need to be closed. Switching to the bag mode causes the APL valve to be connected to the breathing system. Some modern anesthesia machines do not have a bag/ventilator selector switch. Turning the ventilator ON causes electronically controlled valves to direct gases into the proper channels.

B. Gas Flows through Circle Breathing Systems

1. **General Principles**

a. This section will examine the gas flow through the classic circle system. Newer anesthesia machines have different arrangements of components, so there may be some differences in gas flow. Once the gas flows through

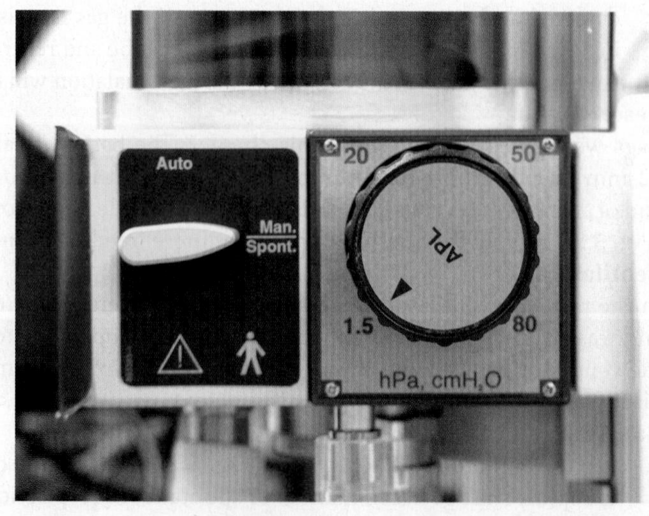

Figure 5.27 This bag/ventilator selector switch and the adjustable pressure-limiting valve are on the front of the ventilator.

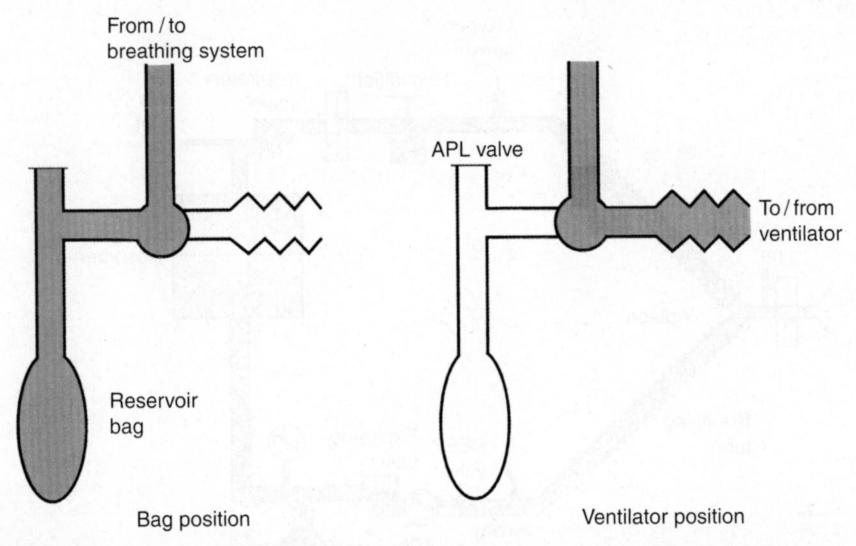

Figure 5.28 Bag/ventilator selector switch. In the bag position, the reservoir bag and the adjustable pressure-limiting (APL) valve are connected to the breathing system. In the ventilator position, the APL valve and the bag are excluded from the breathing system. On most new machines, putting this in the ventilator position turns ON the ventilator.

the classic breathing system are understood, it should be easy to determine the gas flows through other systems.

b. For the purposes of this discussion, we refer to fresh gas from the anesthesia machine as dry gas. Rebreathed gases are exhaled gases that may or may not have had the carbon dioxide removed. These gases have a higher humidity level than fresh gas. Retrograde gas flow indicates that gas is flowing in a direction opposite to the flow directed by the unidirectional valves. Retrograde flow is important, because dry gas flowing through the absorber can potentially desiccate the absorbent. It is doubtful that very much dry gas reaches the absorber during clinical anesthesia, even though some retrograde flow does occur. Problems created by desiccated absorbent were discussed earlier in this chapter.

2. **Classic Circle System**

The classic circle system is shown in **Figure 5.29.** It has the ventilator in proximity to the reservoir bag. The classic circle system is on most Ohmeda anesthesia machines, except for the ADU. It has also been used on North American Drager Narkomed machines, which have a bellows, but not a piston, ventilator.

a. Spontaneous Breathing

1) During spontaneous inspiration (**Fig. 5.30**), the patient draws inspiratory gas from the reservoir bag and through the absorber, where it joins with the fresh gas and flows to the patient.

2) During exhalation (**Fig. 5.31**), exhaled gases pass into the reservoir bag until it is full. Then, excess gases are vented through the APL valve. Since the inspiratory unidirectional valve is closed, fresh gas entering the breathing system flows retrograde toward the absorber, pushing the gas in the absorber toward the APL valve. The first gas to be vented through the APL valve will be previously exhaled gas containing carbon dioxide that was in the tubing between the APL valve and the absorber. If the fresh gas flow is high, some gas that was in or had passed

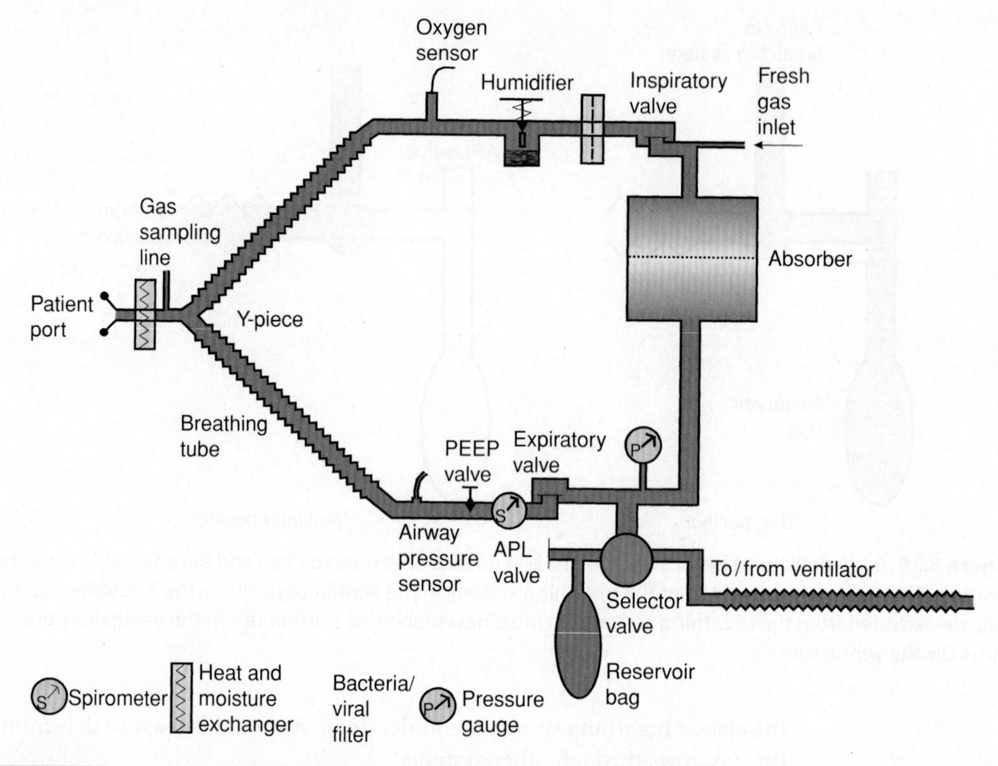

Figure 5.29 Classic circle breathing system. Not all these components may be present in a given system. For example, a heat and moisture exchanger and a humidifier would not be used at the same time. PEEP, positive end-expiratory pressure; APL, adjustable pressure limiting.

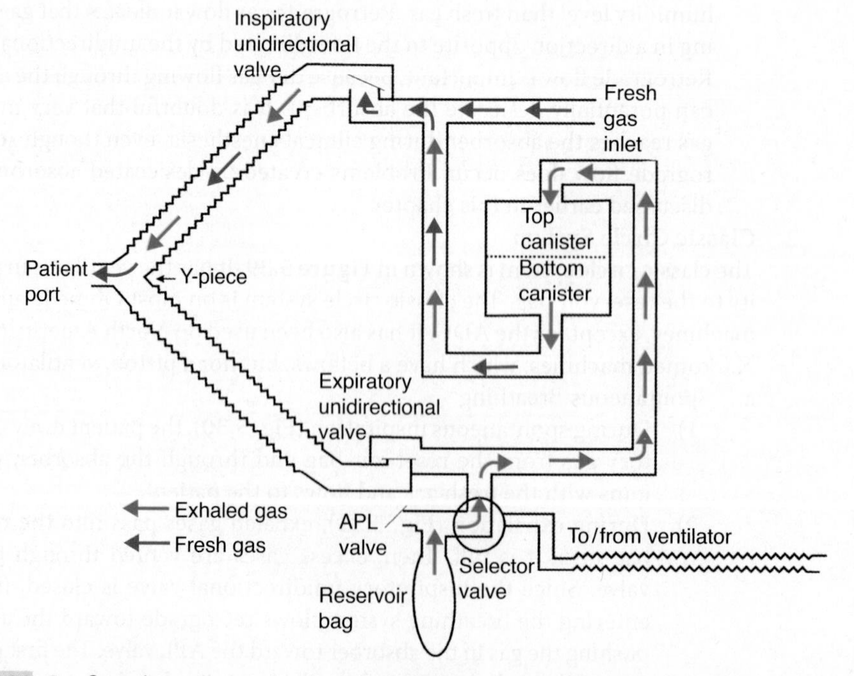

Figure 5.30 Gas flow through the classic circle breathing system during spontaneous inspiration. APL, adjustable pressure limiting.

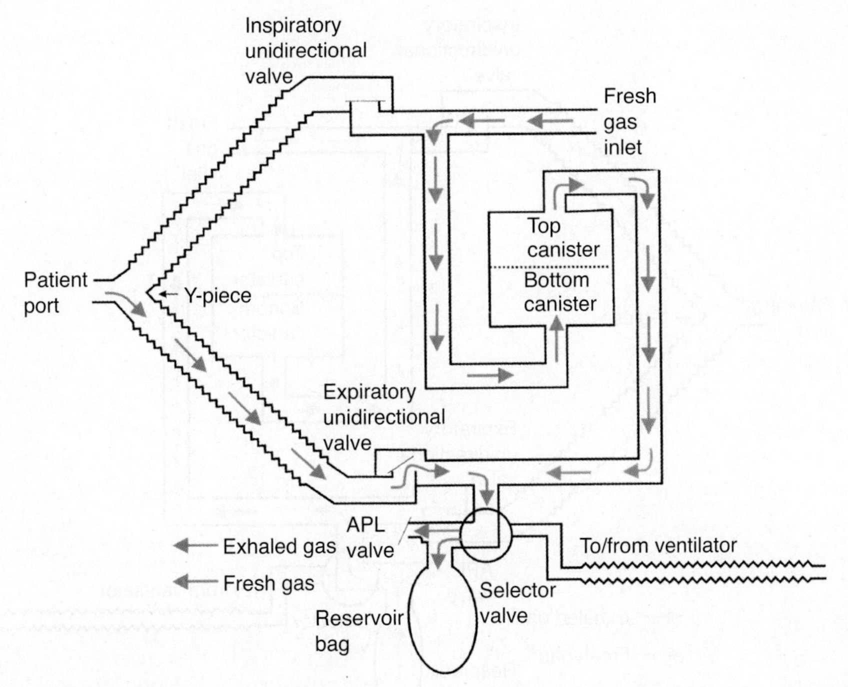

Figure 5.31 Gas flow through the classic circle breathing system during spontaneous exhalation. APL, adjustable pressure limiting.

through the absorber will flow retrograde and into the reservoir bag or be vented through the APL valve. If the fresh gas flow is high enough, fresh gas may enter the outlet from the absorber. Low fresh gas flows may result in no retrograde fresh gas flow through the absorber.

b. Manual Ventilation

1) During manual ventilation, excess gases are vented through the partially open APL valve during inspiration (**Fig. 5.32**). The gas flowing through the absorber and ultimately to the patient will be a mixture of fresh gas and exhaled gases that has had carbon dioxide removed.

2) During exhalation with manually controlled ventilation (**Figs. 5.33** and **5.34**), exhaled gases flow into the reservoir bag. Fresh gas flows retrograde through the absorber. If the fresh gas flow is low (**Fig. 5.33**), fresh gas does not enter the absorber. If the fresh gas flow is high (**Fig. 5.34**), some fresh gas may enter the absorber.

c. Mechanical Ventilation

1) During inspiration, gas flows from the ventilator through the absorber and inspiratory unidirectional valve to the patient. The gas in the ventilator bellows consists of exhaled gas with carbon dioxide. As the ventilator cycles, the gas in the ventilator passes through the absorber and is added to the fresh gas that is entering the breathing system. The inhaled mixture is a combination of fresh gas and previously exhaled gas from which the CO_2 has been removed.

2) During exhalation (**Fig. 5.35**), exhaled gases will flow into the ventilator bellows. Fresh gas will flow retrograde through the absorber. Excess gases are vented through the spill valve in the ventilator during the latter part of exhalation. The longer the exhalation time and the

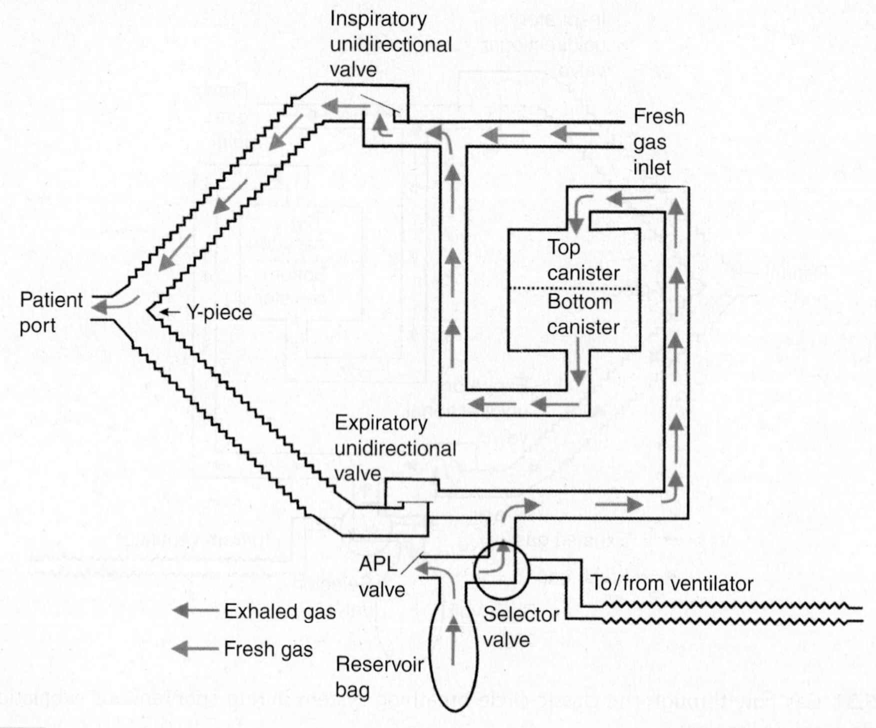

Figure 5.32 Gas flow through the classic circle breathing system during inspiration with manual ventilation. APL, adjustable pressure limiting.

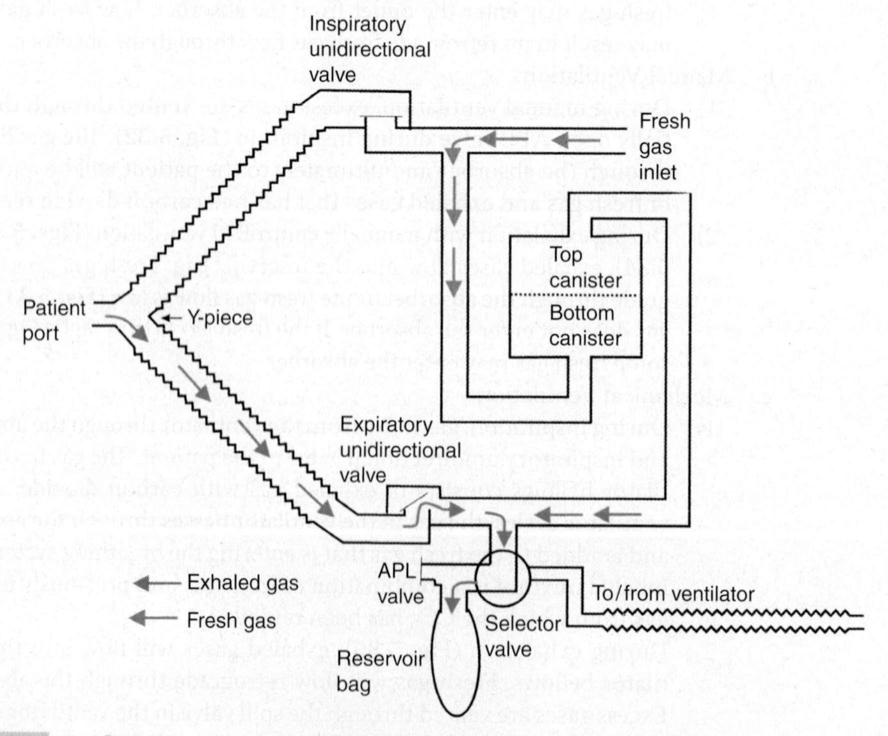

Figure 5.33 Gas flow through the classic circle breathing system during exhalation with manual ventilation and a low fresh gas flow. APL, adjustable pressure limiting.

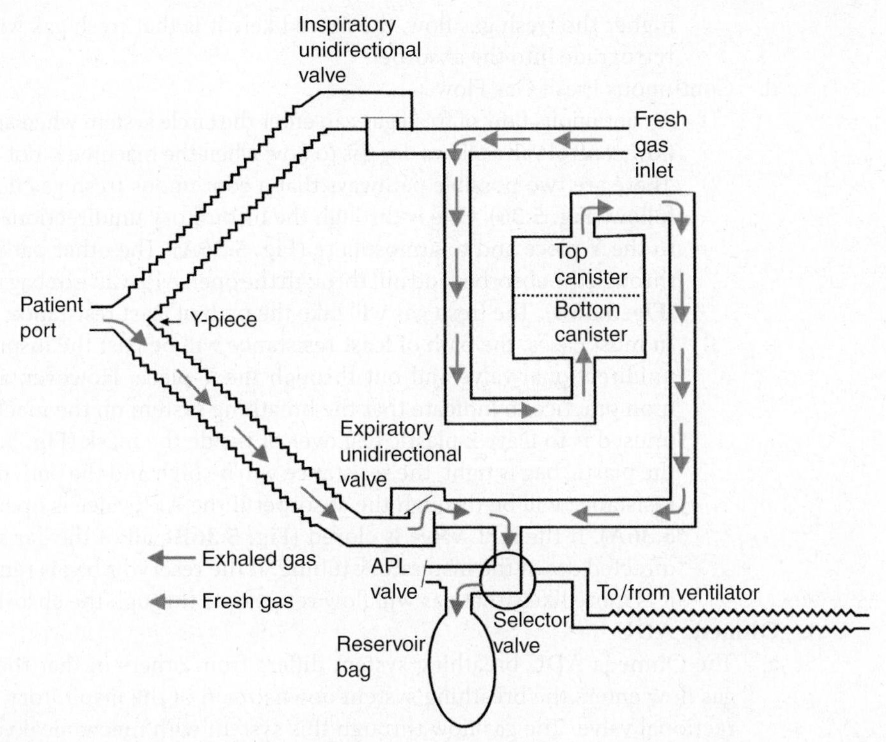

Figure 5.34 Gas through the classic circle breathing system during exhalation with manual ventilation and a high fresh gas flow. APL, adjustable pressure limiting.

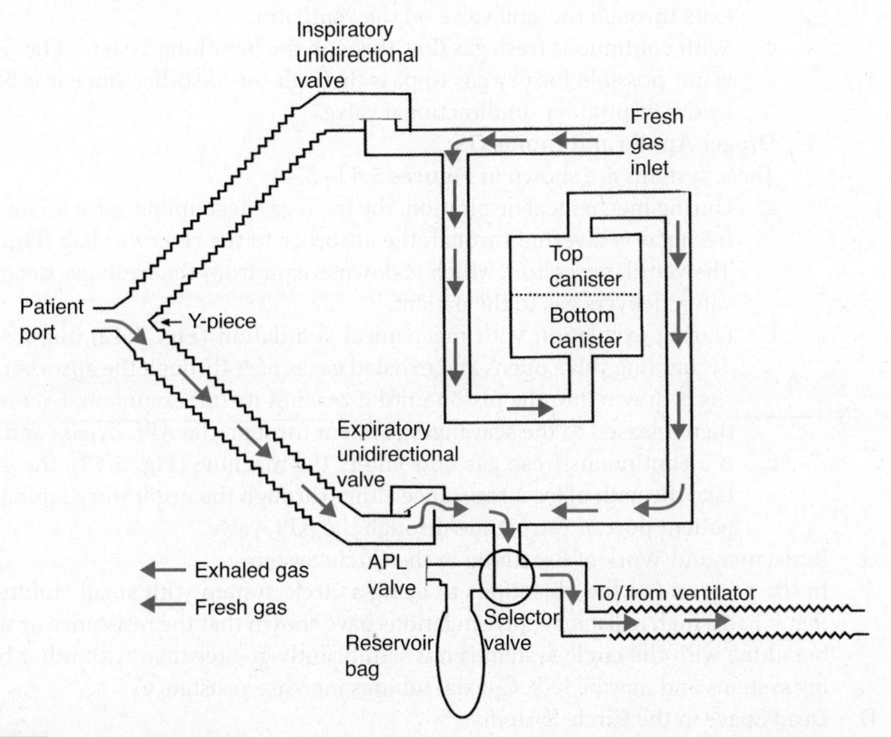

Figure 5.35 Gas through the classic circle breathing system during exhalation with mechanical ventilation. APL, adjustable pressure limiting.

higher the fresh gas flow, the more likely it is that fresh gas will pass retrograde into the absorber.

d. Continuous Fresh Gas Flow
 1) A continuous flow of fresh gas can enter the circle system when an open flow control valve allows dry gas to flow when the machine is not in use.
 2) There are two possible pathways that a continuous fresh gas flow can follow (**Fig. 5.36**). One is through the inspiratory unidirectional valve to the Y-piece and to atmosphere (**Fig. 5.36A**). The other pathway is through the absorber and out through the open APL valve or bag mount (**Fig. 5.36B**). The fresh gas will take the path of least resistance.
 3) In most cases, the path of least resistance will be past the inspiratory unidirectional valve and out through the Y-piece. However, a common practice to indicate that the breathing system on the machine is unused is to leave a plastic bag over or inside the mask (**Fig. 5.37**). If the plastic bag is tight, the resistance will be high and the path of least resistance will be through the absorber if the APL valve is open (**Fig. 5.36A**). If the APL valve is closed (**Fig. 5.36B**), all of the gas will be directed down the inspiratory tubing. If the reservoir bag is removed, it is more likely that gas will flow retrograde through the absorber.

3. **Ohmeda ADU**
 a. The Ohmeda ADU breathing system differs from others in that the fresh gas flow enters the breathing system downstream of the inspiratory unidirectional valve. The gas flow through this system with mechanical ventilation and inspiration is shown in **Figure 5.38.**
 b. During exhalation (**Fig. 5.39**), a mixture of fresh and exhaled gases enters the ventilator, raising the bellows to the top of the housing. Excess gas then exits through the spill valve on the ventilator.
 c. With continuous fresh gas flow through the breathing system (**Fig. 5.40**), it is not possible for dry gas to pass through the absorber since it is blocked by the inspiratory unidirectional valve.

4. **Drager Apollo and Fabius GS**
 These systems are shown in **Figures 5.41–5.43**.
 a. During mechanical inspiration, the fresh gas decoupling valve is closed and fresh gas is diverted through the absorber to the reservoir bag (**Fig. 5.41**). The ventilator piston, which is downstream from the fresh gas decoupling valve, delivers gas to the patient.
 b. During exhalation with mechanical ventilation (**Fig. 5.42**), the fresh gas decoupling valve opens and exhaled gases pass through the absorber. Fresh gas is drawn into the piston until it reaches its full excursion. Excess gas is then released to the scavenging system through the APL bypass and valve.
 c. If a continuous fresh gas flow enters the machine (**Fig. 5.43**), the gas will take the path of least resistance either through the inspiratory tubing to the patient port or retrograde through the APL valve.

C. Resistance and Work of Breathing in the Circle System
In the past, one of the objections to using a circle system with small children was that it had a high resistance. Investigations have shown that the resistance or work of breathing with the circle system is not significantly greater than with other breathing systems and may be less. Coaxial tubings increase resistance.

D. Dead Space in the Circle System
In the circle system, the dead space extends from the patient port of the Y-piece to the partition between the inspiratory and exhalation tubings. A Y-piece with

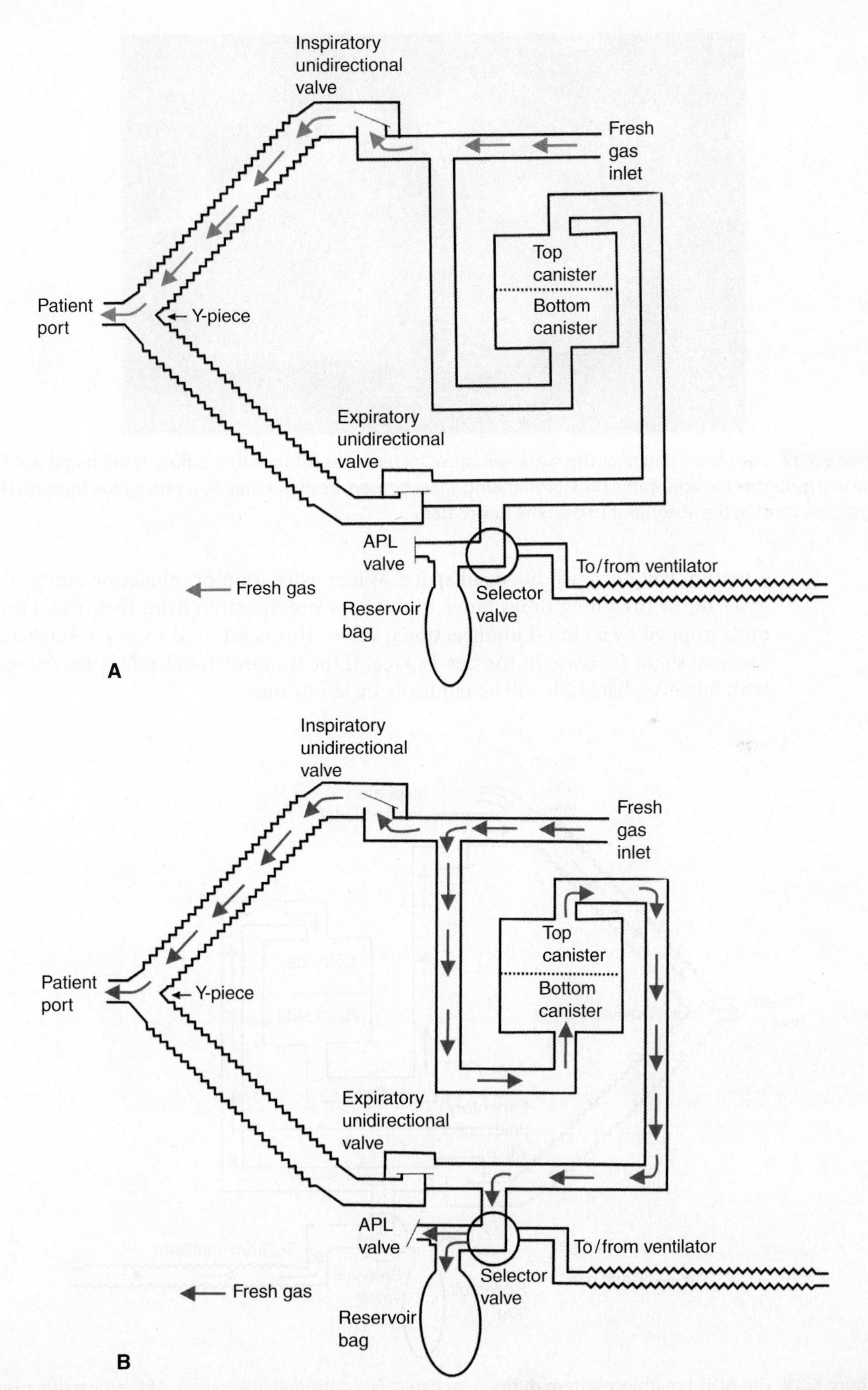

Figure 5.36 Possible paths of gas flow through the classic circle breathing system during a period of non-use, with a continuing fresh gas flow. APL, adjustable pressure limiting.

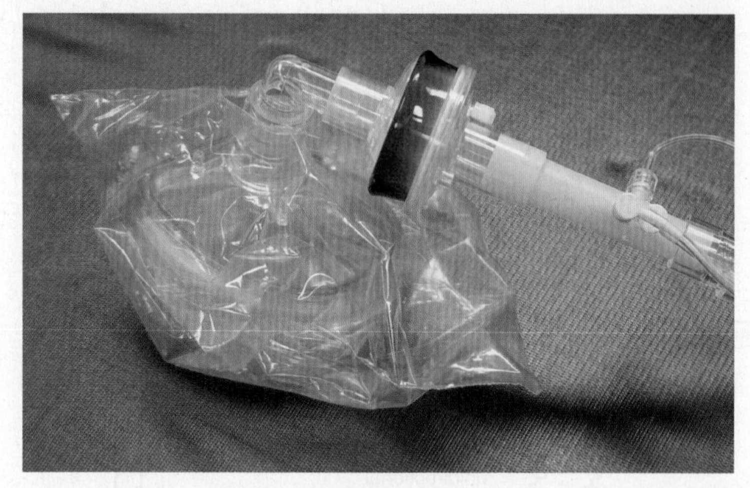

Figure 5.37 The plastic bag over the mask will cause increased resistance to gas flow. If the bag is not on the bag mount or the adjustable pressure-limiting valve is open, fresh gas may flow retrograde through the absorber, causing the absorbent to become desiccated.

a septum will decrease the dead space. When exhalation or inhalation starts, the gases in the breathing tubes move in the opposite direction from their usual flow until stopped by a closed unidirectional valve. This is referred to as *backlash* and causes a slight increase in the dead space. If the unidirectional valves are competent, however, backlash will be clinically insignificant.

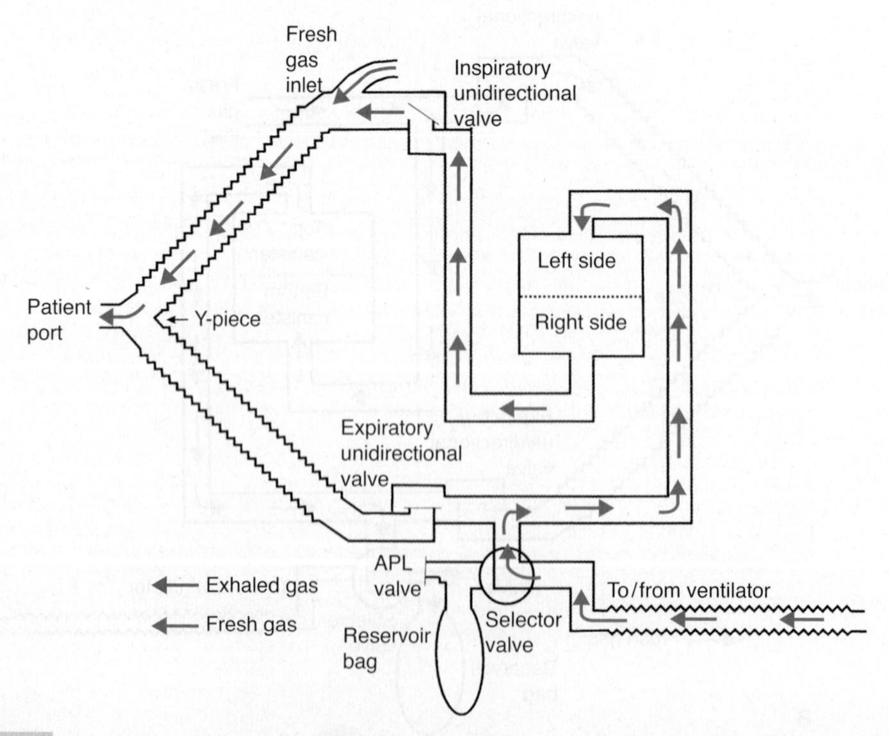

Figure 5.38 The ADU breathing system during mechanically controlled inspiration. APL, adjustable pressure limiting.

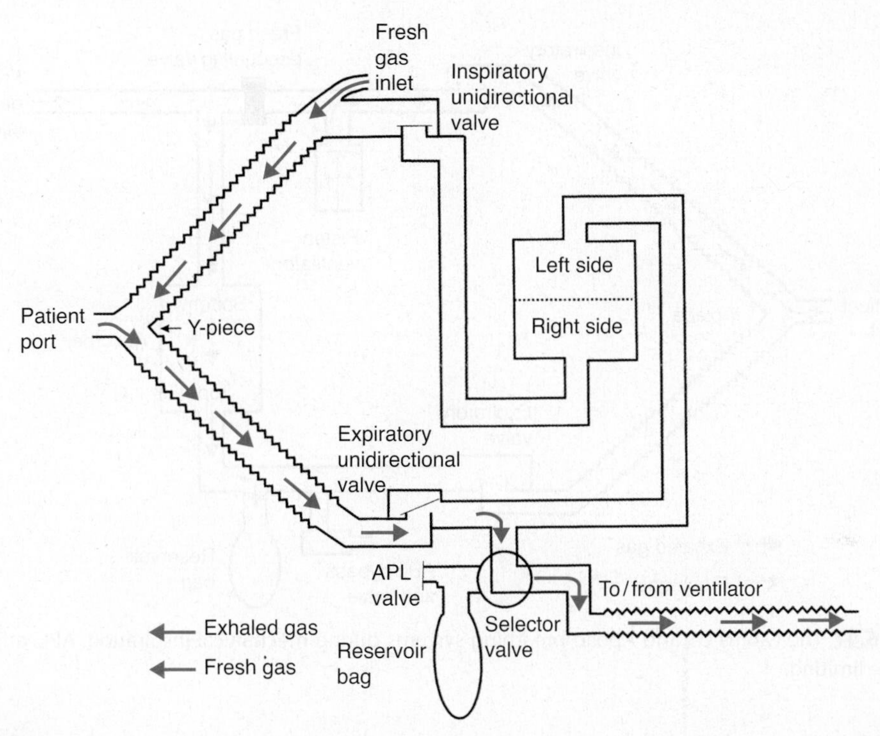

Figure 5.39 The ADU breathing system during mechanically controlled ventilation. APL, adjustable pressure limiting.

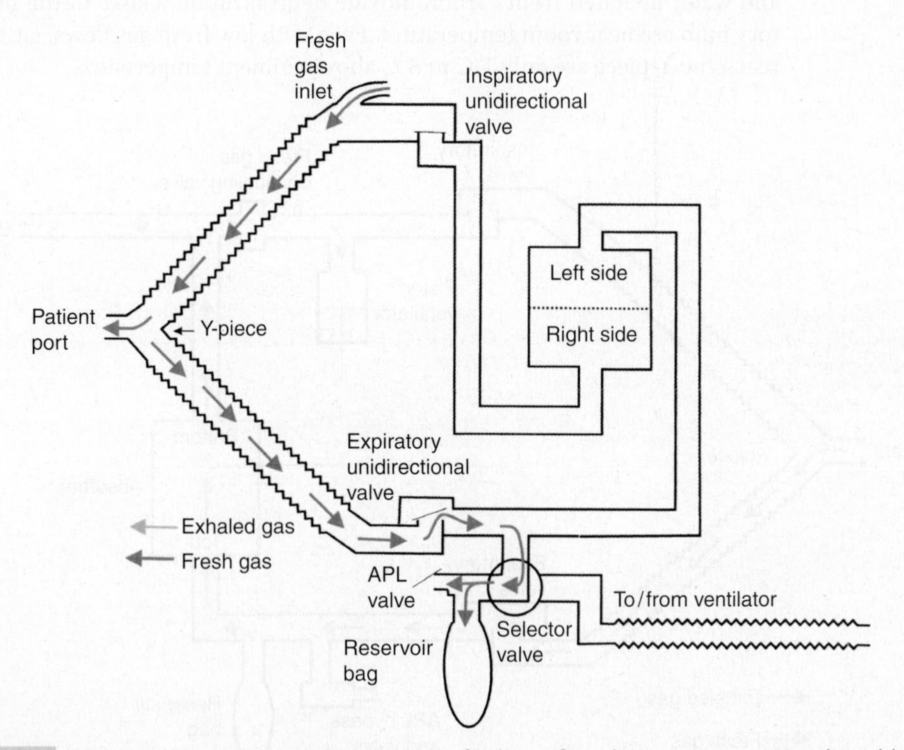

Figure 5.40 ADU breathing system with continuous fresh gas flow during nonuse. APL, adjustable pressure limiting.

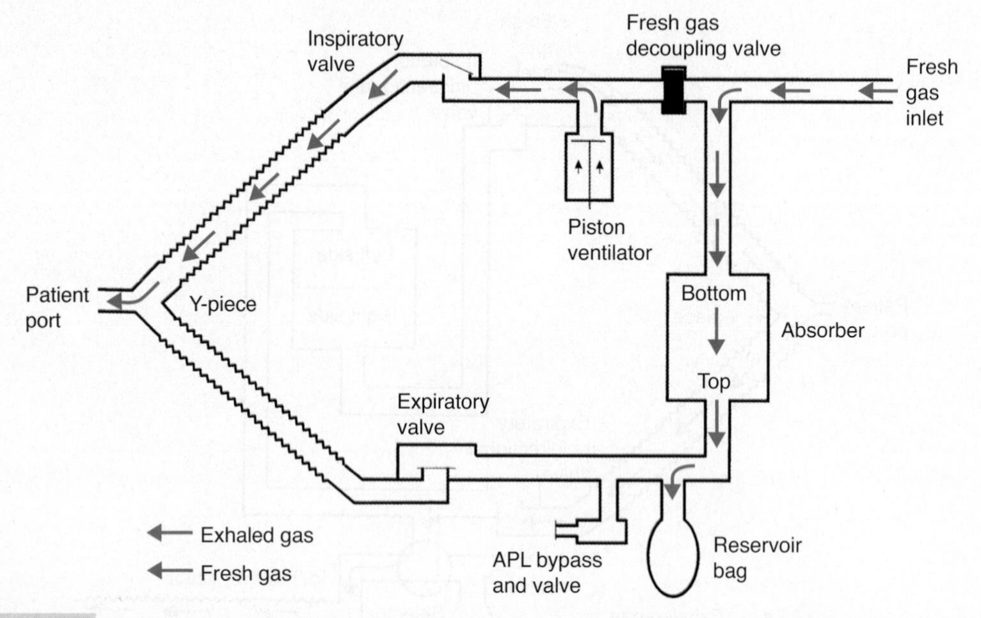

Figure 5.41 The Fabius GS and Apollo breathing systems during mechanical inspiration. APL, adjustable pressure limiting.

E. Heat and Humidity

1. In the circle system, moisture is available from exhaled gases, the absorbent, and water liberated from carbon dioxide neutralization. Gases in the inspiratory limb are near room temperature. Even with low fresh gas flows, gases that reach the Y-piece are only 1°C to 3°C above ambient temperature.

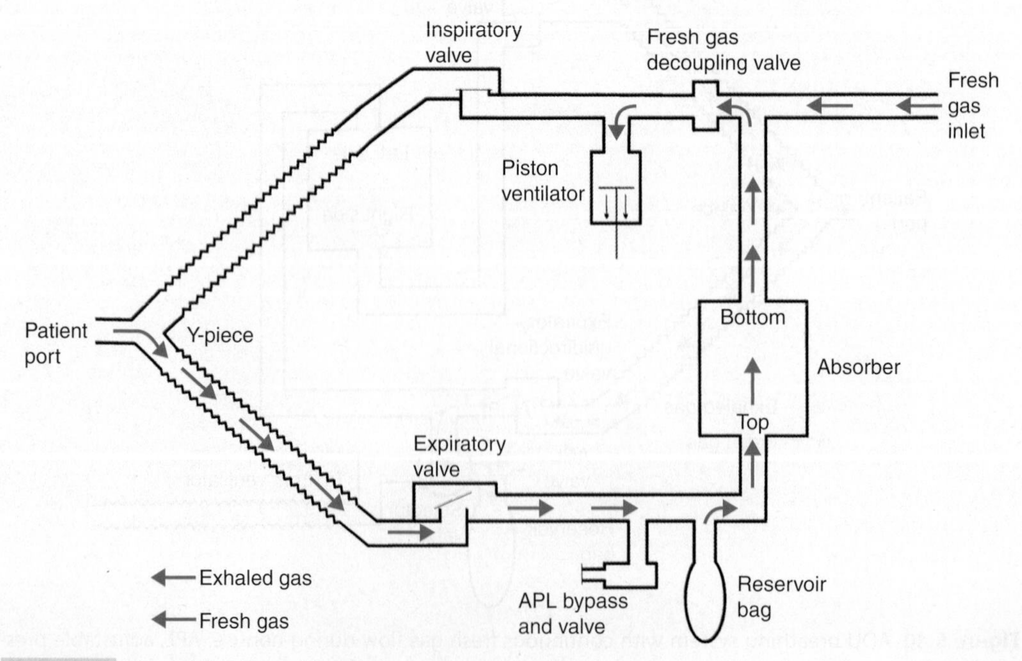

Figure 5.42 The Fabius GS and Apollo breathing systems during mechanical mid exhalation. APL, adjustable pressure limiting.

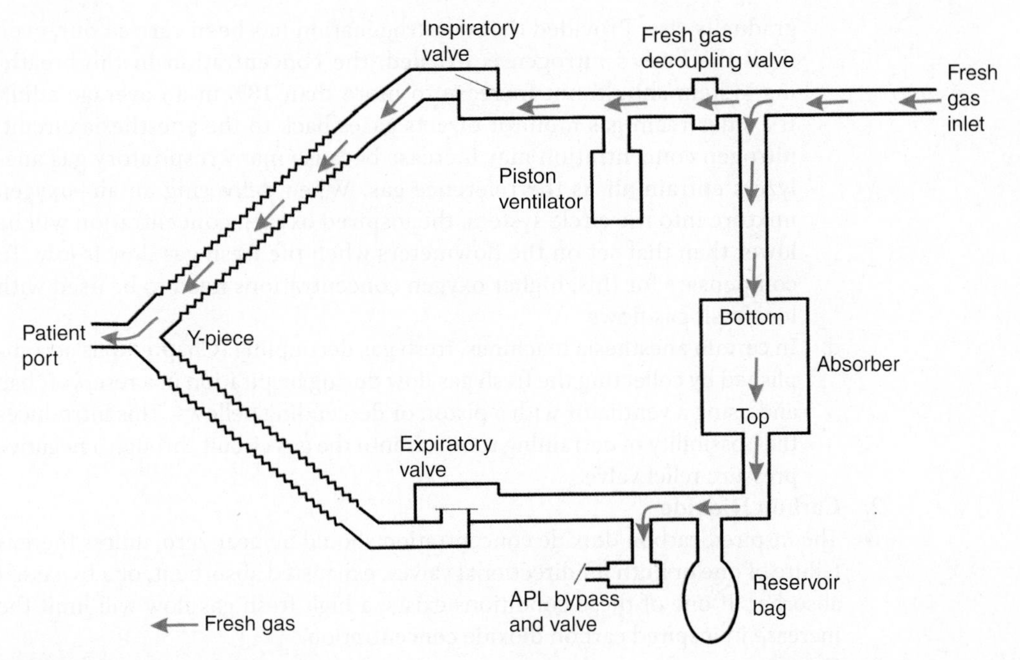

Figure 5.43 The Fabius GS and Apollo breathing systems with continuous fresh gas flow during nonuse. APL, adjustable pressure limiting.

2. The humidity in a standard adult circle system increases gradually with use and then stabilizes. A fresh gas flow of 0.5 to 2 L/minute will result in a humidity level between 20 and 25 mg H_2O/L after 60 minutes. Prior system use will result in an initially higher humidity level that stabilizes in the same period of time at the same final humidity level. Higher humidity will result from lower fresh gas flows, increasing ventilation, locating the fresh gas inlet upstream of the absorber, wetting the tubings, and using a humidifier, smaller canisters, or coaxial breathing tubes. Using an HME (Chapter 9) will result in decreased humidity in the circle system but increased humidity in the inspired gases.

F. Relationship between Inspired and Delivered Concentrations

In a system with no rebreathing, gas and vapor concentrations in the inspired mixture will be close to those in the fresh gas. With rebreathing, however, the concentrations in the inspired mixture may differ considerably from those in the fresh gas. The larger the breathing system's internal volume, the greater the difference between inspired and delivered concentrations.

1. **Nitrogen**
   a. Nitrogen is important, because it hinders building up of high concentrations of nitrous oxide and may cause low inspired oxygen concentrations. Before any fresh gas is delivered, the concentration of nitrogen in the breathing system is approximately 80%. Nitrogen enters the system from exhaled gases and leaves through the APL valve, ventilator spill valve, and leaks.
   b. Using high fresh gas flows for a few minutes to eliminate most of the nitrogen in the system and much of that in the patient is called *denitrogenation*. There is no set time or flow that will produce adequate denitrogenation in all cases. A tight mask fit is necessary for proper denitrogenation, because air will be inspired around a loose-fitting mask.
   c. After denitrogenation, nitrogen elimination from the patient will proceed at a slower rate. In a closed system, the nitrogen concentration will

gradually rise. Provided that denitrogenation has been carried out, even if all the body's nitrogen is exhaled, the concentration in the breathing system should not increase to more than 18% in an average adult. If a sidestream gas monitor directs gases back to the anesthesia circuit, nitrogen concentration may increase because many respiratory gas analyzers entrain air as the reference gas. When delivering an air–oxygen mixture into the circle system, the inspired oxygen concentration will be lower than that set on the flowmeters when the fresh gas flow is low. To compensate for this, higher oxygen concentrations need to be used with low fresh gas flows.

d. In certain anesthesia machines, fresh gas decoupling (Chapter 6) is accomplished by collecting the fresh gas flow during inspiration in a reservoir bag and using a ventilator with a piston or descending bellows. This introduces the possibility of entraining room air into the gas circuit through a negative pressure relief valve.

2. **Carbon Dioxide**

The inspired carbon dioxide concentration should be near zero, unless there is failure of one or both unidirectional valves, exhausted absorbent, or a bypassed absorber. If one of these conditions exists, a high fresh gas flow will limit the increase in inspired carbon dioxide concentration.

3. **Oxygen**

The concentration of oxygen in the inspired mixture is affected by the uptake and elimination of oxygen and other gases by the patient, the arrangement of the components, ventilation, fresh gas flow, the volume of the system, and the concentration of oxygen in the fresh gas. Because so many of these variables are unpredictable and uncontrollable, it is absolutely essential to use an oxygen analyzer in the breathing system. Oxygen analyzers are discussed in Chapter 17.

4. **Anesthetic Agents**

a. The following influence the concentration of an anesthetic agent in the inspired mixture: uptake by the patient, uptake by breathing system components, arrangement of system components, uptake and elimination of other gases by the patient, the breathing system volume, concentration of the fresh gas flow, degradation by the absorbent, and fresh gas flow. It is not possible to predict the inspired concentration accurately unless a high fresh gas flow is used. The greatest variation occurs during induction, when anesthetic uptake is high and nitrogen washout from the patient dilutes the gases in the circuit. For this reason, most authors recommend that anesthesia administration be started with high fresh gas flows. The time interval until there is some equilibration between inspired and end-expired agent concentrations varies with the agent, being minimal with desflurane, intermediate with sevoflurane, and greatest with isoflurane. Several devices are now available to measure the inspired anesthetic agent concentration (Chapter 17).

b. High flows are also commonly used at the end of a case to increase anesthetic agent elimination. The elimination rate may be increased by bypassing the absorber.

c. When malignant hyperthermia is suspected, increasing the fresh gas flow is the most important measure that will aid in washing out anesthetic agents from the patient. Using a charcoal filter, or changing the anesthesia machine and breathing system, is of little or no benefit.

G. Circle System with Low Fresh Gas Flows. *Low-flow anesthesia* has been variously defined as an inhalation technique in which a circle system with absorbent is used with a fresh gas inflow that is less than the patient's minute volume, less than 1 or 1.5 L/minute, 3 L/minute or less, 0.5 to 2 L/minute, less than 4 L/minute, 500 mL/minute, 500 to 1000 mL/minute, or 0.5 to 1 L/minute. *Closed-system* anesthesia is a form of low-flow anesthesia in which the fresh gas flow equals uptake of anesthetic gases and oxygen by the patient, breathing system, and gas sampling device. No gas is vented through the APL valve.

1. **Equipment**
   a. A standard anesthesia machine can be used, but it must have flowmeters that will provide low flows. The minimum mandatory oxygen flow on many older machines makes a closed system difficult to accomplish.
   b. Standard calibrated vaporizers capable of delivering high concentrations can be used. The oxygen concentration must be monitored. Anesthetic agent monitoring is useful.
2. **Induction**
   Most commonly, induction is accomplished by using high flows to allow denitrogenation, establish anesthetic agent concentrations, and provide oxygen well in excess of consumption. During intubation, the vaporizer should be left ON and the fresh gas flow turned to minimum or OFF. After gas exchange has stabilized, lower fresh gas flows are used.
3. **Maintenance**
   During maintenance, gas flows and vaporizer settings should be adjusted to maintain a satisfactory oxygen concentration and the desired level of anesthesia. If a rapid change in any component of the inspired mixture is desired, the fresh gas flow should be increased. If, for any reason, the circle system integrity is broken, high flows with desired inspired concentrations should be used for several minutes before returning to low flows. If closed-system anesthesia is used, it is recommended that higher flows be used for 1 to 2 minutes at least once an hour to eliminate gases such as nitrogen and carbon monoxide that have accumulated in the system.
4. **Emergence**
   Recovery from anesthesia will be slower if low flows are used. High flows are usually needed at least briefly to eliminate nitrous oxide. Coasting, in which anesthesia administration is stopped toward the end of the operation and the circuit is maintained closed with enough oxygen flow to maintain a constant end-tidal volume from the ventilator or reservoir bag, can be used.
5. **Advantages**
   a. Economy
      Significant economy can be achieved with lower nitrous oxide and oxygen flows, but the greatest savings occurs with the potent volatile agents. These savings are partly offset by increased absorbent usage, but this cost is relatively small. Individual feedback and education regarding volatile agent use may be effective in encouraging anesthesia providers to reduce fresh gas flows.
   b. Reduced Operating Room Pollution
      With lower flows, there will be less anesthetic agent into the operating room. Using low-flow techniques does not eliminate the need for scavenging, because

high flows are still necessary at times. Since less volatile agent is used, vaporizers have to be filled less frequently so that exposure to anesthetic vapors during filling is decreased.

c. Reduced Environmental Pollution
   Fluorocarbons and nitrous oxide attack the earth's ozone layer, and nitrous oxide contributes to the greenhouse effect. With low flows, these ecological hazards are reduced.
d. Estimating Anesthetic Agent Uptake and Oxygen Consumption
   In a closed system without significant leaks, the fresh gas flow is matched by the patient's uptake of oxygen and anesthetic agents. Changes in volume may be attributed principally to the uptake of oxygen or nitrous oxide because the volume contributed by the potent inhalational agents is usually not significant.
e. Buffered Changes in Inspired Concentrations
   The lower the fresh gas flow, the longer it takes for a change in the fresh gas flow concentration to cause a comparable change in the inspired concentration.
f. Heat and Humidity Conservation
   With lower gas flows, inspired humidity will be increased and the rate of fall in body temperature reduced. The incidence of shivering is lowered.
g. Less Danger of Barotrauma
   High pressures in the breathing system take longer to develop with lower flows.

6. **Disadvantages**
   a. More Attention Required
   With closed-system anesthesia, fresh gas flow into the system must be kept in balance with uptake. This requires frequent adjustments.
   b. Inability to Quickly Alter Inspired Concentrations
   Using low fresh gas flows prevents rapid changes in fresh gas concentrations in the breathing system that occurs with high fresh gas flows. As a result, it may be more difficult to control acute hemodynamic responses. This is a significant disadvantage only if the user insists on using low flows at all times. The clinician who uses low flows should accept that when it is necessary to change inspired concentrations rapidly, higher flows should be used.
   c. Danger of Hypercarbia
   Hypercarbia resulting from exhausted absorbent, incompetent unidirectional valves, or the absorber being in the bypass position will be greater when low flows are used.
   d. Accumulation of Undesirable Gases in the System
      1) Accumulation of undesirable gases is likely only a problem with closed-circuit anesthesia, because low flows provide a continuous system flush. With closed-system anesthesia, flushing with high fresh gas flows once for an hour will decrease the concentration of most of these substances. Alternately, a diverting gas monitor with the sample gas scavenged instead of being returned to the circle system can be used to remove small amounts of gas.
      2) Carbon monoxide from the interaction of desiccated absorbent and anesthetic agent was mentioned earlier in this chapter. Since low-flow anesthesia tends to preserve the moisture content of the absorbent, it may protect against carbon monoxide production resulting from

desiccated absorbent. If desiccated absorbent is present, low flows tend to increase the amount of carbon monoxide present in the system. Carbon monoxide produced from hemoglobin breakdown or exhaled by smokers can accumulate in the closed-circle system.

3) Acetone, methane, and hydrogen can accumulate during low-flow anesthesia. However, dangerous levels are reached only after hours of closed-system anesthesia. Methane can disturb infrared analyzers. The common intoxicant ethanol can also accumulate.
4) The safety of using sevoflurane with low flows is still under investigation. At the time of writing, the FDA was still recommending that sevoflurane should not be used with fresh gas flows of less than 2 L/minute. This recommendation has been revised to suggest that flow rates of 1 L/minute are acceptable but should not exceed 2 minimum alveolar concentration (MAC)-hours. Some investigators feel that restricting the use of low fresh gas flows with sevoflurane cannot be justified.
5) If oxygen is supplied from an oxygen concentrator (Chapter 1), there will be an accumulation of argon with low fresh gas flows.
6) Even with initial denitrogenation, nitrogen will accumulate in the closed breathing circuit. If oxygen is being supplied by an oxygen concentrator (Chapter 1), concentrator malfunction can cause nitrogen to appear in the product gas. Infrared monitors (Chapter 17) add air to the sample gas after the sample is analyzed. If the gas exhausted is returned to the breathing system, nitrogen accumulation will be greater.
7) Acrylic monomer is exhaled when joint prostheses are surgically cemented. High flows should be used to prevent this chemical from being rebreathed.

e. Uncertainty about Inspired Concentrations

One of the effects of rebreathing is that the inspired concentrations cannot be accurately predicted. However, absolute or near-absolute knowledge of inspired anesthetic agent concentrations is not necessary for safe anesthesia administration, because patients' responses to drugs vary widely.

f. Faster Absorbent Exhaustion

The lower the fresh gas flow, the faster the absorbent is exhausted.

H. Circle System for Pediatric Anesthesia

1. It was once believed that small patients required special breathing circuits and ventilators. However, studies show that adult circle systems can be used even in small infants and with low fresh gas flows. In the past, special pediatric circle systems with small absorbers were used. These are no longer commercially available. What is referred to as a pediatric circle system today is usually a standard absorber assembly with short, small-diameter breathing tubes and a small bag. This allows a rapid and easy changeover from an adult to a pediatric system and allows anesthesia providers to use equipment with which they are familiar.
2. It is important not to add devices with large dead space or resistance between the Y-piece and the patient. Use of an HME/filter (Chapter 9) in this location can cause the dead space to be unacceptably high for the spontaneous breathing infant.
3. One problem with the circle system is its large volume. Gas compression and distention of the tubings make it difficult to determine the actual minute ventilation that the patient is receiving, unless measurements are performed at the Y-piece.

SUGGESTED READINGS

Baum JA. Interaction of inhalational anaesthetics with CO_2 absorbents. Best Pract Res Clin Anesthesiol 2003;17:63–76.

Baxter AD. Low and minimal flow inhalational anaesthesia. Can J Anaesth 1997;44:643–653.

Coppens MJ, Versichelen LFM, Rolly G, et al. The mechanisms of carbon monoxide production by inhalational agents. Anaesthesia 2006;61:462–468.

Dorsch J, Dorsch S. The breathing system: general principles, common components and classifications. In: Understanding Anesthesia Equipment. Fifth edition. Philadelphia: Wolters Kluwer/Lippincott Williams & Wilkins, 2008:191–208.

Dorsch J, Dorsch S. Mapleson breathing systems. In: Understanding Anesthesia Equipment. Fifth edition. Philadelphia: Wolters Kluwer/Lippincott Williams & Wilkins, 2008:209–222.

Dorsch J, Dorsch S. The circle system. In: Understanding Anesthesia Equipment. Fifth edition. Philadelphia: Wolters Kluwer/Lippincott Williams & Wilkins, 2008:223–281.

Jellish WS, Nolan T, Kleinman B. Hypercapnia related to a faulty adult co-axial breathing circuit. Anesth Analg 2001;93:973–974.

Kharasch ED, Powers KM, Artu AA. Comparison of Amsorb, Sodalime and Baralyme degradation of volatile anesthetics and formation of carbon monoxide and compound A in swine in vivo. Anesthesiology 2002;96:173–182.

Olympio MA. Carbon dioxide absorbent desiccation safety conference convened by APSF. APSF Newslett 2005;20:25, 27–29.

Pond D, Jaffe RA, Brock-Utne JG. Failure to detect CO_2-absorbent exhaustion: seeing and believing. Anesthesiology 2000;92:1196–1198.

Stabernack CR, Brown R, Laster MJ, et al. Absorbents differ enormously in their capacity to produce compound A and carbon monoxide. Anesth Analg 2000;90:1428–1435.

Stevenson G, Tobin M, Horn B, Chen E, Hall S, Cote C. An adult system versus a Bain system: Comparative ability to deliver minute ventilation to an infant lung model with pressure-limited ventilation. Anesth Analg 1999;88:527–530.

Woehick H, Dunning M, Connolly LA. Reduction in the incidence of carbon monoxide exposures in humans undergoing general anesthesia. Anesthesiology 1997;87:228–234.

6 Anesthesia Ventilators

A VENTILATOR (BREATHING MACHINE) IS a device designed to provide or augment patient ventilation. Newer anesthesia ventilators have more features and ventilatory modes than earlier models and are an integral part of the anesthesia workstation.

A ventilator replaces the reservoir bag in the breathing system. It is usually connected to the breathing system by a bag/ventilator selector switch (Chapter 5). On most new workstations, turning the switch to the ventilator position or a ventilatory mode selection switch turns the ventilator ON. Other ventilators have an ON–OFF switch.

I. Definitions

A. *Barotrauma*: Injury resulting from high airway pressure.

B. *Compliance*: Ratio of a change in volume to a change in pressure. It is a measure of distensibility and is usually expressed in milliliters per centimeter of water (L or mL/cm H_2O). Most commonly, compliance is used in reference to the lungs and chest wall. Breathing system components, especially breathing tubes and the reservoir bag, also have compliance.

C. *Continuous Positive Airway Pressure* (CPAP): Airway pressure maintained above ambient. This term is commonly used in reference to spontaneous breathing.

D. *Exhaust Valve*: Valve in a ventilator with a bellows that allows driving gas to exit the bellows housing when it is open.

E. *Expiratory Flow Time*: Time between the beginning and end of expiratory gas flow.

F. *Expiratory Pause Time*: Time from the end of expiratory gas flow to the start of inspiratory flow.

G. *Expiratory Phase Time*: Time between the start of expiratory flow and the start of inspiratory flow. It is the sum of the expiratory flow and expiratory pause times.

H. *Fresh Gas Compensation*: A means to prevent the fresh gas flow from affecting the tidal volume by measuring the actual tidal volume and using this information to adjust the volume of gas delivered by the ventilator.

I. *Fresh Gas Decoupling*: A means to prevent the fresh gas flow from affecting the tidal volume by isolating the fresh gas flow so that it does not enter the breathing system during inspiration.

J. *Inspiratory Flow Time*: Period between the beginning and end of inspiratory flow.

K. *Inspiratory Pause Time*: The portion of the inspiratory phase time during which the lungs are held inflated at a fixed pressure or volume (i.e., the time during which there is zero flow). It is also called the *inspiratory hold, inflation hold,* or *inspiratory plateau.* The inspiratory pause time may be expressed as a percentage of the inspiratory phase time.

L. *Inspiratory Phase Time*: Time between the start of inspiratory flow and the beginning of expiratory flow. It is the sum of the inspiratory flow and inspiratory pause times.

M. *Inspiratory:Expiratory Phase Time Ratio* (*I:E Ratio*): Ratio of the inspiratory phase time to the expiratory phase time.

N. *Inspiratory Flow Rate*: Rate at which gas flows to the patient.

O. *Inverse Ratio Ventilation*: Ventilation in which the inspiratory phase time is longer than the expiratory phase time.

P. *Minute Volume*: Sum of all tidal volumes within 1 minute.

Q. *Peak Pressure*: Maximum pressure during the inspiratory phase time.

R. *Plateau Pressure*: Resting pressure during the inspiratory pause. Airway pressure usually falls when there is an inspiratory pause. This lower pressure is called the *plateau pressure.*

S. *Positive End-Expiratory Pressure* (PEEP): Airway pressure above ambient at the end of exhalation. This term is commonly used in reference to controlled ventilation.

T. *Resistance*: Ratio of the change in driving pressure to the change in flow rate. It is commonly expressed as centimeters of water per liter per second (cm H_2O/L/second).

U. *Sigh*: Deliberate increase in tidal volume for one or more breaths.

V. *Spill Valve*: The valve in an anesthesia ventilator that allows excess gases in the breathing system to flow to the scavenging system after the bellows or piston is filled during exhalation.

W. *Tidal Volume*: Volume of gas entering or leaving the patient during the inspiratory or expiratory phase time.

X. *Ventilatory (Respiratory) Rate or Frequency*: Number of respiratory cycles per minute.

Y. *Volutrauma*: Injury due to overdistention of the lungs.

Z. *Work of Breathing*: Energy expended by the patient and/or ventilator to move gas in and out of the lungs. It is expressed as the ratio of work to volume moved, commonly as joules per liter. It includes the work needed to overcome the elastic and flow-resistive forces of the both the respiratory system and the apparatus.

II. Components

A. Driving Gas Supply

1. Many currently available anesthesia ventilators are pneumatically powered but electrically controlled. The driving (drive, power) gas is oxygen, air, or a mixture of air and oxygen. It is usually less expensive to use air. Some ventilators can switch between driving gases so that if the pressure in the primary driving gas supply is lost, the other gas will automatically be used.
2. Some ventilators use a device called an *injector* (Venturi mechanism) to increase the driving gas flow. An injector is shown in **Figure 6.1.** As the gas flow meets a restriction, its lateral pressure drops (Bernoulli principle). When the lateral pressure drops below atmospheric, air will be entrained. The result is an increase in the total gas flow leaving the injector and decreased driving gas consumption.

CLINICAL MOMENT A significant gas flow is necessary to drive a bellows. The amount will vary, depending on the ventilator and the settings. Using a gas cylinder to power a pneumatic ventilator will quickly deplete the gas supply.

B. Controls

The ventilator controls regulate the flow, volume, timing, and the pressure that moves the bellows or piston.

C. Alarms

1. Newer ventilators use the alarm standard format, which divides the alarms into three categories: high, medium, and low priority. These are discussed in Chapter 18.

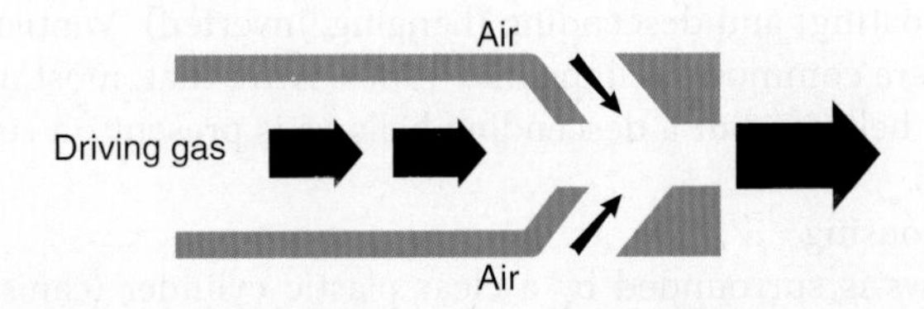

Figure 6.1 Injector (Venturi mechanism). Gas flows through the constricted area at a high velocity. The pressure around it drops below atmospheric pressure, and air is entrained. The net result is an increase in total gas flow leaving the outlet of the injector.

CLINICAL MOMENT Alarm messages that appear on the ventilator screen are color coded for the appropriate category. The anesthesia provider must know where to look for alarm messages and know what the messages mean.

2. A high-pressure alarm is required. On modern ventilators, the high-pressure alarm threshold is adjustable by the user. There is usually a default around 50 cm H_2O.
3. There must be an alarm to indicate that the pressure in the breathing system has not reached a minimum value within a certain time period (low-airway-pressure alarm).

CLINICAL MOMENT To prevent frequent alarms, some clinicians set the low-airway-pressure alarm threshold as low as possible. Many hazardous situations may be missed if this is done. The low-pressure alarm threshold should be set just below the peak airway pressure. If the peak pressure becomes lower, the alarm threshold must be reset.

D. Pressure-Limiting Mechanism

1. A pressure-limiting mechanism (pressure-limiting valve, maximum limited pressure mechanism) is designed to limit the inspiratory pressure. An adjustable mechanism carries the hazard of operator error. If it is set too low, insufficient pressure for ventilation may be generated; if it is set too high, excessive airway pressure may occur. With volume-controlled ventilation, setting the pressure limit 10 cm H_2O above the peak pressure attained with the desired tidal volume and flow rate will avoid most barotrauma.

CLINICAL MOMENT A pressure-limiting mechanism may be of benefit when mechanically ventilating a patient with a supraglottic airway device using pressure-controlled ventilation. Many supraglottic device manufacturers recommend a peak pressure of 20 to 30 cm H_2O, depending on the device, to avoid gastric inflation.

2. Pressure-limiting devices work in one of two ways. When the maximum pressure is reached, one type holds the pressure at that level until the start of exhalation, at which time the pressure decreases. The other type terminates inspiration when the pressure limit is reached so that the pressure drops immediately.

E. Bellows

The bellows is an accordion-like device attached at either the top or bottom of the bellows assembly (**Fig. 6.2**). Latex-free bellows are available. There are two types of bellows, distinguished by their motion during exhalation: ascending (standing, upright, floating) and descending (hanging, inverted). Ventilators with descending bellows were common until the mid-1980s. After that, most new ventilators had an ascending bellows, but a descending bellows is present on some recent anesthesia ventilators.

F. Bellows Housing

The bellows is surrounded by a clear plastic cylinder (canister, bellows chamber or cylinder, pressure dome) that allows the bellows movement to be observed. A scale on the side of the housing provides a rough approximation of the tidal volume being delivered.

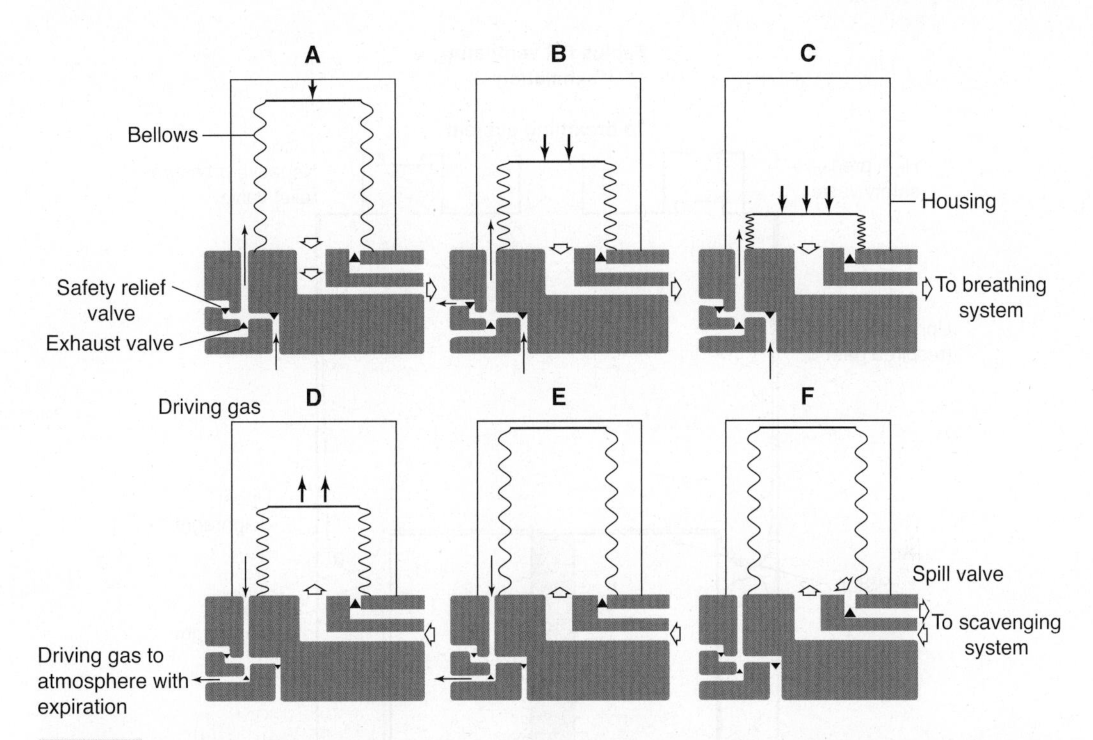

Figure 6.2 Functioning of the bellows-in-box ventilator. **A:** Beginning of inspiration. Driving gas begins to be delivered into the space between the bellows and its housing. The exhaust valve (which connects the driving gas pathway with atmosphere) is closed. The spill valve (which vents excess breathing system gases to the scavenging system) is also closed. **B:** Middle of inspiration. As driving gas continues to flow into the space around the bellows, its pressure increases, exerting a force that causes the bellows to be compressed. This pushes the gas inside the bellows toward the breathing system. The exhaust and spill valves remain closed. If the pressure of the driving gas exceeds the opening pressure of the safety relief valve, the valve will open and vent driving gas to atmosphere. **C:** End of inspiration. The bellows is fully compressed. The exhaust and spill valves remain closed. **D:** Beginning of expiration. Breathing system (exhaled and fresh) gases flow into the bellows, which begins to expand. The expanding bellows displaces driving gas from the interior of the housing. The exhaust valve opens, and driving gas flows through it to atmosphere. The spill valve remains closed. **E:** Middle of expiration. The bellows is nearly fully expanded. Driving gas continues to flow to atmosphere. The spill valve remains closed. **F:** End of expiration. Continued flow of gas into the bellows after it is fully expanded creates a positive pressure that causes the spill valve at the base of the bellows to open. Breathing system gases are vented through the spill valve into the scavenging system.

G. Exhaust Valve

The exhaust valve (exhalation valve, ventilator relief valve, compressed gas exhaust, bellows control valve) is connected to the inside of the bellows housed on pneumatically powered ventilators. It is closed during inspiration. During exhalation, it opens to allow driving gas inside the housing to be exhausted to atmosphere. With a piston ventilator, there is no need for an exhaust valve.

H. Electrically Driven Piston

1. Many of the newer ventilators utilize an electrically driven piston inside a cylinder to supply pressure to the breathing system. These ventilators do not have a bellows or bellows housing. They do not require a drive gas. The computer determines the amount the piston must move to deliver the required tidal volume. At the end of inspiration, the piston retracts and the cylinder is filled with fresh and exhaled gas that has passed through the CO_2 absorber.

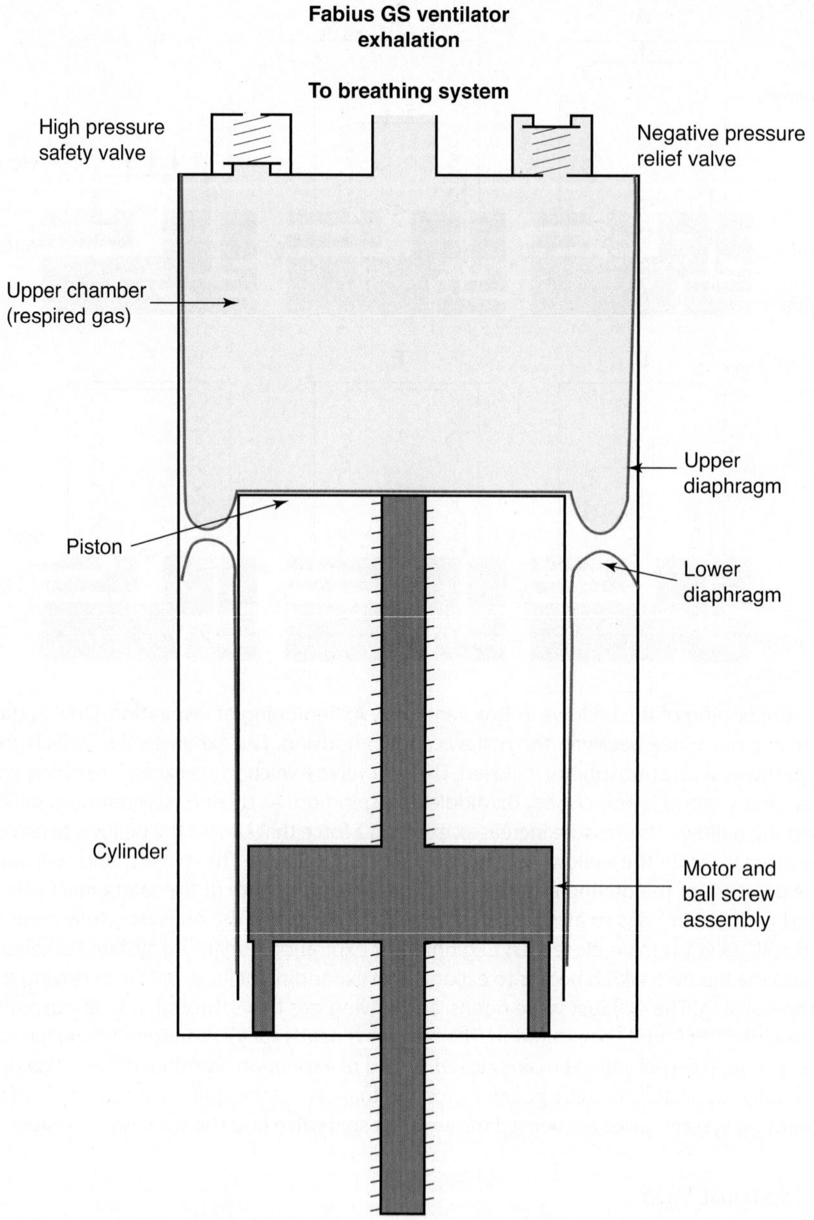

Fabius GS ventilator
exhalation

To breathing system

High pressure
safety valve

Negative pressure
relief valve

Upper chamber
(respired gas)

Upper
diaphragm

Piston

Lower
diaphragm

Cylinder

Motor and
ball screw
assembly

Figure 6.3 Piston assembly. As the piston moves downward, the upper diaphragm moves downward with it, creating a space for respired gases.

2. A piston assembly is shown in **Figures 6.3** and **6.4.** Electrical power is used to move the piston. Two rolling diaphragms seal the piston. High- and negative-pressure relief valves connect with the space containing respired gases.

I. Spill Valve

1. Because the adjustable pressure-limiting (APL) valve is isolated from the breathing system during ventilator operation, a spill valve is used to direct excess gases in the breathing system to the scavenging system. This valve is closed during inspiration. During exhalation, it remains closed until the bellows is fully expanded or the piston is fully retracted, at which time the valve

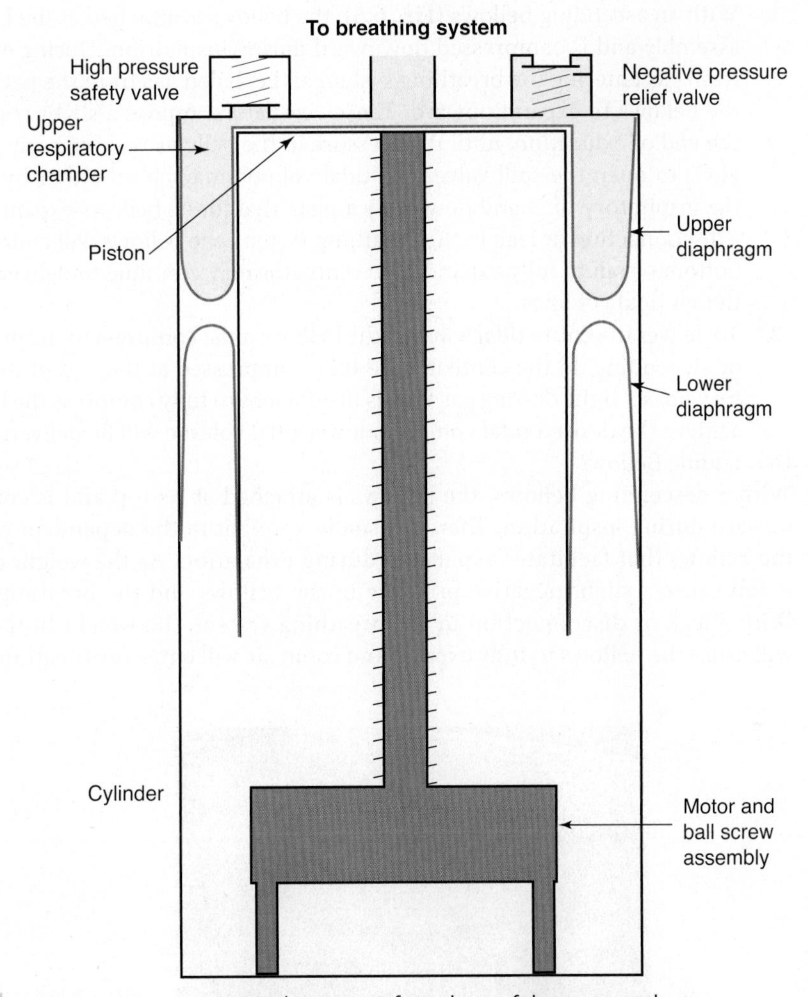

Figure 6.4 As the piston moves upward, gases are forced out of the space at the top.

opens to vent excess gases. With an ascending bellows, the spill valve has a minimum opening pressure of 2 to 4 cm H_2O. This enables the bellows to fill during exhalation. This amount of PEEP is applied to the breathing system. It is not applied with a piston or hanging bellows ventilator.

2. With a piston ventilator, excess gas is vented either through a spill valve, which may not be in the ventilator, or through an electronically controlled APL valve, which acts as a spill valve.

J. Ventilator Hose

On older ventilators, a tubing connects the ventilator to the breathing system. On most new ventilators, a separate hose is not present and the connection between the ventilator and the breathing system is internal.

K. Positive End-Expiratory Pressure Valve

PEEP valves are discussed in Chapter 5. Modern ventilators have integral electrically operated PEEP valves. A standing bellows causes a small amount (2 to 4 cm H_2O) of PEEP.

III. Relationship of the Ventilator to the Breathing System

A. Ascending Bellows

1. With an ascending bellows (**Fig. 6.5**), the bellows is attached at the base of the assembly and is compressed downward during inspiration. During exhalation, fresh gas entering the breathing system and exhaled gas from the patient cause the bellows to expand upward. These ventilators impose a slight resistance at the end of exhalation, until the pressure in the bellows rises enough (2 to 4 cm H_2O) to open the spill valve. The tidal volume may be set either by adjusting the inspiratory time and flow or by a plate that limits bellows expansion. With a disconnection or leak in the breathing system, the bellows will collapse to the bottom or fail to fully expand. The ventilator may continue to deliver less than the set tidal volumes.
2. To deliver the entire tidal volume, the bellows must compress to the proper level or, depending on the ventilator, be fully compressed at the end of the inspiratory phase. If the driving gas flow is insufficient to fully compress the bellows or achieve the desired tidal volume, a lower tidal volume will be delivered.

B. Descending Bellows

With a descending bellows, the bellows is attached at its top and is compressed upward during inspiration. There is usually a weight in the dependent portion of the bellows that facilitates expansion during exhalation. As the weight descends, it can cause a slight negative pressure in the bellows and the breathing system. With a leak or disconnection in the breathing system, the weight in the bellows will cause the bellows to fully expand and room air will enter the breathing system.

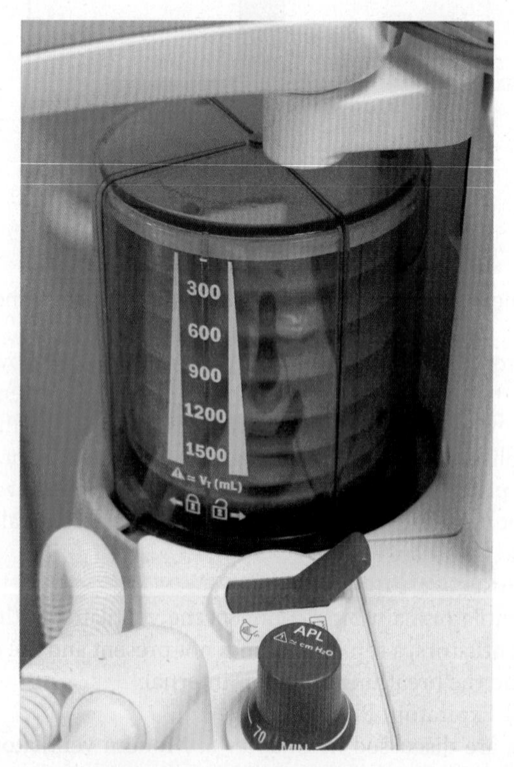

Figure 6.5 Bellows assembly of the 7900 ventilator. The Bag/Vent switch, which also turns the ventilator ON or OFF, is between the bellows assembly and the adjustable pressure-limiting valve.

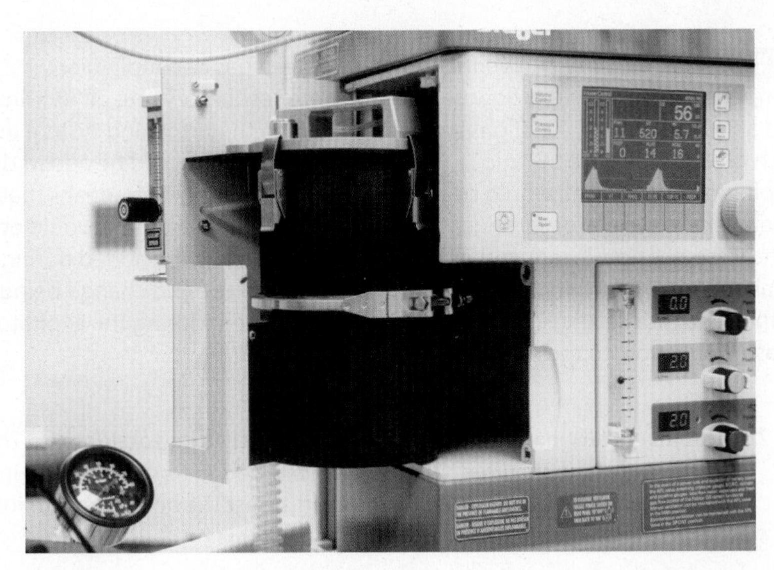

Figure 6.6 Drager Fabius GS ventilator. When the door is opened, the piston ventilator, which is inside a metal case, will swing out.

All or part of the next inspiration will then be lost into the room. Newer ventilators with hanging bellows employ sophisticated software to detect disconnections or leaks and trigger appropriate alarms. A negative-pressure relief valve prevents the patient from being exposed to negative pressure.

C. Electrically Driven Piston

Instead of a bellows in a box, some ventilators have an electrically driven piston in a cylinder (**Fig. 6.6**). By eliminating the need for a drive gas circuit (an additional source of compressible volume), a more stable flow can be provided. In the piston ventilators presently available, during inspiration, the reservoir bag is isolated from the ventilator and collects the fresh gas entering the breathing system. During exhalation, the reservoir bag acts to modulate pressure increases in the system. The bag can be seen to expand during inspiration and contract during exhalation, even though the piston is actually ventilating the patient. Air entrainment can occur if there is a disconnection with a piston ventilator. In this case, the machine may not alarm and the patient will continue to be ventilated, but air will be entrained, resulting in lower concentrations of oxygen and anesthetic agents.

IV. Factors that Affect the Delivered Tidal Volume

A. Fresh Gas Flow

1. Older ventilators do not have a means to adjust the fresh gas flow added to the breathing system during inspiration. This causes the delivered tidal and minute volumes to change when the fresh gas flow, I:E ratio, or respiratory rate is altered. Increased fresh gas flow increases the tidal volume as a result of the amount of fresh gas entering the breathing system during the inspiratory phase. Ventilator settings that prolong the inspiratory time (and thereby increase the I:E ratio) cause an increased tidal volume. As respiratory rate increases, the increase in tidal volume from fresh gas flow is less, although the effect on minute volume remains the same. Slowing the respiratory rate has the opposite effect. The bellows excursion remains unchanged.

CLINICAL MOMENT With a ventilator without fresh gas decoupling or compensation, a fresh gas flow of 10 L/minute, a respiratory rate of 10/minute, and an I:E ratio of 1:2, 1 L of gas would be added to the breathing system during each breath. Since the I:E ratio is 1:2, 333 mL of fresh gas would be added during inspiration and 667 mL would be added during exhalation. This means that whatever the ventilator setting, a 333-mL increase in tidal volume would occur. If the fresh gas flow is reduced by half, only 166 mL would be added during inspiration, so the tidal volume would decrease in spite of no change being made to the ventilator settings. Fresh gas entering the system during the expiratory phase would flow to the scavenging system.

2. Manufacturers have reengineered their ventilators to eliminate the effect of fresh gas on the inspired volume. One method is to measure the inspired and exhaled gas flows to the patient and then adjust the bellows excursion to deliver the set tidal volume (fresh gas compensation).

CLINICAL MOMENT Fresh gas compensation will not be able to adjust for high gas flows into the breathing system when the oxygen flush is activated during inspiration.

CLINICAL MOMENT With ventilators that adjust the bellows excursion to compensate for the fresh gas flow, a high fresh gas flow will cause the bellows to remain at the top of the ventilator housing.

3. The other method to deliver a set tidal volume and exclude the added fresh gas flow is to prevent the fresh gas from entering the breathing system during inspiration. This is called fresh gas decoupling. The decoupling valve diverts the fresh gas into the reservoir bag during inspiration, preventing the fresh gas flow being added to the tidal volume. The valve opens during exhalation.

B. Compliance and Compression Volume
1. Decreases in compliance in the breathing system can be accompanied by decreases in tidal volume as more of the inspiratory gas flow is expended to expand the components. Gas compression losses depend largely on the breathing system volume and the pressure during inspiration.
2. Advanced technology now allows the ventilator to compensate for changes in breathing system compliance and gas compression by altering the delivered inspiratory volume. Breathing system compliance and gas compression are determined automatically during the checkout procedure before use. For accurate compensation, the breathing system must be in the configuration that is to be used after the checkout procedure is performed. Changes in the circuit configuration (such as lengthening the breathing tubes or adding components) will cause the compensation to be inaccurate. Some ventilators measure inspired volumes at the patient connection and adjust the ventilator excursions accordingly.

CLINICAL MOMENT If the ventilator is in the standby mode after a previous case and the breathing system is changed, the data from the previous checkout will be used to deliver accurate tidal volumes. To provide accurate ventilation, the electronic checkout needs to be performed at least once a day and whenever the breathing system is altered.

C. Leaks

A leak around the tracheal tube or supraglottic device will cause a decrease in tidal volume. Diverting gas monitors (Chapter 17) may decrease the volume delivered to the patient.

V. Ventilation Modes

A. Overview

1. A major difference between the older and newer anesthesia ventilators is the additional ventilation modes that are available on newer ones. Many ventilators offer dual modes to gain the advantages of both modes. Ventilator settings must be carefully individualized in each mode to avoid hypoventilation, hyperventilation, volutrauma, or barotrauma. It is important when switching from one mode to another to ensure that the settings are appropriate. Tidal volume, flow, and pressure should be carefully monitored.
2. A ventilator can deliver gas by generating flow or pressure. With flow generators, the flow pattern can be constant (square wave) or nonconstant (accelerative or decelerative). A pressure generator may produce a constant or varying pressure. See pressure- and flow-volume loops in Chapter 18.
3. Features of some commonly used ventilatory modes are shown in **Table 6.1.** The terminology used to describe ventilator modes has not been agreed upon. Some manufacturers have coined proprietary terms for their ventilator modes.

B. Volume Control Ventilation

1. The most commonly used mode in the operating room is volume control (volume) ventilation, in which a preset tidal volume is delivered. The tidal or minute volume and the respiratory rate are set by the anesthesia provider and delivered by the ventilator independent of patient effort. It is time-initiated, volume-limited, and cycled by volume or time.
2. Flow rate is constant during inspiration. If the inspiratory flow is too low to provide the set tidal volume within the inspiratory time period, the bellows or piston will not complete its excursion and an inadequate tidal volume will result. If the flow is higher than is needed to provide the tidal volume, the tidal volume will be reached before the end of the inspiratory tine. This will result in an inspiratory

Table 6.1 Ventilatory Modes

Mode	Initiation	Limit	Cycle
Volume-controlled ventilation	Time	Volume	Volume/time
Pressure-controlled ventilation	Time	Pressure	Time
Intermittent mandatory ventilation	Time	Volume	Volume/time
Synchronized intermittent mandatory ventilation	Time/pressure	Volume	Volume/time
Pressure support ventilation	Pressure/flow	Pressure	Flow/time

pause. The inspiratory phase may be terminated before the tidal volume has been delivered if the peak airway pressure reaches the high pressure limit.

3. Typically, the waveform shows steadily increasing pressure during inspiration. Changes in compliance or resistance are reflected in changes in peak inspiratory pressure and the difference between peak and plateau pressure. For a given set tidal volume, the pressure in the breathing system is determined by the breathing system resistance and compliance and the patient. Peak pressure is also influenced by resistance. Plateau pressure reflects compliance. The pressure–volume and flow–volume loops associated with volume-controlled ventilation are shown in Figures 18.4 and 18.5.
4. Adding PEEP decreases the tidal volume delivered. The PEEP effect is greater when tidal volumes are small. On newer ventilators with integral PEEP, ventilation may be better maintained when PEEP is added.

C. Pressure Control Ventilation

Pressure control (pressure-limited, pressure-controlled, pressure-preset control, or pressure) ventilation is available on many newer anesthesia ventilators. With this mode, the operator sets the maximum inspiratory pressure at a level above PEEP. The ventilator quickly increases the pressure to the set level at the start of inspiration and maintains this pressure until exhalation begins.

1. Gas flow is highest at the beginning of inspiration and then decreases. Increased resistance may change the shape of the flow-versus-time waveform to a flatter, more square-shaped pattern as tidal volume delivery shifts into the latter part of inspiration. This allows the ventilator to preserve tidal volume with increased resistance until resistance becomes severe. The pressure–volume and flow–volume loops show special characteristics with pressure-controlled ventilation (Figs. 18.11 and 18.12).
2. Tidal volume is determined partly by the rise time and set pressure. Tidal volume fluctuates with changes in resistance and compliance and with patient–ventilator asynchrony. If resistance increases or compliance decreases, the tidal volume will decrease.

CLINICAL MOMENT Since the tidal volume can be variable, it is important that a respirometer and/or pressure–volume and flow–volume loops be used during pressure-controlled ventilation.

CLINICAL MOMENT It has been postulated that a decrease in tidal volume with pressure-controlled ventilation would detect a partially occluded tracheal tube. Studies have shown that tidal volume does not decrease until the occlusion is nearly complete.

3. Unlike most intensive care unit ventilators, an anesthesia ventilator in the pressure-controlled mode operates with a preset I:E ratio, so increasing the respiratory rate shortens the inspiratory time and lowers the tidal volume. An increase in PEEP causes a reduction in tidal volume. Tidal volume is not affected by fresh gas flow because excess gas is vented through the spill valve.
4. On some ventilators, the inspiratory flow is adjustable (**Fig. 6.7**). It may also be possible to change the inspiratory rise time. For patients with good compliance, inspiratory flow should be high to ensure that the inspiratory pressure is rapidly

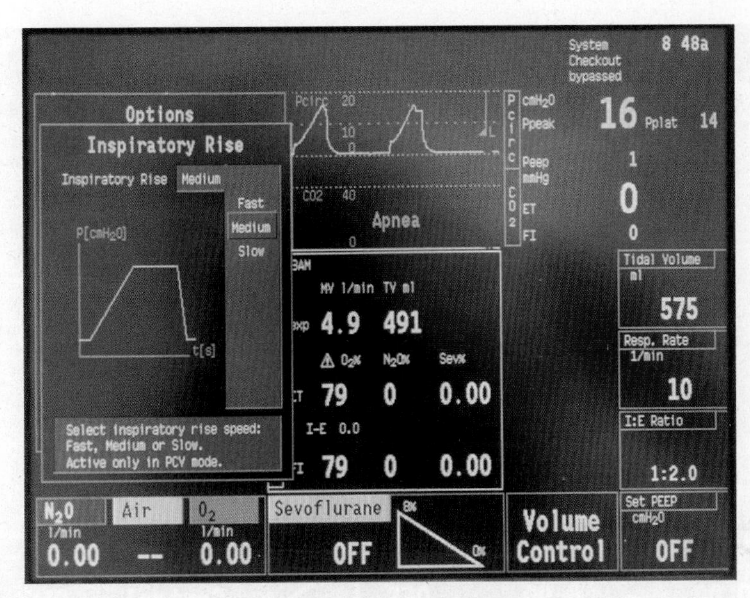

Figure 6.7 The inspiratory rise can be displayed on the left part of the screen. It is changed by using the rotary mouse.

attained. Limiting the maximum inspiratory flow is useful to avoid overshooting the target pressure, especially when compliance is low.

5. Pressure-controlled ventilation should be considered whenever it is important to avoid high airway pressures. It is often used with supraglottic airway devices and patients with narrow or partially obstructed tracheal tubes to provide ventilation at relatively low pressures. Limiting the peak inflating pressure delivered by the ventilator may reduce ventilator-induced lung injury. In obese patients, patients with lung injury, or during single-lung ventilation, pressure-controlled ventilation may improve oxygenation and produce greater tidal volumes than volume-controlled ventilation without using higher pressures. It may be useful if there is an airway leak (e.g., uncuffed tube, supraglottic airway device, bronchopleural fistula). If there is a large leak, the cycling pressure limit may not be reached, causing a prolonged inspiration.

D. Intermittent Mandatory Ventilation

With intermittent mandatory ventilation (IMV), the ventilator delivers mechanical (mandatory, automatic) breaths at a preset rate and permits spontaneous, unassisted breaths with a controllable inspiratory gas mixture between mechanical breaths. The ventilator has a secondary source of gas flow for spontaneous breaths. This utilizes either continuous gas flow within the circuit or a demand valve that opens to allow gas to flow from a reservoir. This mode is often used for weaning patients from mechanical ventilation. The IMV rate is gradually reduced, allowing increased time for the patient's spontaneous breaths.

E. Synchronized Intermittent Mandatory Ventilation

Synchronized intermittent mandatory ventilation (SIMV) synchronizes ventilator-delivered breaths with the patient's spontaneous breaths. If patient inspiratory activity is detected, the ventilator synchronizes its mandatory breaths so that the set respiratory frequency is achieved.

1. The time between the end of each mandatory breath and the beginning of the next is subdivided into a spontaneous breathing time and a trigger time. During the trigger time, the ventilator verifies whether the airway pressure has dropped

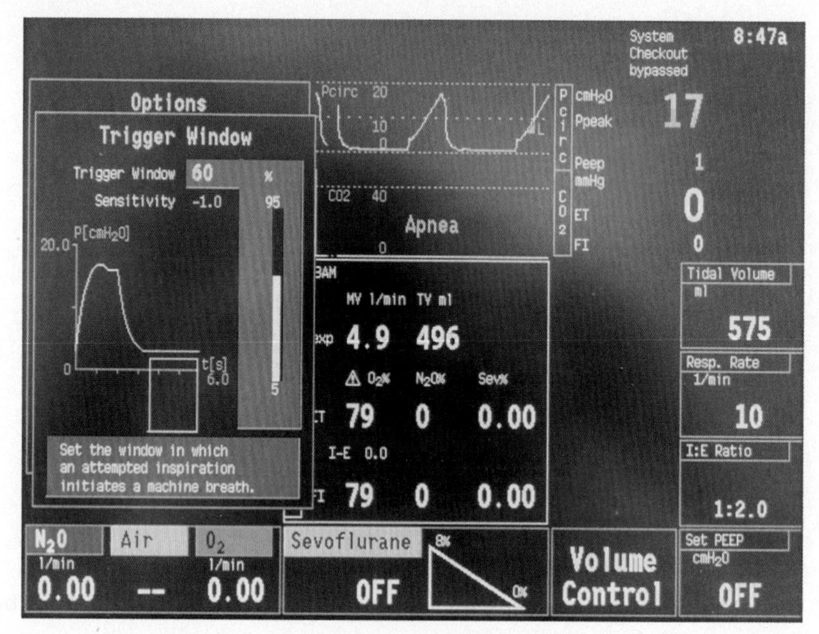

Figure 6.8 The trigger window can be displayed on the left part of the screen. It is changed by using the rotary mouse.

a minimum amount below the pressure measured at the end of the expiratory phase. If a drop is not sensed, the ventilator delivers a breath. The trigger window may be adjustable (**Fig. 6.8**).

2. A mandatory tidal volume and a minimum mechanical ventilation rate must be selected. This determines the minimum minute ventilation. When setting the ventilator rate, the patient's spontaneous rate should be considered. If the SIMV rate is set too high, the patient may become apneic. Setting an I:E ratio is not required in SIMV. The I:E ratio will change as the patient's respiratory rate and rhythm changes.
3. SIMV is used to facilitate emergence from anesthesia as the patient transitions from controlled to spontaneous ventilation. It ensures a minimal amount of ventilation while freeing the anesthesia provider from ventilating the patient by hand. It reduces the incidence of patient–ventilator disharmony in which the patient tries to fight the ventilator and the need for sedation or narcosis to tolerate mechanical ventilation. SIMV can be combined with pressure support ventilation (PSV).

F. Mandatory Minute Ventilation

Mandatory minute ventilation is a method of mechanical ventilation in which the amount of ventilatory support is automatically adjusted so that the set minute ventilation is reached. The ventilator circuitry monitors exhaled volume and, if it falls below a predetermined level, provides the difference between the selected and actual minute volume.

G. Pressure Support Ventilation

Pressure support (pressure-assisted or assisted spontaneous) ventilation is now used on many anesthesia ventilators. It is designed to augment the patient's spontaneous breathing by applying positive pressure to the airway in response to patient-initiated breaths.

1. A supported breath may be pressure- or flow-initiated. Flow triggering imposes less inspiratory workload than pressure triggering and is used more frequently. When the user-selected flow or subbaseline pressure caused by a spontaneous

breath is reached, flow from the ventilator begins and the set pressure is quickly reached. The ventilator then modulates the flow to maintain that pressure. The flow decreases until it falls below a predetermined fraction of the initial rate (usually 5% or 25%) or a fixed flow (usually 5 L/minute) or after a specific duration of time. At this point, flow is terminated and exhalation begins.

2. The airway pressure needed to initiate inspiration is determined by the pressure support setting. The rise time is usually adjustable. Flow delivery is determined by the pressure support setting, the pressure generated by the respiratory muscles, and airway resistance. Because the pressure is reached early in inspiration and is maintained throughout the inspiratory phase, the pressure waveform has a square shape.
3. PSV has the disadvantage that ventilation will cease if the patient fails to make any respiratory effort. To avoid this potentially disastrous situation, most ventilators have a backup or "apneic" SIMV rate (assist/control ventilation).
4. The anesthesia provider must set the trigger sensitivity and the inspiratory pressure (usually from 5 to 10 cm H_2O). The trigger sensitivity should be set so that it will respond to inspiratory effort without autocycling in response to artifactual changes in airway pressure. On some ventilators, the trigger window can be changed (**Fig. 6.8**). The initial inspiratory flow is usually not adjustable but can be changed on some ventilators by adjusting the inspiratory rise time (**Fig. 6.7**). The optimal initial inspiratory flow is highest in patients with low compliance, high resistance, and most active ventilatory drive. Sighs in conjunction with PSV may counteract the tendency for lung collapse associated with a low tidal volume.
5. Tidal volume is determined by the pressure support level, lung characteristics, and patient effort. The desired tidal volume should be calculated and the pressure support level adjusted so that the desired volume is delivered. If the exhaled volume is inadequate, the inspiratory pressure should be increased or the inspiratory rise time decreased (if adjustable). A very high inspiratory flow (due to a high set pressure) may decrease tidal volume by prematurely terminating inspiration. Undesired hyperventilation can be treated by adjusting the trigger sensitivity, pressure level, or trigger window or, if these seem adequate, by additional sedation.
6. PSV has proved useful both in preoxygenating obese patients by increasing the functional residual capacity and during weaning from mechanical ventilation. It can be useful with a supraglottic airway device to keep the airway pressure low. This mode has been shown to improve gas exchange and ventilation and lower the work of breathing during spontaneous breathing. It has been used to improve ventilation during fiber-optic intubation in patients with an anticipated difficult intubation, during an inhalation induction, and with monitored anesthesia care.
7. An advantage of PSV is the synchrony between the patient and the ventilator. The patient controls rate, volume, and inspiratory time. This may increase patient comfort. Peak and mean airway pressures are lower than with volume-controlled ventilation. Asynchrony may occur in patients who have airflow obstruction (e.g., chronic obstructive pulmonary disease). If there is a leak around the device, PSV will be able to compensate for the leak to some extent, as the airway pressure is maintained irrespective of the volume.
8. Too high an inspiratory flow may cause patient discomfort. PSV will deliver a variable minute volume in a patient with a changing respiratory drive.

Inappropriate ventilator triggering caused by a leak, patient movement, or cardiac contractions can occur with PSV. The use of PEEP may affect the delivered pressure support with some anesthesia ventilators.

VI. Pediatric Ventilation

A. In the past, pediatric ventilation has caused uneasiness among anesthesia providers because the large amount of space in the absorber, tubings, and the ventilator resulted in relatively large loss of volume from gas compression and breathing system compliance. Experience has shown that volume-controlled ventilation of infants with newer ventilators is safe and effective, although the delivered tidal volume may be somewhat imprecise. Pressure-controlled ventilation can also be used with pediatric patients. Some ventilators have a pediatric mode that is tailored to small infants and children.

B. Newer ventilators compensate for fresh gas flow as well as gas compression and circuit compliance. These ventilators can deliver small tidal volumes in the volume-controlled mode accurately in patients requiring small tidal volumes and who have low compliance (1).

VII. Magnetic Resonance Imaging Ventilators

Standard ventilators with ferrous material cannot be used in the magnetic resonance imaging (MRI) unit, because the electromagnetic environment will interfere with the controls and the ventilator can interfere with the radiofrequencies of the MRI system. Anesthesia ventilators suitable for use in an MRI unit are available.

VIII. General Hazards

A. Hypoventilation

1. **Ventilator Failure**

a. Although most anesthesia ventilators perform reliably for long periods of time, some may occasionally fail to work properly. Some problems are insidious and result in less-than-total failure. A malfunction may not be readily apparent, and a false sense of security may be generated by the sound that the ventilator makes.

b. Causes of ventilator failure include disconnection from or failure of the power source (electricity or driving gas) and internal malfunctions. A setting between two numbers on a dial may cause cycling failure. On some ventilators with fresh gas flow compensation, a very high fresh gas flow can cause ventilator standstill. Problems with the electric motor or fluid entering the electronic circuitry may cause the ventilator to stop functioning.

c. If the bellows housing is not tightly secured, driving gas can leak, causing a reduction in the tidal volume. The housing may become dislocated by a hitting ceiling column or other object. Operating room personnel may attempt to move a ventilator by grabbing the housing, loosening it, or causing it to break.

d. A malfunction in a computer-controlled ventilator may interrupt cycling. A cycling failure may sometimes be solved by turning the anesthesia machine OFF and then ON but often requires reference to the operation manual or a call to the manufacturer.

e. Low maximum flow rates and variability in flow rates with increased airway pressure with older anesthesia ventilators can reduce the tidal volume that can be delivered. Although this is usually not a problem in patients with normal lungs, it can become important in patients with expiratory airflow obstruction, for whom a prolonged expiratory phase may be necessary to avoid auto PEEP.

2. **Breathing System Gas Loss**
   a. Older anesthesia ventilators had no means of compensating for gas loss in the breathing system. New computer-controlled ventilators can compensate for small leaks. A ventilator may cycle but fail to occlude the exit port of the spill valve, blowing part or all of the tidal volume into the scavenging system.
   b. If breathing system gas is lost and an ascending bellows ventilator is in use, the bellows may not return to its fully expanded position. This usually is obvious. However, with a closed scavenging system, the bellows may remain expanded if there is a disconnection. A descending bellows ventilator may appear to function normally with the loss of breathing system gas.
3. **Incorrect Settings**
   a. In a crowded anesthetizing area, ventilator switches or dials may be inadvertently changed as personnel move about. If an anesthesia machine is turned OFF and then turned back ON, the ventilator may default to different settings than were being used. The anesthesia provider may fail to adjust settings for a new patient. For ventilators that provide a control for limiting the peak inspiratory pressure, setting that pressure too low may result in an inadequate tidal volume being delivered.
   b. It is essential that there be sufficient inspiratory time for the desired tidal volume to be delivered. Insufficient inspiratory time may be indicated by a bellows that does not make a full excursion, causing a decrease in the tidal volume.
4. **Ventilator Turned OFF**
   There are times during anesthetic delivery when the ventilator must be turned OFF, such as during radiological procedures in which movement would compromise image quality. The operator may forget to turn it back ON.
5. **Flow Obstruction**
   As will be pointed out in Chapter 10, restricted or occluded gas flow can occur at a variety of sites and can be caused by a variety of mechanisms. With obstruction to flow, the bellows excursion will be reduced but not totally eliminated. The pressure shown on the system pressure gauge will vary, depending on the locations of the obstruction and the gauge.
6. **Positive End-Expiratory Pressure**
   Adding PEEP may decrease the tidal volume delivered with some ventilators. The effect is more pronounced with low tidal volumes but less if lung compliance is low.

B. Hyperventilation
   1. If ventilator settings for a patient with low compliance are not modified prior to the next anesthetic delivery for a patient with high compliance, the result may be excessive tidal volume.
   2. With a hole in the bellows or a loose connection between the bellows and its base assembly, driving gas from the housing can enter the bellows, causing an unexpectedly high tidal volume. This can be accentuated by a high inspiratory flow rate. A small hole in the bellows may not cause a change in the tidal volume.

C. Hyperoxia
   A hole or tear in the bellows when oxygen is the driving gas can result in an increase in the inspired oxygen concentration and lower-than-expected anesthetic concentrations. If the tear is small, there may be no effect.

D. Excessive Airway Pressure

1. Excessive airway pressure can develop very rapidly, especially if high fresh gas flows are being used. Quick action may be required to prevent injury.
2. Because the ventilator spill valve is closed during inspiration and the APL valve in the breathing system is closed or isolated, activating the oxygen flush during the inspiratory phase can result in barotrauma. Fresh gas decoupling reduces this danger by diverting the oxygen to the reservoir bag, which greatly enlarges. Ventilators that compensate by altering the bellows excursion may not always be able to prevent excessive airway pressure if the oxygen flush is used during inspiration.

CLINICAL MOMENT It is potentially very dangerous to activate the oxygen flush during mechanical ventilation. If there is a decoupling valve that prevents fresh gas from entering the breathing system during inspiration, this will not be a problem. If the ventilator compensates for gas inflow during inspiration, it will not be able to fully compensate for the additional volume and excessive airway pressure may result.

3. A hole in the bellows or a loose connection between the bellows and its base may allow driving gas to enter the bellows, resulting in a higher-than-expected pressure during inspiration. Pressure on the ventilator spill valve can result in excess pressure.
4. Sufficient time for full exhalation must be allowed. Insufficient expiratory time may be indicated by a bellows that does not fully expand. This situation carries the risk of air trapping and auto (occult, intrinsic) PEEP.
5. A properly set pressure-limiting mechanism should reduce the risk of barotrauma. Some ventilators have adjustable high-pressure alarms. On others, the alarm limit is not adjustable.

CLINICAL MOMENT When there is high airway pressure, a disconnection should be made immediately at the tracheal tube and manual ventilation instituted. Taking time to find the problem source may harm the patient.

E. Negative Pressure during Expiration

Negative pressure is considered undesirable under most circumstances because of adverse effects on pulmonary function and increased risk of air embolism and negative pressure pulmonary edema. A ventilator with a weighted hanging bellows can generate subatmospheric pressure during the early part of expiration if expiratory flow is not impeded. This will be accentuated if the fresh gas flow is low. Newer ventilators with a hanging bellows have a negative pressure valve to admit air if negative pressure develops.

F. Alarm Failure

1. Although low-pressure alarms have significantly advanced patient safety, they can fail. If the low-airway-pressure alarm threshold is adjustable, it should be set just below the peak inspiratory pressure. Cases have been reported in which resistance (from tracheal tube connectors, Y-pieces, filters, and other components, or the patient port of the breathing system being pressed against the patient or a pillow) coupled with high inspiratory flow rates created sufficient

back pressure to create a false-negative alarm condition when the low-pressure-alarm threshold was set too low.

2. Using a PEEP valve in the breathing system may cause the low-pressure alarm not to be activated if the PEEP valve raises the pressure above the alarm threshold.

G. Electromagnetic Interference

Ultrahigh-frequency radios and certain cell phones may interfere with anesthesia ventilators. Effects include faulty readings, misleading alarm messages, modified ventilation parameters, and output interruption and are usually temporary.

H. Loss of Electrical Power

Most ventilators in use today are electrically powered. If there is a power failure, there must be battery backup for at least 30 minutes. A message on the computer screen will note the changeover to battery power and give an indication of battery life (Figs. 3.2 and 3.3). When all electrical energy is consumed, most anesthesia machines will default to a manual/spontaneous breathing mode. The anesthesia provider may need to initiate this move. Without the ventilator or machine monitors, most machines will provide oxygen to the breathing system and sometimes volatile agent. Backup systems that will prolong electrical activity are available.

CLINICAL MOMENT Since anesthesia machines handle electrical power loss in different ways, the user needs to determine how a particular machine will react to a power outage and develop a plan of action if this occurs. This information is in the user manual.

IX. Advantages

Using a ventilator allows the anesthesia provider to devote time and energy to other tasks and eliminates the fatigue resulting from squeezing a bag. A ventilator produces more regular ventilation with respect to rate, rhythm, and tidal volume than manual ventilation.

X. Disadvantages

A. Probably, the greatest disadvantage of using a ventilator is the loss of contact between the anesthesia provider and the patient. The feel of the bag can reveal disconnections, changes in resistance or compliance, continuous positive pressure, and spontaneous respiratory movements. With mechanical ventilation, these may go undetected for a considerable period of time. Close attention must be paid to the respiratory monitors.

B. A ventilator may induce a false sense of security in the user if it continues to make the appropriate sounds even when it malfunctions.

C. Some anesthesia ventilators do not include all the newer modes of ventilation, and some cannot develop high enough inspiratory pressures or flows to ventilate certain patients. It may be necessary to take a critical care ventilator into the operating room to provide adequate ventilation for critically ill patients.

D. Components that are subject to contamination, especially those on older ventilators, may not be easy to remove or clean.

E. Some ventilators lack user friendliness. There is room for improvement in the design and grouping of controls.

F. Some ventilators are disturbingly noisy or too quiet.

G. Some ventilators require relatively high driving gas flows. Gas consumption increases with increased minute volume and, with some ventilators, an increased I:E ratio. A ventilator with a piston will not consume driving gas.

REFERENCE

1. Bachiller PR, McDonough JM, Feldman JM. Do new anesthesia ventilators deliver small tidal volumes accurately during volume-controlled ventilation. Anesth Analg 2008;106:1392–1400.

SUGGESTED READINGS

Abramovich A. Descending bellows drives question. Fresh gas decoupling minimizes complexity. Response. APSF Newslett 2005;20:34–35.

Ciochetty DA. Descending bellows drives question. Fresh gas decoupling minimizes complexity. APSF Newslett 2005;20:34.

Dorsch J, Dorsch S. Anesthesia ventilators. In: Understanding Anesthesia Equipment. Fifth edition. Philadelphia: Wolters Kluwer/Lippincott Williams & Wilkins, 2008:310–371.

Hess DR. Ventilator waveforms and the physiology of pressure support ventilation. Respir Care 2005;50:166–186.

Klemenzson G, Perouansky M. Contemporary anesthesia ventilators incur a significant "oxygen cost." Can J Anesth 2004;51:616–620.

Macnaughton P, Mackenzie I. Modes of mechanical ventilation. In: Mackenzie I, ed. Core Topics in Mechanical Ventilation. West Nyack, NY: Cambridge University Press, 2008:88–114.

Malhotra A, Kacmarek RM. Mechanical ventilation. In: Hagberg CA, ed. Benumof's Airway Management. Second edition. St Louis: Elsevier, 2007:1079–1122.

Olympio MA. Modern anesthesia machines offer new safety features. APSF Newslett 2003;18:24–27.

7 Manual Resuscitators

I. Introduction

Breathing systems that use nonrebreathing valves have largely disappeared from anesthesia practice. However, these valves are still used in small portable manual resuscitators, which are used primarily for patient transport and emergency situations. They can also be used to administer anesthesia.

II. Components

A typical manual resuscitator is shown diagrammatically in **Figure 7.1**. It has a compressible self-expanding bag, a bag inlet valve, and a nonrebreathing valve. The bag inlet and nonrebreathing valve are combined in some units.

A. Self-expanding Bag

The self-expanding (ventilating or ventilation, self-inflating, self-refilling) bag is constructed so that it remains inflated in its resting state. Some bags collapse like an accordion for storage. During exhalation, the bag expands. If the volume of oxygen from the delivery source is inadequate to fill the bag, the difference is made up by room air. The rate at which the bag reinflates will determine the maximum minute volume.

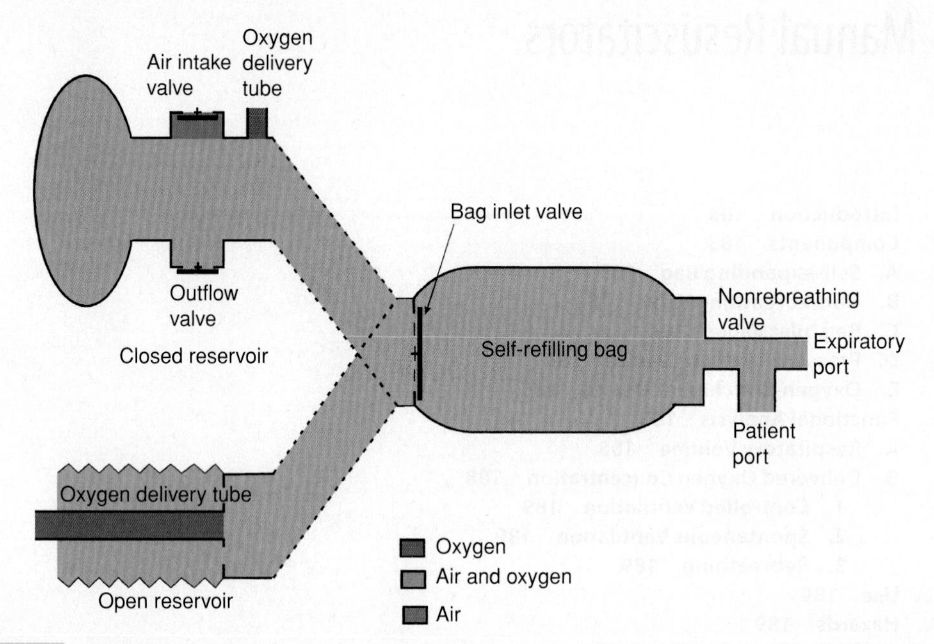

Figure 7.1 Components of a manual resuscitator. The nonrebreathing valve directs the gas from the bag to the patient during inspiration. During expiration, the nonrebreathing valve directs exhaled gases from the patient to the atmosphere through the expiratory port and the bag inlet valve opens to allow the bag to fill.

B. Nonrebreathing Valve

1. There is a nonrebreathing valve connected to the bag. The valve is T-shaped and has three ports. Gas from the self-expanding bag enters the valve through the inspiratory port. As the bag is squeezed, the valve directs the gas through the patient port. This port is usually at right angles to the other ports and has concentric 15- and 22-mm fittings to connect it to a mask, tracheal tube, or supraglottic airway device. The third port is the expiratory port though which the patient's exhaled gases are released to atmosphere. During inspiration, this port is closed to prevent inspired gases from being lost to atmosphere. Other parts that may be associated with the nonrebreathing valve include a pressure-limiting valve, an expired gas deflector, a positive end-expiratory pressure (PEEP) valve, and a 19- or 30-mm connector to attach to a scavenging system.
2. Quite a few valves have been used over the years. The most commonly used today is called the fishmouth valve (**Figs. 7.2** and 7.3), so called because when the bag is squeezed, the inspiratory portion of the valve opens much like a fish's mouth. There is a flap on the valve that closes the expiratory port, directing all the gas from the bag to the patient port. During exhalation, the exhaled gases close the fishmouth valve and the flap is pushed away from the expiratory port. The exhaled gases then pass from the valve to the air or scavenging system.

C. Bag Inlet Valve

The bag inlet (refill) valve is a one-way valve that is opened by negative pressure inside the bag. This valve is usually located at the opposite end of the bag from the nonrebreathing valve. When the bag is squeezed, the valve closes. This prevents gas from escaping through the inlet. A simple flap (**Fig. 7.4**) is most commonly used.

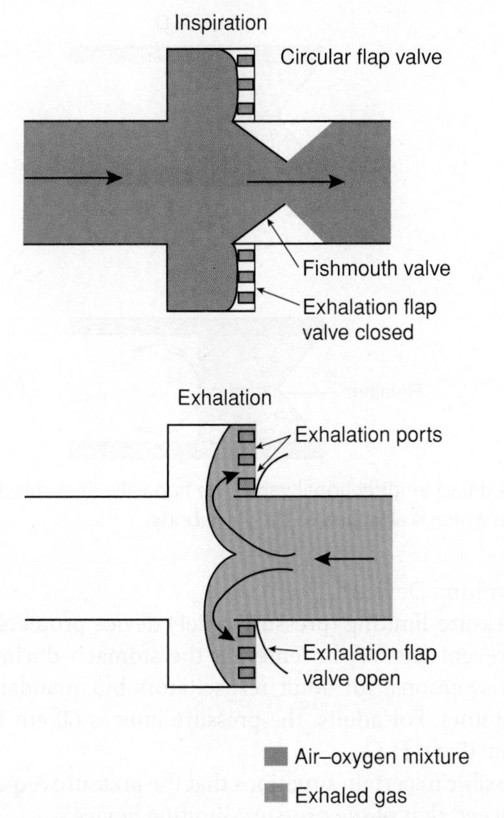

Figure 7.2 Fishmouth-flap nonrebreathing valve. The circular flap and fishmouth valves are attached around the periphery. When the bag is squeezed, the flap valve is seated against the exhalation ports and the fishmouth portion of the valve opens. During expiration, the fishmouth closes and the flap falls away from the exhalation channel. A second flap valve over the exhalation ports prevents air from being inspired during spontaneous respiration.

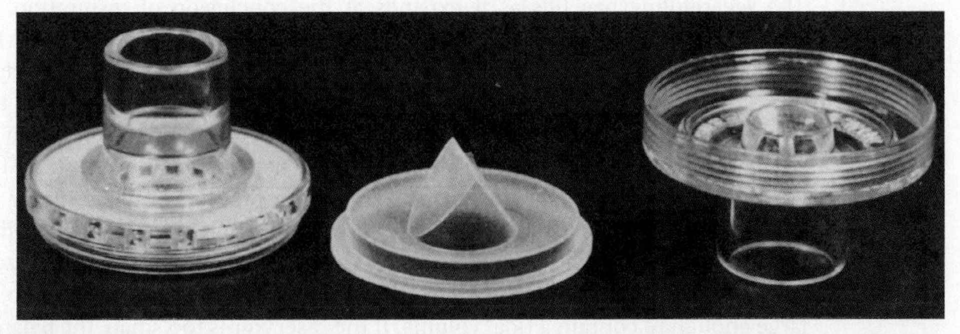

Figure 7.3 Components of the fishmouth-flap nonrebreathing valve. **Left:** The patient connection with the expiratory flap. **Center:** The fishmouth valve with its concentric flap. **Right:** The part of the housing closest to the bag.

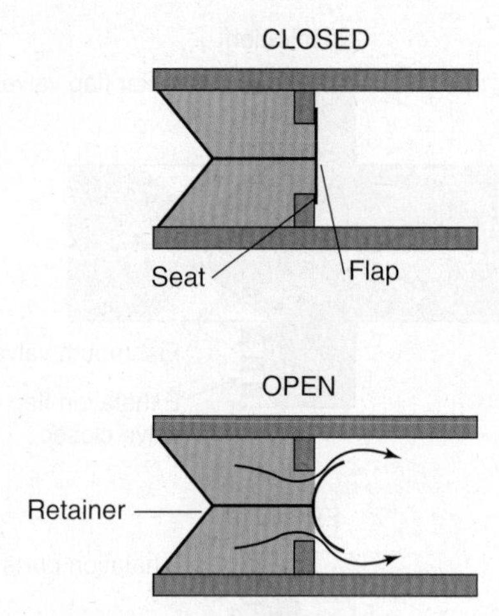

Figure 7.4 Center-mounted flap unidirectional valve. The flap valve is secured by a tab at the center. The tab is secured by a retainer, which is attached to the valve body.

D. Pressure-Limiting Device

1. The pressure-limiting (pressure-relief) device protects against barotrauma and may prevent gases from entering the stomach during mask ventilation. This device is optional for adult resuscitators but mandatory for infant and child resuscitators. For adults, the pressure limit is 60 cm H_2O, and for infants and children 45 cm H_2O.
2. It is possible in certain situations that the pressure required to ventilate a patient may exceed that of the pressure-limiting device.

CLINICAL MOMENT If the pressure-limiting device does not allow a high enough pressure for adequate ventilation, an override device will be needed. The user must become familiar with the operation of this device prior to use in an emergency.

E. Oxygen-Enrichment Device

1. The self-refilling bag fills as it expands at the conclusion of inspiration. In most cases, room air does not have a high enough oxygen concentration for the patient's needs. Therefore, a way to deliver additional oxygen is needed. The simplest method is to attach the oxygen tubing from a flowmeter to the inlet valve on the bag. While this will increase the oxygen concentration to some extent, the flow from the flowmeter may be considerably less than the flow needed to fill the bag. The balance of the inflow to the bag will be made up of room air. To increase the oxygen concentration further, a reservoir is needed (**Fig. 7.5**). Oxygen will accumulate in the reservoir when the bag is squeezed. The reservoir size may limit the inspired oxygen concentration. It needs to be large enough to contain a tidal volume. If the reservoir is too small, the balance of gas entering the bag will be air.
2. There are two types of reservoir: open and closed (**Figs. 7.6** and **7.7**). The open reservoir opens to the atmosphere. It may be a corrugated breathing tube. The open end allows air to enter if there is an inadequate amount of oxygen in the tubing.
3. The closed reservoir is usually a bag with a valve that will let in room air if the bag becomes empty.

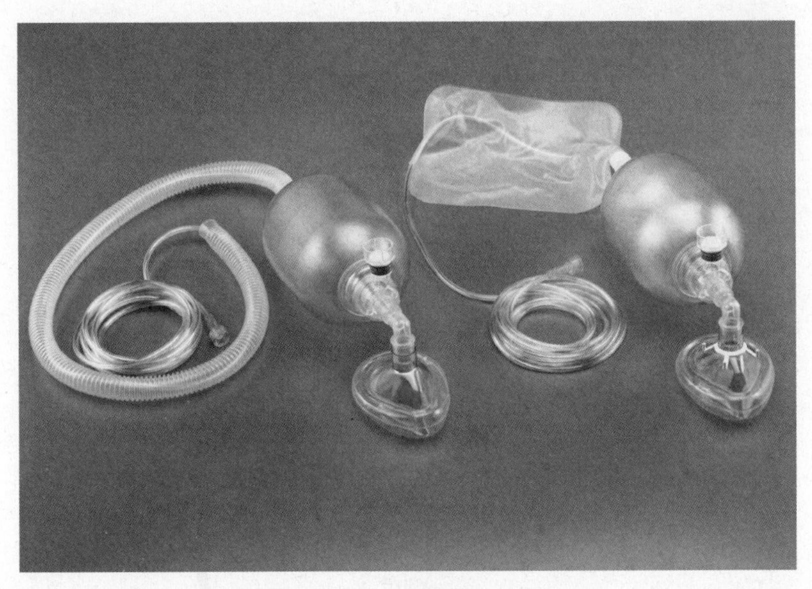

Figure 7.5 **Left:** A resuscitator with an open reservoir. **Right:** A resuscitator with a closed reservoir.

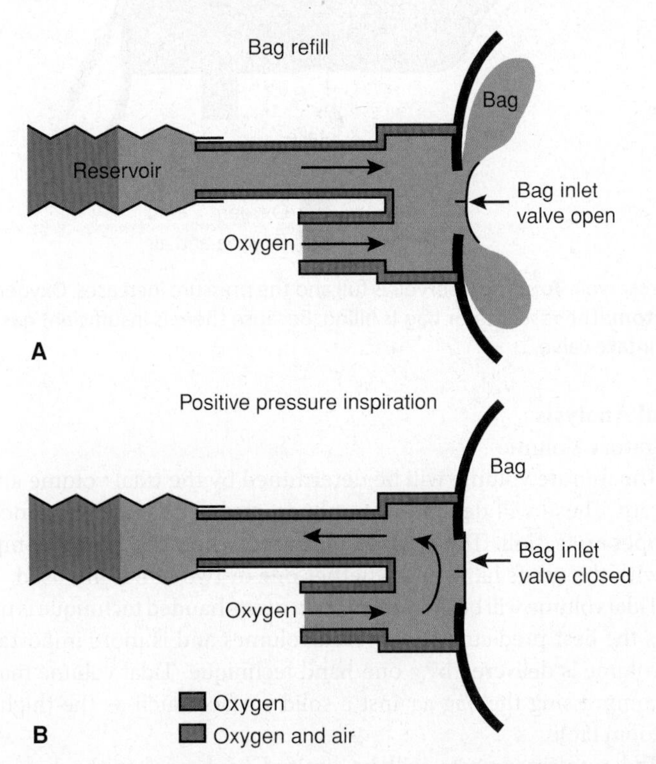

Figure 7.6 Open reservoir. **A:** The bag is filling. Oxygen from the delivery tubing as well as that in the reservoir flows into the bag. If the volume entering the bag exceeds that in the reservoir and is flowing through the delivery tubing, room air will make up the difference. The size of the reservoir is, therefore, important. **B:** The bag inlet valve is closed. Oxygen from the delivery tubing flows into the reservoir. Because the reservoir is open to atmosphere, some oxygen will be lost if the flow is high.

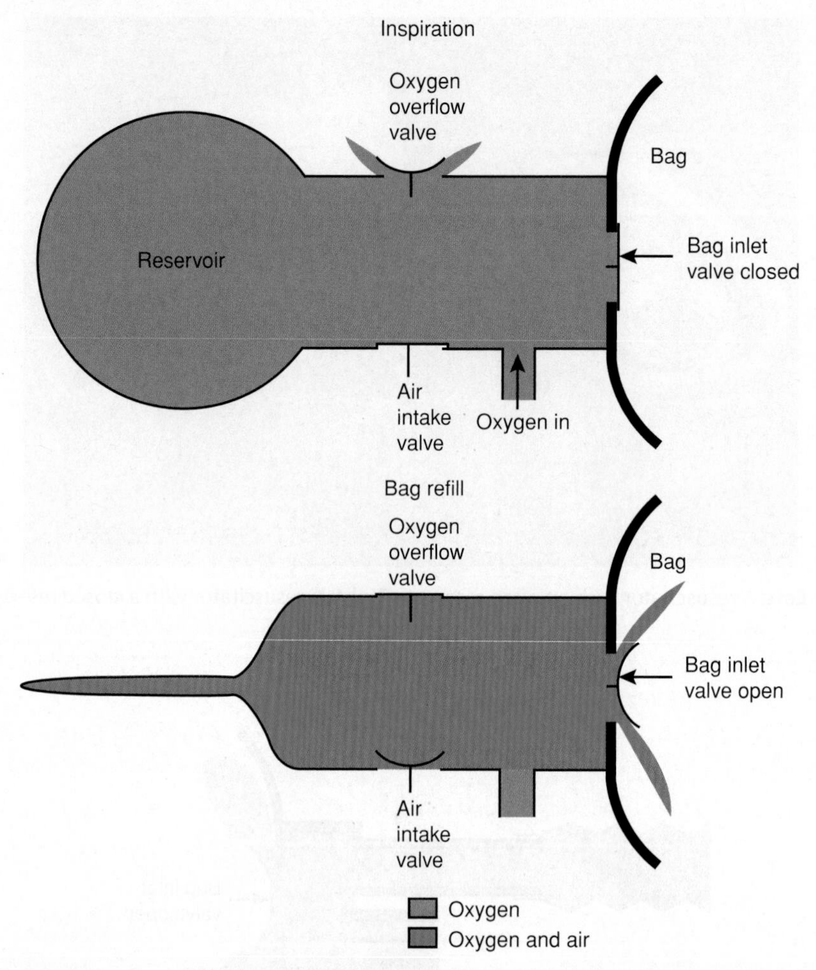

Figure 7.7 Closed reservoir. **Top:** The reservoir is full and the pressure increases. Oxygen flows through the overflow valve. **Bottom:** The resuscitator bag is filling. Because there is insufficient gas in the reservoir, air enters through the intake valve.

III. Functional Analysis

A. Respiratory Volume

1. The minute volume will be determined by the tidal volume and the respiratory rate. These will depend not only on resuscitator performance but also on the operator's skill. The volume delivered when the bag is compressed will vary with the user's hand and whether one or two hands are used.
2. Tidal volume will be increased when a two-handed technique is used. Grip strength is the best predictor of delivered volumes and is more important when the tidal volume is delivered by a one-hand technique. Tidal volume may be increased by compressing the bag against a solid surface, such as the thigh or the operating room table.
3. The respiratory rate will be limited by how fast the bag reexpands, which depends on the bag construction and the size of the bag refill valve inlet. The maximum compression rate may be reduced at low temperatures.

B. Delivered Oxygen Concentration

The ASTM standard requires that a resuscitator for adults be capable of delivering an inspired oxygen concentration of at least 40% when connected to an oxygen source supplying not more than 15 L/minute and at least 85% with an oxygen-enrichment device supplied by the manufacturer.

The delivered oxygen concentration is limited by reservoir size and the oxygen flow. If the reservoir volume is greater than the bag volume and the oxygen flow is greater than the minute volume, the delivered oxygen concentration may approach 100%. If the tidal volume is greater than the reservoir volume plus the volume of oxygen delivered during inspiration, air will be drawn into the unit and reduce the delivered oxygen concentration.

1. **Controlled Ventilation**
   The delivered oxygen concentration will be determined by the minute volume, the reservoir (if present) size, the oxygen flow, and the technique used to squeeze and release the bag. If the bag is allowed to fill at its most rapid rate, all of the oxygen in the reservoir may be exhausted and air drawn in. If bag filling is manually retarded, the delivered oxygen concentration will be higher. This may be useful when low oxygen flows must be used or when the reservoir is small or not present, but it limits the respiratory rate. Furthermore, it may cause the nonrebreathing valve to jam in the inspiratory position. Activating the pressure-limiting device may cause the delivered oxygen concentration to decrease.
2. **Spontaneous Ventilation**
   With spontaneous ventilation, inspired gas may come from the exhalation port as well as from the bag. The inspired oxygen concentration can vary from 25% to 100%.

CLINICAL MOMENT The self-expanding bag is not a good choice for spontaneously breathing patients because the negative pressure during inspiration may not be adequate to open the inspiratory port. In this case, the patient may inspire room air through the exhalation port.

3. **Rebreathing**
   If the nonrebreathing valve is competent, inhaled and exhaled gases should not mix. If the inspiratory limb valve is incompetent, a back leak will allow exhaled gases to pass back into the resuscitator.

IV. **Use**

A. A bag and a mask that are the appropriate size for the patient should be selected. For adults, an oxygen flow of 10 to 15 L/minute is most commonly used. For children and infants, lower flows are recommended. Higher flows than those recommended by the manufacturer can result in significant levels of auto-PEEP.

B. If anesthetic gases are to be administered, the transfer tube from a scavenging system (Chapter 8) should be attached to the expiratory port.

C. A manual resuscitator can be adapted for manual ventilation during magnetic resonance imaging by inserting an extension tube that is long enough to cover the distance between the patient and the person squeezing the bag between the nonrebreathing valve and the bag. An extension must not be placed between the patient and the nonrebreathing valve, because this will cause the dead space to be increased.

V. **Hazards**

A. High Airway Pressure

High airway pressure is a hazard mainly if the patient is intubated. A dangerously high pressure is less likely when a mask or supraglottic device is used.

B. Nonrebreathing Valve Sticking in the Inspiratory Position
This complication is possible if the nonrebreathing valve has a disc and a spring that pushes it onto a seat, preventing exhaled gases from reentering the bag. If the nonrebreathing valve sticks in the inspiratory position, the patient will be attempting to exhale against a closed outlet and continued inflow will quickly cause a continuous and dangerous increase in pressure. A variety of other conditions can cause this, including interrupting manual ventilation to observe for spontaneous respiratory efforts, manually restricting bag refill, the valve contaminated with foreign material, a small squeeze or bump on the bag causing the valve to lock up, patient coughing, improper assembly, attaching an oxygen inlet nipple without vent holes directly to the resuscitator, failure of the expiratory flap valve to open, and a kink in the reservoir tail.

C. High Oxygen Inflow
Infant resuscitators are especially prone to obstruction with high flows because the bag is small. A case has been reported in which the pressure monitoring port was connected to an oxygen source. This distorted the valve and resulted in excessive pressure.

D. Pressure-Limiting Device Failure
Pressure-limiting devices can malfunction, opening well above an acceptable pressure.

E. Excessive Resistance
Some nonrebreathing valves offer high resistance to flow so that high negative pressures must be generated during spontaneous breathing.

F. Rebreathing
Rebreathing of exhaled gases can occur if the valve on the inspiratory limb from the bag is not competent or is improperly assembled. The fishmouth valve can become unseated, allowing rebreathing and/or insufficient pressure during inspiration. Extension tubing should not be placed between the patient and the valve.

G. Hypoventilation

1. Studies show that it is more difficult to achieve satisfactory ventilation with a resuscitation bag and a face mask than with a supraglottic airway device.
2. A defective nonrebreathing valve may have forward leak so that during inspiration a part of the volume expelled from the bag escapes through the expiratory port. Venting through the pressure-relief device may result in hypoventilation. The seal at the rear of the bag may not seat, allowing gas to exit. Hypoventilation can be caused by a disconnection or broken pieces on the resuscitator. It may be possible to misassemble the resuscitator so that when the bag is squeezed, the contents are exhausted to atmosphere. The bag may become detached from the nonrebreathing valve. If the fishmouth valve sticks or is absent, ventilation will not be possible.
3. Pediatric bags will not provide adequate volumes when used with adults. Using an intermediate size bag may result in adequate ventilation, with reduced risk of gastric inflation when using a face mask.
4. The operator is an important factor in determining the effectiveness of ventilation. Squeezing the bag may require considerable physical effort, and performance may deteriorate as the operator becomes fatigued. Operators with small hands may have difficulty delivering adequate tidal volumes. Squeezing the bag using one hand instead of two tends to lower the delivered volume. Adequate tidal volumes are frequently not delivered when a mask is used, unless two persons participate, one holding the mask and one squeezing the bag.

5. Because resuscitators are used away from the hospital, it is possible that they will be subjected to low temperatures. In this situation, the maximum cycling rate is often reduced and the units may become inoperable or incapable of delivering satisfactory ventilation.
6. If the pressure-relief device is set incorrectly, it may open at a low pressure, causing hypoventilation. Decreased tidal volume may be seen with increased resistance or decreased compliance.

H. Low Delivered Oxygen Concentration
1. Low delivered oxygen concentrations may be the result of insufficient oxygen flow, a detached or defective oxygen tubing, or problems with the oxygen-enrichment device. A defect in the nonrebreathing valve may result in oxygen not flowing to the patient. The reservoir may be too small for the tidal volume. Low temperatures may result in low inspired oxygen concentrations being delivered.
2. During spontaneous ventilation, the patient may inhale room air from the expiratory port as well as oxygen-enriched gas from the bag.

I. High Resistance
Some nonrebreathing valves offer high resistance to flow so that high negative pressures may be generated during spontaneous ventilation. The work of breathing may be quite high.

J. Contamination
Because these devices are often used with patients who have respiratory infections, they frequently become contaminated. Oxygen flowing through the valve may aerosolize bacteria and spread them into the surrounding air. For these reasons and because these devices are difficult to clean, disposable units have become popular. Filters (Chapter 5) may be used to avoid contamination of the device.

K. Foreign Body Inhalation
Part of the inside of the bag or parts of the nonrebreathing valve may break off and be inhaled.

VI. Checking Manual Resuscitators

A. Before use, the resuscitation bag should be visually inspected for signs of wear such as cracks or tears. After the bag has been inspected, it should be checked for leaks. The patient port should be occluded and the bag squeezed. Pressure should build up rapidly to a point at which the bag can no longer be compressed. If there is a pressure-limiting device, it can be checked by connecting a pressure manometer between the patient port and the bag by using a T-fitting. If there is an override mechanism on the pressure-limiting device, this should be checked. This check also determines that the refill valve will close when the bag is squeezed.

B. To check that the bag refill valve opens, the bag should be squeezed and then the patient port occluded and the bag released. The bag should expand rapidly.

C. If the resuscitator has a closed reservoir, its function can be checked by performing several compression release cycles with no oxygen flow into the reservoir. The reservoir should deflate, but the resuscitation bag should continue to expand.

D. A reservoir bag from a breathing system is placed over the patient port. Squeezing the resuscitation bag should cause the reservoir bag to inflate. After the reservoir bag has become fully inflated and the resuscitation bag has been released, the bag should deflate easily. This tests the inspiration and exhalation parts of the valve and the exhalation pathway for patency.

VII. Advantages

A. The equipment is inexpensive, compact, lightweight, and portable yet rugged.

B. The equipment is easy to use.

C. The equipment is simple with a small number of parts. Disassembly and reassembly are usually easily performed.

D. Dead space and rebreathing are minimal if the nonrebreathing valve functions properly.

E. With proper attention to the oxygen-enrichment device, oxygen flow, and ventilation technique, it is possible to administer close to 100% oxygen with most resuscitators.

F. During emergency situations in which connection to a gas source is not readily available, the resuscitator can be used with room air until a source of oxygen becomes available.

G. The operator has some feel for pressures and volumes delivered. Barotrauma may be less likely with these devices than with gas-powered resuscitators, which do not allow the operator to sense when the patient's lungs are fully inflated.

VIII. **Disadvantages**

A. Some of the valves are noisy and can stick, particularly when wet.

B. There may be considerable heat and humidity loss from the patient with prolonged use. Consideration should be given to using a heat and moisture exchanger (Chapter 9) with prolonged transport.

C. The feel of the bag is different from that in other breathing systems. The user's hands must be retrained.

D. The valve must be located at the patient's head. Its bulk may be troublesome, and its weight may cause the tracheal tube to kink or be displaced.

CLINICAL MOMENT During infant resuscitation, manual resuscitators are unreliable as free-flowing oxygen delivery devices.

CLINICAL MOMENT Do not use a manual resuscitator to delivery oxygen to a spontaneously breathing patient.

SUGGESTED READINGS

Dorsch J, Dorsch S. Manual resuscitators. In: Understanding Anesthesia Equipment. Fifth edition. Philadelphia: Wolters Kluwer/Lippincott Williams & Wilkins, 2008:282–295.

Mazzolini DGJ, Marshall NA. Evaluation of 16 adult disposable manual resuscitators. Respir Care 2004;49:1509–1514.

Martell RJ, Soder CM. Laerdal infant resuscitators are unreliable as free-flow oxygen delivery devices. Am J Perinatol 1997;14:347–351.

8 Controlling Trace Gas Levels

I. Introduction

A. Before scavenging was instituted, excess anesthetic gases and vapors were discharged into room air. Operating room personnel were exposed to these, with little concern about any detrimental effects that could result from such exposure. In more recent times, questions about possible hazards from exposure to trace amounts of anesthetic gases and vapors have been raised. (For the remainder of this chapter, anesthetic gases and vapors will be referred to as *gases*, because most vapors behave as gases.)

B. A trace level of an anesthetic gas is a concentration far below that needed for clinical anesthesia or that can be detected by smell. Trace gas levels are usually expressed in parts per million (ppm), which is volume/volume (100% of a gas is 1,000,000 ppm; 1% is 10,000 ppm).

C. Reported trace gas concentrations in operating rooms vary greatly, depending on the fresh gas flow, ventilation system, length of time that an anesthetic has been administered, measurement site, anesthetic technique, and other variables. Trace gas levels tend to be higher with pediatric anesthesia, in dental operatories, and in poorly ventilated postanesthetic care units (recovery rooms).

II. Personnel Health Risks

A. The evidence that trace anesthetic gases are harmful is at present suggestive rather than conclusive. The hazard, if it exists, is not great and is more properly regarded as disquieting than alarming. Researchers who have systematically examined the published data have concluded that reproductive problems in women were the only health effect for which there was reasonably convincing evidence. While it is reassuring to note from studies that anesthesiologists have a mortality rate less than that expected for physicians or the general population, reproductive problems are not reflected in mortality data and high cure rates may be responsible for the low mortality. One study showed an increased rate of early retirement as a result of ill health and a high rate of deaths while working among anesthesia personnel.

B. A cause and effect relationship between occupational exposure and the problems described has not been firmly established. If there is an increased risk, it may be related to other factors such as mental and physical stress; strenuous physical demands; disturbed night rest; the need for constant alertness; long and inconvenient working hours that often interfere with domestic life; irregular routine; exposure to infections, solvents, propellants, cleaning substances, lasers, methylmethacrylate, radiation, or ultraviolet light; preexisting health and reproductive problems; hormonal or dietary disturbances; the physical or emotional makeup of those who choose to work in operating rooms; socioeconomic factors; or some other as yet undefined factor.

III. Control Measures

A. Scavenging System

A scavenging system consists of five basic parts (**Fig. 8.1**): a gas collecting device, which captures gases at the site of emission; a transfer tubing, which conveys the collected gases to the interface; the interface, which provides positive (and sometimes negative) pressure relief and may provide reservoir capacity; the gas disposal tubing, which conducts the gases from the interface to the gas disposal system; and the gas disposal system, which conveys the gases to a point where they are discharged.

1. **Gas Collecting Device**

A gas collecting device is a part of the adjustable pressure-limiting (APL) valve in a breathing system or the spill valve on an anesthesia ventilator. Collection devices are also fitted to pump oxygenators. Gas monitors (Chapter 17) have a mechanism to either route gas that has passed through the monitor to the scavenging system or return monitored gas to the breathing system (**Fig. 8.2**).

2. **Transfer Tubing**

The transfer tubing conveys gas from the collecting assembly to the interface. It is commonly a length of tubing with a connector at either end. The inlet and outlet fittings can be either 19 or 30 mm so that it cannot be interconnected

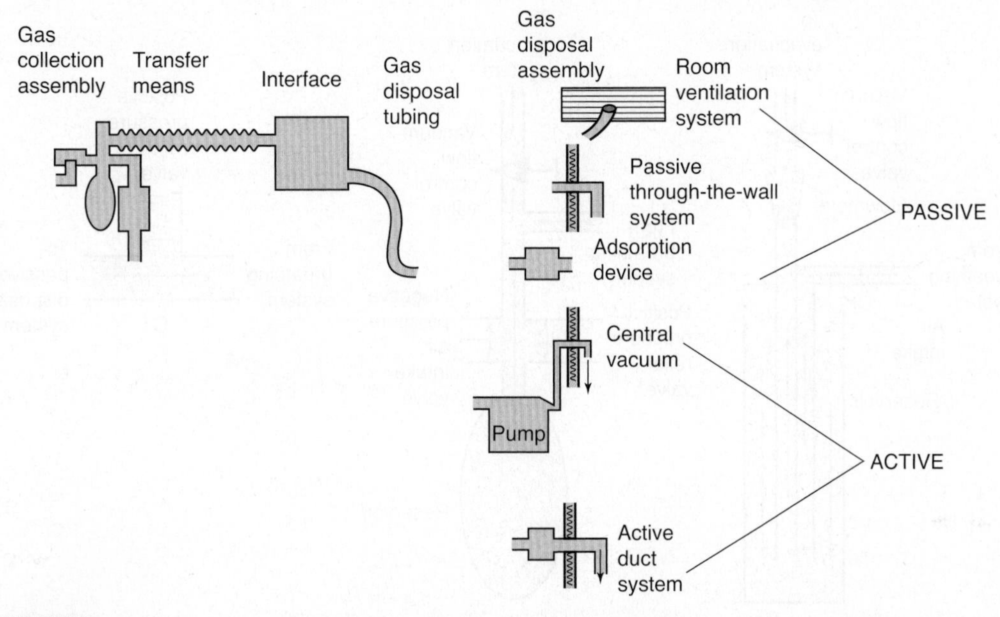

Figure 8.1 Complete scavenging system. The gas collecting assembly may be an integral part of the breathing system, ventilator, gas monitor, or extracorporeal pump oxygenator. The interface may be an integral part of the gas collecting assembly or some other portion of the scavenging system.

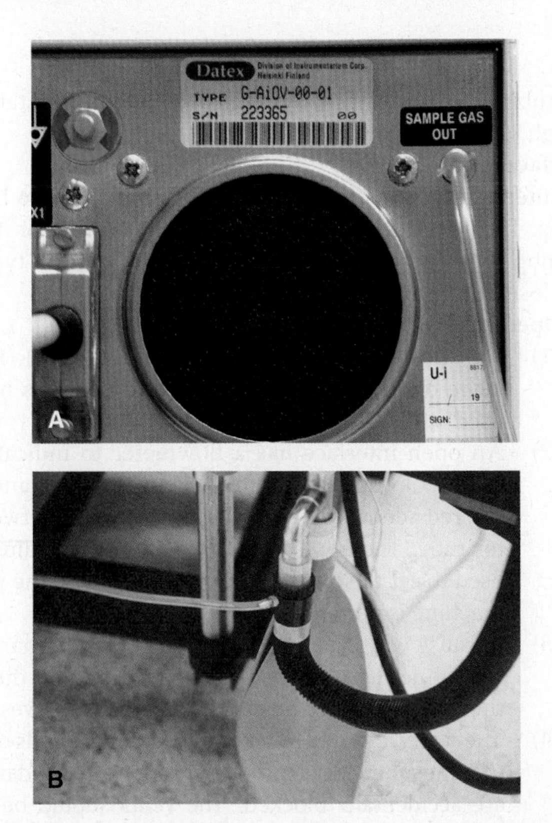

Figure 8.2 **A:** Gas monitor with sample gas outlet (at *upper right*). **B:** Connection of transfer tubing near the interface.

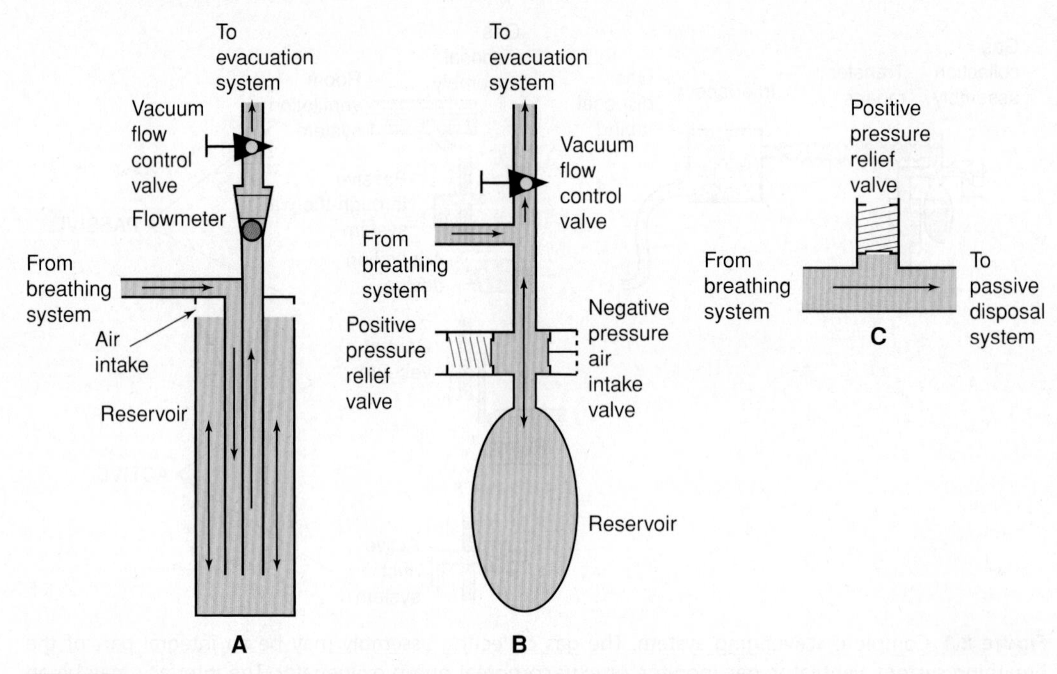

Figure 8.3 **A:** An open interface. Note the air intake ports at the top of the reservoir. These provide positive and negative pressure relief. **B,C:** Closed interfaces. *A* and *B* are active systems. *C* is a passive system.

with tubing in the breathing systems. It should be resistant to kinking and short enough to not touch the floor.

3. **Interface**

   The interface receives gas from the collecting device by way of the transfer tubing. The interface is designed to prevent positive or negative pressure from reaching the breathing system. There are two basic types of interface: open and closed.

   a. Open Interface

      1) An open interface (air break receiver unit) (**Fig. 8.3A**) has one or more openings to atmosphere and contains no valves. It should be used only with an active disposal system.
      2) An open interface has a flowmeter to indicate that the vacuum is turned ON and flow is adequate (**Figs. 8.3A** and **8.4**). Vacuum is considered adequate if the indicator is between two lines on the flowmeter tube. There is usually a vacuum flow adjustment control that is used to set the optimal flow and turn OFF the vacuum flow when the machine is not in use.
      3) Because waste gases are intermittently discharged while the vacuum is continuous, a reservoir is needed to hold the gas surges that enter the interface until the disposal system removes them.
      4) The safety afforded by an open system depends on the vents being open to atmosphere. It is important to have redundant outlets in case some are accidentally blocked. The vents should be checked and cleaned regularly. Plastic bags and surgical drapes should be kept away from the vents.

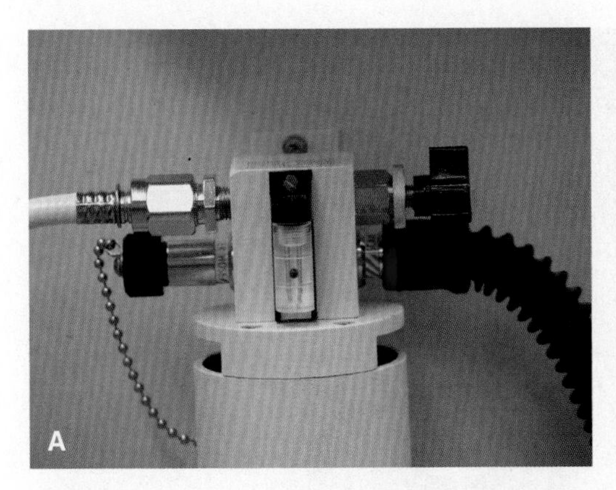

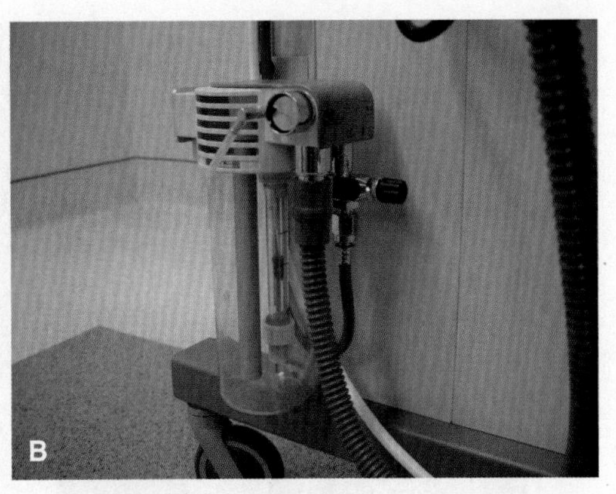

Figure 8.4 Open interfaces. The open ports at the top of the canister provide positive and negative pressure relief. The flow control valve is used to regulate the scavenging flow. The flowmeter indicates whether or not the flow is within the range recommended by the manufacturer. The float should be between the two markings on the flowmeter. Inside the canister, one tube conducts waste gases to the bottom and the other tube conducts gases from the bottom to the disposal system.

CLINICAL MOMENT Be certain to check that the flow to an open interface is turned ON and is adequate before beginning an anesthetic administration. This should be part of the routine checkout procedure.

b. Closed Interface

1) A closed interface (**Figs. 8.3B, C**) makes its connection(s) to atmosphere through valve(s). A positive pressure relief valve is always required to allow gases to be released into the room if there is obstruction or a malfunction in the scavenging system downstream from the interface. If an active disposal system is to be used, a negative pressure relief (pop-in, air inlet relief) valve is necessary to allow air to be entrained when the pressure in the reservoir falls below atmospheric pressure. A reservoir is not required with a closed interface unless an active disposal system is used. If an active disposal system is used, a distensible bag is present both to handle gas surges and to monitor scavenging system function.

CLINICAL MOMENT If the interface has a reservoir bag, it should be observed intermittently during a case. If the bag fully distends, the vacuum flow should be increased. If it remains fully collapsed, the vacuum flow should be decreased.

CLINICAL MOMENT If the valves for a closed interface fail to function properly, either positive pressure or negative pressure may be transmitted to the breathing system. These valves should be checked for proper function during the initial machine checkout (see Chapter 26).

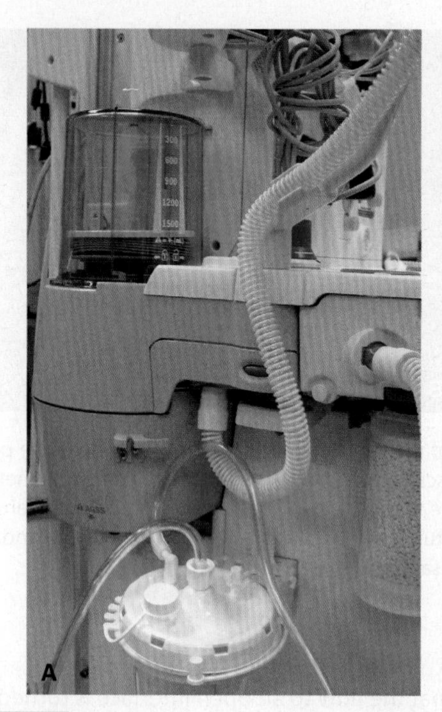

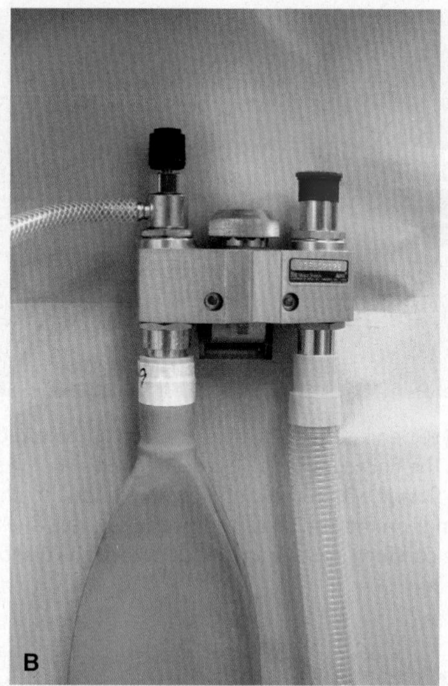

Figure 8.5 Closed interfaces. Note the wide-bore flexible transfer tubing that is different in appearance from the breathing system tubes.

2) A closed interface with a positive pressure relief valve should be used only with a passive disposal system. An example is shown in **Figure 8.3C.** The positive pressure relief valve remains closed unless there is an obstruction downstream of the interface.
3) Examples of the closed interfaces are shown in **Figures 8.3B, C** and **8.5.** If an active disposal system is used, the negative pressure relief valve should close during high peak flow rates from the gas collecting assembly and open when the vacuum flow into the gas disposal assembly is greater than the flow of gases entering the gas collecting assembly from the breathing system.

4. **Gas Disposal Tubing**

   The gas disposal tubing (receiving hose, disposal tubing) connects the interface to the disposal system (**Fig. 8.1**). In most active systems, this will be a hose to the vacuum piping system. To avoid misconnections, it should be different in size and appearance from the breathing system hoses. It should be resistant to collapse and free of leaks. With a passive gas disposal system, it is important that the hose be as short and wide as practical to minimize resistance.

5. **Gas Disposal System**

   The gas disposal system (elimination system or route, disposal exhaust route, disposal assembly) removes waste gases from the anesthetizing location. The gases must be vented to the outside at a point that is isolated from personnel and any intake from the air.

   a. Passive Systems

   Passive systems utilize the positive pressure of gases that leave the interface. The pressure is raised above the atmospheric pressure by the patient's exhaled gases, by manually squeezing the reservoir bag, or by a ventilator releasing excess gas through its spill valve. Passive systems are simpler than active systems but may not be as effective in lowering trace gas levels.

1) Room Ventilation System
There are two types of ventilation systems used in operating rooms: nonrecirculating (one-pass, single-pass, 100% fresh air) and recirculating. A nonrecirculating system takes in exterior air, filters it, and adjusts the humidity and temperature. The processed air is circulated through the room and then all of it is exhausted to atmosphere. This type of ventilation system can be used for waste gas disposal by securing the disposal tubing to a convenient exhaust grille. Air flowing into the grille removes the gases. The nonrecirculating systems are expensive to operate and are not often used today.

2) Piping Directly to Atmosphere
Piping directly to the atmosphere is also known as a through-the-wall system. Excess gases are vented through the wall, window, ceiling, or floor to the outside. This type of system is not suitable for an operating room that is far from an outside wall.

b. Active Gas Disposal Systems
Active disposal systems utilize flow-inducing devices such as fans or negative pressure relief valves from the vacuum system to move the gases from the interface to the outside. There will be a negative pressure in the gas disposal tubing. Active systems are usually more effective in keeping pollution levels low. They allow smaller bore tubing to be used, and excessive resistance is not a problem. They also aid in room air exchange. They are not automatic and must be turned ON and OFF. If they are not turned ON, air pollution will occur; if they are not turned OFF when not in use, there will be needless energy waste. Active systems are more complex than passive ones. Their use requires that the interface have negative pressure relief.

1) Piped Vacuum
   (i) The central vacuum system is a popular method for gas disposal. Newer facilities have a separate system for gas scavenging with a different connection (**Fig. 8.6**). The system should be capable of providing a flow of high volume (30 L/minute), but only slight negative pressure is needed. The flow is controlled at the interface. This will conserve energy, reduce the load on the central pumps, and reduce the noise level. This is done by observing the reservoir bag and the positive and negative pressure relief valves on the interface or adjusting the flow to levels recommended by the manufacturer (**Fig 8.4**).
   (ii) The disadvantages of this type of system may include an inadequate number of vacuum outlets for scavenging and other uses, inconveniently located outlets, and vacuum system overload.

2) Active Duct System
   (i) The other type of active disposal assembly is a dedicated evacuation system that leads to the outside and employs flow-inducing devices (fans, pumps, blowers, etc.) that can move large volumes of gas at low pressures. The negative pressure helps to ensure that cross contamination between operating rooms does

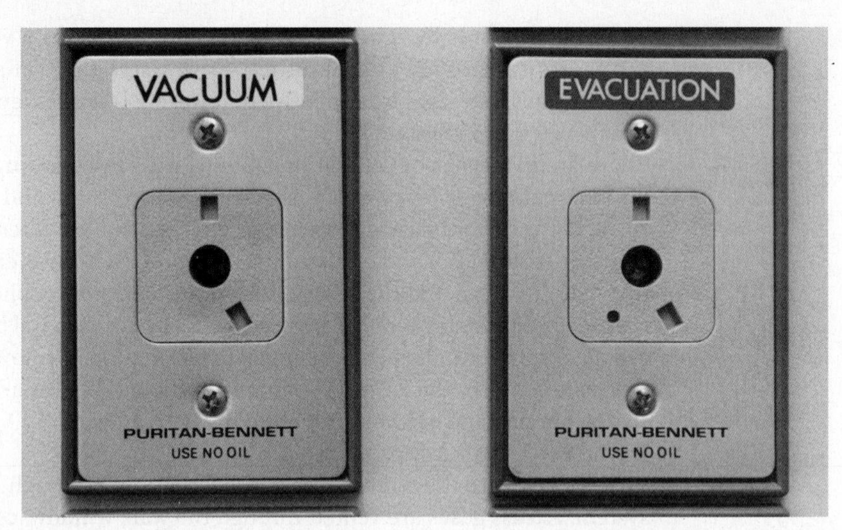

Figure 8.6 Inlet for anesthetic gas evacuation (at *right*). A probe attached to the gas transfer disposal tubing is inserted into this inlet.

not occur and prevents atmospheric conditions from affecting the outflow from the system.

(ii) The advantages of the active duct system are that resistance is not a problem and wind currents do not affect the system. Disadvantages include those present in any active system: added complexity and the need for negative pressure relief and reservoir capacity in the interface. It requires a special installation, which should be considered during renovation or when a new anesthetizing location is being designed. The flow-inducing device means added energy consumption and requires regular maintenance.

B. Altered Work Practice

Simply adding equipment to collect and dispose of excess gases is not enough to reduce trace anesthetic gases in the operating room environment. Work practices need to be altered to prevent these gases from entering the room. Adhering to the following practices will significantly reduce contamination. Most can be followed without compromising safety, and some are beneficial to the patient. Trace gas monitoring can be used to demonstrate to personnel the techniques needed to avoid polluting room air. Adhering to good work practices should not distract from patient comfort and safety.

1. **Checking Equipment Before Use**

a. Before starting an anesthetic administration, all components of the scavenging system should be securely connected and made patent. If an active gas disposal assembly is to be used, the flow should be turned ON.

b. Leaks in the anesthesia machine and the breathing system can contribute to operating room contamination. The preuse checkout (Chapter 26) should reveal these leaks so that they can be corrected.

c. Nitrous oxide should be turned ON only momentarily during the preuse equipment checkout. Most tests should be conducted by using oxygen or air.

2. **Good Airway Equipment Fit**
   a. Obtaining a good mask fit requires skill but is critical to maintain the lowest possible levels of anesthetic gases in the room, especially during assisted or controlled ventilation when higher pressures will magnify the leak between the patient and the mask. An active scavenging device near the mask can reduce room pollution from a poor fit. Pollution is also a problem with supraglottic airway devices, although lower levels of anesthetic gases are found with these devices than with face masks.
   b. Using cuffed tracheal tubes will reduce environmental contamination from waste anesthetic gases. Only small leaks should be permitted around uncuffed tubes. When using an uncuffed tube, contamination can be reduced by placing a suction catheter in the mouth and using a throat pack.
3. **Preventing Anesthetic Gas Flow Directly into the Room**
   a. Nitrous oxide and other agents should not be turned ON until the mask is fitted to the patient's face. Turning the gas flow (but not the vaporizer) OFF during intubation is also a good practice. This maintains postintubation concentrations close to preintubation levels and decreases operating room pollution. The patient connection port on the breathing system can be blocked during intubation, but care should be taken that part of the blocking device does not become dislodged and enter the breathing system. The fresh gas flow should be turned OFF or the APL valve opened to prevent the bag from overfilling.
   b. Disconnections can be prevented by making certain that all connections are tight before use. Disconnections for activities such as taping the tracheal tube or positioning the patient should be kept to a minimum. If it is necessary to make a disconnection, releasing anesthetic gases into the room can be minimized if the reservoir bag is first gradually emptied into the scavenging system and then the fresh gas flow is turned OFF. Alternately, the patient port can be occluded and the APL valve opened so that the gases will enter the scavenging system. If a ventilator (which has its own spill valve) is being used, the APL valve does not need to be opened.
4. **Washing Out Anesthetic Gases at the End of a Case**
   At the end of a case, 100% oxygen should be administered before extubation or the face mask or supraglottic device is removed to flush most of the anesthetic gases into the scavenging system.
5. **Preventing Liquid Agent Spills**
   It is easy to spill liquid agent when filling a vaporizer, so care should be exercised. Using an agent-specific filling device (Chapter 4) will reduce spillage. Devices that reduce spillage when using funnel fill vaporizers are available. The connections for filling and draining a vaporizer should be kept tight. Vaporizers should be filled before or after the cases for the day when no other operating room personnel are in the room.
6. **Avoiding Certain Techniques**
   Insufflation techniques, in which an anesthetic mixture is introduced into the patient's respiratory system during inhalation without a supraglottic airway device or tracheal tube, are sometimes used for laryngoscopy and bronchoscopy. High anesthetic flow rates are required to avoid dilution with room air

and result in a cloud of anesthetic gases escaping into the room air. Local scavenging can be used to remove the anesthetic gases if an insufflation technique is used.

7. **Disconnecting Nitrous Oxide Sources**
   a. Nitrous oxide and oxygen pipeline hoses leading to the machine should be disconnected at the end of the operating schedule. The disconnection should be made as close to the wall terminal unit as possible and not at the back of the anesthesia machine so that if there is a leak in the hose, no gases will escape into the room.
   b. When cylinders are used, the cylinder valve should be closed at the end of the operating schedule. Gas remaining in the machine should be "bled out" and evacuated through the scavenging system.
8. **Low Fresh Gas Flows**
   Using low fresh gas flows will reduce the pollution resulting from disconnections in the breathing system and from inefficient scavenging. Low gas flow anesthesia is discussed in Chapter 5.
9. **Intravenous Agents and Regional Anesthesia**
   Using intravenous techniques or regional anesthesia significantly reduces trace gas exposure.
10. **Keeping the Scavenging Hose Off the Floor**
    A scavenging hose on the floor can be obstructed or damaged by equipment rolling over it, thus reducing scavenging.

C. Leak Control
   1. Some leaks are unavoidable, but they can be minimized. Leak control may require replacing equipment that cannot be made gas-tight.
   2. Most anesthesia machines are serviced at regular intervals. Unfortunately, this servicing does not always identify or correct all leak points. Leaks in some equipment develop fairly frequently, so quarterly servicing is not sufficient. In-house monitoring and maintenance can minimize leakage.

IV. Scavenging Equipment Hazards

A. Misassembly
Most scavenging components have 19- or 30-mm connectors rather than the 15- and 22-mm ones found in breathing systems. This will not completely prevent misconnections, because there may be other apparatus in the room that will accept 19- or 30-mm connectors and sometimes a 19- or 30-mm connector can be fitted onto a 22-mm one. The safety provided by 19- and 30-mm connectors can be bypassed by using cheater adapters or tape for making connections.

B. Pressure Alterations in the Breathing System
When a scavenging system malfunctions or is misused, positive or negative pressure can be transmitted to the breathing system. This is more likely to occur with closed interfaces. Measures to prevent these untoward incidents include employing collapse-resistant material in all disposal lines, making the transfer means easy to disconnect, incorporating positive and negative pressure relief valves in the interface, regularly checking the valves for proper function, using an open interface, and using airway pressure monitors (Chapter 18).

1. **Positive Pressure**
   a. Positive pressure in the scavenging system can result from an occlusion in the transfer or gas disposal tubing. This may be caused by an anesthesia machine or other equipment rolling onto the tubing. Ice, insects, water, or other foreign matter may clog the scavenging system external outlet. Other

causes are defective components and a misassembled connection to the exhaust grille.

b. Positive pressure may result even when a positive pressure relief mechanism is incorporated into the interface. The positive pressure relief mechanism may be incorrectly assembled, may not open at a low enough pressure, or may be blocked. Transfer tubing obstruction or misconnection may occur. Because these problems are on the patient side of the interface, disconnecting the transfer means from the gas collecting assembly may be necessary to prevent a dangerous increase in pressure. All tubings that conduct scavenged gas should be off the floor or protected so that they cannot become obstructed.

2. **Negative Pressure**

a. If an active disposal system is in use and the APL valve is fully open, there is a danger that subambient pressure will be applied to the breathing system. Monitoring expired volume (but not airway pressure) may fail to detect a disconnection in the breathing system because the scavenging system may draw a considerable flow.

CLINICAL MOMENT Some APL valves when fully open do not offer any resistance to negative pressure being transmitted to the scavenging system. Slightly closing the APL valve may be necessary to prevent gas from being evacuated from the breathing system.

b. The negative pressure relief mechanism may malfunction. Another problem is using an interface designed for a passive system (which has no means to prevent subatmospheric pressure) in an active scavenging system. A restrictive orifice is incorporated into the vacuum hose fitting in some scavenging systems that use the central vacuum system. This orifice limits gas evacuation, regardless of the pressure applied by the central vacuum source. If this orifice is omitted or becomes damaged, excessive vacuum will be applied to the interface and the negative pressure relief mechanism capacity may be exceeded.

c. Ways to prevent negative pressure from being transmitted to the breathing system include making provision of one or more negative relief mechanisms in the interface with an active disposal system, adjusting the flow through the gas disposal system to the minimum necessary, and protecting the openings to atmosphere from accidental occlusion.

C. Loss of Monitoring Input

A scavenging system may mask the strong odor of a volatile anesthetic agent, delaying overdose recognition. Anesthetic agent monitoring (Chapter 17) should largely overcome this problem.

D. Alarm Failure

A case has been reported in which negative pressure from being transmitted to the scavenging system interface prevented the ventilator bellows from collapsing when a disconnection in the breathing system occurred. The low airway pressure alarm in the ventilator was not activated. In another case, room air was drawn into the breathing system through a disconnection, preventing the low minute volume alarm from sounding.

SUGGESTED READINGS

American Society of Anesthesiologists. Waste Anesthetic Gases: Information for Management in Anesthetizing Areas and the Postanesthesia Care Unit (PACU). Park Ridge, IL: American Society of Anesthesiologists, 1999. www.ASAhq.org/publications.

Barker JP, Abdelatti MO. Anaesthetic pollution. Potential sources, their identification and control. Anaesthesia 1997;52:1077–1083.

Dorsch J, Dorsch S. Controlling trace gas levels. In: Understanding Anesthesia Equipment. Fifth edition. Philadelphia: Wolters Kluwer/Lippincott Williams & Wilkins, 2008:373–401.

Nilsson R, Björdal C, Anderson M, et al. Health risks and occupational exposure to volatile anaesthetics—a review with a systematic approach. Clin Nurs 2005;14:173–186.

9 Humidification Devices

I. General Considerations

A. Terminology

1. *Humidity* is a general term used to describe the amount of water vapor in a gas. It may be expressed in several ways.
2. *Absolute humidity* is the mass of water vapor present in a volume of gas. It is commonly expressed in milligrams of water per liter of gas.
3. The maximum amount of water vapor that a volume of gas can hold is the humidity at saturation. This varies with the temperature. The warmer the temperature, the more water vapor that can be held. **Table 9.1** shows the absolute humidity of saturated gas at various temperatures. At a body temperature of 37°C, it is 44 mg H_2O/L.
4. *Relative humidity,* or *percent saturation,* is the amount of water vapor at a particular temperature expressed as a percentage of the amount that would be held if the gas were saturated.
5. Humidity may also be expressed as the pressure exerted by water vapor in a gas mixture. **Table 9.1** shows the vapor pressure of water in saturated gas at various temperatures.

B. Interrelationships

1. If a gas saturated with water vapor is heated, its capacity to hold moisture increases and it becomes unsaturated (has <100% relative humidity). Its absolute humidity remains unchanged. Gas that is 100% saturated at room temperature and warmed to body temperature without additional humidity will absorb water by evaporation from the surface of the respiratory tract mucosa until it becomes saturated.
2. If a gas saturated with water vapor is cooled, water will condense (rain out). The absolute humidity will fall, but the relative humidity will remain at 100%.
3. If an inspired gas is to have a relative humidity of 100% at body temperature, it must be maintained at the body temperature after leaving the humidifier or heated above the body temperature at the humidifier and allowed to cool as it flows to the patient. Cooling will result in condensation (rainout) in the breathing system.
4. The specific heat of a gas is low. As a consequence, it quickly assumes the temperature of the surrounding environment. Inhaled gases quickly approach body temperature, and gases in corrugated tubes rapidly approach room temperature.
5. The heat of vaporization of water is relatively high. Water evaporation, therefore, requires considerably more heat than is needed to warm gas. Likewise, water condensation yields more heat than gas cooling.

Table 9.1 Water Vapor Pressure and Absolute Humidity in Moisture-Saturated Gas

Temperature (°C)	mg H_2O/L	mm Hg
0	4.84	4.58
1	5.19	4.93
2	5.56	5.29
3	5.95	5.69
4	6.36	6.10
5	6.80	6.54
6	7.26	7.01
7	7.75	7.51
8	8.27	8.05
9	8.81	8.61
10	9.40	9.21
11	10.01	9.84
12	10.66	10.52
13	11.33	11.23
14	12.07	11.99
15	12.82	12.79
16	13.62	13.63
17	14.47	14.53
18	15.35	15.48
19	16.30	16.48
20	17.28	17.54
21	18.33	18.65
22	19.41	19.83
23	20.57	21.07
24	21.76	22.38
25	23.04	23.76
26	24.35	25.21
27	25.75	26.74
28	27.19	28.35
29	28.74	30.04
30	30.32	31.82
31	32.01	33.70
32	33.79	35.66
33	35.59	37.73
34	37.54	39.90
35	39.57	42.18
36	41.53	44.56
37	43.85	47.07
38	46.16	49.69
39	48.58	52.44
40	51.03	55.32
41	53.66	58.34
42	56.40	61.50

II. Considerations for Anesthesia

A. Humidification during Anesthesia

1. Gases delivered from the anesthesia machine are dry and at room temperature. As gases flow to the alveoli, they are brought to body temperature (by heating or cooling) and 100% relative humidity (by evaporation or condensation). In the unintubated patient, the upper respiratory tract (especially the nose) functions as the principal heat and moisture exchanger. During normal nasal breathing, the temperature in the upper trachea is between 30°C and 33°C, with a relative humidity of approximately 98%, providing a water content of 33 mg/L.
2. Tracheal tubes and supraglottic airway devices bypass the upper airway, modifying the pattern of heat and moisture exchange so that the tracheobronchial mucosa must assume a greater role in heating and humidifying gases.

B. Effects of Inhaling Dry Gases

The importance of humidification in anesthesia remains uncertain. It is of greatest benefit in pediatric patients, patients at increased risk for developing pulmonary complications, and patients undergoing long procedures.

1. **Damage to the Respiratory Tract**
   a. As the respiratory mucosa dries and its temperature drops, secretions thicken, ciliary function is reduced, surfactant activity is impaired, and the mucosa becomes more susceptible to injury. If secretions are not cleared, atelectasis or airway obstruction can result. Thickened plugs may provide loci for infection. Dry gases can cause bronchoconstriction, further compromising respiratory function. Humidifying gases may decrease the incidence of respiratory complications (coughing and breath holding) associated with an inhalation induction.
   b. There is no agreement on the minimum humidity necessary to prevent pathological changes. Recommendations have ranged from 12 to 44 mg H_2O/L. Exposure duration is important. It is unlikely that a brief exposure to dry gases will damage the tracheobronchial tree. As time increases, the likelihood that significant tracheobronchial damage will occur becomes greater.
2. **Body Heat Loss**
   Body temperature is lowered as the airways bring the inspired gas into thermal equilibrium and saturate it with water. Using a humidification device can decrease the heat loss that occurs during general anesthesia and may provide some heat input, but controlling inspired gas temperature and humidity is not an efficient method of maintaining body temperature. Means to increase body temperature are discussed in Chapter 24.
3. **Tracheal Tube Obstruction**
   Thickened secretions in a tracheal tube increase its resistance and can result in complete obstruction.

C. Consequences of Excessive Humidity

An increased water load can cause ciliary degeneration and paralysis, pulmonary edema, altered alveolar-arterial oxygen gradient, decreased vital capacity and compliance, and a decrease in hematocrit and serum sodium levels.

III. Sources of Humidity

A. Carbon Dioxide Absorbent

The reaction of an absorbent with carbon dioxide liberates water (Chapter 5). Water is also contained in the absorbent granules. Since the reaction is exothermic, heat is produced. If the absorbent granules become desiccated, they may react with certain anesthetics and produce extreme heat (see Chapter 5).

B. Exhaled Gases
   1. Some rebreathing occurs in a tracheal tube, supraglottic airway device, face mask and connections to the breathing system. Almost half of the humidity in the expired gas is preserved in this manner.
   2. In systems that allow rebreathing of exhaled gases (Chapter 5), the humidity and temperature of inspired gases depend on the relative proportions of fresh and expired gases. This will depend on the system and the fresh gas flow. As the flow of the fresh gas is increased, the temperature and humidity of inspired gases are reduced.

C. Moistening the Breathing Tubes and the Reservoir Bag
Rinsing the inside of the breathing tubes and the reservoir bag with water before use increases the inspired humidity.

D. Low Fresh Gas Flows
Using low fresh gas flows with a circle breathing system will conserve moisture. This is discussed in more detail in Chapter 5.

E. Coaxial Breathing Circuits
Coaxial circle systems, when combined with low flows, will increase the humidity more quickly than a system with two separate limbs because the inspiratory flow is heated somewhat by the exhaled gases in the circle system, but this is not very efficient in terms of improvement in heat or humidity. The Bain system (see Chapter 5) does not meet optimal humidification requirements because of the high fresh gas flow required.

IV. Heat and Moisture Exchangers

A heat and moisture exchanger (HME) conserves some exhaled water and heat and returns them to the patient in the inspired gas. Many HMEs also perform bacterial/viral filtration and prevent inhalation of small particles. When combined with a filter for bacteria and viruses, it is called a *heat and moisture exchanging filter* (HMEF).

A. Description
HMEs are disposable devices, with the exchanging medium enclosed in a plastic housing. They vary in size and shape. Typical ones are shown in **Figure 9.1.** Each has a 15-mm female connection port at the patient end and a 15-mm male port at the breathing system end. The patient port may also have a concentric 22-mm male fitting (**Figs. 9.1C, D**). There may be a port to attach the gas sampling line for a respiratory gas monitor (**Figs. 9.1B, D**) or an oxygen line. The dead space inside an HME varies. Pediatric and neonatal HMEs with low dead space are available. Most modern HMEs are one of two types, hydrophobic or hygroscopic.

   1. **Hydrophobic**
      a. Hydrophobic HMEs have a hydrophobic membrane with small pores. The membrane is pleated to increase the surface area. A hydrophobic HME provides moderately good inspired humidity. Hydrophobic HME performance may be impaired by high ambient temperatures.
      b. Hydrophobic HMEs are efficient bacterial and viral filters. A pleated hydrophobic filter will consistently prevent the hepatitis C virus from passing, whereas a hygroscopic filter may be ineffective. At usual ventilatory pressures, they allow water vapor but not liquid water to pass through. They are associated with small increases in resistance even when wet.
   2. **Hygroscopic**
      a. Hygroscopic HMEs contain wool, foam, or a paper-like material coated with moisture-retaining chemicals. The medium may be impregnated with

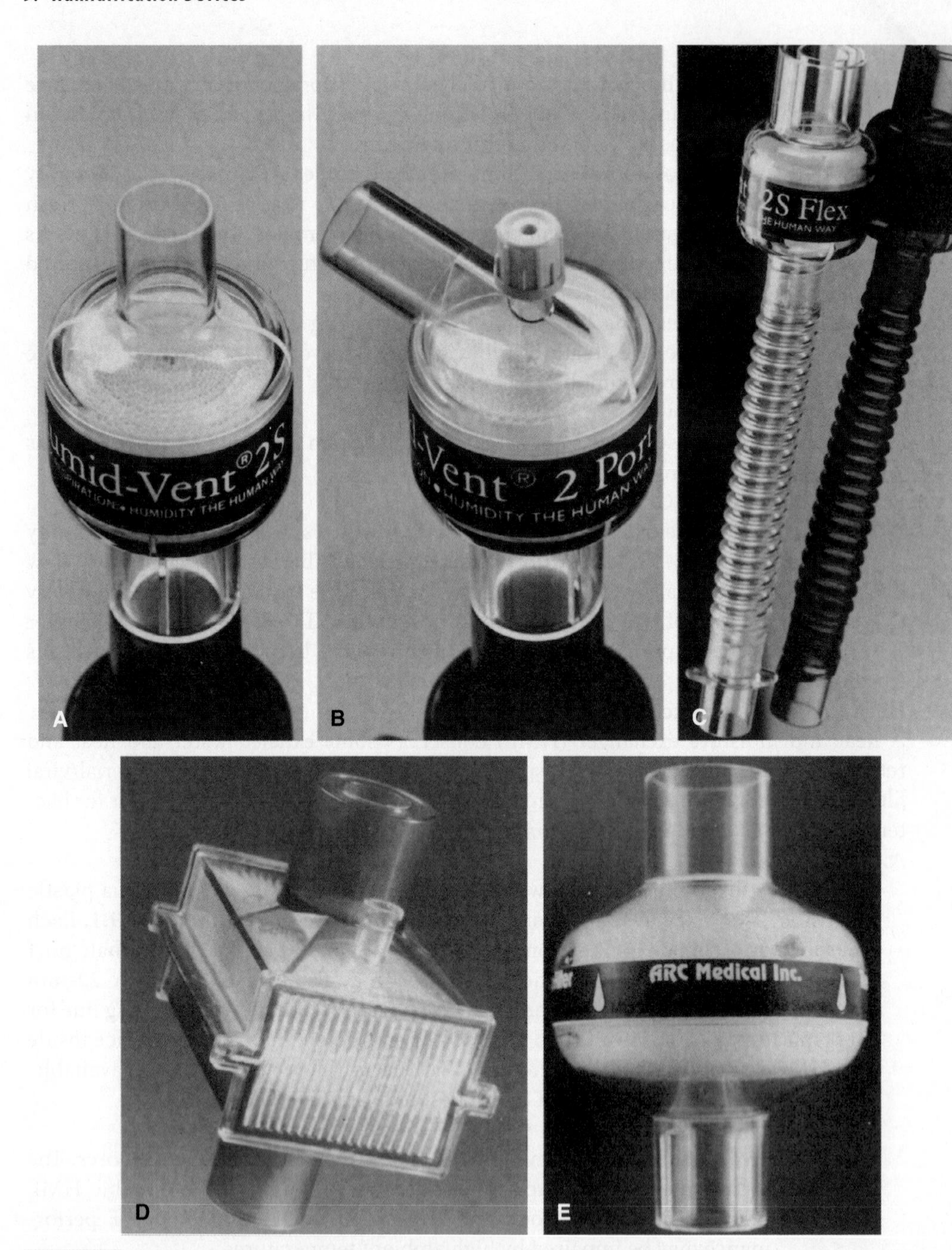

Figure 9.1 Heat and moisture exchangers. **A,E:** Straight variety. **B:** Right angle HME with a port for aspiration of respiratory gases on the breathing system side. **C:** The flexible tube attached to the HME extends the distance between the patient and the breathing system and allows the angle between the breathing system and the patient to be altered. Because this HME has significant dead space, it should be used only with high tidal volumes and controlled ventilation with monitoring of inspired and exhaled carbon dioxide. **D:** Hydrophobic HME with respiratory gas aspiration port. (Photographs C, D, and E courtesy of Gibeck Respiration, Pall Corporation, Post Washington, NY, and ARC Medical Inc., Tucker, GA.)

a bactericide. Composite hygroscopic HMEs consist of a hygroscopic layer plus a layer of thin, nonwoven fiber membrane that has been subjected to an electrical field to increase its polarity. This improves filtration efficiency and hydrophobicity.

b. Most studies have shown that composite hygroscopic HMEs are more efficient at moisture and temperature conservation than hydrophobic ones. They will lose their airborne filtration efficiency if they become wet, and microorganisms held by the filter medium can be washed through the device. Their resistance can increase greatly when they become wet.

B. Indications

1. An HME can be used to increase inspired heat and humidity during both short- and long-term ventilation. HMEs may be especially useful when transporting intubated patients, because transport ventilators frequently have no means for humidifying inspired gases.
2. An HME can be used to supply supplemental oxygen to an intubated patient or a patient with a supraglottic airway by connecting oxygen tubing to the gas sampling port.

C. Contraindications

Contraindications include patients with thick, copious, or bloody secretions and patients experiencing a leak that prevents exhaled gas from traversing the HME (e.g., bronchopleural cutaneous fistula and leaking or absent tracheal tube cuff). HMEs should be used with caution when weaning a patient from a respiratory support.

D. Factors Affecting Moisture Output

1. **Heat and Moisture Exchanger Type**
   Composite hygroscopic HMEs have better heat and moisture exchanging properties than do hydrophobic ones.
2. **Initial Humidity**
   Increasing the humidity of the gas entering the HME from the breathing system will increase the inspired humidity.
3. **Inspiratory and Expiratory Flows**
   The faster a gas passes through the HME, the less time there is for moisture to evaporate or deposit. A large tidal volume may cause the humidity in the inspired gas to fall.
4. **System Continuity**
   A leak around the tracheal tube will result in decreased inspired humidity.

E. Use

1. The HME selected should be of an appropriate size for the patient's tidal volume. If a small HME is used in a large patient, the HME will be inefficient. Connecting more than one HME in series will improve performance. Care should be taken that the units are pushed firmly together and that the increase in dead space is not excessive. Added dead space can especially be a problem with small patients.
2. The greatest inspired relative humidity occurs with the HME positioned next to the tracheal tube, mask, or supraglottic airway device. Some gas monitors (Chapter 17) are particularly sensitive to water. If the sampling line is on the anesthesia machine side of the HME, the monitor will be exposed to less moisture.
3. An HME can be used with any breathing system. With the Mapleson systems, dead space can be reduced by utilizing the gas sampling port as the

fresh gas inlet. Oxygen can be administered through the gas sample port on the HME. An HME may be used for a patient who has undergone tracheostomy.

4. An HME may be used as the sole source of humidity or may be combined with another source such as an unheated humidifier but should not be used with a heated humidifier.
5. If a nebulizer or metered-dose inhaler (Chapter 5) is used to deliver medication, it should be inserted between the HME and the patient or the HME be removed from the circuit during aerosol treatment.
6. An HME should be replaced if it is contaminated with secretions.

F. Advantages

HMEs are inexpensive, easy to use, small, lightweight, reliable, simple in design, and silent during operation. They have low resistance when dry. They do not require water, an external source of energy, a temperature monitor, or alarms. There is no danger of overhydration, hyperthermia, skin or respiratory tract burns, or electrical shock. Their use may increase the correlation between esophageal and core temperatures. They act as a barrier to large particles, and some are efficient bacterial and viral filters, although their role in reducing nosocomial infections remains controversial. They may reduce problems caused by humidity in the breathing system such as obstructed lines and ventilator malfunction.

G. Disadvantages

1. The main disadvantage of HMEs is the limited humidity that these devices can preserve. Their contribution to temperature preservation is not significant. Temperature management is discussed in Chapter 24. Active heating and humidification are more effective than an HME in retaining body heat, alleviating thick secretions, and preventing tracheal tube blockage. The difference is more apparent when intubation lasts for several days.
2. Placing an HME between the breathing system and the patient increases dead space. This may necessitate an increase in tidal volume and can lead to dangerous rebreathing. It also increases the work of breathing during both inspiration and exhalation. The increased work of breathing and the added dead space can be especially troublesome in small patients.
3. HME and HMEF components occasionally enter the breathing system and cause increased resistance.

H. Hazards

1. **Excessive Resistance**
   a. Using an HME increases resistance, although usually it is not a major component of the total work of breathing. Resistance increases with use. Heavy viscous secretions can greatly increase resistance.

CLINICAL MOMENT An HME should not be used with a heated humidifier, because the humidifier can cause a dangerous increase in resistance. Nebulized medication increases the resistance of hygroscopic HMEs.

   b. With a Mapleson system, increased resistance may cause fresh gas to be diverted down the expiratory limb.
   c. High resistance may result in sufficient back pressure to prevent the low-airway-pressure alarm from being activated if there is a disconnection between the patient and the HME.

CLINICAL MOMENT If increased resistance is suspected during controlled ventilation, the peak pressure should be measured with and without the HME in place. Spontaneously breathing patients, especially pediatric patients, should be observed for signs of increased work of breathing.

2. **Airway Obstruction**
   a. An HME can become obstructed by fluid, blood, secretions, a manufacturing defect, or nebulized drugs. Parts may become detached and block the breathing system. The weight of the HME may cause the tracheal tube to kink.
   b. If an HME is used for long-term ventilation, occlusion of the tracheal tube may occur.
3. **Inefficient Filtration**
   Liquid can break through a hygroscopic HME, resulting in poor filtration.
4. **Foreign Particle Aspiration**
   Parts of the HME may become detached. The parts may then be inhaled by the patient.
5. **Rebreathing**
   The HME dead space may cause excessive rebreathing, especially with small tidal volumes. Special low-volume devices are available for pediatrics. Even these small devices may be too large for small infants. HMEs should not be used for mask ventilation of small infants.
6. **Leaks and Disconnections**
   Adding an HME to a breathing system increases the potential for disconnections and leaks.
7. **Hypothermia**
   Patient warming is discussed in Chapter 24. HMEs are a means to conserve heat, but the amount preserved by this method is small.
8. **Dry Carbon Dioxide Absorbent**
   HMEs decrease the amount of humidity available to the absorbent. The extent to which HMEs will lead to desiccation of the absorbent, if any, is unclear. The effect of dry carbon dioxide absorbents on the production of compound A and carbon monoxide is discussed in Chapter 5. In addition, dry absorbent will absorb some volatile agents. This can impede anesthetic induction with these agents.

V. Humidifiers

A humidifier (vaporizer or vaporizing humidifier) passes a stream of gas over water (passover), across wicks dipped in water (blow-by), or through water (bubble or cascade). Humidifiers may be heated or unheated. Unheated humidifiers cannot deliver more than about 9 mg H_2O/L.

A. Description

Humidifiers have a disposable or reusable humidification chamber that holds the water. There may be a reservoir that adds water as needed (**Fig. 9.2**). There may be a heating element to warm the water (**Fig. 9.3**). Humidified gas passes to the patient through the inspiratory tube. If this tube is not heated, water will condense in the tube as the gas cools and a water trap will be needed. Some humidifiers have a heated wire in the delivery tube to prevent cooling and humidity loss. Heating or insulating the inspiratory tube allows better control of the temperature and humidity delivered to the patient. A temperature monitor at the patient end of the circuit controls the amount of heat necessary to maintain proper humidification.

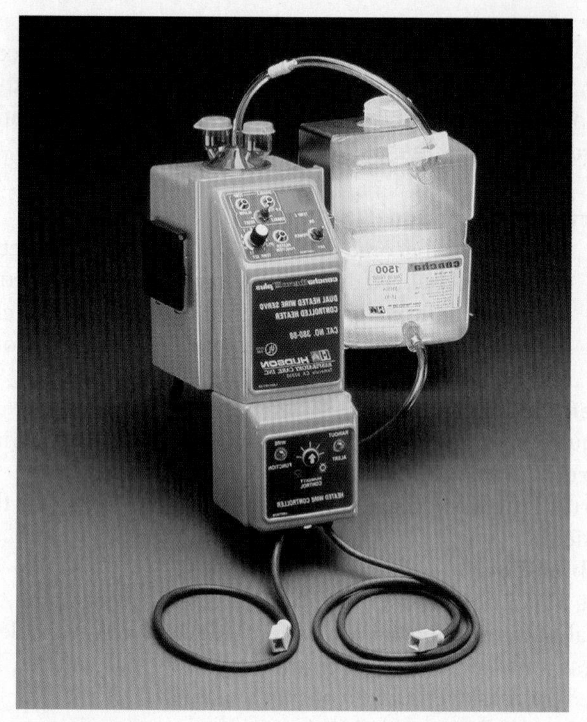

Figure 9.2 Heated humidifier with separate water reservoir. (Photograph courtesy of Hudson RCI, Research Triangle Park, NC.)

B. Use

1. In the circle system, a heated humidifier is placed in the inspiratory limb downstream of the unidirectional valve by using an accessory breathing tube. A heated humidifier must not be placed in the expiratory limb. If a filter is used in the breathing system, it must be placed upstream of the humidifier to prevent it from becoming clogged with water.

CLINICAL MOMENT Do not use a heated humidifier with an HME.

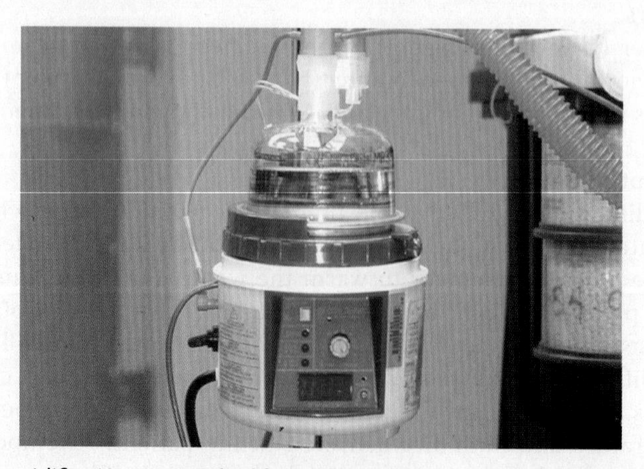

Figure 9.3 Heated humidifier. Heat is supplied from a heated plate below the humidification chamber. The heating wire at the left fits inside the delivery tube.

2. The humidifier must be located lower than the patient to avoid water running down the tubing into the patient's respiratory tract. The condensate must be drained periodically, or a water trap must be inserted into the most dependent part of the tubing to prevent blockage or aspiration.
3. The heater wire in the delivery tube should not be bunched but strung evenly along the length of the tube. The delivery tube should not rest on other surfaces or be covered with sheets, blankets, or other materials. A boom arm or tube tree may be used for support.

C. Advantages

Most heated humidifiers are capable of delivering saturated gas at body temperature or above, even with high flow rates. A heated humidifier can produce more effective humidification than an HME. Some (but not all) can be used for spontaneously breathing and tracheotomized patients.

D. Disadvantages

1. Humidifiers are bulky and somewhat complex. These devices involve high maintenance costs, electrical hazards, and increased work (temperature control, refilling the reservoir, draining condensate, cleaning, and sterilization). Their use is associated with higher costs than HMEs.
2. Compared with other warming modalities (Chapter 24), the heated humidifier offers relatively little protection against heat loss during anesthetic administration.

E. Hazards

1. **Infection**

   Bacterial growth can occur in water stored in a reservoir or the condensate in the delivery tube. The use of a heated circuit reduces the amount of condensate, which may reduce the risk of infection.

2. **Breathing System Problems**
   a. Reported breathing system problems include sticking valves, leaks, disconnections, incorrect connections, obstructed fresh gas line or inspiratory limb, noise, and clogged filters and HMEs.
   b. The delivery tubing may melt, resulting in an obstruction or leak. Fires have been reported. A charred breathing system may result in fumes entering the patient's lungs. Overheated breathing circuits with melting may be caused by defects in or damage to the heated wire; bunched heated wire coils within the breathing system; electrical incompatibility between the heated wire breathing circuit and the humidifier; operating the device outside the specified range of flows or minute volumes; or covering the delivery tube with sheets, blankets, or other materials. Problems may occur because of a circuit that is not compatible with the humidifier. While some circuits may be fitted to other manufacturers' humidifiers, they may not conform to the specifications of the humidifier being used. Electrical connectors for heated wire circuits that are physically compatible may not be electrically interchangeable.

CLINICAL MOMENT When there is no gas flow to the breathing system, turn the heated humidifier OFF. If the flow through the system is interrupted when a heated humidifier is ON, the temperature at the patient end will drop. This causes the heated humidifier to increase heat output, which could cause the adjacent breathing tube to melt.

c. Changes in Breathing System
Adding a humidifier may change the volume and compliance of the breathing system significantly. This can result in the delivery of a less accurate tidal volume from the anesthesia ventilator.

CLINICAL MOMENT If any humidifier is to be used, it should be added to the breathing system before the system is checked. Automated checkout programs needs to compensate for the added volume in order to program the ventilator for more accurate function.

3. **Water Aspiration**
There is danger of liquid water entering the trachea and asphyxiating the patient or causing a burn in the respiratory tract. These risks can be decreased by installing a water trap in both the inspiratory and exhalation sides in the most dependent portion of the breathing tube, draining condensate frequently, and placing the humidifier and breathing tubes below the patient.
4. **Overhydration**
A heated humidifier can produce a positive water balance and even overhydration. Although most anesthetics have a short-term effect so that this is usually not significant, it can be a problem with infants.
5. **Thermal Injury**
   a. Delivering overheated gases into the trachea can cause hyperthermia or damage to the tissues lining the tracheobronchial tree. Skin burns have been reported from administering heated oxygen nasally or when delivering continuous positive airway pressure. Burns can also occur when tissue is in contact with heated breathing circuits.
   b. Overheating inspired gas may be caused by omitting, misplacing, dislodging, or not fully inserting the airway temperature probe or by turning the humidifier ON with a low gas flow. A temporary increase in inspired gas temperature may occur following a period of interrupted flow or an increased flow rate.
6. **Increased Work of Breathing**
A heated humidifier increases resistance. Most cannot be used with spontaneously breathing patients.
7. **Monitoring Interference**
   a. A humidifier may add enough resistance to prevent a low airway pressure alarm from being activated if the sensor is upstream of the humidifier. Some flow sensors are affected by condensation, producing a false positive alarm. Pressure and flow monitoring are discussed in Chapter 18.
   b. High humidity can cause problems with sidestream (aspirating) respiratory gas monitors (Chapter 17).
8. **Equipment Damage or Malfunction**
   a. Some ventilators are sensitive to rainout caused by water condensation. Signs include increased resistance to exhalation, inaccurate pressure and volume measurements, autocycling, and ventilator shutdown. To prevent these problems, a water trap should be used if water is likely to condense in the breathing system. These need to be inspected regularly and emptied as needed. The humidifier needs to be placed lower than the patient and the ventilator.

b. Anesthesia gas monitors are sensitive to water. They commonly have water traps, but these can be overwhelmed with heated humidification.

VI. Nebulizers

A. Description

1. A nebulizer (aerosol generator, atomizer, nebulizing humidifier) emits water in the form of an aerosol mist (water vapor plus particulate water). The most commonly used ones are the pneumatically driven (gas-driven, jet, high-pressure, compressed gas) and ultrasonic nebulizers. Both can be heated. In addition to providing humidification, nebulizers may be used to deliver drugs.
2. A pneumatic nebulizer works by pushing a jet of high-pressure gas into a liquid, inducing shearing forces and breaking the water up into fine particles. An ultrasonic nebulizer produces a fine mist by subjecting the liquid to a high-frequency, electrically driven, ultrasonic resonator. The oscillation frequency determines the size of the droplets. There is no need for a driving gas. Ultrasonic nebulizers create a denser mist than pneumatic ones.

B. Use

Because a high flow of gas must be used with a pneumatic nebulizer, it should be placed in the fresh gas line. An ultrasonic nebulizer can be used in the fresh gas line or the inspiratory limb.

C. Hazards

1. Nebulized drugs may obstruct an HME or filter in the breathing system. Overhydation can occur. If the droplets are not warmed, hypothermia may result. Infection can be transmitted because microorganisms can be suspended in the water droplets.
2. There are reported cases in which a nebulizer was connected directly to a tracheal tube without provision for exhalation. In one case, this resulted in a pneumothorax.

D. Advantages

Nebulizers can deliver gases saturated with water without heat and, if desired, can produce gases carrying more water.

E. Disadvantages

Nebulizers are somewhat costly. Pneumatic nebulizers require high gas flows. Ultrasonic nebulizers require a source of electricity and may present electrical hazards. There may be considerable water deposition in the tubings, requiring frequent draining, installing water traps in both the inspiratory and exhalation tubes, and posing the dangers of water draining into the patient or blocking the tubing.

SUGGESTED READINGS

Carson KD. Humidification during anesthesia. Respir Care Clin N Am 1998;4:281–299.

Dellamonica J, Boisseau N, Goubaux B, Raucoules-Aimie M. Comparison of manufacturers' specifications for 44 types of heat and moisture exchanging filters. Br J Anaesth 2004;93:532–539.

Demers RR. Bacterial/viral filtration; Let the breather beware! Chest 2001;120:1377–1389.

Dorsch J, Dorsch S. Humidification equipment. In: Understanding Anesthesia Equipment. Fifth edition. Philadelphia: Wolters Kluwer/Lippincott Williams & Wilkins, 2008:296–309.

Lawes EG. Hidden hazards and dangers associated with the use of HME/filters in breathing circuits. Their effect on toxic metabolite production, pulse oximetry and airway resistance. Br J Anaesth 2003;91:249–264.

Lessard MR. Should we use breathing filters in anesthesia? Can J Anesth 2002;49:115–120.

Peterson BD. Heated humidifiers. Structure and function. Respir Care Clin N Am 1998;4:243–259.

Whitelock DE, de Beer DAH. The use of filters with small infants. Respir Care Clin N Am 2006;12:307–320.

Wilkes AR. Heat and moisture exchangers. Structure and function. Respir Care Clin N Am 1998;4:261–279.

10 Hazards of Anesthesia Machines and Breathing Systems

ALTHOUGH ENORMOUS STRIDES HAVE BEEN made in anesthesia apparatus safety, problems continue to be reported. Human error is more frequent than equipment failure. This chapter examines hazards of anesthesia machines and breathing systems from the perspective of their effect on the patient. Many examples are given, but this should not be considered a complete listing of all possible dangers. Many hazards involve older apparatus that may have been modified or is no longer sold or serviced by the manufacturer. Hazards are discussed in more detail in their related chapters.

I. Hypoxia

A. Hypoxic Inspired Gas Mixture

1. Incorrect Gas Supplied

a. Piping System

Reported pipeline problems include the wrong gas supplied, construction errors, crossovers in connected equipment, and incorrect gas hose or gas outlet connectors.

b. Cylinder

There may be an incorrect label or color. The pin index system may be overridden, or the cylinder contents may be incorrect.

c. Machine Crossover

If the anesthesia machine has been serviced or modified, there may be a plumbing crossover error that allows nitrous oxide to be delivered through the oxygen flowmeter.

2. **Hypoxic Mixture Set**
    a. Flow Control Valve Malfunction
    Wear or damage to the flow control valve may cause increased or decreased oxygen flow with a slight touch on the control.
    b. Incorrect Flowmeter Setting
    The minimum oxygen ratio device (Chapter 3) may malfunction, the oxygen flow may be inadvertently lowered, air may be used instead of oxygen, or the oxygen flowmeter may be incorrectly read (**Fig. 10.1**).
3. **Oxygen Loss to Atmosphere**
A leak may occur downstream of the oxygen flowmeter
4. **Air Entrainment**
If the pressure in the breathing system falls below atmospheric pressure, air may be drawn into the system. Subatmospheric pressure may be caused by a faulty scavenger interface, a hanging bellows or piston ventilator with low fresh gas flow, or an open adjustable pressure-limiting (APL) valve without sufficient resistance. Suction applied to an enteric tube placed in the trachea or through a bronchoscope may cause air to enter the lower airway.

II. **Hypoventilation**

A. Insufficient Gas in the Breathing System

1. **Low Inflow**
    a. Pipeline Problems
    There may be a loss of the pipeline supply, a leak or blockage in a pipeline hose, or a malfunctioning check valve at the anesthesia machine pipeline inlet.

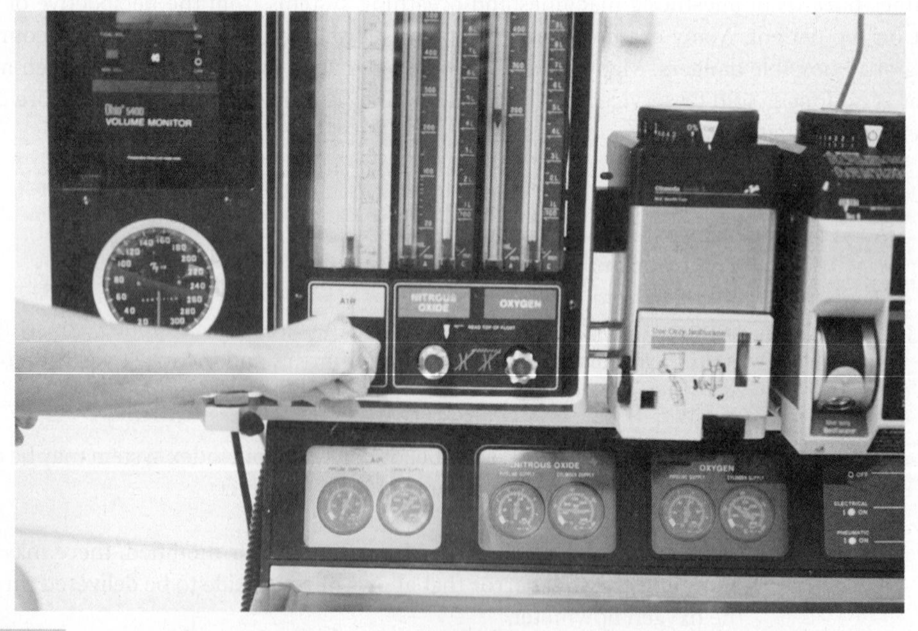

Figure 10.1 A dangerous practice. The flow control knob may look like a good thing to grab to for someone moving an anesthesia machine. Flows may be altered in the process.

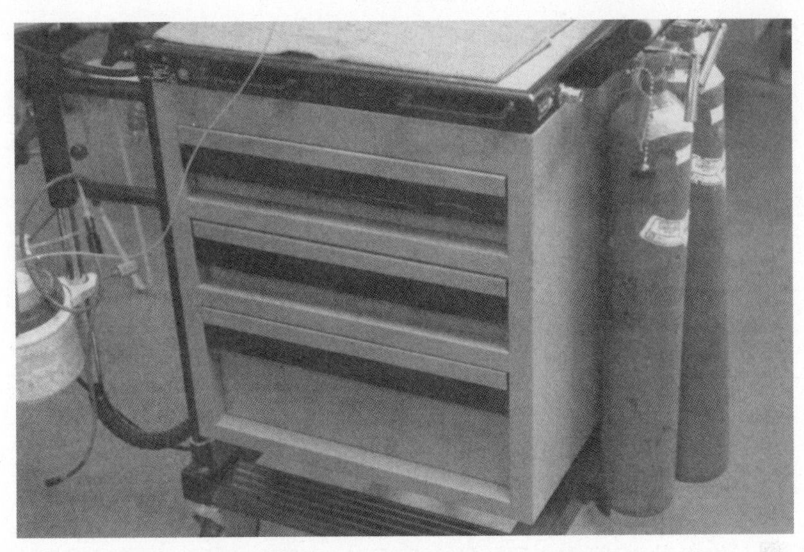

Figure 10.2 A sure sign that a cylinder is not correctly fitted in its yoke is that it hangs at an angle to the machine rather than perpendicular to the floor.

CLINICAL MOMENT If the pipeline supply fails, open the oxygen cylinder, turn OFF the pneumatic ventilator, and ventilate manually. If opening the cylinder does not repressurize the system, the problem is in the anesthesia machine or the cylinder is either empty or not properly connected. Use a manual resuscitator to ventilate the patient until the problem can be determined or the anesthesia apparatus replaced.

b. Cylinder Problems

A cylinder may be empty, incorrectly installed on the machine (**Fig. 10.2**), or have an inoperative valve. The retaining screw may be inserted into the pressure relief device. There may be no handle to open the cylinder valve.

CLINICAL MOMENT If the dust protection cap is not removed before a cylinder is installed on a machine, a portion of the cap may be pushed into the cylinder valve port, preventing gas from exiting the cylinder (**Fig. 10.3**).

CLINICAL MOMENT If the yoke-retaining screw is inserted into the pressure relief device, it may cause it to rupture and release the cylinder contents.

c. Machine Problems

Obstruction may occur in a component such as the oxygen flush, yoke, flow control valve, or vaporizer connection. Leaks may occur in a cylinder; check valve; flowmeter; machine piping; defective vaporizer connection (often apparent only after the vaporizer is turned ON); a loose, defective, or absent vaporizer filler cap (**Fig. 10.4**); or a leaking pressure relief device.

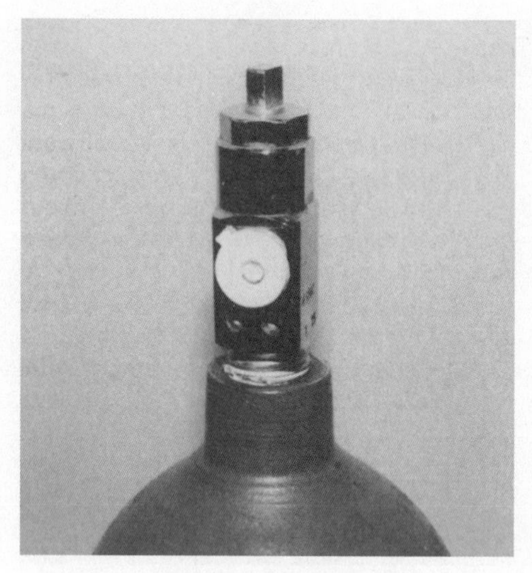

Figure 10.3 Failure to remove the dust protection cap from a cylinder before installing it on a machine can cause a portion of the cap to be pushed into the cylinder valve port, and this can block the exit of gas from the cylinder.

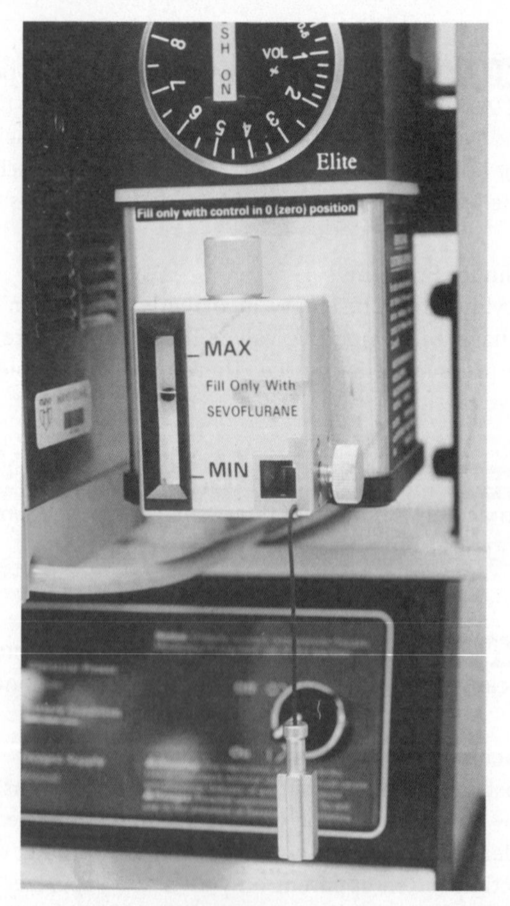

Figure 10.4 When the block on the filling block is not in place, there will be a leak when the vaporizer is turned ON.

d. Gas Supply Switched OFF
The anesthesia machine may be turned OFF or the ON–OFF switch may be in the STANDBY position.
e. Fresh Gas Supply Problems
The hose from the wall to the anesthesia machine may be completely or partially disconnected, leaking, or obstructed. Fresh gas from the machine may be diverted to an auxiliary machine outlet.

2. **Excessive Outflow**
a. Breathing System Leaks
Leaks can occur in an absorber, ventilator, humidifier, breathing tube, or monitoring device. A defective APL valve may not close.
b. Disconnections
Disconnections can occur between breathing system components or airway devices such as tracheal tubes or supraglottic devices. Surgical drapes may hide a disconnection.
c. Negative Pressure Applied to Breathing System
Negative pressure can come from a malfunctioning air inlet valve in a closed scavenging interface or blocked holes in an open interface, allowing negative pressure to be transferred through the APL valve to the breathing system. Suction applied to a bronchoscope working channel or an enteric tube placed in the trachea can cause negative pressure in the breathing system.
d. Improper APL Valve Adjustment
If the APL valve is opened too much for manually controlled or assisted ventilation, the bag will be empty when it is squeezed.

3. **Blocked Inspiratory and/or Expiratory Pathway**
Blockage in the breathing system may come from manufacturing defects, foreign bodies, misconnections, blood or secretions, or kinked or twisted tubes or reservoir bag. The bag/ventilator selector switch may be in the wrong position. An add-on positive end-expiratory pressure (PEEP) valve or humidifier could be installed in a reverse direction. Obstruction can result if the seals on a disposable absorbent package are not removed (**Fig. 10.5**).

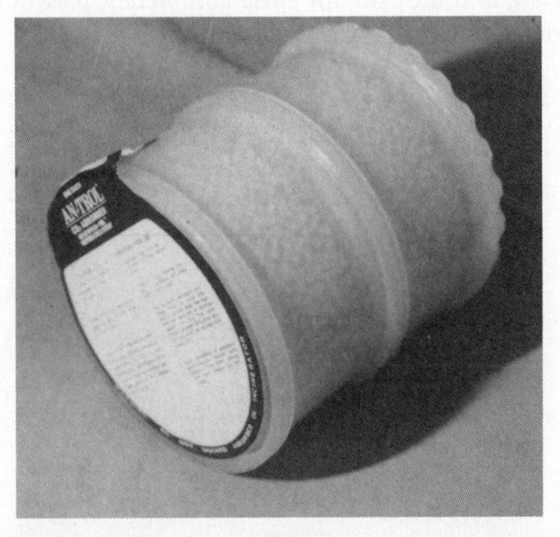

Figure 10.5 Prepacked absorbent container. Failure to remove the label from the top and/or the bottom will result in obstruction to flow through the absorber.

4. **Ventilator Problems**
Possible ventilator problems include cycling failure, leaks of driving or breathing system gas, inappropriate settings, or the ventilator may be turned OFF.

B. Detecting Hypoventilation
Useful monitors include those that measure airway pressure, respiratory volume, carbon dioxide, and oxygen. The low-temperature alarm on a heated humidifier may indicate gas flow loss.

CLINICAL MOMENT If hypoventilation is occurring, the first step is to switch to manual ventilation. If obstruction to ventilation is present, use a resuscitation bag. If ventilation is still difficult, the problem is probably in the airway device or further down the respiratory tract.

If inadequate fresh gas flow is the problem, increase it. If this does not solve the problem, use the manual resuscitation bag and possibly another oxygen source. Call for help to determine the problem.

III. Hypercapnia

A. Hypoventilation
Hypoventilation is the most common cause of hypercapnia. Inspired CO_2 will be zero as a result of hypoventilation.

B. Inadvertent Carbon Dioxide Administration
If a machine has a cylinder and a system for CO_2 administration, it may be inadvertently turned ON or turned to a higher flow than desired.

C. Rebreathing without Carbon Dioxide Removal

1. **Absorbent Failure or Bypass**
The absorbent may be unable to absorb CO_2 or channeling may have occurred. With newer absorbers with which the absorbent can be changed without interrupting ventilation, the absorber may not be properly attached or may not be reattached. When the absorber is not properly attached, it is bypassed.
2. **Unidirectional Valve Problems**
Unidirectional valves must close properly to maintain correct gas flow in the circle system. If they do not close completely, part of the gas flow will reverse direction, causing CO_2 to be rebreathed (**Fig. 10.6**).

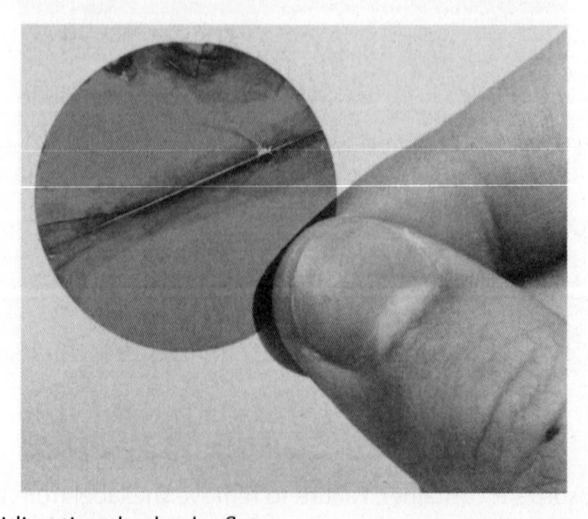

Figure 10.6 Damaged unidirectional valve leaflet.

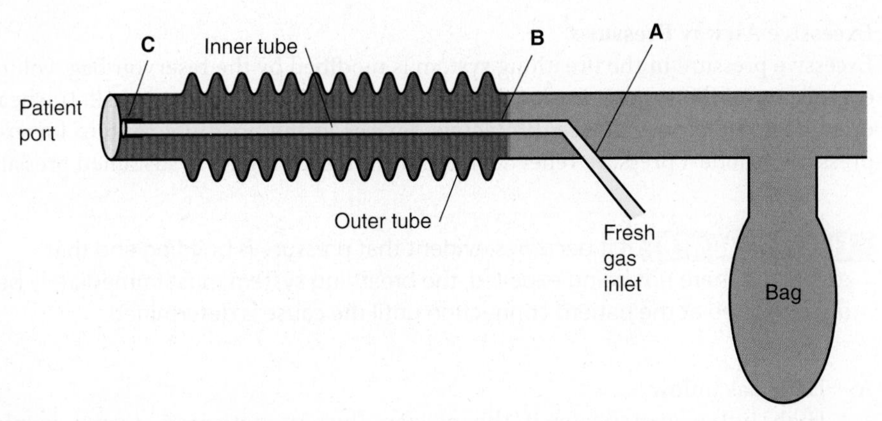

Figure 10.7 Possible problems with the inner tube of the Bain system that can result in hypercarbia. The fresh gas supply tube can become detached (*A*), the inner tube can become kinked or develop a leak (*B*), and the inner tube may not extend to the patient port (*C*).

3. **Nonrebreathing Valve Problems**
   Improperly assembled or defective nonrebreathing valves may stick or allow exhaled gas to reenter the bag.
4. **Inadequate Fresh Gas Flow to a Mapleson System**
   Mapleson systems require a minimum fresh gas flow to eliminate CO_2. If the flow is insufficient, the patient may become hypercapnic.
5. **Coaxial System Problems**
   In a coaxial system (Mapleson or circle), if the inner tube is not properly connected at either end or has an opening between the ends, dead space will increase and the patient will inspire additional CO_2 (**Figs. 5.23** and **10.7**).
6. **Excessive Dead Space**
   If a connector or a heat and moisture exchanger is placed between the patient and the breathing system, the dead space will be increased (**Fig. 10.8**). Added dead space is especially important with pediatric patients.
7. **Hyperventilation**
   Hyperventilation can be caused by a tear or hole in the bellows where driving gas mixes with the gas of the breathing system to increase the tidal volume.

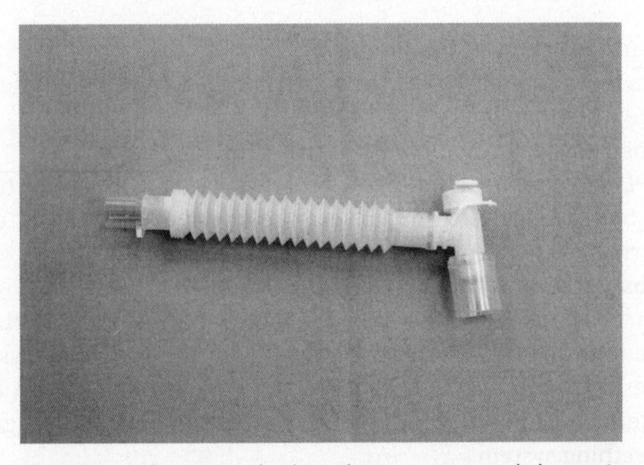

Figure 10.8 Increased dead space between the breathing system and the patient can result in serious hypercarbia in pediatric patients and spontaneously breathing adults.

IV. Excessive Airway Pressure

Excessive pressure in the breathing system is modified by the reservoir bag, volume and compliance of the system, fresh gas flow, and leaks around the face mask, tracheal tube, or supraglottic airway device. Protective devices in the breathing system for excessive pressure include a pressure relief device and alarms for high and sustained pressure.

CLINICAL MOMENT If it becomes evident that pressure is building and that excess gases are not being expelled, the breathing system must immediately be disconnected at the patient connection until the cause is determined.

A. High Gas Inflow

High inflow can occur if the oxygen flush is activated during inspiration. Ventilators that compensate for inspired gas flow by altering the bellows excursion may be unable to compensate for that much additional gas. Piston ventilators close the breathing system to fresh gas entering the system during the inspiratory phase. The reservoir bag greatly increases in size if the oxygen flush is activated.

CLINICAL MOMENT Do not activate the oxygen flush during inspiration.

B. Low Outflow

1. **Obstruction in the Expiratory Limb**

   An obstruction that occurs upstream from the reservoir bag excludes the bag, which acts to buffer pressure changes. Such an obstruction may be caused by a foreign body, torsion at the neck of the reservoir bag, a manufacturing defect, or a reversed PEEP valve.

CLINICAL MOMENT An obstruction between the patient and the reservoir bag will prevent the reservoir bag from filling. Often the reaction is to use the oxygen flush to fill the bag. This is very dangerous because the oxygen flush gas may only go to the patient with resultant barotrauma.

2. **Ventilator Outlet Problem**

   Anything that obstructs the ventilator spill valve when the ventilator is in service will block the release of excess gas.

3. **Obstructed Adjustable Pressure-Limiting Valve**

   APL valve obstruction can occur. Subambient pressure from the scavenging system may close some valves. The operator may fail to open the APL valve during pauses in manual or assisted ventilation.

4. **Obstruction in the Scavenging System**

   An obstruction in the transfer tubing between the APL or spill valve and the interface will obstruct outflow from the breathing system. If the positive pressure-relief valve in a closed scavenging interface is obstructed when the interface bag is fully distended, this will impede excess gas from leaving the breathing system.

5. **Nonrebreathing Valve Problems**
Some disc valves may stick, closing the exhalation channel and preventing outflow. This is mostly a problem with high inflow or a quick squeeze or bump on the bag.

C. Misconnected Oxygen Tubing
Connecting an oxygen delivery tube from a flowmeter directly to a tracheal tube or supraglottic airway device without a gas outlet will result in increased pressure in the patient's airway.

D. Unintended PEEP
An add-on PEEP valve may be in the circuit, or the PEEP on the ventilator may be turned ON. Water in the ventilator tubing may cause PEEP in the breathing system.

V. **Inhaled Foreign Substances**

A. Absorbent Dust
Dust can enter the breathing system after a canister is filled. This is less of a problem if prepackaged absorbent is used.

B. Medical Gas Contaminants
Oils, hydrocarbons, water, metallic fragments, and higher oxides of nitrogen may be found in medical gases.

C. Parts from Breathing System Components and Foreign Bodies
Parts from any breathing component could break off and move toward the patient.

D. Carbon Monoxide
Carbon monoxide from the reactions between anesthetic agents and desiccated absorbents is discussed in Chapter 5.

CLINICAL MOMENT If a filter is used between the patient connection port of the breathing system and the patient, particulate contaminants can be trapped.

VI. **Anesthetic Agent Overdose**

A. Tipped Vaporizer
High agent concentrations may be delivered when the vaporizer is first turned ON if the vaporizer has been tipped or agitated when not attached to the anesthesia machine. Some vaporizers have a mechanism to isolate the vaporizing chamber when the vaporizer is not attached to the machine.

CLINICAL MOMENT If a vaporizer has been tipped, it should be attached to the anesthesia machine and turned ON with a 5 L/minute gas flow through it for at least 10 minutes.

CLINICAL MOMENT If a vaporizer is dropped, the manufacturer's service department should be contacted. It may need to be returned for inspection and service.

B. Vaporizer or Nitrous Oxide Inadvertently Turned ON
Someone helping to move a machine could turn a vaporizer ON, change the vaporizer setting, or alter the flow control valve for an anesthetic gas.

C. Incorrect Agent in the Vaporizer
If an agent is inadvertently placed in a vaporizer designed for an agent with a lower vapor pressure and/or a higher minimum alveolar concentration, a hazardously high concentration of the agent will be delivered.

D. Improper Vaporizer Installation
Concentration-calibrated vaporizers are not designed to be placed in the fresh gas line between the anesthesia machine and the breathing system. Gas flow through the vaporizer could be reversed, which could increase the vapor output when it is turned ON. There will be too much resistance for the oxygen flush to function properly if the vaporizer is between the machine outlet and the breathing system.

E. Overfilled Vaporizer
If the bottle adaptor for an agent-specific filling device is loosened and the concentration dial turned ON during filling, the vaporizer can be overfilled. Tipping the vaporizer backward during filling may allow it to be overfilled.

F. Vaporizer Interlock Failure
If the vaporizer interlock fails, more than one vaporizer could be turned ON at the same time. Agent monitors may or may not detect multiple volatile agents.

VII. Inadequate Anesthetic Agent Delivery

A. Decreased Nitrous Oxide Flow
Inadequate nitrous oxide flow can occur from problems in the nitrous oxide pipeline system.

B. Unexpectedly High Oxygen Concentration
Unexpectedly high oxygen concentrations can result from a connection between nitrous oxide and oxygen in the pipeline system if the pressure in the oxygen system is higher than that in the nitrous oxide system. Using the oxygen flush frequently will dilute anesthetic agents.

C. Faulty Vaporizer
A vaporizer leak or incorrect mounting may lower the delivered anesthetic agent concentration. An overfilled vaporizer can cause a lower than expected output or none at all.

D. Empty Vaporizer
Liquid may be visible in the sight tube even if the vaporizer is empty.

E. Incorrect Agent in Vaporizer
If a vaporizer that is designed for use with a highly volatile agent is filled with an agent of lower volatility, the output concentration will be low.

F. Incorrect Vaporizer Setting
The vaporizer setting may be incorrect. The dial may be altered during the procedure. The anesthesia provider may forget to turn the vaporizer ON after filling it. Turning an electronic anesthesia machine OFF and then turning it ON again may cause the vaporizer setting to default to zero.

G. Anesthetic Agent Breakdown
Desiccated absorbents can react with sevoflurane, lowering the delivered concentration to such an extent that it is difficult to keep the patient asleep.

CLINICAL MOMENT If there is a large discrepancy between the vaporizer setting and the agent concentration in the breathing system, anesthetic breakdown should be suspected.

H. Improper Vaporizer Mounting
If a vaporizer is improperly mounted, fresh gas may not pass through the vaporizer.

CLINICAL MOMENT If a vaporizer is improperly mounted, the entire fresh gas flow may be lost when the vaporizer is turned ON. A common problem is that the vaporizer is pushed upward, breaking the seal between the vaporizer and the "O" rings. Make certain that the vaporizer is correctly seated, is perpendicular to the anesthesia machine table, and lines up properly with other vaporizers.

VIII. Inadvertent Exposure to Volatile Agents

Should an episode of malignant hyperthermia occur and the department has a machine from which vaporizers have been removed and that has been thoroughly flushed of volatile agents, it should be substituted for the machine in use. A fresh breathing system should be used. If the department does not have such a machine, the following measures should be taken to reduce the inhaled concentration of volatile anesthetic:

A. Change the breathing system tubes and bag.
B. Change the fresh gas supply hose.
C. Change the absorbent.
D. Use very high oxygen flows.
E. Insert a charcoal filter, if available, on the inspiratory port of the absorber.
F. Avoid using a contaminated ventilator.
G. If possible, remove vaporizers from the machine.

IX. Electromagnetic Interference

Although appropriate medical device design and testing for electromagnetic compatibility (EMC) can reduce potential electromagnetic interference (EMI) risks in the clinical environment, testing and design cannot ensure that a device will not experience problems. Under certain circumstances, EMI can still occur, even if the device conforms to current EMC standards. Periodical testing of wireless transmitting devices and medical equipment is required to ensure a safe environment.

SUGGESTED READINGS

Caplan RA, Vistica MF, Posner KL, Cheney FW. Adverse anesthetic outcomes arising from gas delivery equipment. A closed claims analysis. Anesthesiology 1997;87:741–748.

Domino KB, Posner KL, Caplan RA, Cheney KW. Awareness during anesthesia. A closed claim analysis. Anesthesiology 1999;90:1053–1061.

Dorsch J, Dorsch S. Hazards of anesthesia machines and breathing systems. In: Understanding Anesthesia Equipment. Fifth edition. Philadelphia: Wolters Kluwer/Lippincott Williams & Wilkins, 2008:404–430.

Eisenkraft JB. Hazards of the anesthesia workstation (ASA Refresher Course #212). Orlando, FL: American Society of Anesthesiologists, 2008.

Fasting S, Gisvold SE. Equipment problems during anaesthesia—are they a quality problem? Br J Anaesth 2002;89:825–831.

Morray JP, Geiduschek JM, Ramamoorthy C, et al. Anesthesia-related cardiac arrest in children. Anesthesiology 2000;93:6–14.

Russell WJ, Webb RK, van der Walt JH, Runciman WB. Problems with ventilation: an analysis of 2000 incident reports. Anaesth Intensive Care 1993;21:617–620.

Singh S, Loeb RG. Fatal connection: death caused by direct connection of oxygen tubing into a tracheal tube connector. Anesth Analg 2004;99:1164–1165.

Webb RK, Russell WJ, Klepper I, Runciman WB. Equipment failure: an analysis of 2000 incident reports. Anaesth Intensive Care 1993;21:673–677.

11 Latex Allergy

CONCERN ABOUT LATEX ALLERGY IN the medical community has increased, as healthcare personnel have seen an increase in reactions among both patients and themselves. Latex is the second most common cause of intraoperative anaphylaxis, exceeded only by muscle relaxants.

I. Origin of Sensitivity

A. Natural latex is obtained from the sap of a rubber tree. During the manufacturing process, many chemicals are added to the latex, depending on the requirements of the finished product. These substances may also be allergenic. There may be as many as 240 potentially allergenic substances in a finished latex product.

B. The increased incidence of latex allergy is believed to be due both to changes in the manufacturing processes and to increased use of latex-containing products. Adoption of universal and standard precautions (Chapter 27) has greatly increased latex exposure. Latex sensitization can occur from contact via the skin or mucous membranes, inhalation, ingestion, parenteral injection, or wound inoculation.

II. Latex-Containing Products

A. Latex is ubiquitous in the home, workplace, and healthcare setting but is not always obvious. In the operating room suite, it may be found in gloves; tracheal tubes; Combitubes; face masks; mask straps; airways; wrappers; laryngoscope bulb gaskets; skin temperature monitors; rubber suction catheters; arm boards; bite blocks; teeth protectors; breathing tubes; oxygen tubing; reservoir bags; ventilator hoses and bellows; resuscitation bags (black or blue, reusable); blood pressure cuffs and tubing; stethoscope tubing; intravenous tubing injection ports; tourniquets; syringe plungers; rubber-shod clamps; intravenous bag and tubing ports; medication vial needle ports; tape and other adhesives (e.g., Esmarch bandages, adhesive bandages); dental dams; elastic bandages (Ace wraps); dressings (e.g., Coban, Moleskin, Micropore); rubber pads; protective sheets; drains; electrode pads; rubber aprons; circulating fluid warming blankets; some cast materials; goggles; pulmonary artery catheter balloons; epidural catheter adapters; intravenous medication pump cassettes; electrocardiogram electrodes and pads; finger cots; ostomy bags; intestinal and stomach tubes; rubber bands; chest tube drainage tubing; condom urinals; urinary and nephrostomy catheters; gastrostomy tubes; bulb syringes; adhesive drapes; nipples; instrument mats; specimen traps; catheter bag straps; dilating catheters; and the elastic in items ranging from surgical masks, head coverings, hats, and booties to diapers. Allergic reactions have been attributed to drugs that had been prepared in a latex-containing syringe for a considerable time before use or a bottle with a latex stopper between the drug and the diluent.

B. Well-washed rubber products such as ventilator bellows pose less risk than new items. There is a decrease in latex proteins in gloves that are autoclaved. The risk of latex sensitization may be increased by sterilizing products with ethylene oxide.

C. Gloves have very high allergen levels compared with most other latex-containing medical products. Latex gloves are the biggest contributors to the aeroallergens inside the operating room. Some gloves contain powder. Latex proteins from the gloves bond with this powder. When a glove is put on or removed, the powder may spray into the air. It can then be inhaled by personnel, inoculate an open wound, or contaminate the instruments on the surgical field. The powder can remain suspended in the air for hours.

D. Even in operating rooms where laminar airflow devices are used, latex aeroallergens are present in high quantities. Allergens are carried throughout the environment by ventilation systems as well as on clothing and equipment. Switching to low-allergen gloves has been found to reduce the levels of these aeroallergens.

E. Latex is found in many products outside the healthcare setting. These include toys; condoms; expandable fabrics (waistbands); diaphragms; balloons; hot water bottles; erasers; rubber bands; shoe soles; motorcycle and bicycle handgrips; bathing suits, caps, and goggles; racquet handles; pacifiers; baby bottle nipples; bungee cords; chewing gum; cosmetic applicator sponges; fish tanks; bike helmets; automobile tires; raincoats; computer mouse pads; earphones; household rubber gloves; and carpet padding to name but a few. The American Latex Allergy Association (www.latexallergyresources.org) provides resources to consumers, including information on many latex-free consumer products now available.

III. Clinical Signs and Symptoms

Reactions to latex include a spectrum of non–immune and immune-mediated responses. Signs and symptoms may be local or systemic and vary widely in the severity and time of occurrence. Most adverse reactions to latex occur within 60 minutes after induction. Symptoms can progress quickly from mild to severe. In some cases, life-threatening reactions are the first to appear.

There are three types of reactions to latex: irritant contact dermatitis, type IV delayed hypersensitivity, and type 1 immediate hypersensitivity.

A. Irritant Contact Dermatitis

This is the most common type of glove-related reaction. It results from the direct action of latex and other irritant chemicals and consists of itching, redness, scaling, drying, and cracking. The rash is usually limited to the exposed skin area. Soaps, mechanical irritation from scrubbing, and excessive sweating often exacerbate it.

CLINICAL MOMENT While contact dermatitis is not a true allergy, the disruption in skin integrity may enhance absorption of latex allergens and accelerate the onset of allergic reactions, so it should be avoided and treated vigorously.

B. Type IV Delayed Hypersensitivity
   1. *Hypersensitivity* is an immune response that leads to tissue damage. Once sensitized, an individual's exposure to an antigen can cause a reaction. It may take years for latex sensitivity to develop.
   2. A type IV reaction (allergic contact dermatitis, delayed hypersensitivity) is a T-cell–mediated response characterized by a skin rash that appears up to 72 hours after initial contact and may progress to oozing skin blisters. Unlike irritant contact dermatitis, allergic contact dermatitis often spreads beyond the area of contact with the allergen. Flushing, itching, rhinitis, dizziness, sinus symptoms, conjunctivitis, and eyelid edema may also be present.
   3. Not all individuals who develop type IV hypersensitivity progress to type I hypersensitivity, but most individuals with type I sensitivity previously have had type IV symptoms.

C. Type I Immediate Hypersensitivity
   1. This is the most severe reaction and may lead to significant morbidity and mortality. Symptoms usually appear shortly after exposure but can occur hours later. They run the entire spectrum from mild (skin redness, hives, itching, rhinitis, scratchy throat, itchy or swollen eyes) to more severe (facial edema, faintness, nausea, abdominal cramps, diarrhea, cough, hoarseness, chest tightness) to life-threatening (laryngeal edema, bronchospasm, anaphylaxis). A survey of anaphylaxis during anesthesia showed that cardiovascular symptoms, cutaneous symptoms, and bronchospasm were the most common clinical features.

CLINICAL MOMENT An anaphylactic reaction can occur from causes other than latex allergy. If a medication has been injected shortly before the anaphylactic reaction, the anesthesia provider should suspect that the medication caused the reaction.

   2. Anaphylaxis is an immediate, severe, life-threatening allergic response. Failure to recognize latex allergy can delay removal of latex-containing products and delay effective treatment.

IV. Individuals at Risk

A. Identifying patients at high risk for having an allergic latex reaction allows preventive measures to be targeted. Latex anaphylaxis may be decreased by identifying at-risk patients.

B. The reported prevalence of latex allergy varies greatly depending on the population studied and the methods used to detect sensitization. Anyone with frequent exposure to latex-containing materials is at increased risk of developing latex allergy. The greater the exposure to latex in a population, the greater the number of sensitized individuals. Extended or massive exposure in and of itself is neither necessary nor sufficient to cause sensitization if the person is not genetically predisposed to allergy.

C. Children and younger adults are more likely to become latex sensitive than the general population. Some but not all studies have found that women and members of non-Caucasian races are more likely to have latex allergies.

D. The majority of latex-sensitive individuals have a history of atopy (predisposition to multiple allergic conditions) or positive tests in atopy screening. Many have a history of an anaphylactic reaction. Some studies have found a connection between an allergy to an anesthesia-related agent and latex.

E. Many patients with type I latex allergy have a history of allergy to certain foods, including bananas, mangoes, watermelons, avocados, peaches, figs, apples, chestnuts, pineapples, kiwi, passion fruit, apricots, nectarines, papaya, celery, peanuts, cherries, strawberries, plums, potatoes, and tomatoes. There may be cross sensitivity between latex and ficus, grasses, and ragweed. Patients with milk protein allergies may exhibit allergic reactions to latex products containing casein.

F. Individuals with hand dermatitis who wear latex gloves are at increased risk. A history of glove-related symptoms does not reliably indicate latex allergy; conversely, the absence of symptoms does not rule out sensitization.

G. Many latex-sensitive individuals report swelling or itching on the hands or other areas after contact with rubber gloves, condoms, diaphragms, toys, or other rubber products. Other symptoms include swelling or itching at the lips or mouth from blowing up balloons or after dental examinations.

H. Latex allergy incidence is highest for patients requiring multiple surgical procedures and repetitive urinary catheterization. This includes patients with myelodysplasia, congenital orthopedic defects, and congenital genitourinary tract anomalies. Patients with spina bifida have a particularly high incidence of latex allergy. However, adults with spinal cord injuries have a low risk of latex sensitization. Other high-risk groups include patients who undergo repeated esophageal dilations, patients who have frequent vaginal examinations (particularly those going through an in vitro fertilization program) and are examined with a latex-covered ultrasound probe, and patients undergoing barium enema procedures with a latex balloon tip.

I. Approximately 70% of latex-related adverse events reported to the Food and Drug Administration (FDA) involve healthcare workers. Within the medical profession, individuals who frequently use disposable gloves, including surgeons; anesthesia providers; operating room, postanesthesia care unit (PACU), and emergency room personnel; dentists and dental assistants; and laboratory technicians are more likely to become latex-sensitive than other healthcare workers. Adult anesthesiologists change gloves more often than pediatric anesthesiologists and have a higher prevalence of latex sensitization.

J. Other patients at risk for latex allergy include those who use gloves in their daily activities: farmers, food service workers, gardeners, painters, mortuary workers, auto technicians, law enforcement personnel, waste removal workers, hairdressers, and individuals involved in latex product manufacturing.

V. Diagnosing Latex Allergy

A. History

The history should include the risk factors and occupations in which latex exposure is common, as discussed previously in this chapter.

B. Confirmatory Tests

A patient with a history suspicious for latex allergy may be a candidate for confirmatory testing. Immunologic testing is not foolproof, particularly in the case of latex, because of the numerous different latex proteins. Testing requires a variety of latex antigens, and there can be no certainty that a particular antigen will be included in the test solution. Because false-negative results can occur, patients with a strong suspicion of latex allergy should be managed in a latex-safe environment even if immunological testing indicates a negative reaction.

1. **Skin-Prick Test**

The skin-prick test (SPT) is used to detect type I latex allergy. A dilute solution of allergen is placed on the skin, and the skin is pricked or scratched. A wheal-and-flare reaction is considered positive for latex sensitivity.

2. **Intradermal Test**
   With intradermal testing, a small amount of an allergen suspension is injected into the skin. This method is more sensitive than skin pricking, but the risk of anaphylaxis is greater.
3. **Patch Test**
   The patch test is available for diagnosis of type IV delayed hypersensitivity. A standardized patch or a fragment of the latex product is applied to the skin and checked over several days. A positive reaction includes itching, redness, swelling, or blistering where the patch covers the skin.
4. **In Vitro Measurement of Antibodies**
   In vitro tests are used to measure specific antibodies against latex allergens in blood samples.
5. **Challenge Tests**
   Challenge (provocation, use, wear) tests may be used if other tests show equivocal results or the person has a clinical history highly consistent with latex allergy but other tests show negative results. The potentially allergic person handles, wears, or inhales latex proteins and is observed for reactions. Since there may be discrepancies in results, no challenge method has become broadly accepted by clinicians.

VI. **Preventing Latex Reactions**

A. To prevent latex reactions, products that contain latex need to be identified and alternatives obtained before an emergency arises. Manufacturers have made great strides in decreasing latex in a variety of products. If it is not possible to remove a latex product, barriers should be placed between the item and the patient.

B. It is impossible to totally eliminate latex exposure. The goal is to create a latex-safe environment, that is, one in which the presence of latex antigens is minimized. The need for education cannot be overemphasized. The majority of latex reactions in a center with an established protocol are due to human error.

C. Using powderless or latex-free gloves should be a high priority. These help to minimize reactions to latex at little added expense and decrease the amount of aeroallergens in the working environment. When gloves are powdered, pulling them on and off gently will minimize aerosolizing the latex proteins. Oil-based hand creams or lotions should be avoided. They can break down latex and make the protein more likely to stick to the hands.

D. Patients with known or suspected latex allergy should have their records flagged and wear latex-allergy wristbands. Drug prophylaxis is sometimes undertaken. Allergic reactions, including anaphylaxis, may occur even when prophylactic agents are used. While having these drugs already on board may result in a less severe reaction, they may mask the early signs of anaphylaxis, delaying recognition and implementation of more aggressive treatment. Using H_2 blockers may increase the risk of heart block for patients who develop anaphylaxis.

E. If a patient requiring surgery has confirmed latex sensitivity or a convincing history of latex reaction, avoiding latex-containing products is the only effective measure. Even in the absence of known latex allergy, some procedures involving patients with syndromes such as spina bifida should be performed in a latex-safe area. For high-risk patients, avoiding latex products should begin at birth.

F. The FDA requires that all medical products that contain latex that may directly or indirectly come into contact with the body during use bear labels stating that the product contains latex and that latex may cause allergic reactions in some individuals (**Fig. 11.1**). Governmental agencies in many other countries have similar

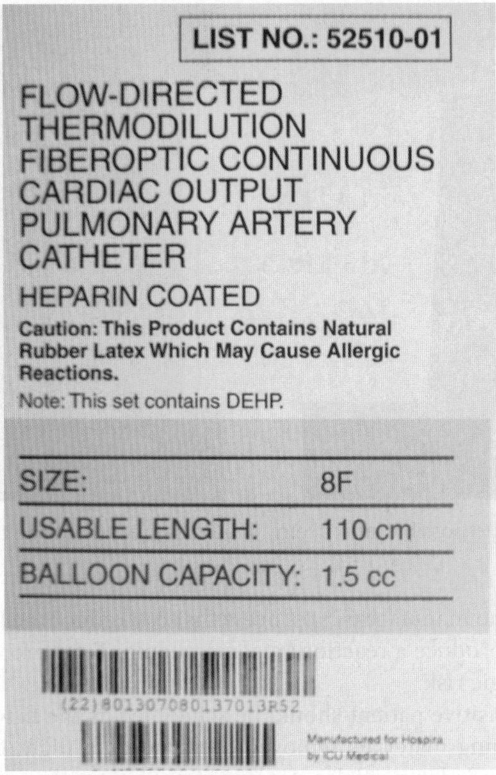

Figure 11.1 Thermodilution catheter clearly marked as containing latex.

requirements. If a product does not have this warning, it is likely that the product is latex-free unless it is a pharmaceutical or is not regulated by the FDA. Drug manufacturers are exempt from the labeling requirement. Manufacturers frequently label devices as latex free (**Fig. 11.2**).

G. The term *hypoallergenic* is no longer used for devices that contain latex. At present, there is no test that can adequately determine the level of latex proteins in a product,

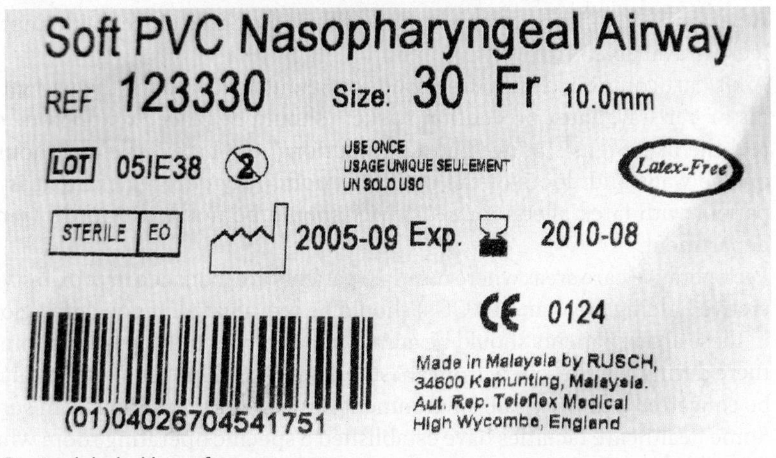

Figure 11.2 Device labeled latex free.

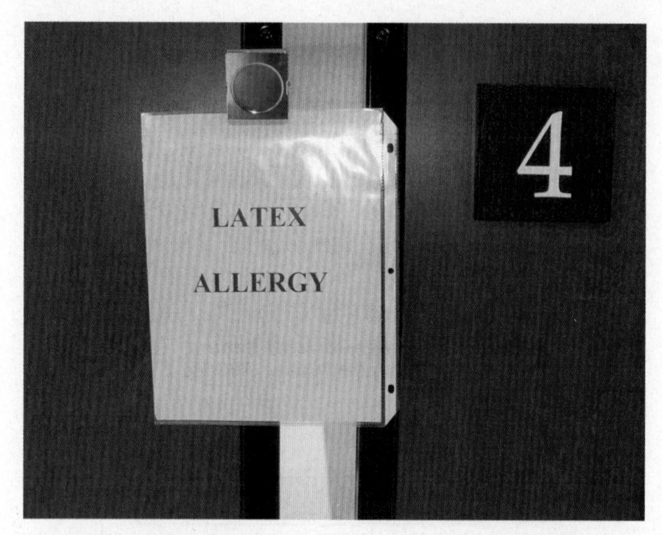

Figure 11.3 A sign indicating possible latex allergy should be placed outside the operating room door.

and there is no manufacturing process that can reduce the level below the minimum required to produce a reaction in some people. Total protein content is not analogous to allergic risk.

H. The latex-sensitive patient should be scheduled as the first case of the day, with all latex-containing materials removed the preceding night to minimize exposure to airborne latex-laden particles. No one should enter that operating room with latex gloves, without scrubbing after taking off latex gloves or while wearing clothing from previous latex exposure.

CLINICAL MOMENT Signs saying "Latex Allergy" or "Latex Alert" (for patients with significant risk factors for latex allergy but no overt signs or symptoms) should be posted inside and outside the operating room as well as in perioperative care areas (**Fig. 11.3**).

I. Latex products should be limited to situations in which it is thought that they are superior to non–latex-containing products. Latex-free gloves with improved fit and feel are available.

J. A kit/cart containing latex-free products should accompany the patient throughout his or her stay. Latex precaution stickers should be placed on doctors' order sheets and the like. Signs stating "Latex Precautions" or "Latex Allergy" should be placed on the walls and doors of the patient's room. Any department that is to receive a patient with latex allergy or sensitivity should be notified prior to transfer to that department.

K. Perioperative care areas where multiple patients are managed in proximity (e.g., preoperative holding areas and PACUs) should be reevaluated. If powdered gloves are used in these areas, patients should be admitted directly to the operating room and remain there during their recovery from anesthesia. If the PACU has an isolation room, it may be converted to a latex-safe environment for patients recovering from surgery.

L. Some healthcare facilities have established a specific operating room where all latex-containing materials are banned. Signs should be posted on all entrances to that room, reminding medical personnel of the situation. Traffic in the room should be kept to a minimum.

M. No latex-containing items (i.e., gowns, hats, boots, and compression stockings) should be placed on the patient. Cords and tubes for all monitoring devices should be placed in stockinettes and secured with non-latex tape.

N. Latex-free intravenous start kits containing tourniquet, bandages, dressings, tapes, and gloves are available. Intravenous tubing without latex injection ports should be used or all latex injection ports taped to prevent inadvertent puncture. Stopcocks or one-way valves should be used for push and piggyback medications. Intravenous fluid or commercially prepared medication bags should be pierced through the intravenous tubing port and not through the latex injection port.

O. Although reactions to rubber syringe plungers have been reported, no problems have so far been reported with medications freshly drawn and immediately administered. If latex-containing syringes are used, drugs should be drawn into the syringe immediately before use. Glass syringes offer an attractive alternative, and totally plastic syringes and special needles are available. It is best to use medication from glass ampules, if available. Although it has been advocated that the contents of a vial should be drawn up after the rubber stopper has been removed, this may not be beneficial and may result in increased microbial contamination and waste. Lyophilized drugs in containers with latex should be reconstituted by using a syringe, not shaken in a multidose vial, and withdrawn using a filter. Vials should be kept upright and not shaken.

P. A filter should be used at the breathing system patient port to protect against airborne latex allergens. It may not be possible to entirely avoid some rubber-containing anesthetic equipment—rubber bellows, diaphragms, valves, and tubings. However, when these parts of equipment do not come into contact with the patient and have been previously washed, no complications should result.

Q. Latex-free equipment including face masks, airways, mask straps, tracheal tubes, bag-valve-mask units, reservoir bags, electrocardiographic electrodes and pads, stethoscopes (tubing or diaphragm), pulse oximetry sensors, esophageal stethoscopes, nasogastric and suction tubes, tape, gas hoses, and breathing tubes should be used. Unfortunately, some latex-free reservoir bags have such poor distensibility that their use may compromise patient safety.

R. If a regional anesthesia catheter adaptor contains latex, it should be replaced with a latex-free adaptor.

S. Latex-free reusable blood pressure instruments and accessories are available in a variety of sizes and models. These include inflating tubing, coiled tubing, sphygmomanometers, and inflation bladders. Wrapping the area under the cuff with soft cotton can prevent contact with any latex in these devices.

T. In some cases, some improvising may be necessary, as with a pulmonary artery catheter.

U. From the surgical point of view, using nonlatex gloves, drains, and catheters is mandatory. Special caution should be taken to avoid latex-based equipment such as instrument mats, rubber-shod clamps, vascular tags, bulb syringes, rubber bands, and adhesive bandages. A nonlatex glove can be used as a Penrose drain, which can be a source of latex hypersensitivity.

V. When latex-sensitive patients or staff have been identified, it is important to provide latex-free items. These should be collected into a cart that can be called into action as the need arises. The American Society of Anesthesiologists and others have made recommendations for the contents of a latex-safe cart. Suggested items are listed in **Table 11.1.** Each item should give information on latex content and should be reviewed for this information before adding the item to the latex-safe cart or before use.

Table 11.1 Suggested Contents of a Latex-Safe Cart

- Latex-free or glass syringes
- Syringe needles
- Intravenous catheters
- Intravenous tubing and extensions made from polyvinylchloride
- Stopcocks (in-line, three-way, and single)
- Latex-free heparin lock caps and T-pieces with side port
- Alcohol wipes in a new box
- Latex-safe adhesive tape from a new box
- Latex-free intravenous tourniquets
- Sterile gauze pads
- Esophageal thermometer
- Disposable blood pressure cuffs of various sizes
- Stethoscope
- Sterile case padding
- Latex-free disposable pulse oximetry finger sensors
- Latex-free electrocardiographic electrodes
- Latex-free resuscitation bags sized for infants, children, and adults
- Nasal oxygen cannula
- Oxygen extension tubing
- Latex-free tracheal tubes, double-lumen tubes, and stylets
- Latex-free oral and nasal airways
- Silicone or PVC supraglottic device
- Plastic face masks and head straps (elastic strap may contain latex)
- Medications for cardiac arrest and emergency situations
- Vinyl gloves for any size staff
- Sterile nonlatex gloves, sizes 6 to 9
- Silicone urinary catheter in assorted sizes
- Urimeter
- Epidural and spinal trays
- Polyvinylchloride suction catheters, size 8 to 14 French
- Anesthesia breathing circuits without latex components
- Anesthesia medications in vials
- In-line, high-efficiency particulate gas filter
- Policy binder with all latex policies and protocols
- Reference guide for latex-containing materials
- Brightly colored signs that warn of latex allergy

VII. Treating Latex Reactions

CLINICAL MOMENT For allergic reactions, the most important step is to stop administration and/or reduce absorption of the offending agent. All potential routes of exposure, including mucosal and inhalational, must be considered.

A. The signs and symptoms of irritant contact dermatitis can often be controlled by removing the irritant. Measures include wearing a soft glove liner and reducing exposure to other irritants (e.g., soaps). Using protective hand cream is contraindicated.
B. Topical corticosteroids can be used for a rash or hives. Topical nasal steroids may be used for rhinitis. Antihistamines and systemic steroids can be used to treat other mild reactions. If the symptoms are more severe, more aggressive treatment is indicated, including antihistamines, systemic steroids, H_2 blockers, oxygen, intravenous fluids, bronchodilators, and epinephrine. If anaphylaxis occurs, artificial airway support, intravascular volume expansion, administration of vasoactive medications, and other life-support techniques may be needed. The crash cart should not have latex-containing items.
C. Latex precautions should accompany the patient throughout the remainder of the postoperative period.
D. The details of any allergic reaction should be clearly documented in the patient's chart. This should include a description of the anesthetic agents and techniques, surgical products used, resuscitative measures required, laboratory evaluation, and the perioperative course. The patient should be referred to an allergist and the patient's record flagged to alert subsequent caretakers.
E. Desensitization by progressive contact has been described. It consists of increasing exposure to latex by wearing latex gloves daily for increasing periods. Sublingual desensitization may result in significant improvement in symptoms.

VIII. Latex Allergy and Medical Personnel

Numerous studies show a high incidence of latex allergy in healthcare workers. Medical personnel who wear latex gloves on a regular basis (surgeons, anesthesia providers, operating room staff, radiologists, housekeeping staff, and laboratory personnel) are at higher risk for developing latex allergies than other healthcare workers. Occupational asthma has been reported in an administrative employee who was exposed to airborne latex allergens.

A. Healthcare Institution Responsibilities
   1. Institutions should provide educational programs and training materials about latex allergy. This includes educating all staff members and not just professional healthcare providers. For example, environmental and nutritional service workers are required to wear gloves. They should be knowledgeable about their glove choices.
   2. Staff should be encouraged to report allergic symptoms. Detecting symptoms early and protecting symptomatic workers from latex exposure are essential to prevent long-term adverse health effects. Prevention strategies should be reevaluated whenever a worker is diagnosed with latex allergy. Studies have shown that economically feasible interventions to reduce latex exposure can successfully allow latex-allergic individuals to continue working as well as decrease the number of new cases of occupational latex allergy.
   3. Using powderless gloves (**Fig. 11.4**) should be encouraged. Using nonlatex gloves for activities that are not likely to involve contact with infectious materials (food

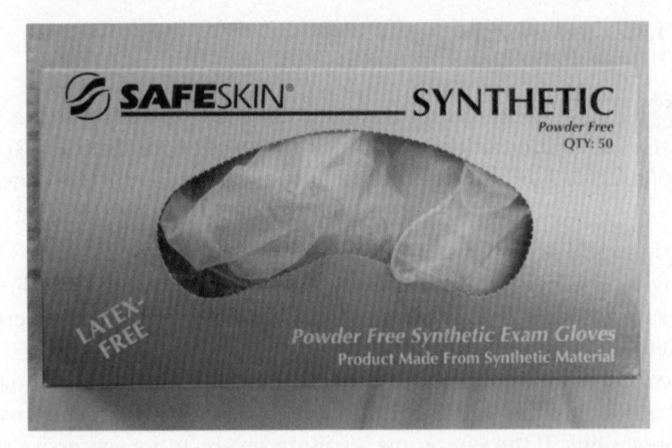

Figure 11.4 Using powderless, latex-free gloves is an important step to reducing the incidence of latex allergic reactions.

handling, housekeeping, and transport) should be promoted. This can greatly reduce the levels of latex antigens in the environment.

4. Wearing nonlatex gloves or using some type of barrier between the latex gloves and the skin should be encouraged. Nonlatex gloves are usually more expensive than gloves containing latex. Newer options in latex-free gloves are more comfortable, resilient, and form-fitting than previous ones.

CLINICAL MOMENT Since anesthesia personnel may change gloves numerous times, it is wise to use nonlatex gloves. When this is not possible, powderless gloves should be used.

5. Facilities should ensure that good housekeeping practices are performed to remove latex-containing dust from the workplace. This can be accomplished by identifying areas that are contaminated with latex dust (carpets, upholstery, and ventilation ducts) for cleaning and changing ventilation filters and vacuum bags frequently.

B. Healthcare Worker Responsibilities

1. Healthcare workers need to take advantage of latex allergy education and training to become familiar with ways to prevent latex allergy and to learn to recognize the signs and symptoms.
2. Workers should protect themselves from latex exposure inside and outside the workplace. Intact skin is an effective barrier, and it is important to maintain good hand care. Cuts and open sores should be covered with a plastic barrier dressing before wearing latex gloves. Oil-based hand creams or lotions should be avoided because they may enhance release of latex protein from the gloves. After removing latex gloves, hands should be washed with a mild soap and thoroughly dried. This will decrease the allergen load.
3. Healthcare workers should avoid wearing work clothes (scrubs) home after working in the operating room. Indirect exposures have caused latex allergy in children and spouses.
4. If signs and symptoms of latex allergy develop, the person should avoid contact with latex-containing products until he or she can be seen by a physician who

is experienced in diagnosing and treating latex allergy. A symptom diary should be kept. Delay and self-treatment can delay diagnosis, allowing the problem to become more serious.

C. The Healthcare Worker with Latex Sensitivity
   1. Depending on the severity of the reaction, latex sensitivity in healthcare workers can be inconvenient or a life-threatening hazard. It can mean the end of a career. Often, healthcare personnel are unaware of their sensitization. The only clue might be the temporal relationship with working. Denial can be a problem.
   2. Anesthesia providers with latex allergy should be counseled both on the risks of continued work in environments with high latex use and on strategies to limit exposure. They should have proper allergy identification, including a medical alert device, and should inform their healthcare providers (including dentist and local hospital). They must carry an allergy kit, including an epinephrine auto-injector device, nonlatex gloves to wear or give to others to wear if they must care for them, and a complete list of medications taken. Friends and family should be given information about latex allergy. The individual must be on the lookout for hidden latex. Consideration should be given to avoiding foods that may contain proteins similar to those present in latex.
   3. Once latex allergy is diagnosed, the only option is to avoid contact with latex and to try to control the symptoms. Almost all the products that healthcare workers encounter in their daily work can be made latex-free. A latex-safe environment also prevents exposure of other workers.
   4. There are many nonlatex gloves available, both sterile and nonsterile. These include vinyl, nitrile, styrene butadiene, and neoprene. Unfortunately, these may not match the physical characteristics of latex gloves such as high elasticity, strength, flexibility, tear resistance, tactile sensation, and barrier integrity. Latex gloves are biodegradable and do not produce hazardous and toxic emissions when incinerated, as do synthetic gloves. Nonlatex glove liners and latex gloves with integral nonlatex layers are available. Coworkers should wear powderless, low-latex gloves. This reduces the exposure to latex by those who are not yet sensitized and may decrease symptoms in sensitized patients.
   5. Healthcare workers with latex sensitivity are not at an increased risk when incidentally exposed to dry, molded, or extruded rubber products in the healthcare environment; however, if direct contact with such objects is routine, exposure should be minimized by covering the object or exposed body part.

SUGGESTED READINGS

American Society of Anesthesiologists. Natural Rubber Latex Allergy: Considerations for Anesthesiologists. Park Ridge, IL: Author, 2005. Available at: www.ASAhq.org/publications.

Dorsch J, Dorsch S. Latex allergy. In: Understanding Anesthesia Equipment. Fifth edition. Philadelphia: Wolters Kluwer/Lippincott Williams & Wilkins, 2008:431–442.

Hepner DL, Castells MC. Latex allergy: an update. Anesth Analg 2003;96:1219–1229.

Hepner DL, Castells MC. Anaphylaxis during the perioperative period. Anesth Analg 2003;97:1381–1395.

Paskawicz J, Chatwani A. Latex allergy: a concern for anesthesia personnel. Am J Anaesthesiol 2001;28:435–441.

Rinaldi PA. Perioperative Management of the Patient with Latex Allergy. Orlando, FL: American Society of Anesthesiologists, 1998. ASA Refresher Course No. 532.

Airway Equipment

12 Face Masks and Airways

I. Face Masks

A face mask allows gases to be administered to the patient without introducing any apparatus into the patient's mouth. The ability to hold a mask and administer positive pressure ventilation through the mask is a basic skill that all anesthesia providers must master. The introduction of supraglottic airway devices (Chapter 13) has led to decreased mask use.

A. Description

1. The majority of anesthesia providers today use disposable plastic masks. These are designed to fit a wide variety of patients. Some masks are ergonomically designed for better hand placement and improved seal.
2. The body is the main part of the mask. Most masks today are transparent to allow observation for vomitus, secretions, blood, the color and position of the lips, and exhaled moisture (**Fig. 12.1**).
3. The cushion is the soft part that contacts the face. Two general types are available. The inflatable cushion is the most common type. It may be filled with air or a firmer substance such as a gel that conforms to the face. The other, cushion type, has a flap that is pressed down onto the face.
4. The connector (orifice, collar, mount) is at the opposite side of the body from the seal. It consists of a thickened fitting with a 22-mm internal diameter (ID). Hooks may be placed around the connector to allow a mask strap to be attached.

B. Specific Masks

1. Masks come in a variety of sizes and shapes. An assortment of masks should be kept readily available because no one mask will fit every face. A number of pediatric masks have been developed to fit the unique anatomy of infants' and children's faces (**Fig. 12.2**).

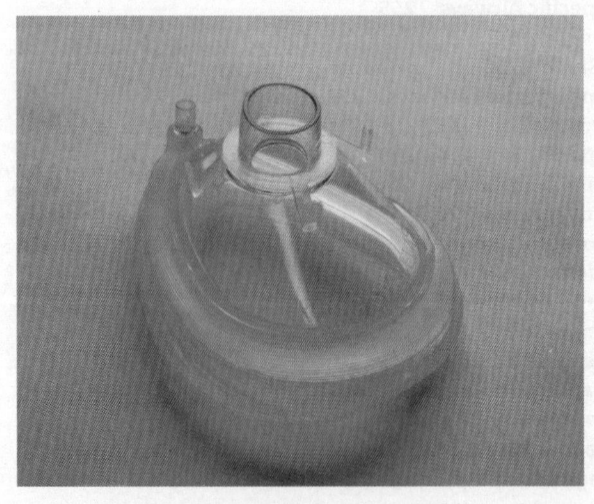

Figure 12.1 Clear disposable mask. (Picture courtesy of King Systems.)

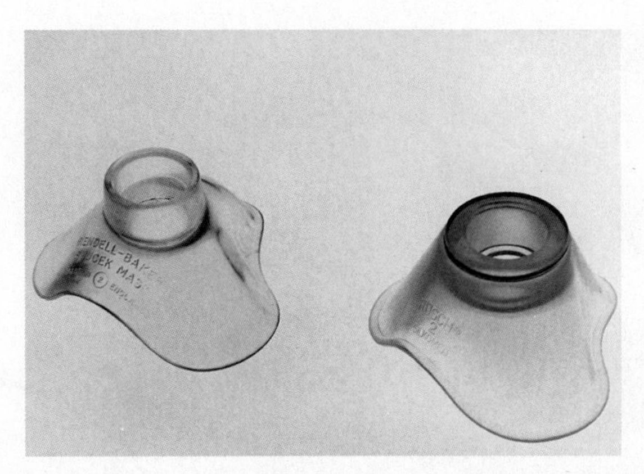

Figure 12.2 Rendell-Baker-Soucek masks. (Courtesy of Rusch, Inc., Research Triangle Park, NC.)

2. Scented masks are useful for inhalation mask inductions. Masks designed for specific functions such as endoscopy are available (**Fig. 12.3**).

C. Techniques of Use

Correct mask use starts with selecting the appropriate size and shape. This may require some trial and error. The smallest mask that will do the job is best because it will cause the least increase in dead space, will usually be easiest to hold, and will be less likely to cause pressure on the eyes. If a seal is difficult to establish, reshaping the mask's malleable perimeter (if possible), altering the amount of air in the seal, or selecting a different mask may be helpful.

CLINICAL MOMENT The best position for laryngoscopy may not be the best option for mask ventilation. It is usually better to elevate the shoulders with the neck in a neutral or slightly extended position and to allow the head to extend off the neck.

CLINICAL MOMENT Simple maneuvers to improve the airway when using a mask include head tilt, chin lift, jaw thrust, and elevation of the shoulders with a towel or blanket.

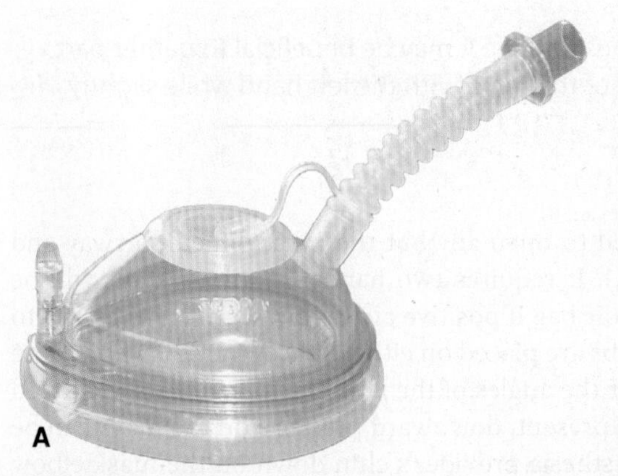

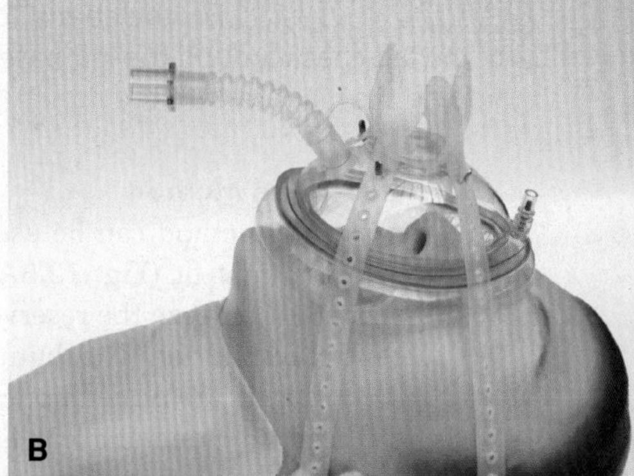

Figure 12.3 Endoscopic masks. (Pictures courtesy of VBM Medical, Inc., Noblesville, NC.)

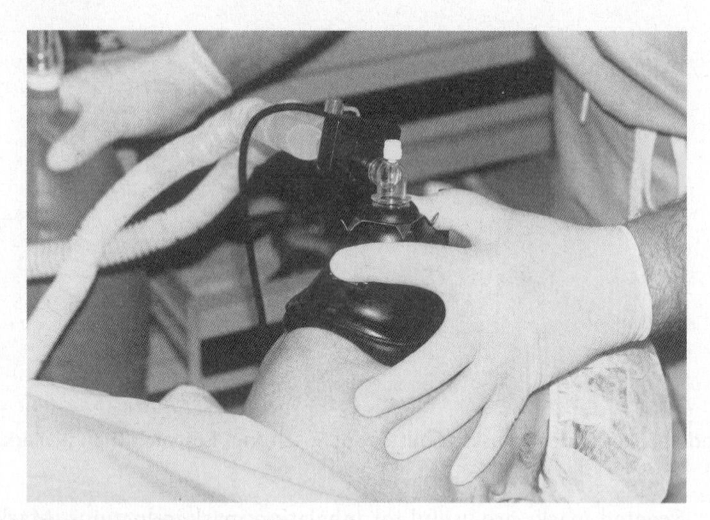

Figure 12.4 Holding the mask with one hand.

CLINICAL MOMENT With a known or presumed neck injury, the risk of neurological catastrophe may need be balanced against the need to change head position in order to provide effective mask ventilation.

1. **One-Hand Method**
   There are several methods of holding a mask to maintain an open airway and a tight seal. A commonly used method is shown in **Figure 12.4.** The thumb and the index finger on the left hand are placed on the mask body on opposite sides of the connector. These fingers push downward to hold the mask on the face and prevent leaks. Additional downward pressure, if required, can be exerted by the anesthesia provider's chin pushing down on the mask elbow. The next two fingers are placed on the jaw, taking care not to push into the soft tissues inside the mandible. The fifth finger is placed under the angle of the jaw and is used to pull the jaw upward. It is important that the applied pressure does not decrease airway patency. Care should be taken to prevent pressure on the eyes. In some cases, it may be necessary to extend the fingers to the right side of the mask to get a good seal.

CLINICAL MOMENT For the edentulous patient, it may be beneficial to gather part of the left cheek around the left base of the mask with the left hand while slightly tipping the mask toward the right.

2. **Two-Hand Method**
   A second method can be used to open any but the most difficult airway and obtain a tight fit (**Fig. 12.5A**). It requires two hands, so an assistant will be needed to squeeze the reservoir bag if positive airway pressure is necessary to control respiration. The thumbs are placed on either side of the mask body. The index fingers are placed under the angles of the jaw. The mandible is lifted and the head extended. If a leak is present, downward pressure on the mask can be increased by pressing the anesthesia provider's chin down on the mask elbow (**Fig. 12.5B**).

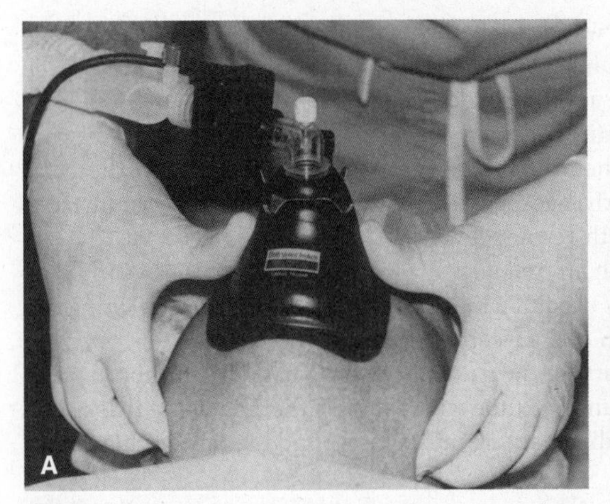

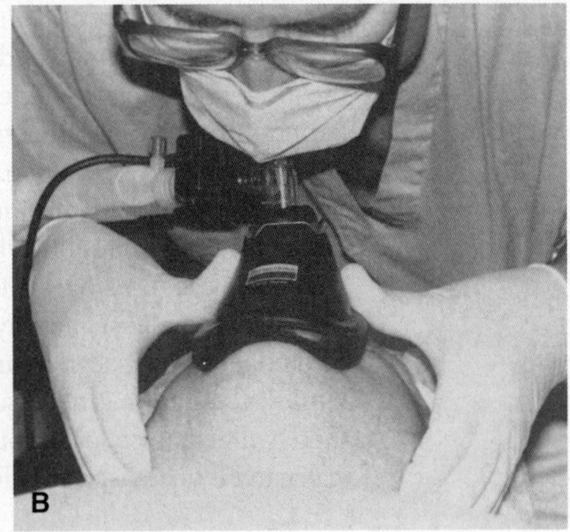

Figure 12.5 **A:** Holding the mask with two hands. Also shown is the Esmarch-Heiberg maneuver, which involves dorsiflexion at the atlanto-occipital joint and protrusion of the mandible anteriorly by exerting a forward thrust on the ramus. **B:** The anesthesia provider's chin on the mask elbow helps to create a better seal between the mask and the patient's face.

3. **Bearded Patient Techniques**
   Achieving a satisfactory mask fit is often difficult when the patient has a beard. One solution is to shave the beard. The beard may be covered with a clear adhesive drape, a defibrillator pad with a hole cut in the middle, plastic cling wrap, or gel and gauze. A small mask can be placed over the nose and the mouth held shut.

CLINICAL MOMENT It may be easier to get a good mask fit if the patient's dentures remain in place. Check to see if they are loose, in which case it may be better to remove them.

4. **Mask Ventilation of a Tracheostomy Stoma**
   A Rendell-Baker-Soucek mask can be used over a tracheotomy stoma to achieve controlled or assisted ventilation. It is placed around the stoma with the nasal portion pointing in a caudal direction so that the mandibular curve rests on the tracheal region and the apex on the suprasternal notch.

D. Difficult Face Mask Ventilation
   1. Difficult mask ventilation is reported in 5% to 6% of anesthetics. A variety of facial characteristics (fat, emaciated, edentulous) and faces with prominent nares, burns, flat noses, or receding jaws or other problems (drainage tube in the nose) are encountered in the clinical practice. Predictors of difficult mask ventilation include male gender, a beard, lack of teeth, over 57 years of age, macroglossia, high body mass index, limited jaw protrusion, abnormal neck anatomy, sleep apnea, snoring, increased Mallampati score, and short thyromental distance.
   2. The edentulous patient presents the most common problem. There is a loss of bone from the alveolar ridge, causing a loss of distance between the points where the mask rests on the mandible and the nose and shrinking at the corners of the mouth. The buccinator muscle loses its tone in these patients. The cheeks sag, creating gaps between them and the mask. Means to improve mask fit

include inserting an oral airway, leaving the patient's dentures in place, packing the cheeks with gauze, and inserting the inferior margin of the mask between the gingiva of the mandible and the lower lip.

3. Patients with facial deformities are particularly challenging. These may be covered by a beard to make them less evident. Mask application with the nasal projection pointed inferiorly has been used for children with certain facial deformities and patients with acromegaly.
4. If the mask is too small with an oral airway in place, the oral airway should be removed and a nasal airway used. If a mask is too long, the mouth opening can be elongated by inserting an oral airway.
5. If mask ventilation is necessary for the patient who has a nasogastric tube in place, there will usually a leak around the tube where it exits the side of the mask. This leak can be decreased by adding denture adhesive around the tube at this point.

CLINICAL MOMENT Mask ventilation often improves when muscle relaxants are administered. Before giving a muscle relaxant, the clinical situation needs to be evaluated carefully because the airway could be lost if the patient cannot be managed with a mask. A tracheal tube, supraglottic airway, or cricothyrotomy may be necessary in this situation.

E. Dead Space

The face mask and its adaptor normally constitute the major part of the mechanical dead space. Dead space may be decreased by increasing the pressure on the mask, changing the volume of the cushion, using a smaller mask, extending the separation between the inspiratory and expiratory channels closer to the mask, or blowing a jet of fresh gas into the mask.

F. Mask Straps

1. For procedures lasting longer than a few minutes, it may be advantageous to use a mask strap to hold the mask firmly on the face. This allows the clinician to attend to other tasks. Particular care needs to be taken to maintain the airway when using a mask strap because obstruction or regurgitation is more likely to go unrecognized than when the mask is being held by the anesthesia provider's hand.
2. A typical mask strap (**Fig. 12.6**) consists of a circle with two or four projections. The head rests in the circle, and the straps attach around the mask connector.

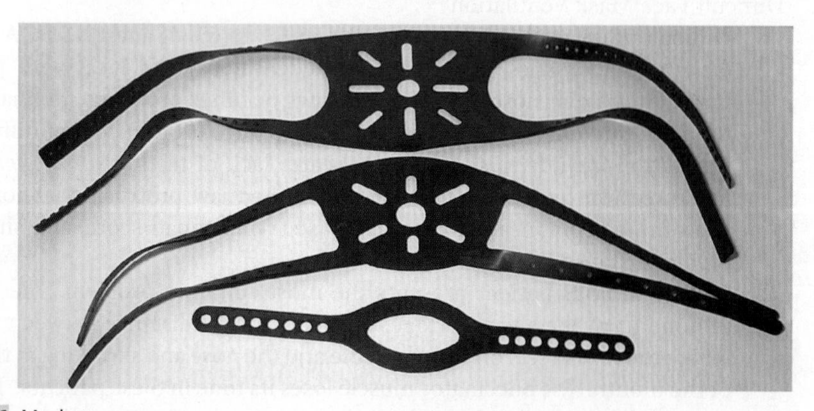

Figure 12.6 Mask straps.

Crossing the two lower straps under the chin may result in a better fit and counteract the pull from the upper straps, making it less likely that the mask will creep above the bridge of the nose and onto the eyes. The best strap application is a matter of individual preference and may be the result of a trial-and-error process.

3. Care must be taken that the straps are no tighter than necessary to achieve a seal in order to avoid pressure damage from the mask or the straps. Straps should be released periodically and the mask moved slightly. Gauze sponges placed between the straps and the skin will help to protect the face. Another risk of using a mask strap is that it will take longer to remove the mask if vomiting or regurgitation occurs. Pressure from mask straps that are too tight can cause alopecia where the strap contacts the back of the head.

CLINICAL MOMENT Holding a mask is a good way to monitor a patient's respiration. The anesthesia provider can feel breath movement and often detect regurgitation should it occur. A mask strap moves the clinician further from the patient, making it more difficult to detect problems.

G. Advantages

Using a face mask is associated with a lower incidence of sore throat and requires less anesthetic depth than using a supraglottic device or a tracheal tube. Muscle relaxants are not required. The face mask may be the most cost-efficient method to manage the airway for short cases.

CLINICAL MOMENT With the advent of the supraglottic airways such as the laryngeal mask, administering anesthesia with a face mask has lost favor. This is unfortunate because the skills learned administering anesthesia with a face mask will serve the anesthesia provider well when an airway emergency occurs. All anesthesia providers must be expert at using a face mask.

H. Disadvantages

With a face mask, one or more of the anesthesia provider's hands are in continuous use, and higher fresh gas flows are often needed. During remote anesthesia (magnetic resonance imaging and computerized tomographic scanning), airway access is difficult. Patients who are managed with a face mask have more episodes of oxygen desaturation, require more intraoperative airway manipulations, and present more difficulties in maintaining an airway than patients with a supraglottic airway device. In spontaneously breathing patients, the work of breathing is higher with a face mask than with a supraglottic airway device or a tracheal tube. Using an airway and/or continuous positive pressure may reduce the work of breathing. Dead space is increased compared with a tracheal tube or a supraglottic device. This increase is probably not significant in adults but can be important in neonates and small children.

I. Complications

1. **Skin Problems**

Dermatitis may occur if the patient is allergic to the mask material. The pattern of the dermatitis follows the area of contact between the mask and the skin. Some masks or mask straps contain latex (see Chapter 11). Cleaning or sterilizing reusable masks can leave a residue that can cause a skin reaction.

Pressure necrosis under the face mask has been reported following prolonged mask application in the presence of hypotension.

CLINICAL MOMENT It is important that a face mask be adjusted periodically, especially if a mask strap is used.

2. **Nerve Injury**
   Pressure from a mask or mask strap may result in injury to underlying nerves. Forward jaw displacement may cause a stretching nerve injury. Fortunately, the sensory and motor dysfunctions reported have been transient. If excessive pressure on the face or extreme jaw displacement must be exerted, tracheal intubation or a supraglottic airway device should be considered. The mask should be removed from the face periodically and readjusted to make certain that continuous pressure is not applied to just one area.
3. **Foreign Body Aspiration**
   The diaphragm on an endoscopic mask may rupture during tracheal tube insertion, and a piece pushed into the patient's tracheobronchial tree. Other parts of a mask or mask strap may be aspirated.
4. **Gastric Inflation**
   When positive pressure ventilation is used with a face mask, gases may be forced into the stomach. It is recommended that the peak inspiratory pressure be kept below 20 cm H_2O.
5. **Eye Injury**
   A corneal abrasion may be caused by a face mask inadvertently placed on an open eye. Chemicals that enter the reusable mask cushion during cleaning and disinfection can be expelled from cracks in the cushion and come into contact with the eye when the mask is applied to the face. Pressure on the medial angles of the eyes and supraorbital margins may result in eyelid edema and conjunctival chemosis, whereas pressure on the supraorbital or supratrochlear nerve may lead to corneal injury, and temporary blindness from central retinal artery occlusion.
6. **Mask Defects**
   A mask with a plastic membrane that occluded the connector has been reported. Another mask had a metal wire sticking out of it.
7. **Cervical Spine Movement**
   Most but not all studies show that mask ventilation moves the cervical spine more than the commonly used tracheal intubation methods. This may be significant in a patient with an unstable cervical spine injury.
8. **Latex Allergy**
   If a face mask contains rubber, a serious reaction can occur in the patient with latex allergy. This is discussed more fully in Chapter 11.
9. **Lack of Correlation between Arterial and End-Tidal Carbon Dioxide**
   The difference between arterial and end-tidal carbon dioxide levels is higher with face mask ventilation than with a tracheal tube or a supraglottic device, particularly with small tidal volumes.
10. **Environmental Pollution**
    Studies show that the use of a face mask is associated with greater operating room pollution with anesthetic gases and vapors than when a tracheal tube or a supraglottic airway device is used. Pollution can be reduced with a close active scavenging device.

11. **User Fatigue**
    Holding a mask securely onto the face and at the same time maintaining the correct jaw position can be difficult and may result in operator fatigue. Failure to maintain the correct jaw position may result in lost airway patency or gastric distention.
12. **Jaw Pain**
    Postoperative jaw pain is more common after mask anesthesia than when a supraglottic airway device is used.

II. Airways

A fundamental responsibility of the anesthesia provider is to maintain a patent airway. Figure 12.7A shows the normal unobstructed airway in a supine patient. It has a rigid posterior wall, supported by the cervical vertebrae, and a collapsible anterior wall consisting of the tongue and the epiglottis. Figure 12.7B shows the most common cause of airway obstruction. Under anesthesia, the muscles in the floor of the mouth and pharynx supporting the tongue relax, and the tongue and epiglottis fall back into the posterior pharynx, occluding the airway. The purpose of an oropharyngeal or nasal airway is to lift the tongue and the epiglottis away from the posterior pharyngeal wall and prevent them from obstructing the space above the larynx. Maneuvers such as dorsiflexion at the atlanto-occipital joint and anterior mandible protrusion may still be necessary to ensure a patent airway. An oral or nasal airway may decrease the work of breathing during spontaneous breathing with a face mask.

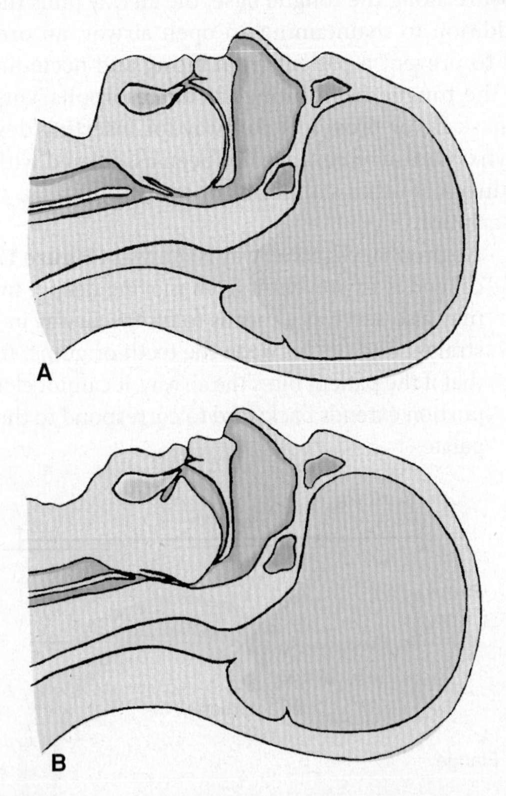

Figure 12.7 **A:** The normal airway. The tongue and other soft tissues are forward, allowing an unobstructed air passage. **B:** The obstructed airway. The tongue and epiglottis fall back to the posterior pharyngeal wall, occluding the airway. (Courtesy of V. Robideaux, MD.)

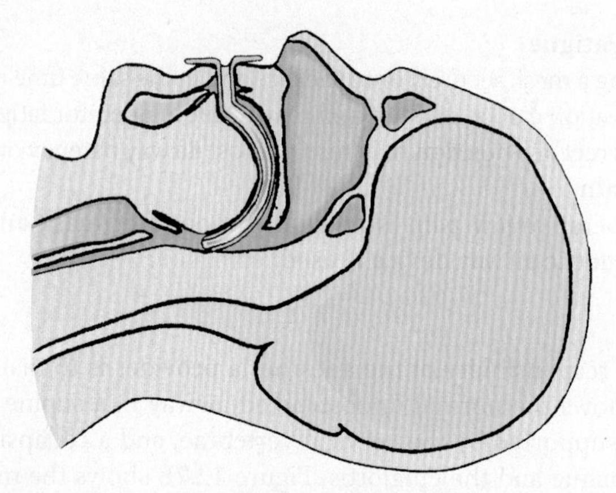

Figure 12.8 Oropharyngeal airway in place. The airway follows the curvature of the tongue, pulling it and the epiglottis away from the posterior pharyngeal wall and providing a channel for air passage. (Courtesy of V. Robideaux, MD.)

A. Types

1. **Oropharyngeal Airways**

Figure 12.8 shows an oropharyngeal (oral) airway in place. The bite portion is between the teeth and lips, and the flange is outside the lips. The pharyngeal end rests between the posterior pharyngeal wall and the tongue base. By exerting pressure along the tongue base, the airway pulls the epiglottis forward.

In addition to maintaining an open airway, an oropharyngeal airway may be used to prevent a patient from biting and occluding an oral tracheal tube, protect the tongue from biting, facilitate oropharyngeal suctioning, obtain a better mask fit, or provide a pathway for inserting devices into the esophagus or pharynx. Oral airways have not been associated with an increased incidence of sore throat or other symptoms or bacteremia.

a. Description

1) An oropharyngeal airway is shown in **Figure 12.9.** The flange at the buccal end is to prevent it from moving deeper into the mouth. The flange may also serve as a means to fix the airway in place. The bite portion is straight and fits between the teeth or gums. It must be firm enough so that if the patient bites the airway, it cannot close the lumen. The curved portion extends backward to correspond to the shape of the tongue and palate.

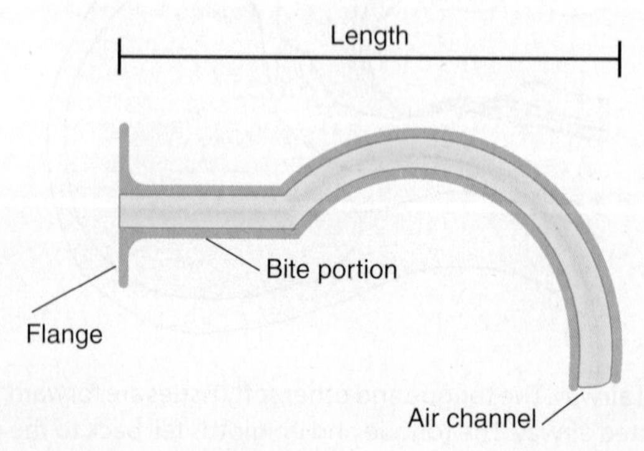

Figure 12.9 Oropharyngeal airway. All oral airways have a flange to prevent overinsertion, a straight bite block portion, and a curved section.

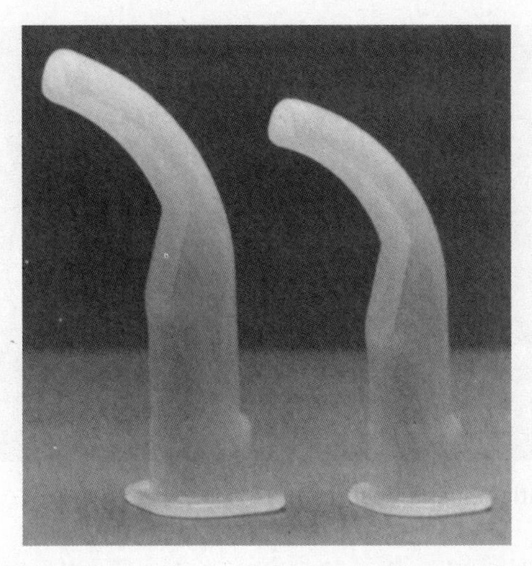

Figure 12.10 Williams airway intubators. (Courtesy of Mercury Medical, Clearwater, FL.)

2) The size of most oral airways is designated by the length in centimeters (**Fig. 12.9**). Airways are sometimes sized by an older system, using numbers from 0 to 6. There may be some variability in airway size among airways with the same number designation from different manufacturers.

b. Specific Airways

1) Several types of oral airways are in use today. They are often used for specific purposes such as fiber-optic–guided intubation.
2) The Patil-Syracuse endoscopic airway was designed to aid fiber-optic intubation. It has lateral channels and a central groove on the lingual surface to allow a fiberscope with a tracheal tube to pass. A slit in the distal end allows the fiberscope to be manipulated in the anteroposterior direction but limits the lateral movement. It is made of aluminum.
3) The Williams airway intubator (**Fig. 12.10**) was designed for blind orotracheal intubations. It can also be used to aid fiber-optic intubations or as an oral airway. The airway is plastic and available in two sizes, nos. 9 and 10, which will admit up to an 8.0- or 8.5-mm-tracheal tube, respectively. The proximal half is cylindrical, whereas the distal half is open on its lingual surface. The airway is removed after intubation. The tracheal tube connector should be removed during intubation because it will not pass through the airway when the airway is removed.
4) The Ovassapian fiber-optic intubating airway (**Fig. 12.11**) has a flat lingual surface that gradually widens at the distal end. At the

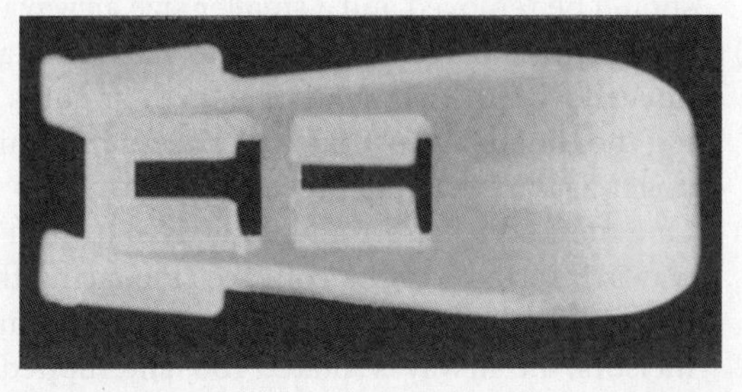

Figure 12.11 Ovassapian fiber-optic intubating airway. (Courtesy of A. Ovassapian, MD.)

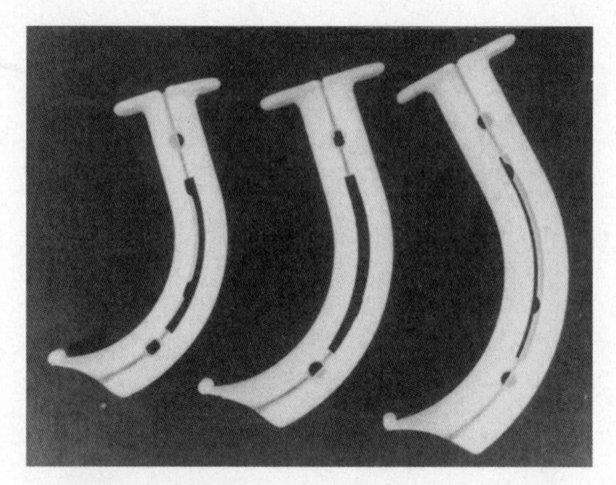

Figure 12.12 Berman intubation pharyngeal airways.

buccal end are two vertical sidewalls. Between the sidewalls are two guide walls that curve toward each other. The guide walls are flexible and allow the airway to be removed from around the tracheal tube. The proximal half is tubular so that it can function as a bite block. The distal half is open posteriorly. It will accommodate a tracheal tube up to 9.0-mm ID. The black line along the middle of the airway helps to identify the midline and facilitates advancing the flexible endoscope.

5) The Berman intubation pharyngeal airway (Berman II) (**Fig. 12.12**) is tubular along its entire length. It is open on one side so that it can be split and removed from around a tracheal tube. It can be used as an oral airway or as an aid to fiber-optic or blind orotracheal intubation. When the fiberscope is in the airway, the tip cannot be bent, limiting scope maneuverability. Partially withdrawing the airway will improve maneuverability.

c. Use

1) Pharyngeal and laryngeal reflexes should be depressed before an oral airway is inserted to avoid coughing or laryngospasm.
2) Selecting the correct size is important. Too small an airway may cause the tongue to kink and force part of it against the roof of the mouth, causing obstruction. Too large an airway may cause obstruction by displacing the epiglottis posteriorly and may traumatize the larynx. The correct size can be estimated by holding the airway next to the patient's mouth. The tip should rest cephalad to the angle of the mandible. The best criterion for proper size and position is unobstructed gas exchange. If the airway repeatedly comes out of the mouth, it should be removed and a smaller size airway used.
3) Wetting or lubricating the airway may facilitate insertion. The jaw is opened with the left hand. The teeth or gums are separated by pressing the thumb against the lower teeth or gum and the index or third finger against the upper teeth or gum.
4) One method to insert an airway is shown in **Figure 12.13.** The airway is inserted with its concave side facing the upper lip. When the junction between the bite portion and the curved section is near the incisors, the airway is rotated 180° and slipped behind the tongue into

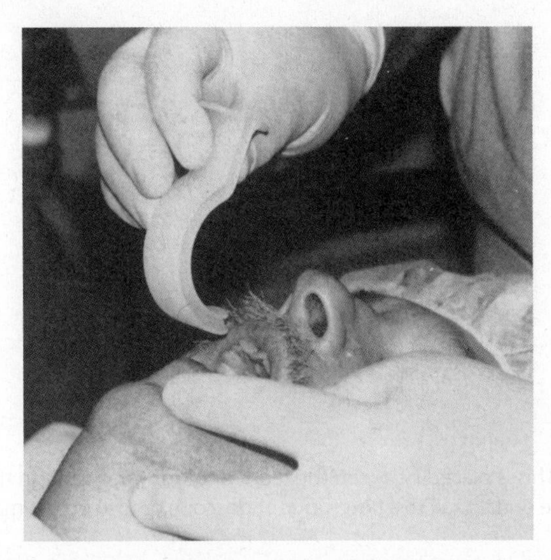

Figure 12.13 Insertion of an oral airway. The airway is inserted 180° from the final resting position.

the final position. If resistance is met during insertion, it can usually be overcome with a jaw thrust.

5) An alternate method to insert an oral airway is shown in **Figure 12.14.** A tongue blade is used to push forward and depress the tongue. The airway is inserted with the concave side toward the tongue. As it is advanced, it is rotated to slide around behind the tongue.

CLINICAL MOMENT While using a tongue blade is an accepted practice, it would be wise to master a technique that does not require an additional device. A tongue blade is not always available in an emergency and its absence may make inserting the airway difficult for an anesthesia provider accustomed to using it.

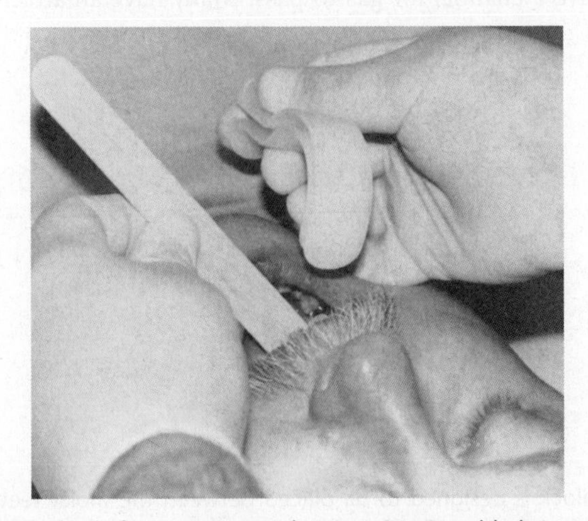

Figure 12.14 Alternative method of inserting an oral airway. A tongue blade is used to displace the tongue forward.

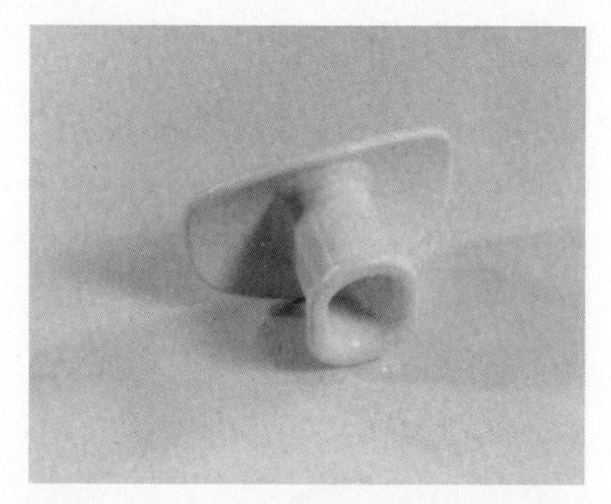

Figure 12.15 Bite block. This is placed between the teeth or gums (preferably in the molar area) to prevent occlusion of a tracheal tube or damage to a fiber-optic endoscope or to keep the mouth open for suctioning.

6) If the airway has been used to facilitate fiber-optic intubation, it may be better to remove the airway after the fiberscope has entered the trachea because the airway might prevent the tracheal tube from passing into the trachea.

2. **Bite Block**
   a. A bite block (gag, mouth prop, or bite protector) is placed between the molar teeth or gums but not the incisors. It is intended to prevent the teeth from biting the tracheal tube, supraglottic airway, fiberscope, or other device. Not only will it protect these devices but it may also avoid dental injury. A bite block is also used during electroconvulsive therapy and in unconscious individuals to protect the tongue and lips (**Fig. 12.17**). An oral airway should not be used for these purposes. It is ineffective and may be harmful to the patient in this role because all the biting power is concentrated on the incisors, which are not designed for this pressure and may break or loosen. Because a bite block does not extend into the pharynx, it is usually less irritating than an oral airway.
   b. A variety of bite blocks have been developed (**Figs. 12.15–12.17**). Some have a channel for gas to pass. Many have an attached string that can be

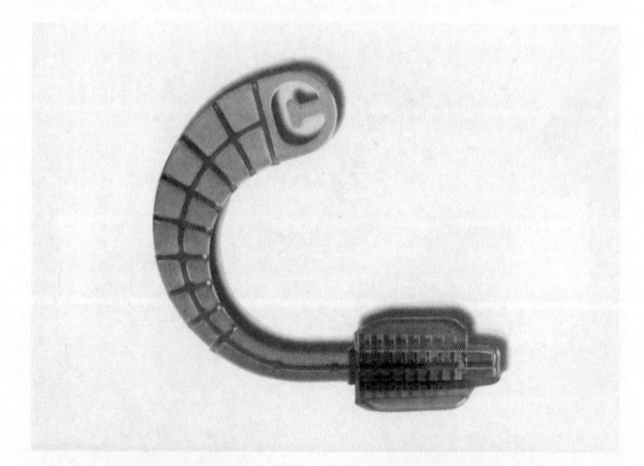

Figure 12.16 This bite block is designed to be placed between the molar teeth, with the flat portion extending toward the side of the face. The flat portion is used to grip for insertion and removal. (Picture courtesy of Hudson RCI, Research Triangle Park, NC.)

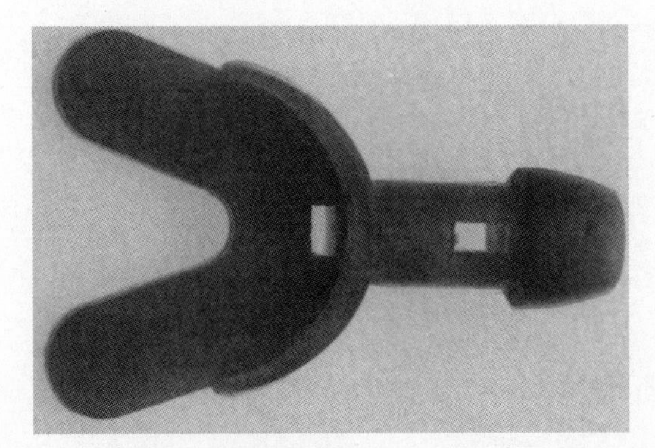

Figure 12.17 Oberto mouth prop, which is used for protecting the teeth during electroconvulsive therapy. (Courtesy of Rusch, Inc.)

pinned to the patient's gown or taped to the skin so that it can be easily retrieved. A bite block may be part of a device used to secure a tracheal tube.

3. **Nasopharyngeal Airways**

A nasopharyngeal airway (nasal airway, nasal trumpet) is shown in position in **Figure 12.18.** When fully inserted, the pharyngeal end should be below the tongue base but above the epiglottis. This airway is usually better tolerated than an oral airway.

a. Description

A nasopharyngeal airway, shown in **Figure 12.19,** resembles a shortened tracheal tube with a flange at the outer end to prevent it from passing completely into the nose. Some airways come with a safety pin that can be inserted into the flange or airway wall. The flange is movable on some models. Many nasal airways have a bevel at the patient end. The nasopharyngeal airway size is designated by the inside diameter in millimeters.

b. Specific Airways

1) The cuffed nasopharyngeal (pharyngeal) airway is similar to a short cuffed tracheal tube. It is inserted through the nose into the pharynx; the cuff is inflated and is then pulled back until resistance is felt.

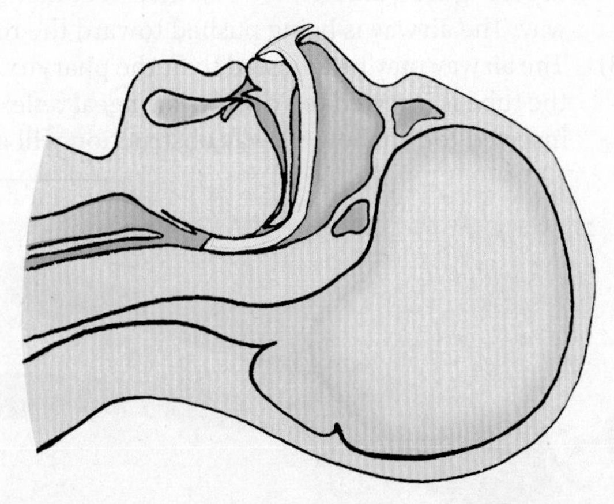

Figure 12.18 The nasopharyngeal airway in place. The airway passes through the nose and extends to just above the epiglottis. (Courtesy of V. Robideaux, MD.)

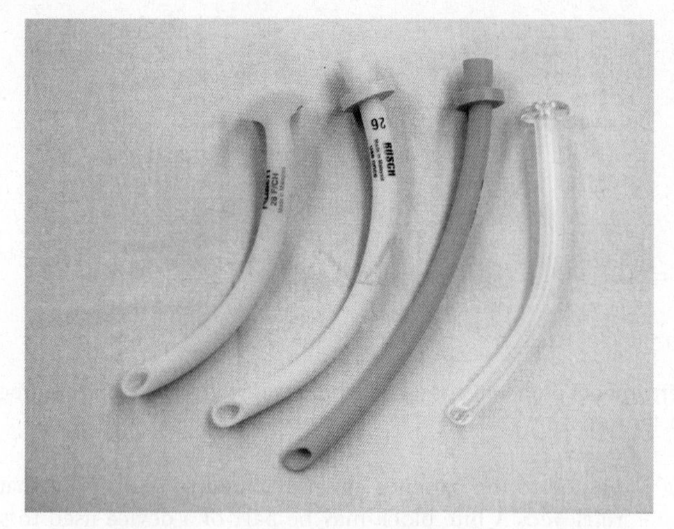

Figure 12.19 Nasopharyngeal airways. The one on the right does not contain latex.

2) The binasal airway (**Fig. 12.20**) consists of two nasal airways joined together by an adaptor that attaches it to the breathing system. It can be used to administer anesthesia or to provide continuous positive airway pressure (CPAP) to babies.

c. Airway Insertion

1) Before insertion, the nasal airway should be lubricated thoroughly along its entire length. Each side of the nose should be inspected for size, patency, and polyps. A vasoconstrictor may be applied to reduce trauma.

2) A simple technique to open and straighten the pathway through the nares is to push upward and posteriorly on the tip of the nose. The nasopharyngeal airway should be inserted as shown in **Fig. 12.21A.** The airway is held with the bevel against the septum and gently advanced posteriorly while being rotated. If resistance is encountered during insertion, the other nostril or a smaller size airway should be used. **Figure 12.21B** shows an incorrect method for inserting the airway. The airway is being pushed toward the roof of the nose.

3) The airway may be adjusted to fit the pharynx by sliding it in or out. If the tube is inserted too deeply, laryngeal reflexes may be stimulated; if inserted too shallow, airway obstruction will not be relieved.

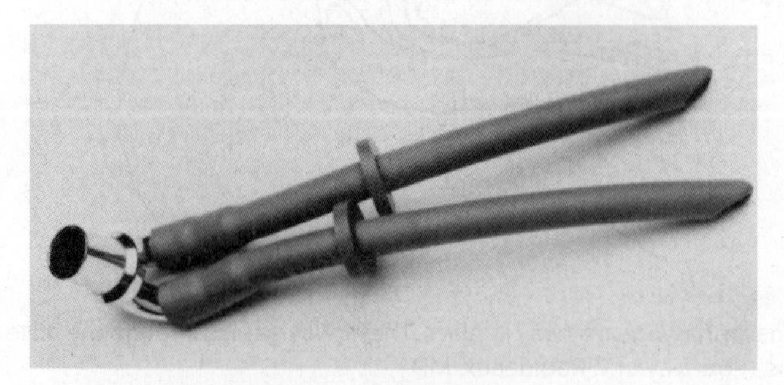

Figure 12.20 Binasal airway. (Courtesy of Rusch, Inc.)

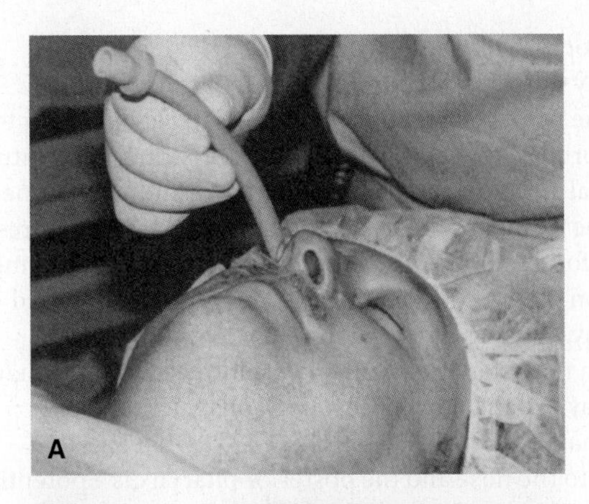

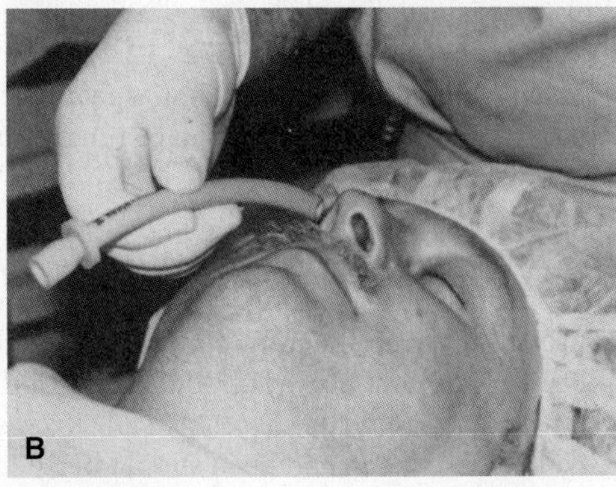

Figure 12.21 Insertion of a nasal airway. **A:** Correct method. The airway is inserted perpendicularly, in line with the nasal passage. **B:** Incorrect method. The airway is being pushed away from the air passage and into the turbinates.

d. Advantages
   1) A nasal airway is better tolerated than an oral airway if the patient has intact airway reflexes. It is preferable to use a nasal airway if the patient's teeth are loose or in poor condition or there is trauma or pathology in the oral cavity. A nasal airway can be used when the mouth cannot be opened.
   2) A nasopharyngeal airway has been used in infants with Pierre Robin syndrome during and after pharyngeal surgery; to apply CPAP; to facilitate suctioning, as a guide for a fiberscope; to treat singultus (hiccups), as a guide for a nasogastric tube; to dilate the nasal passages in preparation for nasotracheal intubation, as a conduit for fiber-optic endoscopy and intubation; and to maintain the airway and administer anesthesia during dental surgery.
   3) A nasopharyngeal airway can be fitted with a tracheal tube connector and used with an anesthesia breathing system. These devices have been used to maintain ventilation during oral fiber-optic endoscopy and to administer CPAP. Environmental gas contamination occurs with this technique.

e. Contraindications
   Contraindications to using a nasopharyngeal airway include anticoagulation; a basilar skull fracture; nasal or nasopharyngeal deformity; or a history of nosebleeds requiring medical treatment.

B. Complications

1. **Airway Obstruction**

   a. The tip of an oral airway can press the epiglottis or tongue against the posterior pharyngeal wall and cover the laryngeal aperture. With a nasopharyngeal airway, neck movement may result in the lumen becoming obstructed. The nasopharyngeal airway lumen may be compressed inside the nose.

   b. A foreign body can enter an airway and cause complete or partial obstruction. The plastic packaging can became stretched over the end of the airway, causing obstruction.

   c. If a nasopharyngeal airway perforates the retropharyngeal space, the space may expand and cause airway obstruction.

2. **Trauma**

   Injury to the nose and the posterior pharynx is a potential complication of nasal airways. Epistaxis is usually self-limiting but can present a serious problem in some patients. An epistaxis airway (**Fig. 12.22**) can be used to control severe nasal and nasopharyngeal bleeding. Pharyngeal perforation and retropharyngeal abscess formation can occur. The lip or tongue may be caught between the teeth and an oral airway.

3. **Tissue Edema**

   Facial, neck, or tongue edema, either unilateral or bilateral, can occur following surgery, especially in the sitting position, and can result in airway obstruction. Pressure from an oral airway may be a contributing factor. To prevent this complication, the oral airway should not be left in place for an extended period. A bite block should be used instead. Excessive head or neck flexion should be avoided. The head and neck should be checked frequently for edema or ecchymoses during long cases. Uvular edema possibly caused by the uvula becoming entrapped between the hard palate and an oropharyngeal airway has been reported. Temporary deafness secondary to uvular and soft palate edema following prolonged nasopharyngeal airway use has been reported. Transient salivary gland swelling may occur with oral airway use.

4. **Ulceration and Necrosis**

   Nose or tongue ulceration can occur if an airway remains in place for a long period of time.

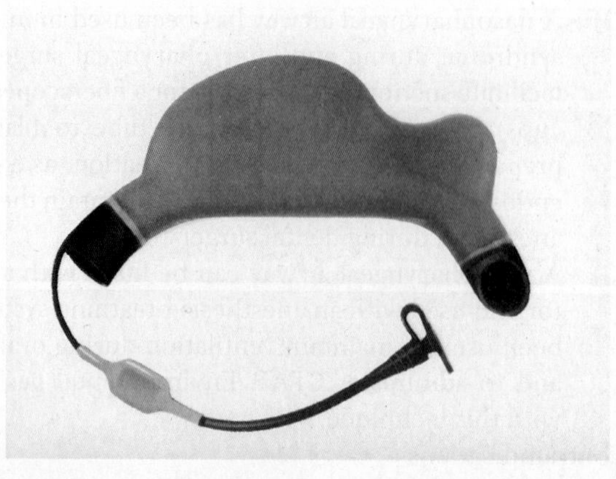

Figure 12.22 Epistaxis airway. This is inserted into the nose and inflated to provide local pressure on the bleeding site. It is available in several sizes. (Courtesy of Rusch, Inc.)

5. **Central Nervous System Trauma**
Using a nasal airway in a patient with a basilar skull fracture can result in the airway entering the anterior cranial fossa.
6. **Dental Damage**
Teeth can be damaged or avulsed if the patient bites down hard on an oral airway. An oral airway should be avoided if there is evidence of periodontal disease, teeth weakened by caries or restorations, crowns, fixed partial dentures, pronounced proclination (the front teeth having a forward inclination and overlapping the lower front teeth), or isolated teeth. In these cases, using a nasopharyngeal airway and/or a bite block between the back teeth may be preferable.
7. **Laryngospasm and Coughing**
Inserting an airway before adequate anesthetic depth is established may cause coughing or laryngospasm, especially if the airway contacts the epiglottis or vocal cords.
8. **Retention, Aspiration, or Swallowing**
Part or all of an airway may become displaced into the pharynx, tracheobronchial tree, or esophagus. Placing a safety pin through the nasal airway flange may prevent it from slipping into the nose but may interfere with suctioning or with the use of a T-piece for oxygen administration.
9. **Devices Caught in Airway**
In one case, an esophageal stethoscope cuff became detached when it was removed from a patient with an oral airway in place. It was thought that the cuff became caught in the airway's side grooves. Another case was reported in which a fiberscope inadvertently traversed a fenestrated oral airway, making it impossible to pass a tracheal tube.
10. **Equipment Failure**
An oral airway may fracture at the connection between the bite portion and the curved section. A defect in the Williams intubating airway that could tear the tracheal tube cuff has been reported.
11. **Latex Allergy**
If an airway contains latex, a severe reaction may occur if the patient is sensitive to latex. Nonlatex oral and nasal airways are available. Chapter 11 provides more details on latex allergy.
12. **Gastric Distention**
A nasopharyngeal airway that is too long for the patient may enter the esophagus, with resultant gastric distention.

SUGGESTED READINGS

Atlas GM. A comparison of fiberoptic-compatible oral airways. J Clin Anesth 2004;16:66–73.

Dorsch J, Dorsch S. Face masks and airways. In: Understanding Anesthesia Equipment. Fifth edition. Philadelphia: Wolters Kluwer/Lippincott Williams & Wilkins, 2008:443–460.

Greenberg RS. Facemask, nasal, and oral airway devices. Anesth Clin N Am 2002;20:833–861.

Kheterpal S, Han R, Tremper KK, Shanks A, et al. Incidence and predictors of difficult and impossible mask ventilation. Anesthesiology 2006;105:885–891.

McGee JP, Vender JS. Nonintubation management of the airway: mask ventilation. In: Hagberg CA, ed. Benumof's Airway Management. Second edition. St Louis, MO: Elsevier, 2007:345–370.

Patil VU. Oxygenation and ventilation of the patient. In: Fundamentals of Airway Management Techniques. A Color Atlas. Skaneateles, NY: Lotus Publishing LLC, 2003:105–130.

Wheeler M, Ovassapian A. Fiberoptic endoscopy-aided techniques. In: Hagberg CA, ed. Benumof's Airway Management. Second edition. St Louis, MO: Elsevier, 2007:405–407.

13 Supraglottic Airway Devices

SUPRAGLOTTIC AIRWAY DEVICES HAVE BECOME standard fixtures in airway management, filling a niche between the face mask and the tracheal tube in terms of both anatomical position and degree of invasiveness. These devices sit outside the trachea but provide a hands-free means of achieving a gas-tight airway.

The first successful supraglottic device, the Laryngeal Mask Airway (LMA)-Classic, became available in 1989. As time went on, additional devices were added to the LMA family. A number of other devices, some of which are similar to the LMA family and others that work under a different concept, have been developed. It is not possible to discuss all of these devices because they are being introduced at a rapid rate whereas others are disappearing. Some that seem to be gaining acceptance and longevity at the time of this writing will be discussed. The LMA family will be discussed in greatest detail because it has been so extensively studied.

I. Laryngeal Mask Airway Family

A. Types

1. LMA-Classic

a. Description

The LMA-Classic (standard LMA, classic LMA, LMA-C, cLMA) has a curved tube (shaft) connected to an elliptical mask (cup) at a 30° angle (**Fig. 13.1**). There are two flexible vertical bars where the tube enters the mask to prevent the tube from becoming obstructed by the epiglottis. An inflatable cuff surrounds the mask's inner rim. An inflating tube and a self-sealing pilot balloon are attached to the wider end of the mask. A black line runs longitudinally along the posterior aspect of the tube. At the machine end of the tube is a 15-mm connector. The LMA is made from silicone and contains no latex. There are eight sizes to fit patients from neonates to adults (**Table 13.1**).

b. Insertion

1) The standard insertion technique uses a midline or slightly diagonal approach with the cuff fully deflated. The head should be extended and the neck flexed (sniffing position). This position is best maintained during insertion by using the noninserting hand to stabilize the occiput

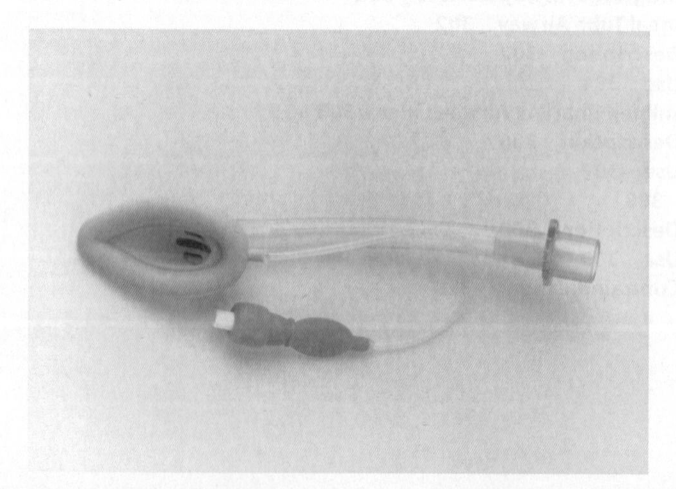

Figure 13.1 LMA-Classic. Note the bars at the junction of the tube and the mask. (Courtesy of LMA North America, San Diego, CA.)

Table 13.1 Available LMA-Classics

LMA Size	Patient Size	Largest Tracheal Tube that can Fit the LMA (ID in mm)	Largest Fiberscope that Fits into a Tracheal Tube (OD in mm)
1	Neonates/infants up to 5 kg	3.5	2.7
1.5	Infants between 5 and 10 kg	4.0	3.0
2	Infants/children between 10 and 20 kg[a]	4.5	3.4
2.5	Children between 20 and 30 kg	5.0	4.0
3	Children 30–50 kg	6.0 cuffed	5.0
4	Adults 50–70 kg	6.0 cuffed	5.0
5	Adults 70–100 kg	7.0 cuffed	5.0
6	Adults >100 kg	7.0 cuffed	5.0

[a]Size 2.5 may be more suitable for children of this size.

(**Fig. 13.2**). The LMA can be inserted without placing the head in the sniffing position. The neutral position may cause a small decrease in successful placement compared with the sniffing position.

2) The jaw may be pulled down by an assistant to more fully open the mouth. The tube portion is grasped as if it were a pen, with the index finger pressing on the point where the tube joins the mask (**Fig. 13.2**).

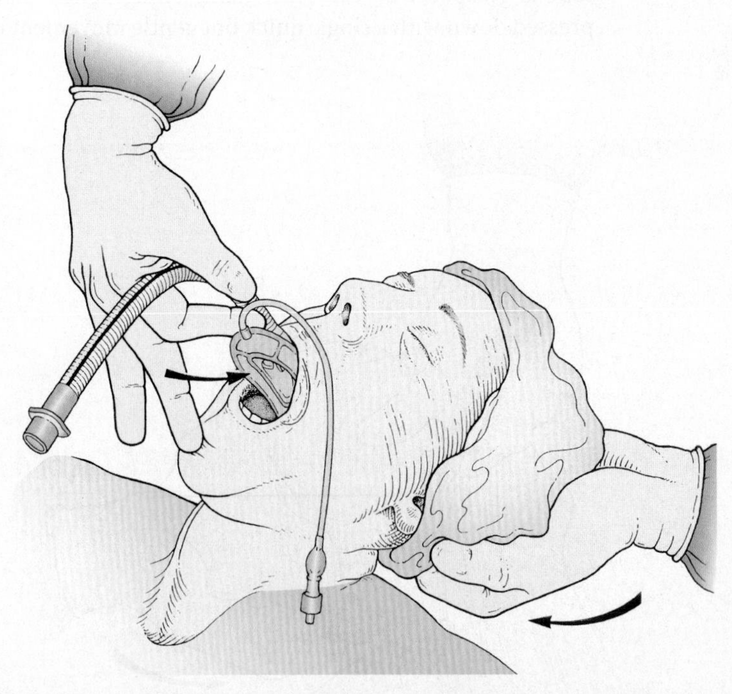

Figure 13.2 Initial insertion of the laryngeal mask. Under direct vision, the mask tip is pressed upward against the hard palate. The middle finger may be used to push the lower jaw downward. The mask is pressed upward as it is advanced into the pharynx to ensure that the tip remains flattened and avoids the tongue. The jaw should not be held open once the mask is inside the mouth. The nonintubating hand can be used to stabilize the occiput. (Courtesy of LMA North America, San Diego, CA.)

With the aperture facing forward (and the black line facing the patient's upper lip), the cuff tip is placed against the inner surface of the upper incisors or gums. At this point, the tube should be parallel to the floor. If the mouth is being held open, the jaw should be released during further insertion. If the patient has a restricted mouth opening, an alternative method is to pass the LMA behind the molar teeth into the pharynx. The tubular part is then maneuvered toward the midline.

3) As the LMA is advanced, the mask portion is pressed against the hard palate using the index finger. This means that the direction of applied pressure is different from the direction in which the mask moves. If resistance is felt, the tip may have folded on itself or impacted on an irregularity or the posterior pharynx. In this case, a diagonal shift in direction is often helpful or a gloved finger may be inserted behind the mask to lift it over the obstruction. If at any time during insertion the mask fails to stay flattened or starts to fold back, it should be withdrawn and reinserted.
4) A change in direction can be sensed as the mask tip encounters the posterior pharyngeal wall and follows it downward. By withdrawing the other fingers as the index finger is advanced and slightly pronating the forearm, it is often possible to insert the mask fully into position with a single movement (**Fig. 13.3**). If this maneuver is not successful, the hand position must be changed for the next movement. The tube is grasped with the other hand, straightened slightly, and then pressed down with a single quick but gentle movement until a definite

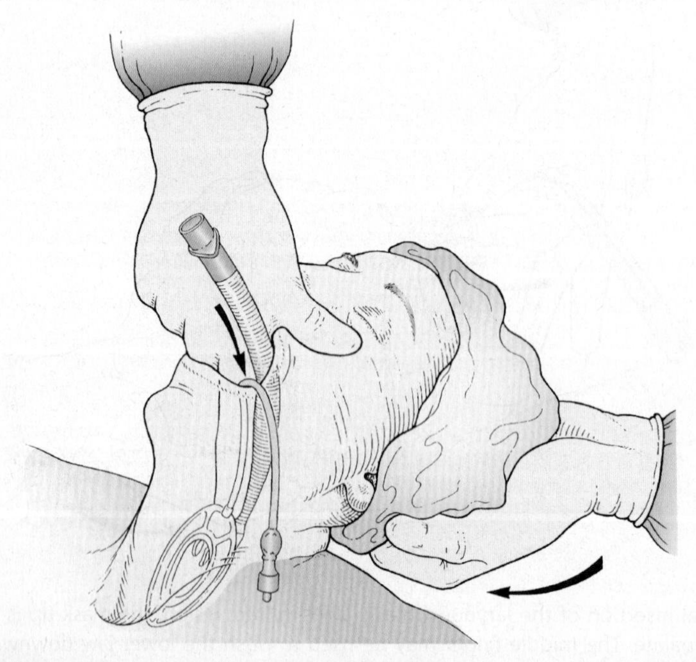

Figure 13.3 By withdrawing the other fingers and with a slight pronation of the forearm, it is usually possible to push the mask fully into position in one fluid movement. Note that the neck is kept flexed and the head is extended. (Courtesy of Gensia Pharmaceuticals, Inc.)

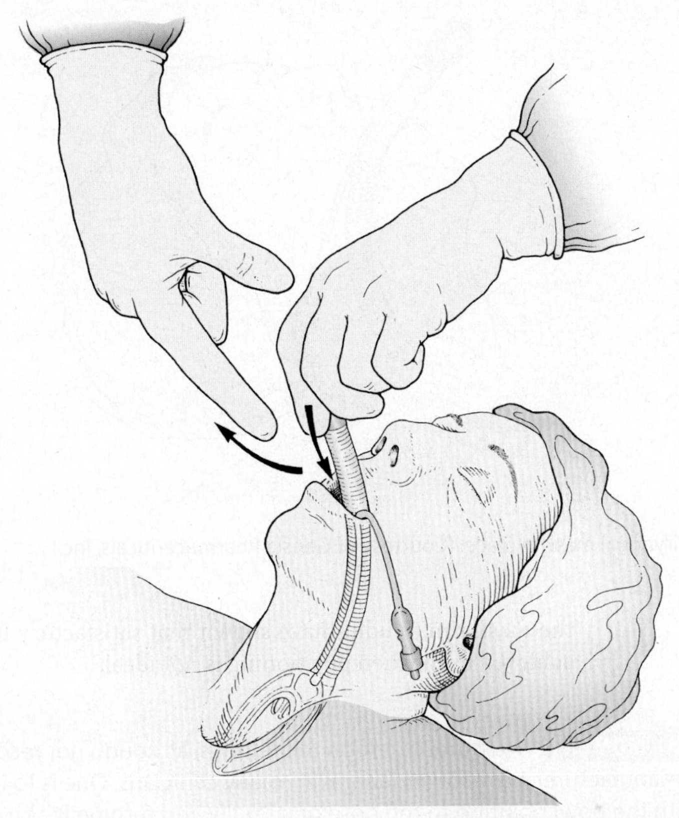

Figure 13.4 The laryngeal mask is grasped with the other hand and the index finger withdrawn. The hand that is holding the tube presses gently downward until resistance is encountered. (Courtesy of Gensia Pharmaceuticals, Inc.)

resistance is felt (**Fig. 13.4**). This may coincide with anterior laryngeal displacement. The longitudinal black line on the shaft should lie in the midline facing the upper lip.

5) If the patient has a high, arched palate, a slightly lateral approach may be needed. The operator should check that the cuff tip is flattened against the palate before proceeding. Difficulty in negotiating the angle at the back of the tongue is most commonly the result of an incorrect angle of approach.

CLINICAL MOMENT If the first insertion attempt is unsuccessful while cricoid pressure is being applied, the pressure should be transiently released while the mask is moving downward during the second attempt.

6) When properly placed, the mask rests on the hypopharyngeal floor. The sides face the pyriform fossae, and the upper border of the cuff is behind the tongue base (**Figs. 13.5** and **13.6**). The epiglottis tip may rest either within the mask bowl or under the proximal cuff at an angle determined by the extent to which the mask has deflected it downward. In some cases, the upper part of the esophagus lies within

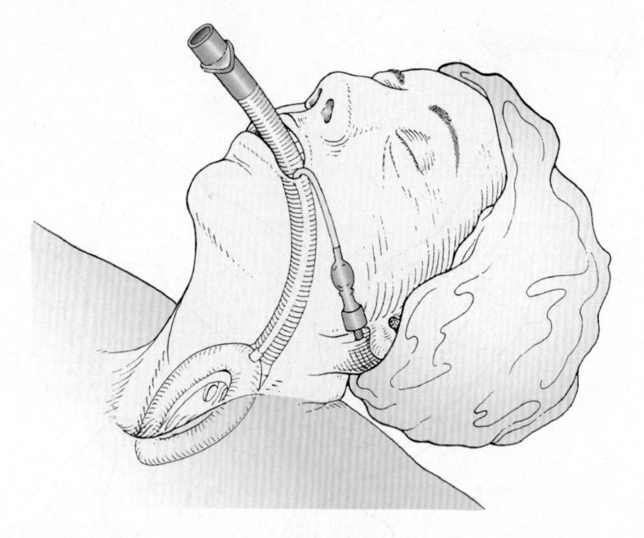

Figure 13.5 The laryngeal mask in place. (Courtesy of Gensia Pharmaceuticals, Inc.)

the mask rim. Studies have shown that satisfactory function may be achieved even when positioning is not ideal.

CLINICAL MOMENT Two other insertion techniques, although not recommended by the manufacturer, have found favor with many clinicians. One is to insert the LMA with the bowl pointing to the nose or laterally and turning it as it is inserted. Another is to partially fill the cuff with air prior to insertion.

c. Tracheal Intubation with the LMA-Classic
   1) The LMA can serve as a conduit through which a tracheal tube, stylet, or fiberscope can be passed. The LMA acts to position the device over the laryngeal aperture.

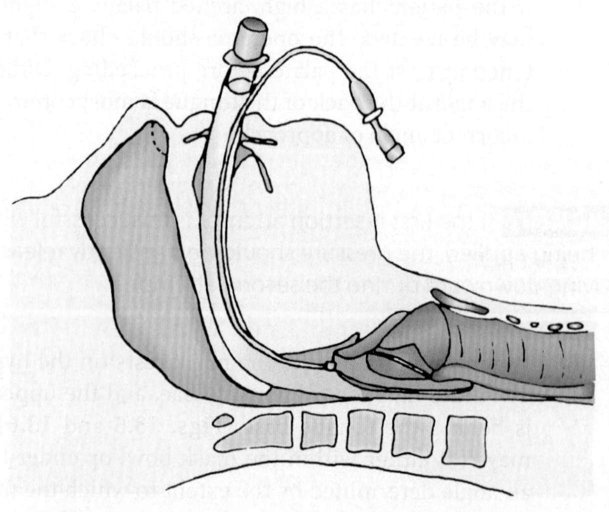

Figure 13.6 Laryngeal mask airway in place. The tip of the mask rests against the upper esophageal sphincter while the sides face the pyriform fossae.

2) Blind intubation through the LMA has been performed in both adults and children. The success rate is variable and depends on the technique, time available, operator experience, number of attempts, and the tracheal tube used. The success rate in patients with limited neck motion is lower than in those with normal anatomy.

CLINICAL MOMENT The tracheal tube that is used for intubation must be long enough so that it can protrude from the end of the LMA.

3) Because a downfolded epiglottis can impair blind intubation, it has been recommended that fiber-optic assessment of epiglottic position should precede intubation through the LMA. If the epiglottis has downfolded, moving the LMA up and down without deflating the cuff may help to reposition the epiglottis. Another maneuver is to withdraw the mask about 5 cm and reinsert it while maintaining a jaw thrust.
4) After the LMA is inserted and fixed into position, the tracheal tube is lubricated and inserted into the LMA tube. Auscultating the end of the tube may be useful during spontaneous breathing. The tracheal tube should be rotated 15° to 90° counterclockwise as it is advanced to prevent the bevel from catching on the bars at the junction of the tube and the mask. Once through the bars, the tracheal tube is rotated clockwise and the neck extended to enable the tip to pass anterior to the arytenoids. The tracheal tube is then advanced until resistance is felt. The head is then flexed, permitting the tube to advance into the trachea.

CLINICAL MOMENT A tracheal tube with a midline bevel may be easier to insert through the LMA and into the trachea.

5) If the tracheal tube does not enter the trachea initially, it is possible that the LMA is not well situated over the laryngeal aperture or the epiglottis is blocking the aperture. Varying degrees of neck flexion and extension at the atlanto-occipital joint may be helpful. If the tube still does not enter the trachea, it should be withdrawn until the bevel is just behind the aperture bars. The LMA cuff should be deflated and the LMA pushed a little farther into the hypopharynx. This maneuver may elevate the downfolded epiglottis. The tracheal tube is then advanced.

CLINICAL MOMENT Smaller tracheal tubes are easier to place than larger ones. If the tube is not large enough, it may be replaced with a larger tube by using a tube exchanger (Chapter 15).

6) The LMA-Classic can be used to aid fiber-optic–guided intubation. The LMA is inserted in the usual manner. The fiberscope surrounded by a well-lubricated tracheal tube that has a fully deflated cuff is advanced over the fiberscope and through the LMA into the trachea. The tracheal tube is advanced until it is in place. The tube should be rotated as it is advanced. It may be useful to position the tracheal tube in the LMA, just proximal to the aperture bars, before inserting the fiberscope.

CLINICAL MOMENT A right-angle bronchoscopic connector with a seal for the fiberscope attached to the tracheal tube allows the fiber-optic scope to be inserted while the patient is being ventilated. With this arrangement, positive end-expiratory pressure (PEEP) can be applied, which often dramatically improves the view by stenting the collapsed upper airway.

d. Removing the LMA after Tracheal Intubation

1) The decision to remove the LMA-Classic after tracheal intubation or to leave it in place depends on the circumstances. Reasons to remove the LMA include concern about pressure on the soft tissues, the need to keep it away from the surgical field, a possible increase in gastroesophageal reflux, and difficulty placing a gastric tube.

2) Many users prefer to leave the LMA-Classic in place after intubation to provide an alternative airway at the conclusion of the anesthetic delivery. If this is option is chosen, the protruding end of the tracheal tube should be firmly secured.

CLINICAL MOMENT In order to remove the LMA without dislodging the tracheal tube, a smaller tracheal tube or other device may be placed at the end of the tracheal tube to act as a pusher (extender) in order to prevent extubation as the LMA is withdrawn.

CLINICAL MOMENT A fiberscope, bougie, jet stylet, or tube changer may be passed through the tracheal tube to facilitate reintubation if extubation occurs as the LMA is being removed.

2. **LMA-Unique**

a. The single-use LMA-Unique (disposable laryngeal mask airway, DLMA) is made of polyvinyl chloride and costs less than a reusable LMA. Sizes are given in **Table 13.2**. While the dimensions are identical to the classic LMA, the tube is stiffer and the cuff is less compliant. It may be helpful to warm

Table 13.2 Sizes of the LMA-Unique

Mask Size	Patient Size (kg)	Maximum Cuff Volume (mL of Air)	Largest Tracheal Tube (ID in mm)[a]	Largest Flexible Endoscope (ID in mm)[b]
1	Up to 5	4	3.5	2.7
1.5	5–10	7	4.0	3.0
2	10–20	10	4.5	3.5
2.5	20–30	14	5.0	4.0
3	30–50	20	6.0	5.0
4	50–70	30	6.0	5.0
5	70–100	40	7.0	5.5

ID, internal diameter.
[a]If the connector is removed, a larger tracheal tube can be inserted.
[b]A larger fiberscope may be accommodated if the aperture bars are removed.

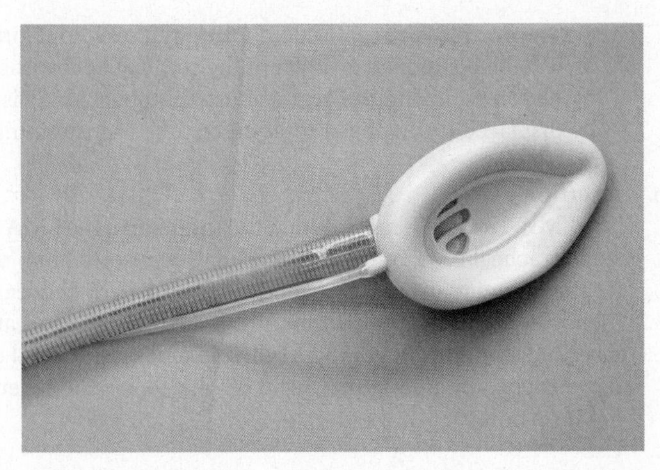

Figure 13.7 LMA-Flexible. The wire-reinforced tube is longer and has a smaller diameter than the standard LMA.

it prior to insertion. Indications are the same as those for the LMA-Classic. It may be a better choice for out-of-hospital or ward use, where it would be difficult to clean and sterilize a reusable LMA. The LMA-Unique is inserted in the same way as the LMA-Classic.

b. Studies comparing the unique LMA and the classic LMA have not found any significant differences in successful insertion or postoperative sore throat. The LMA-Unique had a lower increase in intracuff pressure during nitrous oxide anesthesia than the LMA-Classic. Blindly passing a tracheal tube through the LMA-Unique is associated with a lower success rate.

c. One of the advantages of a single-use LMA is protection against prion infection since it is discarded after use.

3. **LMA-Flexible**

a. Description

1) The LMA-Flexible (wire-reinforced, reinforced LMA, RLMA, FLMA, flexible LMA) (**Fig. 13.7**) differs from the LMA-Classic in that it has a flexible, wire-reinforced tube that is longer and narrower than the tube on the LMA-Classic. It is available in the sizes shown in **Table 13.3**. The cuff dimensions are the same as those for the LMA-Classic. A single-use version is also available.

Table 13.3 Size Comparison between Standard and Flexible Laryngeal Mask Airways

LMA Size	Patient Size (kg)	LMA-Flexible (ID in mm)	LMA-Classic (ID in mm)	LMA-Flexible Tube Length (cm)	Maximum Cuff Inflation Volume (mL)
2	10–20	5.1	7.0	21.5	Up to 10
2.5	20–30	6.1	8.4	23.0	Up to 14
3	30–50	7.6	10.0	25.5	Up to 20
4	50–70	7.6	10.0	25.5	Up to 30
5	70–100	8.7	11.5	28.5	Up to 40
6	>100	8.7	28.5	23.5	Up to 50

LMA, Laryngeal mask airway; ID, internal diameter.

2) The flexible tube can be bent to any angle without kinking. This allows it to be positioned away from the surgical field without occluding the lumen or losing the seal against the pharynx. It is less likely to be displaced during head rotation or tube repositioning than the LMA-Classic.

b. Insertion

The LMA-Flexible is more difficult to insert than the LMA-Classic. A stylet, small tracheal tube, or other device may be inserted into the tube to stiffen it. The manufacturer recommends that it be held between the thumb and the index finger at the junction of the tube and the cuff and positioned by inserting the index finger to its fullest extent into the oral cavity until resistance is encountered. It may be necessary to use the other hand to achieve full insertion.

c. Use

The LMA-Flexible is designed for use with surgery on the head, neck, and upper torso where the LMA-Classic would be in the way.

d. Problems

1) While the LMA-Flexible is more resistant to kinking and compression than the LMA-Classic, it does not prevent obstruction if the patient bites the tube.

2) The spiral reinforcing wire in the LMA-Flexible may become disrupted. Sometimes, the disruption is internal and can be discovered only by looking carefully down the shaft. Defects in the wire may cause obstruction if the tube is bent. Pieces of wire could break off and migrate into the tracheobronchial tree.

3) The smaller tube diameter limits the endoscope or tracheal tube size that can be passed through the LMA-Flexible. Prolonged spontaneous breathing should be avoided because the smaller tube causes increased resistance.

4) The LMA-Flexible is unsuitable for magnetic resonance imaging (MRI) if image quality in the region of the LMA is important. The metallic rings will cause image distortion.

4. **LMA-Fastrach**

The LMA-Fastrach (intubating LMA, ILMA, ILM, intubating laryngeal mask airway) was designed to overcome some of the problems associated with tracheal intubation through the LMA-Classic.

a. Description

1) The LMA-Fastrach (**Fig. 13.8**) has a short, curved stainless steel shaft with a standard 15-mm connector. The tube is large enough to accommodate a cuffed 9-mm tracheal tube and short enough to allow a standard tracheal tube to pass beyond the vocal cords. The metal handle is securely bonded to the shaft near the connector end to facilitate one-handed insertion, position adjustment, and maintain the device in a steady position during tracheal tube insertion and removal. There is a single, movable epiglottic elevator bar in place of the two vertical bars found in the classic and flexible LMAs (**Fig. 13.9A**). A V-shaped guiding ramp is built into the floor of the mask aperture to direct the tracheal tube toward the glottis. The tip is slightly curved to permit atraumatic insertion. **Figure 13.9B** shows a tracheal tube protruding through the LMA tube and into the bowl.

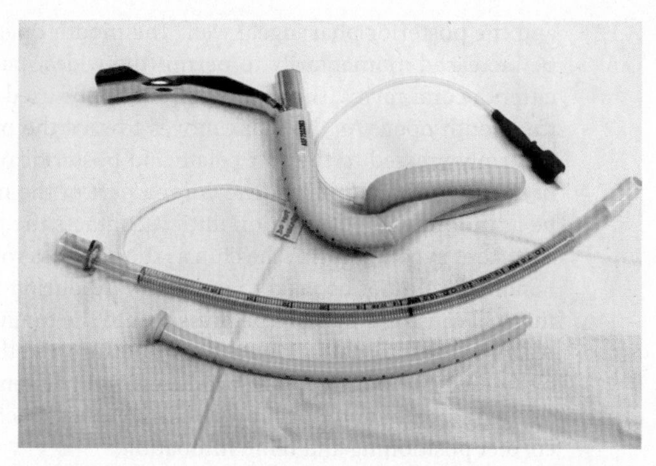

Figure 13.8 **Top:** LMA-Fastrach. The tube is shorter and wider than on the LMA-Classic and has a metal handle. **Middle:** Tracheal tube designed to be used with the LMA-Fastrach. **Bottom:** Stabilizer to allow the LMA to be removed without extubating the patient.

2) The LMA-Fastrach does not contain latex. It is available in sizes 3, 4, and 5. These fit the same size patients as the LMA-Classic. Both reusable and disposable versions are available.

b. Insertion

1) The LMA-Fastrach is designed for use with the patient's head in the neutral position. This includes using a head support, such as a pillow, but no head extension. The insertion technique consists of one-hand movements in the sagittal plane. It does not require placing fingers into the patient's mouth, thus minimizing the risk of injury or infection transmission as well as allowing insertion from almost any position.

2) The LMA-Fastrach should be deflated and lubricated in a manner similar to that of the LMA-Classic. It is held by the handle, which should be approximately parallel to the patient's chest. The mask tip is positioned flat against the hard palate immediately posterior to the upper incisors and then slid back and forth over the palate to spread the lubricant. After the mask is flattened against the hard palate, it is inserted with a rotational movement along the hard palate

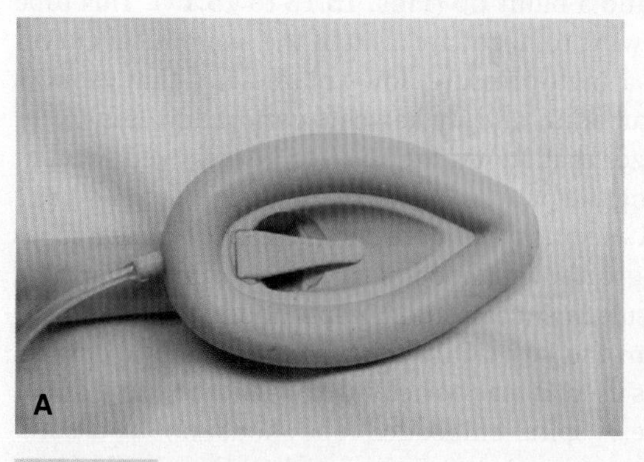

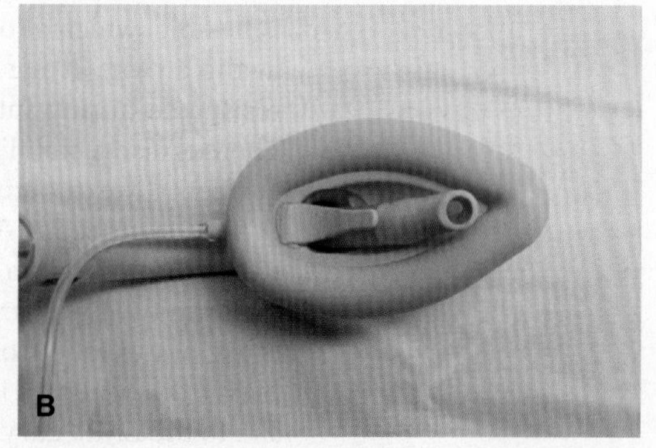

Figure 13.9 LMA-Fastrach. **A:** Note the single, movable epiglottic elevator bar and the V-shaped guiding ramp built into the floor of the mask aperture to direct the tracheal tube toward the glottis. **B:** Tracheal tube emerging from the LMA.

and the posterior pharyngeal wall. The mouth opening may need to be increased momentarily to permit the widest part of the mask to enter the oral cavity. The handle should not be used as a lever to force the mouth open. As the mask moves toward the pharynx, it should be firmly pressed to the soft palate and posterior pharyngeal wall to keep the tip from folding. The curved part of the metal tube should be advanced without rotation until it contacts the patient's chin and then kept in contact with the chin as the device is rotated inward. The handle should not be used to lever upward during insertion because this will cause the mask to be pressed into the tongue.

Aligning the internal LMA-Fastrach aperture and the glottic opening by finding the position that produces optimal ventilation and then applying a slight anterior lift with the LMA-Fastrach handle facilitate correct positioning and blind intubation.

c. Use

1) Although the LMA-Fastrach has been designed to facilitate tracheal intubation, it can also be used as a primary airway device. It is especially useful for the anticipated or unexpected difficult airway. It may be easier to insert the LMA-Fastrach than the LMA-Classic in obese patients.
2) The LMA-Fastrach can be inserted with the same or better success than the LMA-Classic. It is easier to place than the LMA-Classic when manual in-line stabilization is used. The LMA-Fastrach has been used successfully for difficult out-of-hospital airway management. Novice physicians have more success with the LMA-Fastrach than with bag-mask ventilation.

d. Tracheal Intubation

CLINICAL MOMENT Laryngeal or pharyngeal pathology may make intubation through the LMA-Fastrach impossible.

1) Muscle relaxants are not necessary for intubation through the LMA-Fastrach but may increase the success rate.
2) The tracheal tube recommended by the manufacturer for use with the LMA-Fastrach is a silicone, wire-reinforced, cuffed tube with a tapered patient end and a blunt tip (**Figs. 15.15** to **15.17**). This tube is flexible, which allows it to negotiate around the anatomical curves in the airway. It has a high-pressure, low-volume cuff that reduces resistance during intubation and makes cuff perforation less likely. There is also a stabilizer that allows the LMA to be removed without accidentally extubating the patient.
3) When using the LMA-Fastrach, standard curved plastic tracheal tubes are associated with a greater likelihood of laryngeal trauma. Warming a plastic tube will result in success and complication rates similar to those of the tube from the LMA-Fastrach manufacturer. If a curved, plastic tracheal tube is used, it may be helpful to orient the curve opposite to the LMA curve. A spiral-embedded tube should not be used.
4) Whichever tracheal tube is used, it is essential to remove the connector. It is important to lubricate the tracheal tube well and pass it through the LMA several times before use.

5) The tube can be inserted blindly. The patient's head is maintained in the neutral position. The tracheal tube connector should be loosely fitted for easy removal. The tracheal tube should also be lubricated with a water-soluble lubricant and passed into the LMA-Fastrach shaft until the tube tip is about to enter the mask aperture.
6) With the silicone tracheal tube specially designed for the LMA-Fastrach, the longitudinal line should face the LMA handle. The tracheal tube should not be passed beyond the point where the transverse line on the tube is level with the outer rim of the LMA-Fastrach airway tube (**Fig. 15.15**).
7) The LMA-Fastrach handle is grasped with one hand to steady it while the tracheal tube is being inserted and then lifted forward (not levered) a few millimeters like a laryngoscope. This increases the seal pressure and helps to align the axes of the trachea and tracheal tube. It also corrects the tendency for the mask to flex.
8) As it is advanced into the LMA-Fastrach, the tube should be rotated and moved up and down to distribute the lubricant. Ventilation and carbon dioxide monitoring can be performed during tracheal tube insertion by connecting the tracheal tube to the breathing system.
9) The tracheal tube should be advanced gently. The LMA-Fastrach handle should not be pressed downward. If no resistance is felt, it is likely that the epiglottic elevating bar is lifting the epiglottis upward, allowing the tracheal tube to pass into the trachea. When the tracheal tube is thought to be in the trachea, the cuff should be inflated and its position in the trachea confirmed (see Chapter 15).
10) If the tracheal tube fails to enter the trachea, a number of problems may have contributed to the lack of success. The epiglottis may have folded downward, or the tube may have impacted on the periglottic structures. The LMA-Fastrach may be too small or too large for the patient. The larynx may have been pushed downward during insertion. There may have been inadequate anesthesia or muscle relaxation so that the vocal cords closed.
11) If resistance is felt after the tracheal tube leaves the LMA-Fastrach, there are a number of maneuvers that can be carried out to improve the situation. If resistance is felt at 2 cm beyond the 15-cm mark on the tracheal tube, it is likely that the tube has impacted the vestibular wall. Rotating the tracheal tube may overcome the impaction. Another problem at this level may be a downfolded epiglottis. Without deflating the cuff, the LMA-Fastrach should be swung outward 6 cm and reinserted. If resistance is encountered 3 cm beyond the 15-cm mark, the epiglottis may be out of reach of the elevating bar and a larger LMA should be used. If resistance is felt at 15 plus 4 cm or immediately after the tracheal tube leaves the LMA-Fastrachea, the LMA may be too large and a smaller size should be substituted.
12) The blind technique can be time-consuming and may result in trauma or esophageal intubation.
13) Fiber-optic intubation through the LMA-Fastrach has a high success rate. It can be performed when the patient is awake and may be successful in the difficult-to-intubate patient. The epiglottic elevating bar is too stiff to be elevated by a fiberscope without risk of damaging the

tip or directing it downward. It should be lifted by the distal end of the tracheal tube.

The tracheal tube is advanced approximately 1.5 cm past the mask aperture while the intubating metal handle is held to stabilize it. The fiber-optic scope is advanced until the glottis is in view. The tracheal tube is then advanced into the trachea. If difficulties are encountered, the patient's head and neck may be maneuvered or the position of the LMA-Fastrach adjusted by using the metal handle.

CLINICAL MOMENT Fiber-optic intubation through the LMA-Fastrach can be used in patients with unstable necks. It is easier than intubation with a rigid laryngoscope or using only a fiberscope in patients with manual in-line stabilization.

14) After the trachea has been intubated, the decision whether to remove the LMA-Fastrach or to leave it in place needs to be made. The LMA-Fastrach may exert pressure on the mucosa in excess of capillary perfusion pressure. It is usually recommended that the LMA-Fastrach be removed. Alternately, the cuff can be deflated to 20 to 30 cm H_2O and the LMA-Fastrach left in situ. Removing the LMA is associated with a hemodynamic response. Delaying removal for a few minutes may slightly decrease the associated pressor response.

CLINICAL MOMENT Patients in whom the LMA-Fastrach has been left in place after intubation have a high incidence of hoarseness, sore throat, and dysphagia.

15) The tracheal tube needs to be stabilized to prevent extubation while the LMA-Fastrach is removed. The tube connector should be removed. A stabilizer rod (extender) that is placed at the end of the tracheal tube is available from the manufacturer (**Fig. 13.10**).

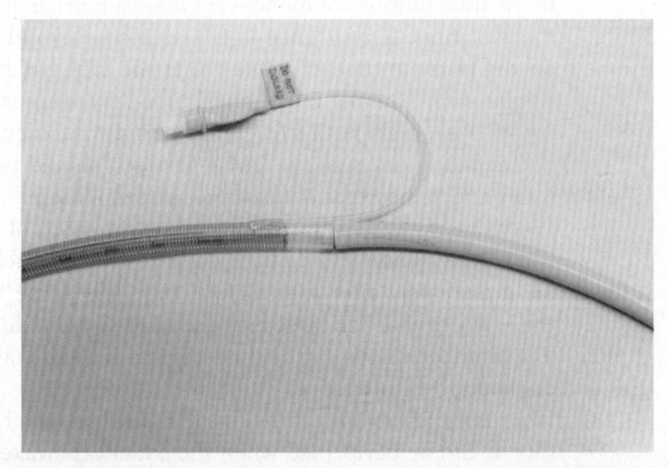

Figure 13.10 To stabilize the tracheal tube and to prevent extubation during LMA-Fastrach removal, a stabilizer rod (extender) is placed at the end of the tracheal tube.

CLINICAL MOMENT A smaller tracheal tube can be inserted at the end of the previously inserted tracheal tube to allow ventilation while the LMA-Fastrach is being removed.

16) The LMA-Fastrach cuff is deflated and swung out of the pharynx into the oral cavity while applying counterpressure to the tracheal tube. The tracheal tube is then firmly grasped while unthreading the inflation tube and the pilot balloon from the LMA-Fastrach. Finally, the tracheal tube connector is replaced.
17) Currently, number 3 is the smallest size available for the LMA-Fastrach. This has been found to work well for intubation of patients weighing more than 30 kg, but for patients under this weight, successful intubation through this device is less certain.

CLINICAL MOMENT The LMA-Fastrach tracheal tube should not remain in place for long periods of time because it has a high-pressure cuff.

18) The LMA-Fastrach requires more time for intubation and results in more esophageal intubations and mucosal trauma than rigid laryngoscopy. Blind intubation through the LMA-Fastrach generates cardiovascular responses similar to tracheal intubation by using direct laryngoscopy.

e. Problems

1) The rigid LMA-Fastrach shaft cannot be easily adapted to a change in the position of the patient's neck. It is more likely to be dislodged than the LMA-Classic with head or neck manipulation.

CLINICAL MOMENT The LMA-Fastrach is unsuitable for use in the MRI unit.

2) A case of obstruction after the LMA-Fastrach was inserted has been reported. Fibroscopy revealed that the epiglottic elevating bar was in the laryngeal aperture, and although it lifted the epiglottis, the arytenoid cartilage was pressed anteriorly by the LMA-Fastrach cuff, partially obstructing the laryngeal aperture. Despite the obstruction, the trachea was intubated successfully.
3) The large diameter of the LMA-Fastrach can cause difficulty during insertion in a patient with a limited mouth opening and may put dentition at risk.

CLINICAL MOMENT Compared with the LMA-Classic, the LMA-Fastrach causes an increased incidence of sore throat, sore mouth, and difficulty swallowing.

4) While the LMA-Fastrach is easier to place than the LMA-Classic and placement is more likely to be successful in patients with immobilized cervical spines, the LMA-Fastrach may exert pressure on the cervical spine. Intubation through the LMA-Fastrach may cause significant

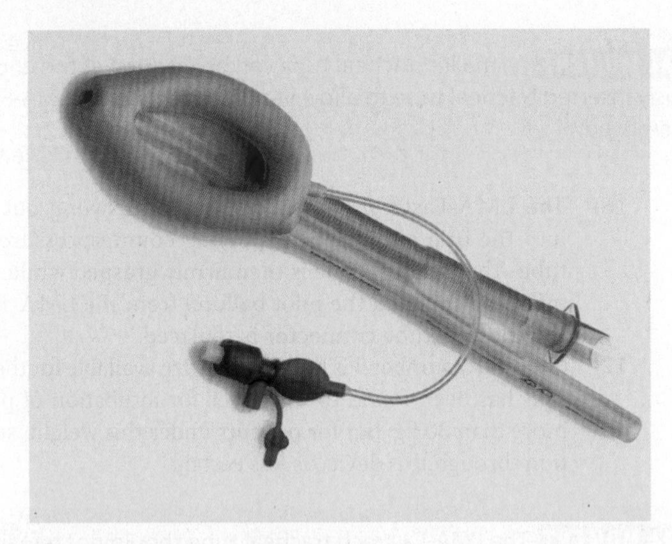

Figure 13.11 LMA-ProSeal. Note the integral bite block and the opening of the drain tube at the tip. (Photograph courtesy of LMA North America.)

motion of the cervical spine. It may be difficult to insert in a patient with a cervical collar, especially if cricoid pressure is used.

5. **LMA-ProSeal**
   a. Description
      1) The LMA-ProSeal (LMA-PROSEAL, PLM) (**Fig. 13.11**) has four main parts: cuff, inflation line with pilot balloon, airway tube, and drain tube. All components are made of silicone and are latex-free. It is available in six sizes (**Table 13.4**). Studies indicate that size 4 is preferable for most adult women and size 5 for most adult men.
      2) The airway (breathing, ventilation) tube of the LMA-ProSeal is shorter and smaller in diameter than the tube on the LMA-Classic and is wire reinforced, which makes it more flexible. There is a locating strap on the anterior distal tube to prevent the finger slipping off the tube and provide an insertion slot for an introducer tool. An accessory vent

Table 13.4 LMA-ProSeal

LMA Size	Patient Size (kg)	Maximum Cuff Inflation Volume (mL)	Maximum Gastric Tube Size (French)	Maximum Fiber-Optic Scope Size (mm)	Length of Drain Tube (cm)	Largest Tracheal Tube (ID in mm)
1.5	5–10	7	10	–	18.2	4.0 uncuffed
2	10–20	10	10	–	19.0	4.0 uncuffed
2.5	20–30	14	14	–	23.0	4.5 uncuffed
3	30–50	20	16	–	26.5	5.0 uncuffed
4	50–70	30	16	4	27.5	5.0 uncuffed
5	70–100	40	18	5	28.5	6.0 cuffed

ID, internal diameter.

under the drainage tube in the bowl prevents secretions from pooling and acts as an accessory ventilation port. The LMA-ProSeal has a deeper bowl than the LMA-Classic and does not have aperture bars. There is a bite block between the airway and drain tubes at the level where the teeth would contact the device.

3) The drain (drainage, esophageal drain, gastric access) tube is parallel and lateral to the airway tube until it enters the cuff bowl, where it continues to an opening in the tip that is sloped anteriorly (**Fig. 13.11**). When the LMA-ProSeal is correctly positioned, the cuff tip lies behind the cricoid cartilage at the origin of the esophagus. It allows liquids and gases to escape from the stomach, reduces the risk of gastric insufflation and pulmonary aspiration, allows devices to pass into the esophagus, and provides information about the LMA-ProSeal position. The drain tube is designed to prevent the epiglottis from occluding the airway tube, eliminating the need for airway bars. A gastric tube, Doppler probe, thermometer, stethoscope, or medication can be passed into the esophagus through the drainage port. A supporting ring around the distal drain tube prevents the tube from collapsing when the cuff is inflated.

4) The LMA-ProSeal has a second dorsal cuff (**Fig. 13.12**). This pushes the mask anteriorly to provide a better seal around the glottic aperture and helps to anchor the device in place. The dorsal cuff is not present on sizes 1½ to 2½. The cuff is softer than that on an LMA-Classic.

5) An optional metal introducer may be used to facilitate placing an LMA-ProSeal (**Fig. 13.13**). It has a curved, malleable, silicone-coated blade with a guiding handle. The distal end fits into the locating strap, and the proximal end fits into the airway tube.

b. Insertion

1) It is recommended that the LMA-ProSeal cuff be deflated into a wedge shape, as with the LMA-Classic. The patient's head should be in the "sniffing" position (lower neck flexion and head extension).

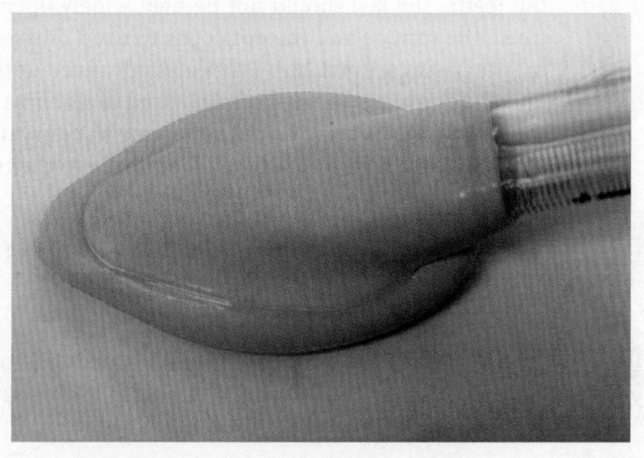

Figure 13.12 Posterior of the LMA-ProSeal, showing the dorsal cuff.

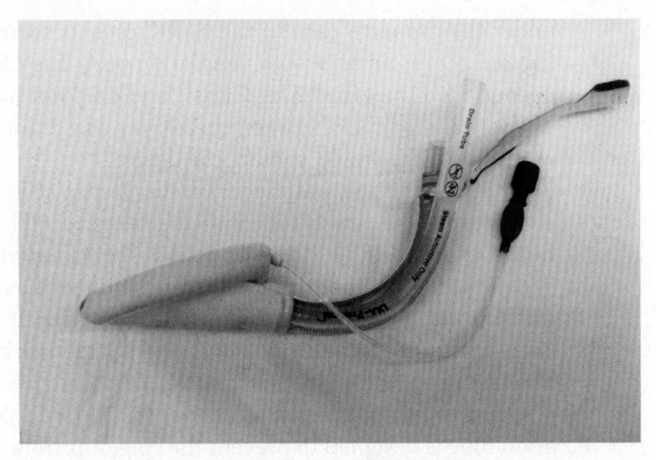

Figure 13.13 The LMA-ProSeal is shown in lateral view with the metal introducer attached in the pocket behind the cuff. The gastric tube channel is above the breathing channel.

CLINICAL MOMENT Cricoid pressure before insertion can hamper proper LMA placement. After placement, cricoid pressure or head flexion often produces a significant increase in airway seal pressure.

2) If the metal introducer is used, the tip is inserted into the strap at the top of the cuff. The airway and drainage tubes are folded into the matching slots on either side of the introducer blade. Lubricant should be placed on the posterior tip. The tip is then pressed against the hard palate and maneuvered to spread the lubricant along the hard palate. If the palate is high, a slightly lateral approach may be needed. The cuff is then slid inward, keeping pressure against the palate.
3) As the LMA-ProSeal is inserted, the introducer is kept close to the chin. The cuff should be observed to make certain that it has not folded over. The introducer is swung inward with a smooth circular movement. The jaw can be pulled downward by an assistant or pushed downward by using the middle finger until the cuff has passed the teeth. The jaw should not be held widely open because this may cause the tongue and the epiglottis to drop downward, blocking the mask's passage. The LMA-ProSeal is advanced until resistance is felt. The nondominant hand should be used to stabilize the airway tube as the introducer is removed by following the curvature backward out of the mouth, taking care to avoid damage to the teeth.

CLINICAL MOMENT The integral bite block should be at the level of the teeth.

CLINICAL MOMENT Insertion in patients with a stereotactic frame or neck collar is probably best performed without the introducer to increase maneuverability.

4) The digital method for insertion is similar to the introducer method except that the tip of the index finger is placed at the junction of the

cuff and the two tubes. As the index finger passes into the mouth, the finger joint is extended and the LMA-ProSeal is pressed backward toward the other hand that exerts counterpressure to maintain the sniffing position. Depending on the patient and the user's finger size, the finger may need to be inserted to its fullest extent before resistance is encountered. The nondominant hand should be used to stabilize the LMA as the finger is withdrawn.

5) The thumb may be used to aid insertion when it is difficult to get access to the patient from behind. The thumb is inserted into the strap. As the thumb enters the mouth, the fingers are stretched forward over the patient's face and the thumb is advanced to its fullest extent. The pushing action exerted by the thumb against the hard palate serves to extend the head. A lateral approach is required more frequently with this method.
6) A bougie, stylet, suction catheter, or airway exchange catheter can be used to assist inserting the LMA-ProSeal. The device is inserted into the esophagus and then threaded through the drain tube, and the ProSeal is advanced over it. The device may be placed in the LMA before it is inserted.
7) After the LMA-ProSeal has been inserted, the cuff should be inflated with enough air to achieve an intracuff pressure of up to 60 cm H_2O. The cuff volume required for the LMA-ProSeal to form an effective seal with the respiratory tract is lower than that for the LMA-Classic. An adequate seal can be obtained in most patients with no air in the cuff; however, the cuff should be inflated with at least 25% of the maximum recommended volume to ensure an effective seal with the gastrointestinal tract. Rotating or flexing the head from the neutral position may increase the leak pressure.
8) To test for proper position, a small amount (1 to 2 mL) of water-based gel or a soap bubble should be placed on the drain tube end and positive pressure applied to the airway tube. If the LMA-ProSeal is properly placed, there should be a slight up/down movement of the lubricant/soap. The soap bubble may move, whereas the lubricant gel may not. If the bolus is ejected, the mask may not be correctly placed.
9) The drain tube should be tested for patency. This can be done by passing a gastric tube, a flexible endoscope, or other device through the drainage tube. Easy passage indicates correct positioning; difficulty suggests that the mask should be repositioned, even if ventilation is satisfactory.

CLINICAL MOMENT Suction should not be applied at the end of the drain tube because this may cause the drain tube to collapse and injure the upper esophageal sphincter. Suction should not be applied to a gastric tube until it has reached the stomach. The gastric tube may be used to reinsert the LMA-ProSeal if it becomes displaced. The drain tube should not be clamped.

CLINICAL MOMENT If the LMA-Proseal is inserted with the cuffs partially inflated, as is often done with the LMA-Classic, the LMA-Proseal may not seat properly and may pop out from the mouth.

c. Tracheal Intubation through the LMA-ProSeal

Tracheal intubation through the LMA-ProSeal requires a long narrow tracheal tube or an airway exchange catheter. After the LMA-ProSeal is removed, a larger tube can be substituted, if necessary.

d. Use

The LMA-ProSeal can be used for spontaneous breathing but is more suited for controlled ventilation. The sealing pressure is higher with the LMA-ProSeal than with the LMA-Classic in adult and pediatric patients, making it a better choice for situations in which higher airway pressures are required, situations in which greater airway protection needed and surgical procedures in which intraoperative gastric drainage or decompression is needed. The LMA-ProSeal has been successfully used in the "cannot intubate, cannot ventilate" situation.

e. Problems with the LMA-ProSeal

1) The LMA-ProSeal is less suitable as an intubation device than the LMA-Fastrach because of the narrower airway tube. The fiberscope and tracheal tube sizes that can be accommodated by the LMA-ProSeal are given in **Table 13.4**. The high resistance associated with the smaller lumen may make it less suitable for spontaneously breathing patients than other devices.
2) The LMA-ProSeal can cause airway obstruction after insertion, either by compressing the supraglottic and glottic structures or by cuff infolding. Removing air from the cuff or placing the patient in the sniffing position may relieve the obstruction. Laryngeal edema may occur after use.
3) Partial upper airway obstruction during spontaneous ventilation may result from air being aspirated through the drain tube into the esophagus. Esophageal insufflation can occur simultaneously with venting from the drainage tube during positive-pressure ventilation when the LMA is malpositioned. This may also result in inadequate ventilation.
4) It may not be possible to insert a gastric tube in some patients. The cause may be using too large a gastric tube, providing inadequate tube lubrication, using a cooled gastric tube, overinflating the cuff, or malpositioning.
5) The LMA-ProSeal is relatively contraindicated for intraoral surgery because it cannot be moved easily around the mouth, the drain tube is vulnerable to occlusion, and the larger proximal cuff could interfere with the surgical field.
6) The LMA-ProSeal has a shorter life span than the LMA-Classic.
7) The bite block will protect the tube only if it is between the teeth. If the tube is the correct size for the patient, the bite block will protect the tube. If the teeth contact the tube, it can become distorted with narrowing and possible obstruction.

6. **LMA Supreme**

a. The LMA Supreme is a single-use, polyvinyl chloride LMA with a mask that has a built-in drain tube and fins in the bowl to protect the airway from epiglottic obstruction. The airway tube has a gentle curve and oblong shape to allow easier insertion and more stable placement.

b. Compared with the LMA-Proseal, the insertion success rate is higher with the LMA Supreme but the LMA-ProSeal is associated with significantly higher leak pressures.

B. Using the LMA Family

1. **Preuse Inspection**

a. Visual Inspection

1) The first step is to examine the airway tube. It should not be discolored, because the operator would not be able to see fluids that may enter the tube. There should be no cuts or tears in the tube, and the spiral wires (if present) should not be kinked.

2) The rest of the LMA's external surface should be examined for damage such as cuts, tears, scratches, or foreign particles. If the drain tube in the LMA-ProSeal bowl is torn or perforated, the LMA should not be used.

3) The interior should be free from obstruction or foreign particles. The LMA-Flexible and the LMA-ProSeal should be examined to make certain that the reinforcing wire is wholly contained within the tube wall.

4) The airway tube should be flexed up to but not beyond 180°. Kinking should not occur. Bending the tube beyond 180° could cause permanent damage.

5) The next test is to examine the mask aperture. The bars or other devices should be gently probed to make certain that they are not damaged and the space between them is free from particulate matter.

6) The connector should fit tightly into the outer end of the airway tube. It should not be possible to remove it easily. If the connector has a crack or surface irregularities or is twisted, it should not be used.

b. Deflation/Inflation

1) The next step is to withdraw air from the cuff so that the walls are flattened against each other. Excessive force should be avoided. The syringe should be removed from the inflation valve and the cuff checked to make certain that it remains deflated. If it reinflates, then there is a faulty valve or a leak in the cuff.

2) The next step is to inflate the cuff with 50% more air than the recommended maximum inflation volume (**Table 13.5**). The cuff should hold the pressure for at least 2 minutes. Any herniation, wall thinning,

Table 13.5 Maximum Test Cuff Inflation Volumes

Size	LMA-Classic or LMA-Unique (mL)	LMA-Flexible (mL)	LMA-Fastrach (mL)	LMA-ProSeal (mL)
1	6	–	–	–
1.5	10	–	–	–
2	15	15	–	–
2.5	21	21	–	–
3	30	30	30	–
4	45	45	45	45
5	60	60	60	60
6	75	75	–	–

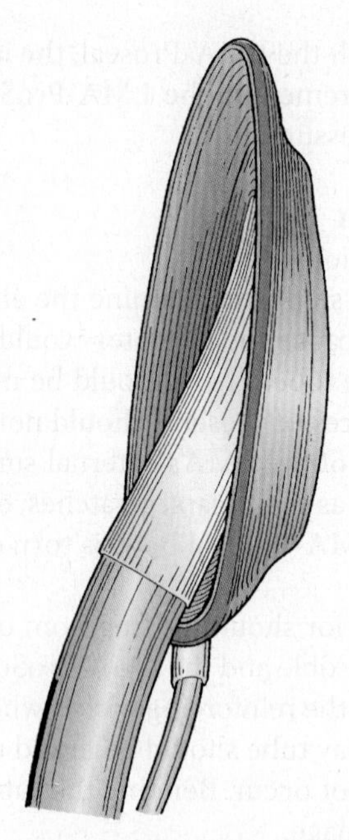

Figure 13.14 The laryngeal mask ready for insertion. The cuff should be deflated as tightly as possible, with the rim facing away from the mask aperture. There should be no folds near the tip. (Courtesy of Gensia Pharmaceuticals, Inc.)

or asymmetry is an indication to discard the LMA. The balloon should be elliptical and not spherical or irregularly shaped. Excessive pilot balloon width indicates weakness and imminent rupture.

2. **Mask Preparation**
   a. The cuff should be fully deflated with a dry syringe to form a flat oval disc (**Fig. 13.14**) by pressing the hollow side down against a clean, hard, flat surface. The deflated cuff should be wrinkle-free.
   b. A cuff-deflating tool is available from the manufacturer (**Fig. 13.15**). This device provides a superior and more consistent shape than hand

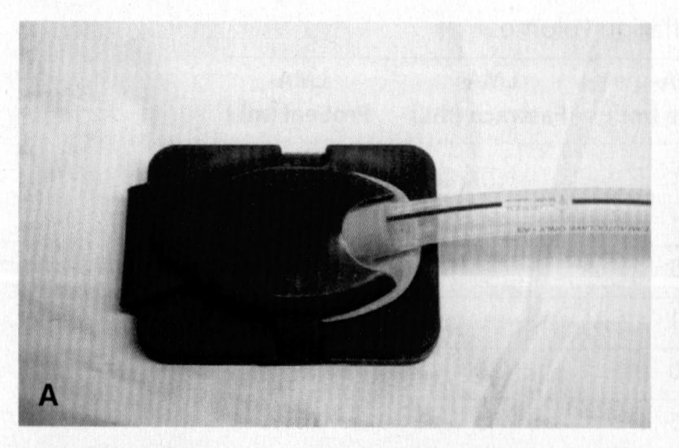

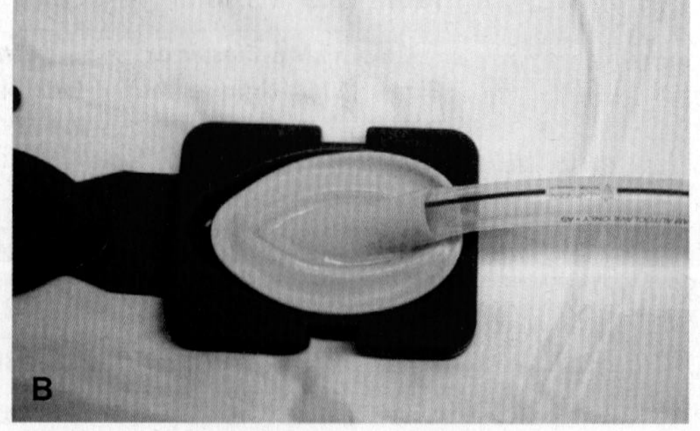

Figure 13.15 The cuff is deflated using a syringe for the laryngeal mask airway (LMA). **A:** The laryngeal mask is inserted into the device. The cuff is deflated by using a syringe. At the same time, the device is compressed. **B:** After cuff deflation, the LMA is ready for insertion.

manipulation or free deflation but does not offer any benefits in terms of residual volume. Using this device will lengthen cuff life.

c. Lubrication should be applied to the posterior cuff surface just before insertion, taking care to avoid getting lubricant on the anterior (bowl) surface. The manufacturer recommends using water-soluble jelly and does not recommend analgesic-containing gels or sprays because this may delay the return of protective reflexes and may provoke an allergic reaction. While some studies show that lubrication with lidocaine gel or spray results in a lower incidence of retching and coughing on emergence from anesthesia, another study showed increased intra- and postoperative problems. Lubricants or sprays that contain silicone may cause the mask to soften and swell.

3. **Cuff Inflation and Assessing Position and Function**

a. The cuff should be inflated to a pressure of approximately 60 cm H_2O. Cuff pressure can be estimated by feeling the tension in the pilot balloon. A spherical pilot balloon is an indication that there is too much gas in the cuff. The cuff should be inflated over 3 to 5 seconds without holding the tube unless the position is obviously unstable (e.g., in edentulous patients with slack tissues). This usually causes slight upward movement of the airway tube, and a slight bulging at the front of the neck is commonly seen. There should be a smooth oval swelling in the neck and no cuff visible in the oral cavity.

CLINICAL MOMENT During insertion and cuff inflation, the front of the neck should be observed to ensure whether the cricoid cartilage moves forward, indicating that the mask has correctly passed behind it.

CLINICAL MOMENT It is difficult to determine intracuff pressure without checking it with a manometer. A manometer can remain attached to the inflation valve and can be used to indicate any increase in intracuff pressure from gas diffusion into the cuff.

b. The recommended *maximum* inflation volumes are given in **Table 13.6**. In practice, it is rarely necessary to use the full volume. Using greater than recommended volumes will not improve the seal against the larynx and may worsen it.

CLINICAL MOMENT A rational approach is to inflate the mask with half the maximum inflation volume and determine the oropharyngeal leak pressure, adding more air if necessary.

CLINICAL MOMENT Cuff size is probably more important than inflating volume in determining the seal, so using a larger LMA may provide a better seal than adding more air to the cuff of a small LMA.

Table 13.6 Maximum Cuff Dimensions

Mask Size	Air Volume (mL)	Maximum Bulge of Cuff Tip (mm)	Maximum Bulge of Wide End of Cuff (mm)	Maximum Transverse Diameter of Cuff (mm)
1	6	7.8	8.6	26.3
1.5	10	9.5	10.2	32.6
2	15	11.5	13.0	39.0
2.5	21	13.0	14.5	45.0
3	30	14.8	16.6	51.2
4	45	17.0	19.0	58.5
5	60	21.1	22.4	68.3

c. If positive-pressure ventilation is to be used, the leak pressure should be greater than 20 cm H_2O (30 cm H_2O with the LMA-ProSeal). If spontaneous respiration is to be used, the leak pressure should be greater than 10 cm H_2O. This is the approximate pressure of fluid at the posterior pharyngeal wall if the oral cavity is flooded.

d. The sealing pressure is determined by observing the pressure gauge in the breathing system as the bag is squeezed and the pressure increases. Several methods can be used to determine the leak pressure. A stethoscope can be placed just lateral to the thyroid cartilage. Another method is to listen over the mouth when the bag is squeezed. Carbon dioxide may be detected by placing the sample line in the oral cavity. Another method is to determine the steady airway pressure after closing the adjustable pressure-limiting (APL) valve in the breathing system. Fresh gas entering the system may mask a leak with this method.

e. It may be possible to improve the seal by adding more air to the cuff (if the maximum recommended volume has not been injected) or by flexing or rotating the head and neck slightly. Higher pressures may be achieved by applying pressure on the front and/or side of the neck, applying continuous forward pressure on the LMA, or lifting the LMA-Fastrach handle.

f. Indications that the LMA is properly positioned include normal breath sounds and chest movements. Pressure–volume loops (see Chapter 18) should be normal in shape and not show a high pressure with little tidal volume during positive-pressure ventilation indicating obstruction or an open loop indicating a leak. Carbon dioxide waveforms should be normal with positive-pressure ventilation. If the patient is breathing spontaneously, normal reservoir bag excursions and no obstructive signs are indications of proper placement. A fiberscope or rigid endoscope can be inserted through the LMA to confirm its position and rule out airway obstruction. Radiography or MRI can also be used to confirm the position. An esophageal detector device (Chapter 15) can be used, although its utility has been questioned.

g. If the airway is obstructed, the cause may be an incorrect mask position, a downfolded epiglottis, a closed glottic sphincter, or an overinflated cuff. In most cases, removing and reinserting the mask will eliminate the obstruction. Another technique is to lift the anterior neck structures by inserting a gloved hand into the mouth, deflate the cuff, and rotate the mask 360°.

In some cases, the epiglottis may be straightened digitally. Jaw manipulation or repositioning the head usually does not relieve airway obstruction. Removing air from the cuff may be helpful.

CLINICAL MOMENT If various manipulations do not quickly provide satisfactory ventilation, the device should be withdrawn and reinserted or a different size LMA or a tracheal tube used.

4. **Fixation**

A bite block or gauze roll should be inserted into the mouth beside the tube to prevent the patient from biting the tube and to improve stability. This is not necessary with the LMA-ProSeal. Various other devices have been used. Failure to use a device may result in tube compression or damage to the teeth.

CLINICAL MOMENT An oropharyngeal airway should not be used, because both the oropharyngeal airway and the LMA are designed to be placed in the midline, and the airway tip might compromise the LMA cuff or cause tube compression.

5. **Intraoperative Management**

a. The manufacturer recommends that cuff pressure be checked periodically with a pressure gauge, transducer, or other device and adjusted to keep the pressure at or below 60 cm H_2O. A pressure gauge may remain attached to the inflation valve in order to detect pressure increases from nitrous oxide diffusion into the cuff. The pilot balloon should be fully compliant. It has been suggested that the logical method to control cuff pressures during nitrous oxide anesthesia may be to take the "just seal" pressure as a control value and withdrawn volume to maintain values close to this pressure.

b. The LMA can be used with controlled (including mechanical) or spontaneous ventilation. If controlled ventilation is used, the peak inspiratory pressure should be kept below 20 cm H_2O (30 cm H_2O with the LMA-ProSeal). Higher pressures may result in a leak around the mask, gastric distention, and operating room pollution. Changes in the ventilatory pattern to reduce tidal volume and using muscle relaxants may result in a lower peak pressure. If higher pressures are required, consideration should be given to exchanging the LMA for a tracheal tube.

CLINICAL MOMENT The peak airway pressure that can be used without gastric insufflation can often be increased if cricoid pressure is applied.

c. Pressure control ventilation (Chapter 6), with or without PEEP, may be the mode of choice for controlled ventilation with the laryngeal mask because it allows a lower peak pressure for the same tidal volume with less leak. For patients breathing spontaneously, pressure support ventilation improves gas exchange and reduces the work of breathing. The work of breathing can also be reduced by using continuous positive airway pressure (CPAP). Tidal volume should be measured during pressure control ventilation to ensure adequate ventilation.

d. Increased leakage, snoring, or other sounds often signal the need for more muscle relaxation, although other causes such as LMA displacement, light anesthesia causing glottic closure, airway obstruction, a leaking cuff, and decreased compliance related to the surgical procedure are other possible causes. Adding air to the cuff will not always correct a leak and may make it worse by increasing tension in the cuff and pushing it away from the larynx. Sometimes removing some air from the cuff is helpful.

e. If regurgitation occurs, the first sign may be the appearance of fluid traveling up the LMA tube. Breath holding or coughing may occur. The patient should be placed in the head-down position, the breathing circuit disconnected, and the airway tube suctioned. It may not be necessary to remove the LMA, although preparations for tracheal intubation should be made and the patient intubated, if indicated.

f. Inserting a nasogastric tube behind the LMA (other than the LMA-Proseal) can be aided by using a nasal airway or a flexible endoscope to displace the LMA forward.

6. **Emergence from Anesthesia**

a. It is important that the bite block or roll of gauze be left in place until the LMA is removed. Cuff deflation should be performed after the LMA is removed. If the cuff remains inflated as the LMA is removed, a greater mass of secretions will be removed, but this technique increases the incidence of bloodstaining (but not sore throat). Taking off the glove that was worn when the LMA was removed and inverting it over the device will minimize the spread of contamination.

b. Removing the LMA while the patient is under deep anesthesia will decrease the incidence of coughing, breath holding, and bronchospasm. This may be highly desirable in some situations, such as after intraocular surgery. It should not be performed in a difficult-to-intubate patient. Deep extubation has been associated with airway obstruction, regurgitation, and laryngospasm. Damage to the LMA is less frequent when the LMA is removed under deep anesthesia.

c. Most studies show that in children, LMA removal when the patient is awake results in a higher incidence of airway problems (laryngospasm, coughing, breath holding, bronchospasm) than LMA removal during deep anesthesia. A similar or higher incidence of airway problems in children with deep removal has been reported by some investigators.

d. The patient should be left undisturbed, except to administer oxygen and perform monitoring, and should not be turned onto his or her side unless there is an indication (such as regurgitation or vomiting) because this may cause the LMA to be prematurely rejected. It is not necessary to remove secretions in the upper pharynx, because they will not enter the larynx provided the cuff is not deflated prior to removal, and the LMA is not removed before the patient is able to swallow effectively.

CLINICAL MOMENT Suctioning through the LMA should not be performed unless there is evidence of gastric contents in the tube.

C. Life Span

With careful use and strict adherence to cleaning and sterilization procedures, a reusable LMA will last for a long time. The recommended maximum number of uses by the manufacturer for the LMA-Classic is 40, but up to 200 uses have been reported. With repeated use, there is a decrease in elastance, an increase in cuff permeability, and a loss in airway tube strength. It may be possible to exchange a malfunctioning inflation valve on an LMA. The LMA-ProSeal has a shorter life span than the LMA-Classic.

D. Useful Situations

The LMA has been used for a wide variety of procedures. It is well suited for outpatient surgery. It has proved useful for patients who need multiple anesthetics over a short period of time. The maximum anesthetic duration for which the LMA can be safely used is not known. The laryngeal mask can be used with low-flow and closed-system anesthesia.

1. **Difficult Face Mask Technique**
   a. For patients in whom mask ventilation is or could be difficult, such as edentulous patients or those with facial injuries or a fragile nose, those with beards or facial contours that are not suited to a face mask, and patients undergoing laser treatment of the face, it may be easier to maintain a satisfactory airway with the LMA.
   b. The LMA may prove useful for patients with facial burns who often require multiple anesthetics. However, it is not appropriate to use the LMA to secure the airway in a patient with upper airway burns.
2. **Difficult or Failed Intubation**
   a. Laryngeal masks have contributed greatly to solving the difficult intubation problem. The LMA is part of the American Society of Anesthesiologists' Difficult Airway Algorithm, the American Heart Association Advanced Cardiac Life Support recommendations, and various international guidelines.
   b. In situations in which the patient cannot be intubated, the LMA may be useful and even lifesaving by using it as the primary means either to maintain the airway or to facilitate tracheal tube passage. For this reason, it is recommended that an LMA be immediately available whenever a "cannot intubate, cannot ventilate" scenario is possible. In the patient whose trachea cannot be intubated because of unfavorable anatomy (but not periglottic pathology), the LMA should be considered as the first option.
   c. The LMA has been used to rescue an airway in patients with laryngeal edema following carotid endarterectomy. This can buy time for a tracheostomy or intubation.
3. **Ophthalmic Surgery**

   The LMA has been used for procedures on the eye. Most studies have shown that intraocular pressure is lower after inserting an LMA than a tracheal tube. Intraocular pressure during emergence from anesthesia is usually lower with an LMA. There is less likelihood that the patient will cough or buck during the anesthesia administration or emergence from anesthesia.
4. **Tracheal Procedures**
   a. Some patients with tracheal stenosis may be managed using the laryngeal mask, although failure in this situation has been reported. The LMA has been used to prevent gas loss from the trachea during a tracheoplasty.
   b. Tracheal compression by a mediastinal mass can cause problems in a manner similar to tracheal stenosis. Both mediastinoscopy and thoracotomy have been performed in this situation with the LMA, but the use of the LMA in a patient with a mediastinal mass is questionable.

5. **Endoscopy**
The LMA has been used to aid fiber-optic laryngotracheoscopy and bronchoscopy in adults and children by directing the fiberscope to the glottis. It has also been used to facilitate bronchoalveolar lavage and to place a bronchial stent. Ventilation can be maintained by using a connector that incorporates a diaphragm opening for the bronchoscope [see (4) in **Fig. 5.2**]. This allows PEEP application, which may improve the bronchoscopic view in the upper airways. The LMA-Flexible is not suitable for fiber-optic examinations because of the narrow tube and because the internal wire may be damaged.
6. **Head and Neck Procedures**
   a. The LMA has been used for a variety of head and neck procedures, including laryngoscopy, microsurgical procedures on the larynx, nasal and pharyngoplastic surgery, myringotomies, adenoidectomy, tonsillectomy, and dental procedures. The LMA has been used in conjunction with a fiber-optic bronchoscope to assist in thyroplasty.
   b. The LMA cuff acts to prevent aspiration of blood, teeth, and secretions from above the mask. Further protection may be provided by inserting an oropharyngeal pack or by positioning a suction catheter in the groove between the mask and the LMA tube.
   c. The LMA has been used in thyroid surgery. The cuff displaces the gland anteriorly, facilitating surgical access. Because damage to the recurrent laryngeal nerve is a complication of thyroid surgery, it may be desirable to stimulate this nerve during and after surgery and observe vocal cord motion by using a fiberscope through the LMA. Tracheal deviation and narrowing should be considered relative contraindications to using the LMA in thyroid surgery.
   d. The LMA is well suited to procedures on the ear. During these cases, it is important that the patient not cough or strain. These problems are less likely with the laryngeal mask. It may be desirable that muscle relaxants not be used so that it will be easier to detect the presence of the facial nerve in the area of dissection. A perceived drawback to using the laryngeal mask in these cases is that often the anesthesia provider is located at the patient's foot. Some clinicians feel uncomfortable with this position when an LMA is in place.

CLINICAL MOMENT If the head position is altered by tilting the bed sideways instead of moving the head, there is less likelihood that the LMA will be displaced.

   e. The LMA has been used for standard and percutaneous dilatational tracheostomy and for inserting a needle into the trachea for jet ventilation. Using the LMA eliminates the need to share the trachea with the surgeon and avoids the possibility of cuff puncture, tube transection, or accidental extubation. It also allows the trachea to be visualized through a fiberscope during the procedure.
7. **Pediatric Patients**
   a. The LMA can be used in children, including small infants. It may be particularly helpful with children in whom unusual anatomy makes tracheal intubation difficult. The LMA has been used in Treacher Collins, Dandy-Walker,

Pierre-Robin, Goldenhar, Freeman-Sheldon, Beckwith-Wiedemann, and Still's syndromes; congenital epulis; and mucopolysaccharidoses. The LMA may not be useful in some patients with Hunter's syndrome.

b. The LMA provides a useful alternative to the tracheal tube when it is necessary to administer anesthesia to a child with an upper respiratory infection. In children with bronchopulmonary dysplasia, the LMA can maintain a satisfactory airway with fewer adverse respiratory effects than a tracheal tube. Children with subglottic stenosis may have respiratory problems if this area is irritated by a tracheal tube. The laryngeal mask has been used in children with this problem who are undergoing surgery that is not related to the airway.

c. The LMA has been used in children who have anesthesia for radiotherapy and MRI examinations, cardiac catheterization, and extracorporeal shock wave lithotripsy and those who require multiple anesthetics over a short period of time. Although difficult to insert, the LMA-Flexible has been used successfully in pediatric dental surgery.

d. Because the epiglottis in children is relatively large and floppy, the likelihood of it being within the mask is greater than in adults. This may make blind intubation or intubation over a bougie or guide wire passed through the LMA difficult.

8. **Professional Singers**

The laryngeal mask may be especially useful for professional singers and speakers in whom the laryngeal complications of intubation would be most serious. The LMA causes less change in vocal function than tracheal intubation. Many singers have heard of the LMA and may request its use.

9. **Remote Anesthesia**

a. Situations in which the anesthesia provider must be away from the patient, including diagnostic imaging and radiotherapy, can often be managed using a laryngeal mask. These procedures are usually associated with minimal or no pain, but they require the patient to remain still. If the patient must be placed in an awkward position and the area of interest is not near the LMA, the LMA-Flexible may be the best choice.

b. MRI poses some special problems. Because some of the inflation valves contain metallic material, it may be necessary to remove the valve and knot the pilot tube. If a nonferrous valve is not available, the valve can be positioned away from the area of interest. If the LMA-Flexible, LMA-Fastrach, or LMA-ProSeal is used, the metal coil produces a large black hole in the image in the area surrounding the airway as well as image distortion in the area surrounding the airway. A reusable silicone LMA may not be suitable if magnetic resonance spectroscopy is performed, because the resonance of some silicone-containing materials compromises interpretation of the scans. The LMA-Unique can be used in this circumstance.

10. **Supplementing Regional Block**

In cases in which surgery outlasts a regional block or only a partial block is achieved, supplementation with light general anesthesia may be desirable. In addition, many patients become restless and cannot tolerate prolonged surgery under regional anesthesia. The LMA can be used in these situations, because it allows a lighter level of anesthesia than would be required with a tracheal tube.

11. **Resuscitation**

The LMA-Classic and the LMA-Fastrach have been used successfully during cardiac arrest. The presence of an LMA does not interfere with palpating the carotid pulse. Since the LMA can be inserted from the patient's front, side, or head, it is useful in entrapment situations. The head can be maintained in the neutral position if cervical trauma is suspected. Better ventilation can be achieved than with a face mask.

CLINICAL MOMENT The LMA should not be considered as a substitute for a tracheal tube in emergency situations in which the patient may have a full stomach or other contraindication to using the LMA if someone present has the ability to place a tracheal tube.

CLINICAL MOMENT The LMA should not be used if the patient is not deeply unconscious or resists insertion. It may not be possible to adequately ventilate patients who require positive-pressure ventilation and who have poorly compliant lungs with pulmonary edema, aspiration, or obstructive pulmonary disease.

12. **Obstetrics**
    a. Because the risk of aspiration is high in the obstetrical patient, the LMA is usually not recommended for elective use. It has been used in healthy parturients undergoing elective Cesarean section and to facilitate tracheal intubation in a parturient.
    b. If intubation cannot be performed, the LMA may be lifesaving. For this reason and because the incidence of failed intubation in the obstetric population is higher than in the general population, laryngeal masks should be kept in every obstetrical operating room. The LMA-ProSeal is probably a better choice than the LMA-Classic.
    c. In the obstetric patient who can be ventilated by using a face mask while cricoid pressure is continuously applied, placing the LMA may have little benefit and might induce vomiting and aspiration. Since cricoid pressure often inhibits LMA placement, cricoid pressure may need to be momentarily released to allow the LMA to be successfully inserted.

13. **Laser Surgery**

The LMA has been used in laser surgery on the face, pharynx, and subglottic areas. Although LMAs, with the exception of the LMA-Unique and the LMA-Fastrach, are more resistant to perforation by lasers than polyvinyl chloride or wire-reinforced tracheal tubes, they can be ignited at clinically used power densities.

14. **Laparoscopy**

The use of an LMA for laparoscopic procedures is controversial, because it does not offer definitive protection from aspiration of gastric contents. Studies suggest that the LMA is safe for gynecologic laparoscopy. It has also been used successfully for laparoscopic cholecystectomy, but aspiration has been reported. If an LMA is used for these procedures, the LMA-ProSeal is recommended.

15. **Lower Abdominal Surgery**
A number of studies indicate that the LMA is safe for lower abdominal procedures such as hysterectomy and retropubic prostatectomy. Adequate anesthetic depth to prevent coughing during peritoneal stimulation needs to be maintained.
16. **Neurosurgery**
a. The LMA has been used for patients undergoing ventriculoperitoneal shunt and intracranial surgery. Hemodynamic stability associated with the LMA may be especially beneficial in patients undergoing procedures in which hypertension must be avoided, such as repairing an intracranial aneurysm, and for the patient with increased intracranial pressure. The LMA can be used to provide a smoother emergence from anesthesia after intracranial or spinal surgery.
b. Cervical spine disease is often associated with head and neck immobility, which can be associated with difficult tracheal intubation. The use of the LMA-Fastrach may enable tracheal intubation without the need to manipulate the head and neck.
17. **Unstable Cervical Spine**
The optimal airway management for the patient with an unstable cervical spine is controversial. While the LMA requires less cervical manipulation during intubation than direct laryngoscopy, its insertion produces flexion and posterior cervical spine displacement despite manual stabilization. Some investigators feel that the LMA should not be used in the patient with an unstable cervical spine unless intubation by standard techniques is unsuccessful.
18. **Extubation**
An LMA can be substituted for a tracheal tube while the patient is still in a deep plane of anesthesia or before antagonism of neuromuscular blockade to facilitate a smoother emergence from anesthesia. The LMA is placed behind or over the tracheal tube, and the cuff is inflated. Correct laryngeal mask position can be confirmed by using a fiberscope or a capnograph. The tracheal tube cuff is then deflated, and the tracheal tube is removed. An exchange catheter or bougie may be used to facilitate reinserting the tracheal tube, if needed.
19. **Extracorporeal Shock Wave Lithotripsy**
Extracorporeal shock wave lithotripsy requires limited diaphragmatic motion to localize the ureteral stone. The LMA in combination with high-frequency jet ventilation can reduce motion and make this procedure more efficient.
20. **Percutaneous Tracheostomy**
Percutaneous tracheostomy is a bedside procedure for inserting a tracheostomy tube. While this procedure is usually performed with a tracheal tube in place, it has also been performed with an LMA.

E. Complications
1. **Aspiration of Gastric Contents**
a. The LMA does not form a watertight seal around the larynx and cannot be relied on to protect the tracheobronchial tree from gastrointestinal tract contents as reliably as a tracheal tube. The overall incidence of gastric content aspiration has been reported as 2.3 to 10.2 per 10,000 cases in adults. The incidence is lower with the LMA-ProSeal.

b. Many reported cases of aspiration with the LMA are associated with patients considered inappropriate for the LMA-Classic, such as gastrointestinal pathology, obesity, airway problems, depressed levels of consciousness, Trendelenburg or lithotomy position, history of reflux, emergency surgery, or trauma. Cases of aspiration in fasted patients with no predisposing factors during elective procedures have been reported. Aspiration is less likely with the LMA-ProSeal, although aspiration may occur if the tube is not correctly placed.
c. Gastroesophageal reflux may be a precursor to aspirating gastric contents. No correlation has been found between pressure and volume inside the cuff and variations in esophageal pH. The incidence of reflux is the same with spontaneous and positive-pressure ventilation. The risk of reflux is increased if the LMA remains in place until the patient can open the mouth on command, as opposed to removal on the first sign of rejection.
d. Regurgitation usually occurs without warning. It is often associated with light general anesthesia. The first indication is often the appearance of gastric fluid in the tube. Fortunately, most of the reported cases have had favorable outcomes because the regurgitated material was not aspirated or the aspiration was relatively mild.
e. A reduction in lower esophageal sphincter tone may occur when a laryngeal mask is used. The upper esophageal sphincter remains competent and can prevent regurgitation in the absence of neuromuscular block. During general anesthesia with the LMA, the pharyngeal reflex is minimal or blocked and does not affect esophageal motility. A study in cadavers found that correctly placed LMAs attenuated liquid flow between the esophagus and the pharynx. The cough reflex is significantly impaired following LMA use.
f. Vomiting is rare while the laryngeal mask is in use. An incidence of 0.4% was reported in a large retrospective study. There was no aspiration in this study.
g. In the event of a failed intubation in a patient for whom there is a significant risk of aspiration and in whom ventilation can be maintained with a face mask while cricoid pressure is applied, it may be safer to continue with the face mask and cricoid pressure rather than try to insert the LMA.

CLINICAL MOMENT Applying cricoid pressure may make the positioning of the LMA more difficult and may decrease the success of ventilation. It is probably a good idea to momentarily relax cricoid pressure while the LMA is being inserted. The LMA does not decrease the effectiveness of cricoid pressure, so cricoid pressure should be reapplied and maintained after the LMA is inserted unless it interferes with ventilation.

h. The incidence of aspiration can be reduced if the LMA is used only for fasting patients who are not at increased risk for gastroesophageal reflux. Gastric distention can be minimized by using the correct size LMA, avoiding cuff under- or overinflation, providing careful positioning and fixation, maintaining adequate anesthetic depth and relaxation throughout surgery, and maintaining low inflation pressures. Using small tidal volumes and low inspiratory flow rates will help to keep peak airway pressure low. The mean pressure at which gastric insufflation occurs is 28 cm H_2O, with a range of 19 to 41 cm H_2O when using size 4 and 5 LMAs. Epigastric auscultation should be performed to ensure that gastric insufflation is not occurring. A gastric tube may be used but may not always be helpful. Using pressure-controlled rather than volume-controlled ventilation (Chapter 6) may result in lower inflation pressures.

i. During spontaneous respiration, it is important to maintain an adequate level of anesthesia because gastric distention resulting from recurrent swallowing can occur when anesthesia is too light. Deglutition frequency may be increased by the LMA. Even in the presence of deep anesthesia and the absence of risk factors, aspiration can occur.

CLINICAL MOMENT If gastric contents are seen in the laryngeal mask, the patient should be placed in the 30° head-down position, the LMA left in situ, anesthesia deepened, and the breathing system disconnected temporarily to allow drainage and suctioning of the airway tube. The lateral position has no advantage, as regurgitated fluid is prevented from escaping via the pharynx. Oxygen should be supplied. Forceful ventilation attempts should be avoided and small tidal volumes delivered. Suctioning should be performed through the LMA, preferably using a fiberscope. The LMA should be replaced with a tracheal tube if aspiration has occurred.

CLINICAL MOMENT If the LMA-ProSeal is being used and unexpected regurgitation occurs, fluid will emerge from the drain tube. It has been shown in cadavers that fluids exit via the drain tube without laryngeal contamination when the mask has been correctly placed, so it may not be necessary to remove the LMA-ProSeal.

2. **Gastric Distention**

Gastric distention, which has been implicated as a factor in aspiration, can occur with positive-pressure ventilation. The incidence of gastric distention increases with increasing airway pressure and tidal volume but is unlikely to occur at airway pressures of less than 20 cm H_2O (30 cm H_2O for the LMA-ProSeal) if the LMA is properly positioned. Using pressure-limited rather than volume-limited ventilation may help to avoid gastric dilatation. Epigastric auscultation is a fairly reliable technique for detecting gastric inflation.

3. **Foreign Body Aspiration**

A foreign body may become entrapped in the LMA tube. Such an object may be subsequently aspirated or cause airway obstruction.

4. **Airway Obstruction**

a. Reported causes of complete or partial airway obstruction while using a laryngeal mask include malpositioning, distal cuff folding, epiglottic folding, cuff herniation, forward displacement of the postcricoid area, aryepiglottic fold infolding, arytenoid cartilage dislocation, laryngeal opening obstruction by the cuff, tube kinking, increased cuff volume, lubricant applied to the mask aperture, the LMA-ProSeal bowl folding inward, a faulty LMA, foreign body, a supraglottic tumor or lingual tonsillar hypertrophy, application of cricoid pressure, firing from a vagal nerve stimulator, mouth gags used for surgery, and laryngospasm.

b. The reported incidence of laryngospasm is 1% to 3% and may occur anytime during the perioperative period. Laryngospasm usually results from inadequate anesthetic depth or lubricant on the mask's anterior surface. Stridor has been reported for as long as 2 days following uneventful LMA use.

c. Biting the tube can cause obstruction and damage to the LMA. This can be avoided by inserting a bite block or gauze roll between the molars and leaving it in place until the LMA is removed. However, a bite block may be deformed. The LMA-ProSeal has a built-in bite block between the two tubes, which may prevent this problem. Oral airways are not satisfactory because they are designed to be in the center of the mouth.

d. Airway obstruction may be caused by the LMA rotating in such a way that the cuff occludes the larynx. Rotation can be detected by checking that the black line faces the upper lip.

e. Applying cricoid pressure or downward pressure on the mandible by the surgeon may cause airway obstruction with the laryngeal mask in place. Changing from single-handed to bimanual cricoid pressure application may resolve the problem.

f. If airway obstruction develops, rapid fiber-optic endoscopy may help to differentiate between the various causes and guide appropriate management. Maneuvers that may help to relieve obstruction include minor jaw or LMA adjustments, mandibular protrusion, and head extension. In most cases, the LMA should be removed and reinserted or a different size LMA should be used.

CLINICAL MOMENT Airway obstruction after the LMA is inserted or during anesthesia administration can be quickly recognized using pressure–volume loops (see Chapter 18).

5. **Trauma**

a. A number of traumatic injuries have been reported with LMA use, including injuries to the epiglottis, posterior pharyngeal wall, uvula, soft palate, tongue, and tonsils; a hematoma above the vocal cords in a patient with a bleeding diathesis; esophageal perforation after blind intubation through the intubating LMA in a patient with a high esophageal pouch; arytenoid and temporomandibular joint dislocation; tongue cyanosis; complete disruption of a cleft soft palate repair; and lingual edema in an infant after prolonged use of an inappropriately large LMA.

b. The incidence of sore throat following LMA use has been reported to be between 0% and 70%. The reported incidence is less than with a tracheal tube but greater than when a face mask is used. Using an insertion aid and cuff deflator may lower the incidence. Inserting the LMA fully or partially inflated will reduce the incidence. Using larger LMAs is associated with a higher incidence of sore throat. Leaving the LMA in place after intubation increases the incidence of sore throat.

c. Studies differ on the effect of intracuff pressure on the incidence of sore throat. Some studies have shown that lowering cuff pressure may decrease the incidence of sore throat, especially in women. Other studies have found no correlation between sore throat and cuff pressure. The pressure on the mucosa beneath the fully inflated cuff may be greater than capillary pressure, raising concerns about ischemic damage to the mucosa or reflex relaxation of the lower esophageal sphincter. Provided the intracuff pressure is kept at or below 60 cm H_2O, pressure on the mucosa will be less than that considered unsafe for prolonged tracheal intubation. There is evidence that the pharynx may adapt to the LMA cuff.

CLINICAL MOMENT Cuff pressures less than 60 cm H_2O will frequently provide a satisfactory seal and should be used, if possible.

d. Blood on the laryngeal mask occurs less often if the laryngeal mask is removed deflated than if it is removed with the cuff partially inflated.
e. Dysphagia is seen more frequently after LMA use than when a tracheal tube or a face mask is used. The incidence of dysphagia may or may not be related to cuff pressure.
f. Vocal cord edema has been reported with the LMA-ProSeal when it was used in a patient with an undiagnosed upper airway infection.

6. **Dislodgment**
   a. Accidental dislodgment can occur. A correctly placed LMA may be forced upward out of the hypopharynx if cricopharyngeal muscle tone is permitted to increase or the cuff becomes overinflated.
   b. If the LMA has come out only a short distance, it can often be pushed back into place. Persistent difficulty in keeping the LMA in position may be solved by using a different size mask, reducing the cuff volume, elevating the mandible, or using a different head position.
7. **Damage to the Device**
   When the reusable LMA is beyond its useful life span, it can break apart (**Fig. 13.16**). The device can be torn on insertion or removal and the tube can be bitten. The connector may become loose after a few autoclave cycles. The cuff can be punctured or the inflating tube severed by a nearby needle or other device.
8. **Nerve Injury**
   Palsies of the hypoglossal, recurrent laryngeal, and lingual nerves have been reported after using an LMA. Local anesthesia applied to the LMA can mimic nerve injury and cause vocal cord paralysis.

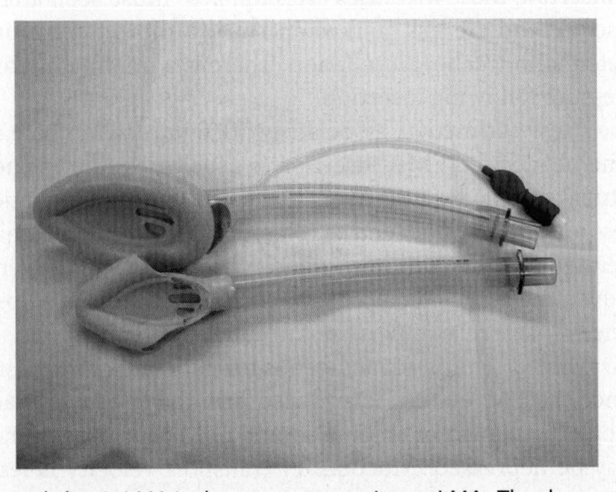

Figure 13.16 Damaged classic LMA is shown next to an intact LMA. The damaged LMA came apart during autoclaving. It had been used past the recommended number of times.

9. **Other**
   a. Transient salivary gland and tongue swelling and sialadenopathy have been described in association with the LMA. Unilateral supraglottic and vocal cord edema have been reported after using an LMA. Hiccups can occur.
   b. An LMA may distort the anatomy and displace mobile landmarks used to cannulate the internal jugular vein or other neck structures, cause spurious diagnosis of a cervical mass, or cause the surgeon to damage local structures. Ultrasound guidance (Chapter 23) is suggested to avoid problems with jugular vein cannulation.
   c. LMA cuff inflation has been found to decrease blood flow through the carotid artery. Venous congestion in the neck can be caused by an overinflated cuff.
   d. The tracheal tube inflating tube may become kinked when inserted through a laryngeal mask.

F. Advantages

1. **Ease of Insertion**

The LMA is relatively easy to insert and has a short learning curve even for nonanesthesia personnel. It can be inserted with the patient in nearly any position, although the prone position is more difficult. It can even be inserted in the patient in a cervical collar.

2. **Smooth Awakening**

The LMA allows a smoother awakening than a tracheal tube, with fewer episodes of desaturation, breath holding, coughing, laryngospasm, and hypertension. Patients with an LMA have better oxygen saturations and less coughing than patients who have an oral airway in place during emergence from anesthesia. Patients who have had an LMA require less analgesia during recovery than those who have been intubated.

3. **Low Operating Room Pollution**

There is less operating room pollution with an LMA than with a face mask. During spontaneous ventilation, trace gas concentrations are comparable with those with a tracheal tube.

4. **Avoiding the Complications of Intubation**
   a. While blood pressure and heart rate usually increase after a laryngeal mask is inserted, these increases are similar to those seen after an oral airway is inserted and are less marked and have a shorter duration than those associated with tracheal intubation. There is a minimal increase in intraocular pressure following insertion.
   b. The stress and anxiety associated with failure to intubate are decreased. The time needed for LMA insertion is usually less than is needed for tracheal intubation. Inadvertent bronchial or esophageal intubation cannot occur.
   c. Less anesthesia is needed to tolerate a laryngeal mask than a tracheal tube. Neither laryngoscopy nor a neuromuscular blocking agent is required, thus preventing associated problems such as trauma to the lips, gums, and teeth. Since muscle relaxants are not needed, complications associated with them are avoided. This is advantageous for patients with myasthenia gravis.
   d. Since the LMA is not introduced into the larynx or trachea, laryngeal or subglottic edema or trauma should not occur. However, laryngeal reflexes may be depressed. Mucociliary transport velocity is less in patients who have a tracheal tube in place than in those who have an LMA. This may have implications for reducing the risk of retained secretions, atelectasis,

and pulmonary infection. The incidence of bacteremia is low when the laryngeal mask is used.

e. Asthmatic patients and other patients with reactive airway disease are at increased risk of developing bronchospasm during manipulations in their airway. Because the LMA is less invasive than a tracheal tube, the risk of bronchospasm is reduced. However, the LMA may be unsuitable for the patient with acute asthma who requires high airway pressures.

5. **Ease of Use**

Because there is no need to support the jaw or hold a face mask, the clinician's hands are free for other tasks. Airway deterioration from user fatigue is eliminated. Intraoperative airway manipulations, difficulty in maintaining a patent airway, and hypoxemia are less common with the LMA than with a face mask.

6. **Avoiding Face Mask Complications**

The LMA avoids many of the complications associated with a face mask (Chapter 12) including dermatitis and injuries to the nose, eyes, teeth, and facial nerves. The incidence of sore jaw is less than when a face mask is used. The LMA provides protection from aspirating nasal and oral secretions. The anesthesia provider's hands are free, minimizing fatigue and potential airway deterioration and allowing the provider to perform other tasks. There are fewer episodes of oxygen desaturation, and gastric inflation is less likely to occur.

7. **Protection from Barotrauma**

Barotrauma is a potential problem with tracheal tubes because of the tight seal inside the trachea. It is less likely to occur with a laryngeal mask because excessive pressure is likely to be vented.

G. Disadvantages

1. **Unsuitable Situations**

a. Relative contraindications to using an LMA include situations associated with increased aspiration risk (full stomach, previous gastric surgery, gastroesophageal reflux, diabetic gastroparesis, pregnancy more than 14 weeks, dementia, trauma, opiate medications, and increased intestinal pressure) unless other techniques for securing the airway have failed. Hiatal hernia is a relative contraindication to LMA use unless effective measures to empty the stomach have been taken.

b. The patient with glottic or subglottic airway obstruction, such as tracheomalacia or external tracheal compression, should not be managed with a laryngeal mask because it cannot prevent tracheal collapse.

c. Supraglottic pathology such as a cyst, abscess, hematoma, vallecular cyst, or tissue disruption can make proper positioning difficult or impossible, although the LMA has proven useful in upper airway obstruction caused by supraglottic edema, thyroglossal tumor, or tonsil hypertrophy. If the mask is pushed behind the epiglottis, ventilation may be possible. It may be more appropriate to use alternative insertion techniques, depending on the nature of the pathology.

d. Major cervical pathology such as a large goiter, swelling in the hypopharynx, neck fibrosis, laryngeal cancer, or a deviated trachea may obstruct the airway and make intubation through an LMA difficult. The LMA-Fastrach may have a higher success rate than the LMA-Classic in these patients.

e. In patients who require high inflation pressures, that is, those with low compliance or high resistance, only the LMA-ProSeal should be used.

f. Some feel that the LMA is relatively contraindicated in situations in which there is restricted access to the airway, especially if there is no guarantee that the LMA can be replaced if it becomes dislodged or intubation becomes necessary. The LMA has been used in the lateral and prone positions.

CLINICAL MOMENT Anesthesia using an LMA in the prone position is highly controversial. Regurgitation is more likely, and higher airway pressures may be needed. The LMA may be more easily displaced in this position.

g. While some anesthesia providers consider prolonged procedures a contraindication to the LMA, time alone has not been shown to be a limiting factor.

2. **Requirement for Paralysis or Obtunded Airway Reflexes**
The LMA should not be inserted unless the jaw and pharynx are fully relaxed. Coughing, gagging, vomiting, biting, laryngospasm, and bronchospasm can occur in inadequately anesthetized patients, especially those with chronic respiratory diseases and heavy smokers.

3. **Lost Airway Management Skills**
The ability to maintain a patent airway while using a face mask is one of the fundamental skills of anesthetic practice. Increasing dependency on the LMA may result in a lack of experience and skills using a face mask for prolonged periods or with a difficult airway. Intubation skills may also be compromised when the LMA is substituted for the tracheal tube.

4. **Less Reliable Airway**
The LMA does not secure a clear airway as effectively as a tracheal tube and does not prevent airway obstruction at the glottic and subglottic levels. Movements of the head, neck, or drapes; insertion of a pack; or similar maneuvers that would be acceptable with a tracheal tube in place may cause LMA displacement.

5. **Unreliable Drug Administration**
During resuscitation, the tracheal tube is sometimes used for drug administration. The LMA is not as reliable a route for administering drugs as the tracheal tube.

II. Other Supraglottic Airways Similar to the Laryngeal Mask

The success of the laryngeal mask has caused a variety of other supraglottic devices to be produced. Some are similar to the LMA, whereas others are distinctly different. Some of these devices have undergone modifications either in materials or in design since their initial introduction, so the reader should make certain that performance studies of a particular device do not relate to an older version of that device. Some devices incorporate a cuff pressure–indicating device in the inflating tube (**Fig. 13.17**).

III. Other Supraglottic Airway Devices

A. Laryngeal Tube Airway

1. **Description**

a. The laryngeal tube airway (laryngeal tube, LT) (**Fig. 13.18**) is a reusable silicone device with a single lumen that is closed at the tip. Single-use versions (LT-D) made of polyvinyl chloride are available. The laryngeal tube

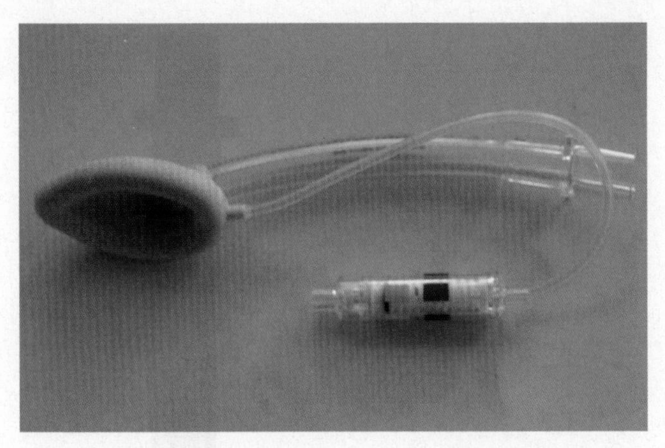

Figure 13.17 This supraglottic device has a cuff pressure–indicating device in the inflating tube. The black line on the white bellows should be at the green line on the housing. Cuff underinflation will result in the indicator line in the yellow section. Cuff overinflation will result in the black line being in the red section.

suction (LTS, Sonda laryngeal tube, SLT) (**Fig. 13.19**) has an additional (esophageal) lumen posterior to the respiratory lumen. It ends just distal to the esophageal cuff.

b. The airway tube is relatively wide and curved. There are three marks on the tube just below the connector to the breathing system. These indicate the range for proper depth placement. The tube size is color coded on

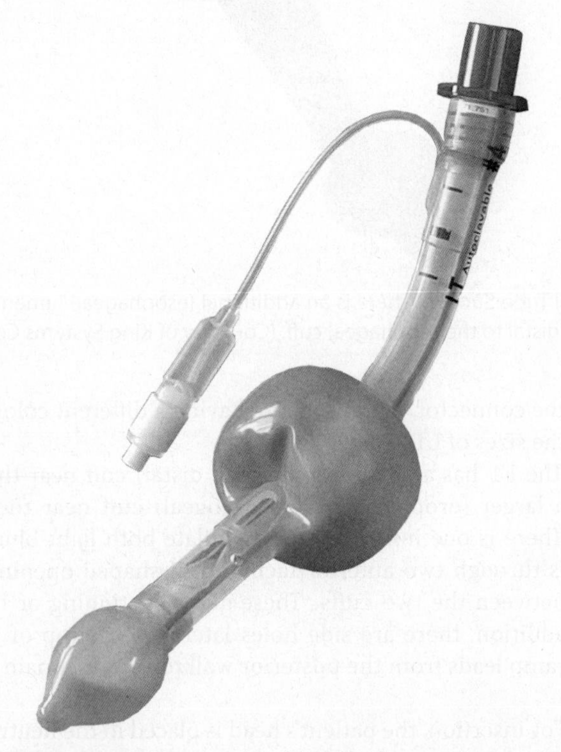

Figure 13.18 Laryngeal Tube Airway. The distal cuff blocks the esophagus. (Courtesy of King Systems Corporation, Noblesville, IN.)

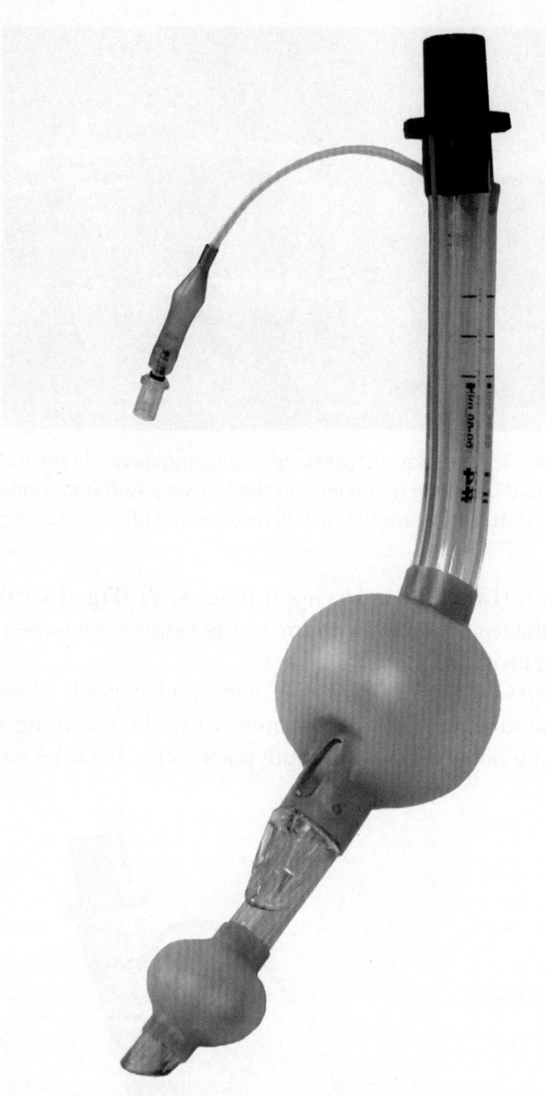

Figure 13.19 Laryngeal Tube Suction. There is an additional (esophageal) lumen posterior to the respiratory lumen that is open distal to the esophageal cuff. (Courtesy of King Systems Corporation.)

the connector, with each size having a different color. **Table 13.7** provides the sizes of LTs available.

c. The LT has a small (esophageal, distal) cuff near the blind distal tip and a larger (oropharyngeal, pharyngeal) cuff near the middle of the tube. There is one inflation tube to inflate both light-blue cuffs. Gas exchange is through two anterior-facing, oval-shaped openings (ventilation holes) between the two cuffs. These allow suctioning or fiberscope passage. In addition, there are side holes lateral to the top of the distal opening. A ramp leads from the posterior wall toward the main ventilatory outlet.

2. **Use**

a. For insertion, the patient's head is placed in the neutral or sniffing position. A jaw thrust may be helpful. Both cuffs should be deflated and a water-based lubricant applied. After the tube is introduced into the mouth, the flat edge

Table 13.7 Sizes of Laryngeal Tubes

Size	Patient	Weight (kg)	Color of Connector	Maximum Cuff Volume (mL)
0	Neonate	<6	Transparent	15
1	Infant	6–15	White	40
2	Child	15–30	Green	60
3	Small adult	30–60	Yellow	120
4	Medium adult	50–90	Red	130
5	Large adult	>90	Violet	150

of the tip is placed against the hard palate, keeping the tube centered. The tube is then slid along the palate and into the hypopharynx until resistance is felt. A malpositioned LT will often bounce back from the intended position. After insertion, the marks on the shaft should be aligned with the teeth. If difficulty is encountered, lateral insertion or using a laryngoscope may be helpful. Cricoid pressure will impede placement.

b. The cuffs should be inflated to a pressure of up to 60 cm H_2O. The proximal cuff will fill first. The volume of air required will depend on the patient. The manufacturer's *maximum* recommended volumes are shown in **Table 13.7**. If a manometer is not available, cuff volume should be adjusted so that there is a slight oropharyngeal leak at the required ventilatory setting and then air is added until the leak just disappears. After insertion and cuff inflation, the airway leak pressure should be measured and epigastric auscultation performed. If gastric inflation is occurring, air should be added to the cuffs. The device may need to be moved up or down to achieve effective ventilation.

c. The LT can be used with either spontaneous breathing or positive-pressure ventilation. Cuff pressure should be monitored continuously. If nitrous oxide is used, cuff pressure will need to be readjusted during use because nitrous oxide will diffuse into the cuff.

d. For tracheal intubation, an airway exchange catheter or tracheal tube mounted on a fiberscope is inserted through the LT and into the trachea. If the view through the fiberscope is not satisfactory, the LT may need to be rotated. A jaw thrust may be helpful.

e. For nasotracheal intubation, the LT is inserted and a fiberscope with a tracheal tube over it is used to identify the glottis, which should be just in front of it. After the tracheal tube is advanced through the nose and the distal cuff has entered the trachea, the LT is removed. An extender such as a small tracheal tube from which the connector has been removed is inserted into the end of the tube in the trachea, with the connector also removed, and it will be necessary to allow the LT to be removed without the tracheal tube being removed from the trachea.

f. The reusable LT must be cleaned and sterilized between uses. It should be autoclaved at 134°C (273°F) and 2.4 bar (35 psi) for 10 minutes. These devices must not be sterilized using formaldehyde, glutaraldehyde, ethylene oxide, or plasma. The manufacturer recommends up to 50 uses for the reusable device.

g. The LT is relatively easy to insert, even by clinicians who have little or no experience. The insertion time is short and the success rate for first-time insertion is high. It is well tolerated during emergence from anesthesia. Because the distal cuff fits over the esophageal inlet, the risk of gastric inflation is low. Satisfactory ventilation with both spontaneous and controlled ventilation can be achieved in most patients.

h. Since the insertion time is short, high ventilation pressures can be used and the distal cuff should seal the esophageal inlet, this device may be especially useful for resuscitation. It has been used in the "cannot intubate, cannot ventilate" situation and in obstetrics after failed intubation.

i. Although one study found that the patient's head and neck stabilization by manual in-line method often made the LT difficult or impossible to insert, it has been successfully used with manual in-line stabilization and a high cervical collar.

j. The incidence of complications such as sore throat, mouth pain, or dysphagia associated with its use is low.

k. Cuff rupture has been reported when a manometer was not used to evaluate cuff pressure.

l. The insertion of the LT by inexperienced personnel was easier than the LMA-Classic. Cases have been reported in which the LMA had failed but the LT was successfully inserted. During controlled ventilation, the LT provides higher sealing pressures and tidal volumes than the LMA-Classic in adults and children and gastric inflation occurs less frequently. When used for spontaneous breathing, the laryngeal mask provided successful airway maintenance in more patients than did the LT. The incidence of complications was similar.

m. In comparison with the LT, the LMA-ProSeal was found to be easier to insert, was inserted successfully on the first attempt more often, and gave a significantly better view of the glottis. During controlled ventilation, the two devices performed equally well in terms of seal pressure. During spontaneous breathing, the LMA-ProSeal was successful more often.

n. In comparing the intubating LMA and LT during manual in-line neck stabilization, placement was easier and quicker and tidal volume was greater with the LMA-Fastrach.

B. Streamlined Pharynx Airway Liner

1. **Description**

a. The Streamlined Liner of the Pharynx Airway (SLIPA™) (**Figs. 13.20** and **13.21**) is a plastic, disposable, uncuffed device that is anatomically shaped to line the pharynx. It forms a seal with the pharynx at the base of the tongue and the entrance to the esophagus by virtue of the resilience of its walls.

b. The distal part of the SLIPA is shaped like a hollow boot with a toe, bridge, and heel. There is an anterior opening for ventilation. The end of the toe rests in the esophageal entrance. The bridge fits into the pyriform fossae at the base of the tongue, which it displaces from the posterior pharyngeal wall. The heel connects to the airway tube, which is rectangular in shape and has a color-coded connector. The heel serves to anchor the SLIPA in a stable position. According to the manufacturer, the SLIPA usually does not need to be fixed in place. The SLIPA has a large-capacity chamber for storing regurgitated liquids. Toward the toe side of the lateral bulges of the bridge are smaller secondary lateral bulges. This feature is meant to relieve pressure at this site and prevent damage to the hypoglossal and recurrent laryngeal nerves.

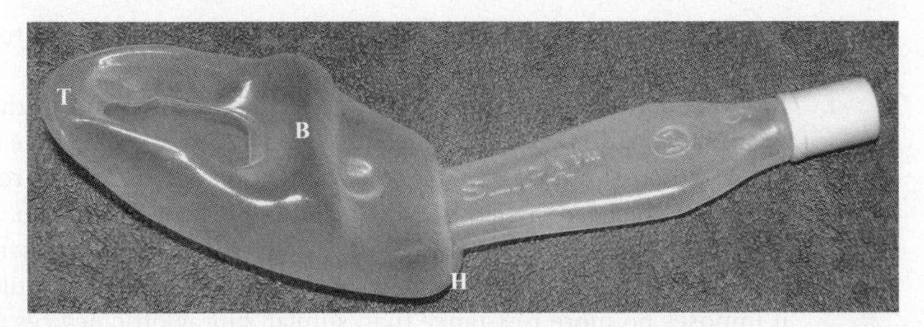

Figure 13.20 Streamlined Pharynx Airway Liner. T, toe; B, bridge; H, heel. (Courtesy of ARC Medical, Inc., Tucker, GA.)

c. The SLIPA is available in six adult sizes that relate to the dimension across the bridge: 47, 49, 51, 52, 55, and 57 mm. To choose the correct size, this dimension should be matched with the width of the patient's thyroid cartilage.

2. **Use**

a. Before insertion, the SLIPA should be examined for defects and water-soluble lubricant be applied. It should be collapsed in the anterior–posterior plane before insertion. After insertion, it spontaneously returns to its preinsertion shape.

b. The head is extended and the device inserted toward the back of the mouth until the heel locates itself in the pharynx. It is helpful if the jaw is lifted forward during insertion. A laryngoscope or gloved fingers can be used to create a space in the pharynx.

c. Airway seal pressure should be checked after insertion. If it is too low, a larger size SLIPA should be tried. If positive-pressure ventilation is used, the epigastrium should be auscultated to make certain that gastric inflation is not occurring.

d. If obstruction is encountered immediately after insertion, a downfolded epiglottis may be the cause. The head should be extended and the jaw pulled forward. If this does not correct the problem, the SLIPA should be removed and reinserted with an accentuated jaw lift. Another maneuver is to momentarily insert the SLIPA deeper so that it will free up the epiglottis. If this does not relieve the obstruction, the likely cause is laryngospasm.

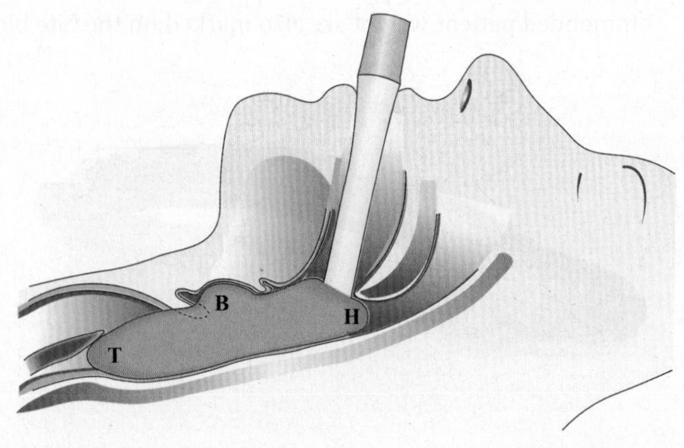

Figure 13.21 Streamlined Pharynx Airway Liner in place. T, toe; B, bridge; H, heel. (Courtesy of ARC Medical, Inc., Tucker, GA.)

e. If regurgitation is suspected, a suction catheter with the curve to one side should be inserted so that it does not touch the vocal cords.
f. It is recommended that the SLIPA be used with the head in the neutral position because twisting the head to one side may dislodge the seal. Partial obstruction during spontaneous ventilation will usually be relieved by extending the head or simply using positive-pressure ventilation.
g. The SLIPA is easy to insert and is associated with a high first insertion success rate even with inexperienced providers. Despite its irregular shape, it imposes no more resistance than similar supraglottic devices. It can be used with both spontaneous breathing and controlled ventilation. It is well tolerated during emergence from anesthesia. The airway sealing pressure is greater than with the LMA-Classic. Because there is no cuff, nitrous oxide has no effect on sealing pressure.
h. The SLIPA provides effective protection against aspiration during positive-pressure ventilation. However, it is possible that the storage capacity of the SLIPA may not be adequate for nonfasted patients. The manufacturer suggests that it may be safe to suction within the device if regurgitated liquid is present.
i. The SLIPA is contraindicated if upper airway anatomy is abnormal or distorted.

C. i-gel

1. **Description**

a. The i-gel (**Fig. 13.22**) is made from a gel-like transparent thermoplastic elastomer. It does not contain latex. It is designed to create an anatomical seal without an inflatable cuff. It is available in three color-coded sizes as shown in **Table 13.8** and **Figure 13.23**. Each i-gel is supplied in a protective cradle. All are single-use devices.
b. The i-gel has a 15-mm connector to attach to the breathing system and a gastric channel that opens at the tip. This channel is used for suctioning, placing a nasogastric tube, and venting from the esophagus. The diameter at the tube center is slightly larger to prevent rotation and aid insertion. Above the cuff is a lip called the epiglottic rest that reduces the possibility that the epiglottis could fold downward and obstruct the airway.
c. There is an integral bite block marked with a black line that signifies the optimum incisor teeth position when the device is in situ. The size and recommended patient weight are also marked on the bite block.

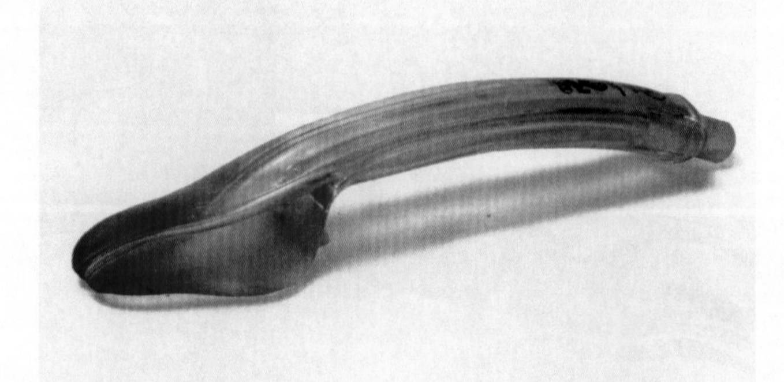

Figure 13.22 The i-gel.

Table 13.8 i-gel Sizing Chart

i-gel Size	Intended Patient	Patient Weight (lb)[a]	Nasogastric Tube Size	Color
3	Small adult	65–130	Up to 12 (FG)	Yellow
4	Medium adult	110–200	Up to 12 (FG)	Green
5	Large adult	200+	Up to 14 (FG)	Orange

[a]Patients with cylindrical necks or wide thyroid-cricoid cartilages may require a larger size than normally recommended on a weight basis. Patients with a broad or stocky neck or smaller thyroid/cricoid cartilage may require a smaller size than would normally be recommended on a weight basis. Patients with central obesity (in whom the main weight distribution is around the abdomen and hips) might require an i-gel of a size commensurate with their ideal body weight.

2. **Use**
   a. After the device has been removed from the cradle, it should be inspected for defects. A small amount of water-soluble lubricant (no silicone-containing gel) should be on the middle of the smooth side of the cradle and the front, back, and sides of the cuff lubricated. The cradle can be used to hold the device until it is time for insertion, but it is not an introducer and should not be placed in the patient's mouth.
   b. The i-gel is inserted by grasping the bite block firmly and positioning the device so that the cuff outlet is facing toward the patient's chin. The patient should be in the sniffing position, with the head extended and the neck flexed. The chin should be gently pressed down. The i-gel should be inserted into the patient's mouth and directed toward the hard palate. It should be glided downward and backward along the hard palate with a continuous gentle push until a definite resistance is felt. At this point, the tip should be located at the upper esophageal opening. The i-gel should be taped from maxilla to maxilla and tied as well as taped if the patient is to be in a lateral or prone position.
   c. The i-gel can be used with spontaneous breathing and positive-pressure ventilation and has been used for resuscitation. An air leak through the gastric channel indicates that the i-gel is not properly seated. The device should be removed and reinserted, with a gentle jaw thrust being applied.
   d. If regurgitation is suspected or fluid is seen in the gastric channel, the patient should be placed in Trendelenburg position and, if possible, turned

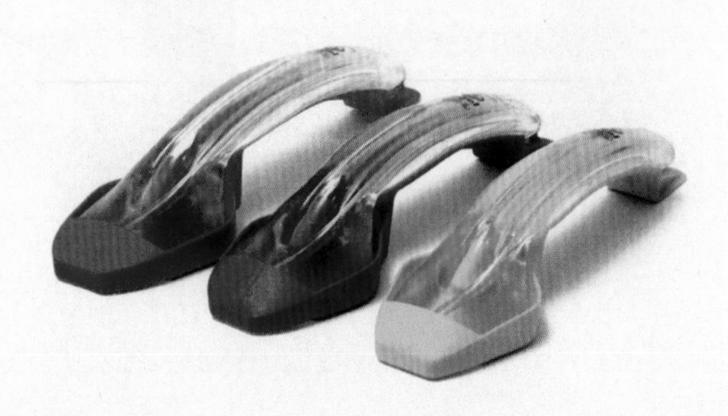

Figure 13.23 The i-gel available in three color-coded sizes.

to a right or left lateral position. The i-gel should be removed thorough suctioning. Tracheal intubation should then be performed.

e. Although reports on the i-gel are few at the time of this writing, there may be a low incidence of sore throat with this device. It has been used for pediatric patients and patients in the prone position. There has been one report of neuropraxia with the i-gel.

3. **Contraindications**

Contraindications include nonfasting patients for routine surgical procedures, patients with a Maliampati score of III or above, trismus or limited mouth opening, and airway pressure above 40 cm H_2O, and patients at increased risk for regurgitation such as hiatal hernia, sepsis, morbid obesity pregnancy, and a history of upper gastrointestinal surgery. The manufacturer suggests limiting its use to 4 hours.

SUGGESTED READINGS

Asai T, Shingu. Review article. The laryngeal tube. Br J Anaesth 2005;95:729–736.

Brimacombe JR. Laryngeal Mask Anesthesia. Principles and Practice. Philadelphia: Saunders, 2005.

Caponas G. Review. Intubating laryngeal mask airway. Anaesth Intensive Care 2002;30:551–569.

Cook TM, Lee G, Nolan JP. The ProSeal™ laryngeal mask airway: a review of the literature. Can J Anesth 2005;52: 739–760.

Cook TM, Silsby J, Simpson TP. Airway rescue in acute upper airway obstruction using a ProSeal™ laryngeal mask airway and an Aintree Catheter™: a review of the ProSeal™ laryngeal mask airway in the management of the difficult airway. Anaesthesia 2005;60:1129–1136.

Dorsch J, Dorsch S. Supraglottic airway devices. In: Understanding Anesthesia Equipment. Fifth edition. Philadelphia: Wolters Kluwer/Lippincott Williams & Wilkins, 2008:461–519.

Ferson DZ, Brain AIJ. Laryngeal mask airway. In: Hagberg CA, ed. Benumof's Airway Management. Second edition. St. Louis: Elsevier, 2007:476–501.

Hagberg CA, Agro FE, Cook TM, Reed AP. New generation supraglottic ventilatory devices. In: Hagberg CA, ed. Benumof's Airway Management. Second edition. St. Louis: Elsevier, 2007:502–531.

Henderson JJ, Popat MT, Latto IP, Pearce AC. Difficult Airway Society guidelines for management of the unanticipated difficult intubation. Anaesthesia 2004;59:675–694.

Hooshangi H, Wong DT. Brief review: the Cobra Perilaryngeal Airway (Cobra PLA®) and the Streamlined Liner of Pharyngeal Airway (SLIPA™) supraglottic airways. Can J Anesth 2008;55:177–185.

Miller DM. A proposed classification and scoring system for supraglottic sealing airways: a brief review. Anesth Analg 2004;99:1553–1559.

14 Laryngoscopes

LARYNGOSCOPES ARE USED TO VIEW the larynx and adjacent structures, most commonly for the purpose of inserting a tube into the tracheobronchial tree. Other uses include placing a device (suction catheter, gastric tube, dilating bougie, gastrointestinal endoscopic equipment, or echocardiographic or temperature probe) into the esophagus, checking the position of a tracheal tube, exchanging a tracheal tube, removing a foreign body, assessing the airway, and documenting recurrent laryngeal nerve status after neck operations.

I. Rigid Laryngoscopes

A. Description

A rigid laryngoscope may be either a single piece or a handle with a detachable blade. The most commonly used type in the United States has a hook-on (hinged, folding) connection between a hinge pin on the handle and a slot on the blade. This allows the blade to be quickly and easily attached or detached. A single-piece laryngoscope has a switch on the handle that controls the power to the lamp.

1. **Handle**
   a. The handle provides a means to hold the laryngoscope. It can provide light by one of several methods. There may be a battery in the handle that provides energy to the bulb when contact with the blade is made. There may be a light bulb in the handle so that when the blade is locked in place, light is transmitted to the blade through a fiber-optic bundle. These handles and blades have a green marking. The handle may connect to a remote light source via a fiber-optic cable. Some handles allow the bulb and battery portion to be removed as a unit. This allows the outer part of the handle to be cleaned and disinfected or sterilized.
   b. Handles are available in different sizes. A short handle is advantageous for the patient with a large chest or breasts or when intubation is necessary in a tight place. While the blade is usually at a 90-degree angle to the handle, there may be an adjustable handle that allows other angles. Some blades have an angle other than 90 degrees where they attach to the base (**Fig. 14.1**).

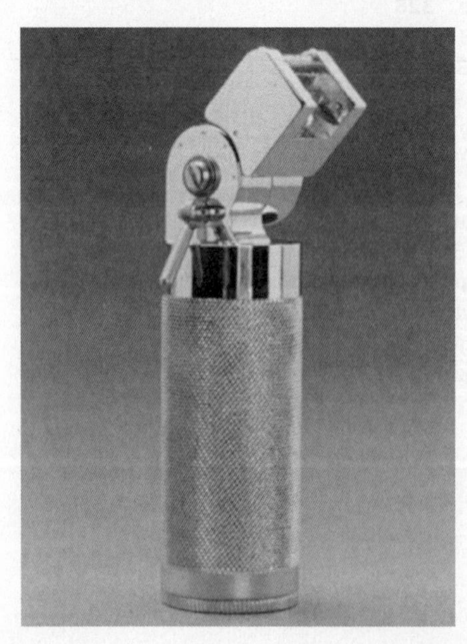

Figure 14.1 Patil-Syracuse handle. With this handle, the blade can be adjusted and locked in four different positions (45°, 90°, 135°, or 180°). (Courtesy of Mercury Medical, Clearwater, FL.)

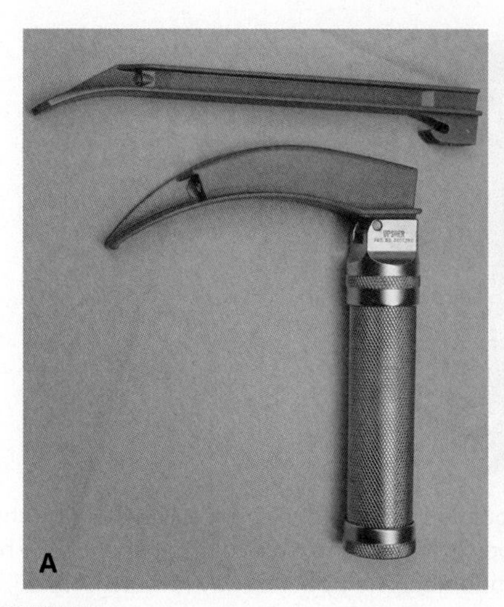

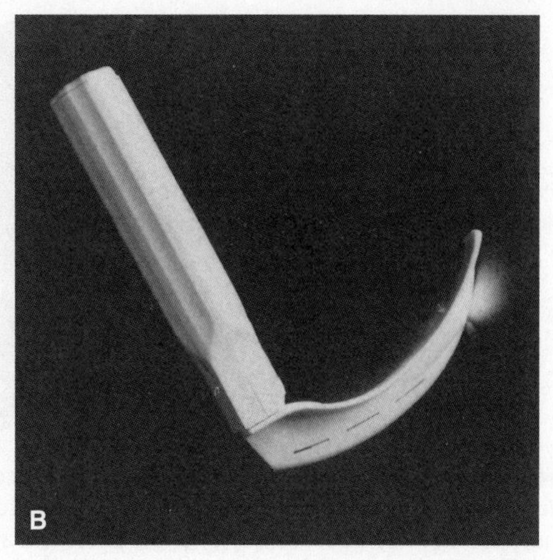

Figure 14.2 **A:** Reusable handle with curved (Macintosh) and straight (Miller) disposable blades. **B:** Disposable handle and blade. (Courtesy of Rusch, Inc., Research Triangle Park, NC, and Vital Signs, Totawa, NJ.)

2. **Blade**
   a. The blade is the component that is inserted into the mouth. When a blade is available in more than one size, the blades are numbered, with the number increasing with size. In general, there are two blade types: straight and curved (**Fig. 14.2**).

CLINICAL MOMENT Neither the straight blade nor the curved blade offers significant advantages to justify one being recommended over the other. It is important that the user be good with one or the other.

   b. The optimal position for laryngoscopy for most adult patients is approximately 35-degree lower cervical spine flexion and 85- to 90-degree head extension at the atlanto-occipital level, the so-called sniffing position. Elevation beyond the sniffing position may improve the laryngeal view in difficult-to-intubate patients. The lower cervical spine portion can be maintained in a flexed position by using a pillow under the head. Atlanto-occipital joint extension is achieved by pressure on the top of the head and/or upward traction on the upper teeth or gums. Intubation is sometimes made easier by extending the operating table head section or removing the pillow from beneath the patient's head and placing it under the shoulders. A 25-degree back elevation has been recommended. In obese patients, considerable shoulder and head elevation may be necessary so that an imaginary horizontal line connects the patient's sternal notch with the external auditory meatus [ramped position, head-elevated laryngoscopy position (HELP)]. A cushion designed to provide an improved position is available (**Fig. 14.3**). In children, it may be unnecessary to flex the lower cervical vertebrae. In neonates, it may be necessary to elevate the shoulders because the head is relatively large.
   c. The laryngoscope handle is held in the left hand. Moistening or lubricating the blade will facilitate insertion if the mouth is dry. In some situations, the

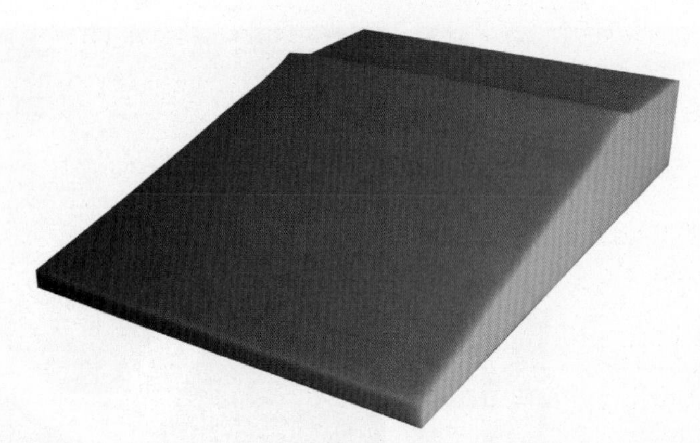

Figure 14.3 Troop elevation pillow. A standard pillow should be used with this. The elevation pillow helps to achieve a better position for ventilation and laryngoscopy in large-framed and obese patients. The head and neck are elevated above the level of the chest and abdomen. The upper airway is more isolated, and the weight of the abdomen is moved away from the diaphragm. This pillow is easier and quicker to use and more stable than a stack of blankets. (Courtesy of Mercury Medical.)

chest will impinge on the handle, making it difficult to insert the blade. In these cases, a short handle may be used, with the blade may be inserted sideways or the unattached blade may be inserted and then attached to the handle. There is a left-handed Macintosh blade for left-handed anesthesia providers.

d. The fingers of the right hand are used to open the mouth. In patients with dentition, optimal mouth opening is often achieved with the thumb on the lower teeth and the index finger pushing on the upper teeth.
e. The blade is inserted at the right side of the mouth and advanced along the side of the tongue toward the right tonsillar fossa. The right hand keeps the lips from getting caught between the teeth or gums and the blade. If the tongue is slippery, placing tape on the lingual blade surface may be helpful. When the right tonsillar fossa is visualized, the blade tip is moved toward the midline. The blade is then advanced behind the base of the tongue until the epiglottis comes into view.

CLINICAL MOMENT While inserting the blade, be careful to not to drag the lips between the teeth and the blade.

f. The straight blade is shown in position for intubation in **Figure 14.4A.** The blade is made to scoop under the epiglottis and lift it anteriorly. The vocal cords should be identified. If the blade is advanced too far, it will elevate the larynx as a whole rather than expose the vocal cords. Occasionally, the blade will expose the esophagus. It should then be withdrawn slowly. If it is withdrawn too far, the epiglottis will be released and flip over the glottis.
g. A straight blade can also be inserted into the vallecula (the angle made by the epiglottis with the base of the tongue) and used in the same manner as a curved blade (see the following text).
h. **Figure 14.3B** shows the curved blade in position. After the epiglottis is visualized, the blade is advanced until the tip is in the vallecula. Traction

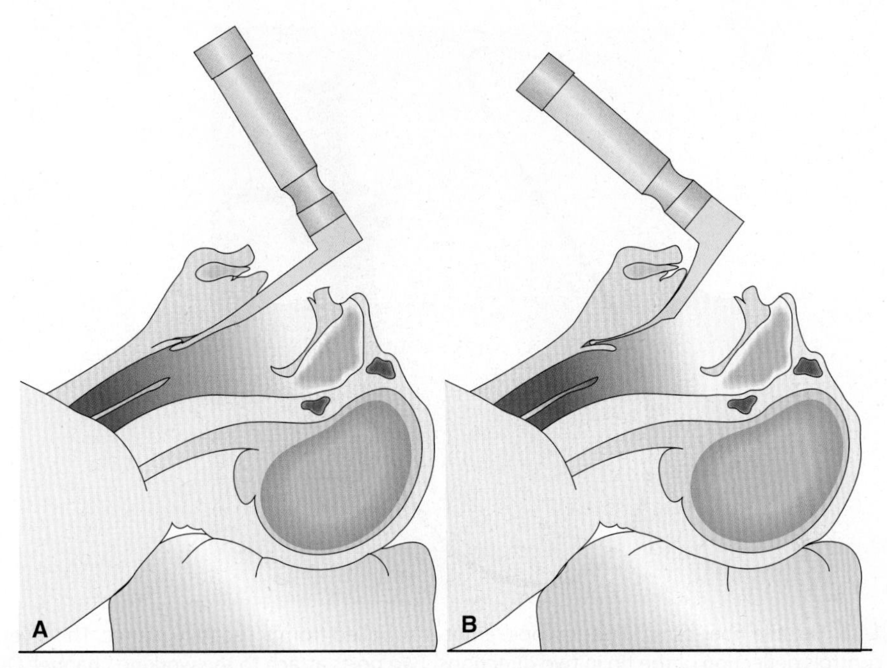

Figure 14.4 **A:** Intubation with a straight laryngoscope blade. The tip of the blade picks up the epiglottis. **B:** Intubation with the curved laryngoscope blade. The epiglottis is below the tip of the blade. A small pillow under the head allows better visualization of the larynx. (Courtesy of Vance Robideaux, MD.)

is then applied along the handle at right angles to the blade to move the tongue base and the epiglottis forward. The glottis should come into view. It is important that the end of the handle opposite the blade is not pulled backward. This will cause the tip to push the larynx upward and out of sight and could cause damage to the teeth or gums.

CLINICAL MOMENT It is important not to use the teeth as a fulcrum, in hope of improving intubating conditions. The best view is usually obtained when the handle is lifted in the same direction that it is pointing.

i. A curved blade can also be used as a straight blade, lifting the epiglottis directly if it is long enough.
j. In cases of difficult laryngoscopy, a left- or right-molar approach often improves the view and may spare the incisor teeth. Unfortunately, difficulty inserting the tracheal tube limits this method's efficiency.
k. Even with correct technique, the larynx will not always be visualized. Displacing the larynx by external **B**ackward, **U**pward, and **R**ightward **P**ressure (BURP) on the thyroid cartilage may improve glottic visualization. Mandibular elevation may also improve the view.

CLINICAL MOMENT When the anesthesia provider is trying to find a good laryngeal view, he or she can manipulate the larynx with the right hand while the left hand holds the laryngoscope. After the best view has been obtained, the anesthesia provider can ask another person to hold the larynx in that position.

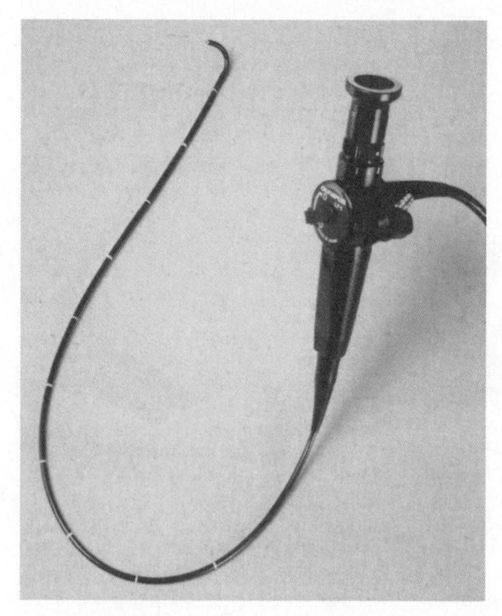

Figure 14.5 Flexible fiber-optic laryngoscope. Light is supplied from a separate source. The lever on the handle controls deflection of the tip in two directions. Two ports attach to the working channel. One is for insufflation or injection, and one is for suctioning. (Courtesy of Olympus Corp., Center Valley, PA.)

II. Endoscopes

The flexible fiber-optic endoscope (fiberscope) (Fig. 14.5) is used to place and evaluate the position of tracheal, double-lumen, tracheostomy and gastric tubes plus supraglottic devices and bronchial blockers, check tube patency, evaluate the airway, and locate and remove secretions and foreign bodies.

A. Description

1. The fiber-optic endoscope light source can be located in either the handle or a remote source. A remote light source connected to the endoscope may provide better light, but a light source in the handle is more portable.
2. The handle (**Fig. 14.6**) houses the batteries if they are used as the power source, or there may be a connector for a fiber-optic cable from a remote light source.

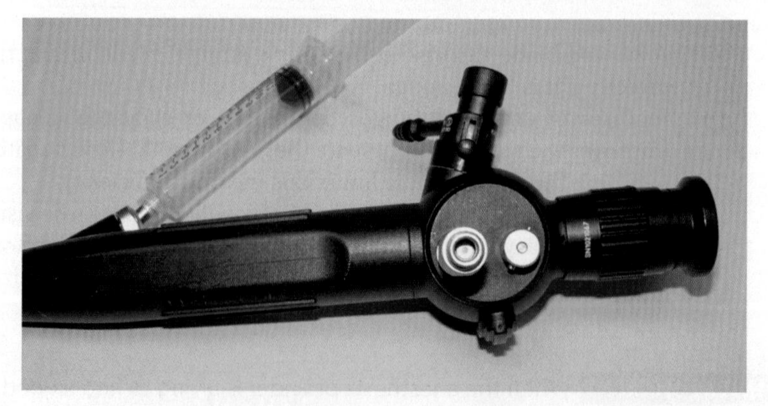

Figure 14.6 Handle of flexible fiberscope. The syringe is attached to the working channel. At the bottom is the lever for controlling the tip. Above it to the left is the connection for the light source. At the top is the connection for suction tubing and the suction control. The eyepiece, to which a camera may be attached, is to the right.

Other parts of the handle include the eyepiece, focusing ring, working channel port (for suctioning or administering oxygen, local anesthetics, or saline), and the tip control lever or knob. By turning the focusing (adjusting) ring, the image can be brought into the best focus. A camera can be attached to the eyepiece for remote viewing. A small television screen may replace the eyepiece. The fiberscope body may or may not be fully submersible.

3. The tip (bending, angulation) control lever or knob may be on the side of the fiberscope body or a thumb-controlled lever system on the back of the handle. By turning this control, the insertion cord tip can be flexed or extended in one plane. A full range of motion can be achieved by rotating the entire instrument. Many fiberscopes have a tip-locking mechanism that fixes the tip in the desired position.
4. The insertion cord (shaft, tube) is the portion that is inserted into the patient. It contains an image-transmitting bundle, one or two light-conducting bundles, two angulation wires, and sometimes a working channel. These are surrounded by a protective wire mesh and vinyl covering. Circular depth marks are usually present. The insertion cord length varies. For tracheal intubation in adults, a 50-cm cord is usually sufficient. Double-lumen or nasotracheal tube insertion may require a length of 55 to 60 cm. The insertion cord needs to be fully submersible in order to facilitate cleaning.
5. The outside diameter of the insertion cord determines the smallest size tracheal tube that the endoscope will pass through. The internal tracheal tube diameter should be at least 1 mm wider than the outside diameter of the insertion cord. The connection between the handle and the insertion cord is usually tapered to hold a tracheal tube.

B. Intubation

1. **General Considerations**
   a. When using a flexible fiber-optic scope for intubation, the type of tracheal tube used is important. The tube will be more likely to advance into the trachea if the largest scope that fits easily inside it is used. A tube with a tip designed to minimize the distance between the fiberscope and the tube's leading edge may pass more easily than a standard tube. A spiral embedded tube may pass more easily than a tube with a preformed curve. Warming a standard tracheal tube may facilitate passage over the endoscope.
   b. Because this instrument is expensive and delicate, great care should be taken to prevent damage. A minor blow can break glass fibers. Care must be taken to avoid forceful bending along the cord.

CLINICAL MOMENT The insertion portion must not be withdrawn or advanced with the tip angulated. Failure to straighten the tip before the scope is removed may result in damage.

   c. Before use, the light should be tested. The tip should either be treated with antifogging solution or be placed in warm water (not saline) for several minutes before use. Alternatively, the tip can be briefly held against the buccal mucosa to warm the lens. Hot air from a convective warming device (Chapter 24) may be directed over the tip. The focusing ring should be adjusted by viewing small print at a distance of 2 to 3 cm. The insertion portion should be coated with a lubricating gel, but the lubricant should not contact the lens. Tubing for suction or oxygen insufflation should be attached to the appropriate port. Oxygen supplied through the working channel will support patient oxygenation, clear secretions, and defog the optics. Control lever function should be assessed. The tracheal tube should be anchored firmly on the wider portion of the insertion cord.

CLINICAL MOMENT Applying suction may cause tissue to be sucked onto the end of the scope, obscuring the view or damaging the tissue.

d. Optimal positioning for fiber-optic laryngoscopy includes extending the cervical spine rather than flexing it as recommended for direct laryngoscopy.
e. The proximal control section is held in one hand with the index finger on the suction/insufflation port and the thumb on the lever that controls tip angulation. The other hand holds the shaft and guides its advance.
f. Because the cables are not strong enough to lift or dislodge tissues, it is important to have an air space at the end of the tip. In the anesthetized patient, visualization is often difficult or impossible unless some means to expand the pharynx is used. This may be accomplished by having a second person pull the tongue and/or elevate the jaw. Occasionally, it may be necessary to lift the larynx by grasping it externally. Alternately, a tongue retractor or rigid or video laryngoscope can be used to push the tongue forward. The awake patient can be asked to stick out his or her tongue, which is then held gently between gauze by an assistant. Special airways have been developed to aid fiber-optic intubation. These are discussed in Chapter 12.
g. Oxygen insufflation or jet ventilation through the working channel can be used to improve oxygenation throughout the procedure.
h. Disorientation in the airway is best resolved by slowly withdrawing the tip and examining the area with gentle up and down tip deflection, rotating the scope as a unit or alternately advancing the tip and withdrawing it slightly. If the view is consistently foggy or hazy, irrigating with saline and suctioning will usually resolve this problem. Adherent secretions may require that the instrument be withdrawn and the tip cleaned with moist gauze.
i. Resistance is frequently encountered when passing the tracheal tube over the fiberscope. Rotating the tracheal tube 90 degrees counterclockwise may be helpful. Other useful maneuvers include applying a jaw thrust, applying external pressure on the larynx, and elevating the epiglottis by using a rigid laryngoscope or the fingers.

CLINICAL MOMENT Since the tip on the standard tracheal tube is on the right side, it will often impact the right side of the vocal cords, preventing it from entering the larynx. Turning the tube 90 degrees will often align the tip with the space between the cords. Using a tube with a tip at the 12 o'clock position may avoid this problem.

j. If the fiberscope tip protrudes through the Murphy eye of the tracheal tube, it may not be possible to slip the tube off the endoscope or to withdraw the fiberscope from the tracheal tube. The fiberscope and tracheal tube may need to be withdrawn as a unit. To avoid this problem, the tracheal tube should be threaded onto the fiberscope before endoscopy or the fiberscope advanced through the tube under direct vision, taking care to pass the fiberscope through the distal opening.

CLINICAL MOMENT The endoscope tip should be in the neutral position as the tracheal tube is advanced and the fiberscope is withdrawn.

k. Various intubation techniques are available. The first is to thread a tracheal or double-lumen tube with the lumen lubricated over the cord until it abuts the handle, advance the flexible portion until the tip enters the trachea or bronchus, and then thread the tube over the endoscope. With the second technique, the tracheal tube is first advanced into the pharynx so that it acts as a guide to bring the endoscope tip close to the laryngeal entrance. The fiberscope is passed through the tube and into the trachea. The tube is then threaded over it. A third technique is to use the fiberscope to place a guide wire or stylet into the trachea. The fiberscope is withdrawn and a tracheal tube is passed over the guide and into the trachea. This may be especially useful in small patients.

2. **Oral Intubation**

a. Oral intubation is considered more difficult than nasal intubation. The tip enters the larynx at an acute angle to the glottis whereas during nasal intubation, it enters at an oblique angle. Oral intubation may be easier if used with an accessory that will protect the instrument from the patient's teeth, guide it into the midline, and keep the tongue from falling backward. These are discussed in Chapter 12. The insertion cord is placed in the midline and advanced under direct vision, curving downward at the posterior pharyngeal wall, seeking the epiglottis. It is important that the tip be kept in the midline as it is advanced. When the epiglottis has been located, the fiberscope tip is deflected downward so that it passes beneath the epiglottis and is then turned upward until the vocal cords are seen. The tip is then passed between the cords and advanced several centimeters. For bronchial intubation, the tip is advanced into the desired mainstem bronchus.

b. With the fiberscope tip in place, the lubricated tube is advanced over the scope, which functions as a stylet. The bevel should face posteriorly. The fiberscope should be used to verify that the tube tip is correctly positioned and then withdrawn, leaving the tube in place.

3. **Nasal Intubation**

Fiber-optic nasotracheal intubation is usually easier than orotracheal intubation because midline positioning is easier to maintain, the patient cannot bite the scope, and the nasopharyngeal anatomy naturally directs the tube into the trachea. It is associated with less cervical spine motion than direct laryngoscopy or other methods to manage the airway. A nasopharyngeal airway may be used to lubricate and dilate the nasal passages, after which it is removed. The fiberscope should be advanced through the tracheal tube before insertion, because it may not be possible to insert a tube loaded over a fiberscope through a narrowed nasal passage after the fiberscope is successfully inserted into the trachea.

C. Advantages

1. Flexible fiber-optic endoscopy is a very reliable approach to difficult airway management. It can be used orally or nasally and when access to the airway is limited. It can be used in any position.
2. The flexible fiberscope can be used to intubate patients who are difficult or impossible to intubate with a rigid laryngoscope. It is especially useful for patients at high risk of dental damage. It can be used in cases in which the patient cannot be placed in the supine position.

CLINICAL MOMENT Insufflating oxygen or jet ventilation through the working channel may provide additional time to pass the tracheal tube into the trachea.

D. Disadvantages

1. The flexible endoscope is more expensive, fragile, and difficult to use and clean than a rigid laryngoscope. Fiber-optic intubation requires more time than intubation with a rigid laryngoscope, so it is of limited use in emergency situations or during a rapid sequence induction. It requires considerable experience and skill maintenance. It does not allow airway structures to be directly manipulated.
2. Intubation with the flexible fiber-optic scope may be difficult or impossible with certain patients. Vision may be impaired or impossible in the presence of blood, secretions, or antacids containing magnesium or aluminum.
3. Gastric distension and rupture, tension pneumothorax, and subcutaneous emphysema have all been reported after oxygen insufflation through the working channel.
4. Laryngeal trauma may occur with fiber-optic intubation. This is frequently associated with difficulty advancing the tracheal tube over the fiberscope.

III. Indirect Rigid Fiber-optic Laryngoscopes

Indirect rigid fiber-optic laryngoscopes are designed to facilitate intubation in difficult-to-intubate patients. They are more rugged in design, control soft tissue better, are more portable and less costly than flexible fiber-optic laryngoscopes, and allow better secretion management.

A. Bullard Laryngoscope

1. **Description**
   a. The Bullard laryngoscope (**Fig. 14.7**) has a rigid metal blade shaped to follow the oropharyngeal contour and rest beneath the epiglottis. Fiber-optic bundles for illumination and operator viewing are housed in a sheath on the posterior aspect of the blade. A viewing arm with eyepiece extends at a 45-degree angle from the handle. A video camera can be attached to the eyepiece for remote viewing.
   b. A working channel extends from the body to the point where the light bundles end at the tip. It can be used for suction, oxygen insufflation, or local anesthetic or saline administration. The end nearest the handle has a Luer-lock connector for attaching a syringe to the working channel.
   c. Three sizes are available: pediatric (for babies); pediatric long (for patients up to 8 to 10 years old), and adult (for adults and children older than 8 to 10 years) (**Fig. 14.8**). The adult version may be useful in younger patients. The handle of the pediatric version may be used with the blade of the adult version to decrease the weight. A plastic tip extender is available.

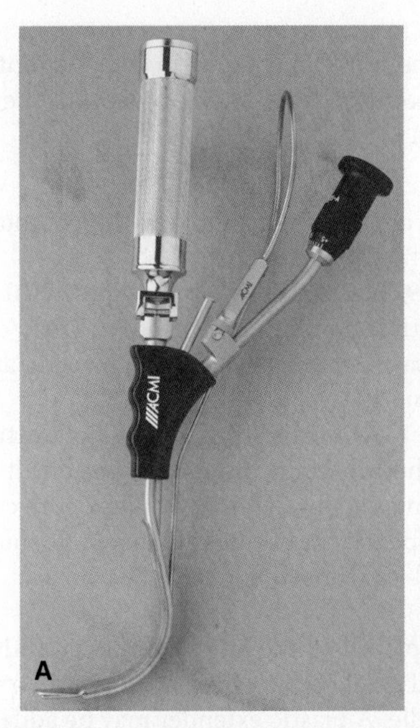

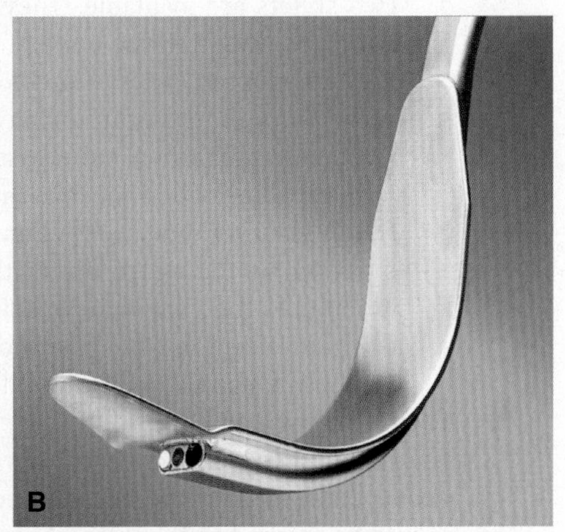

Figure 14.7 **A:** Bullard laryngoscope with a battery handle and a introducing stylet. Between the handle and the stylet is a port for attaching a syringe or inserting a wire. **B:** Patient end. At the left is the light channel. In the middle is the working channel. The image-transmitting bundle is at the right. If an extender is used, it is slipped over the tip.

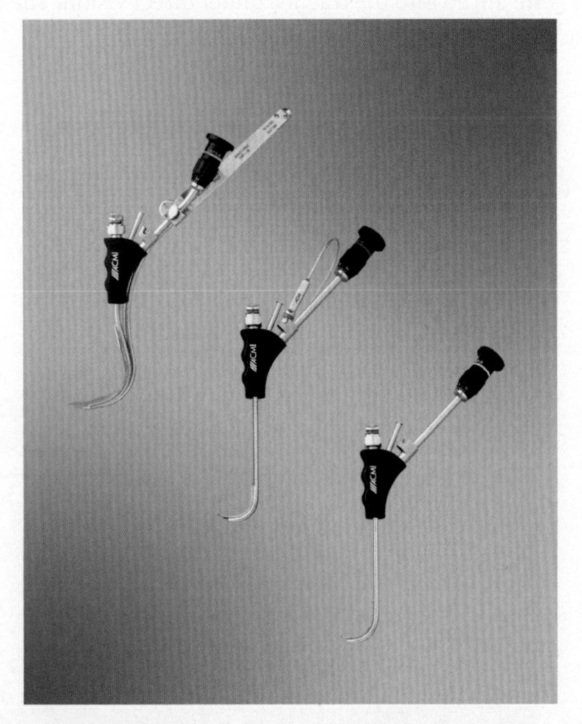

Figure 14.8 Bullard laryngoscopes. The handle contains batteries that power a halogen light bulb. Note that the curve of the blade of the adult version differs from the other two. (Courtesy of Circon ACMI, Stanford, CT, a division of Circon Corp.)

CLINICAL MOMENT The plastic blade extender may be helpful in taller patients. It may also be useful when intubating male patients but is often not helpful or even a hindrance when intubating female patients.

d. Two stylets are available. They are designed to follow the contour of the blade and attach to the body of the laryngoscope.
e. The introducing stylet (**Fig. 14.9**) has a curve of approximately 20 degrees to the left near the tip to bring the end of the stylet into the field of vision and facilitate tracheal tube passage. It attaches near the viewing arm base with a spring-loaded mechanism.
f. The multifunctional stylet (**Fig. 14.10**) consists of a long, hollow tube that is curved at the tip to direct the tube into the field of vision. It may be attached to the viewing arm using a screw clamp. Its hollow core can serve as a guide for a flexible fiberscope, tracheal tube exchanger, or small catheter. It can also be used to instill local anesthetic into the trachea.

2. **Technique of Use**

To use this scope, a tracheal tube is placed on the lubricated stylet. If the introducing stylet is used, the tip is placed through the Murphy eye. Antifog solution should be applied to the vision bundle. A plastic extender may be added for an adult male patient. The scope is introduced in the center of the mouth without looking through the eyepiece. When it is settled in place in the mouth, the operator should look through the eyepiece and see the scope tip above or below the epiglottis. The stylet directs the tracheal tube toward the glottis and the tube is advanced into the trachea under direct vision. The tube is then stabilized as the scope is removed.

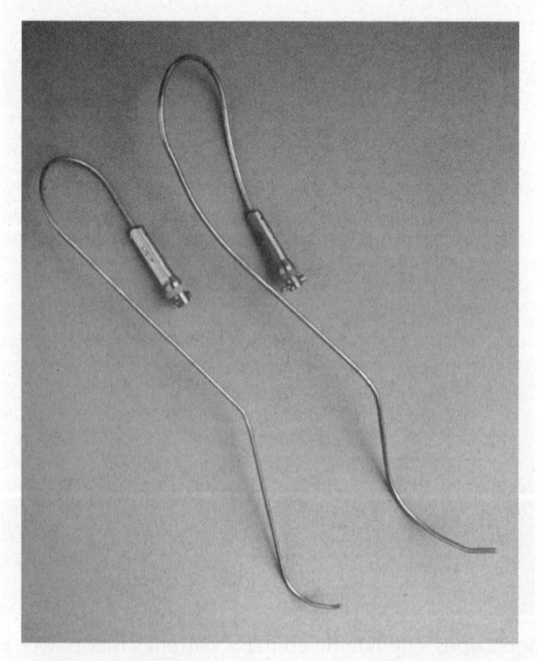

Figure 14.9 Introducing stylets for Bullard laryngoscope. The adult version is on the left and the pediatric version on the right. (Courtesy of Circon ACMI, a division of Circon Corp.)

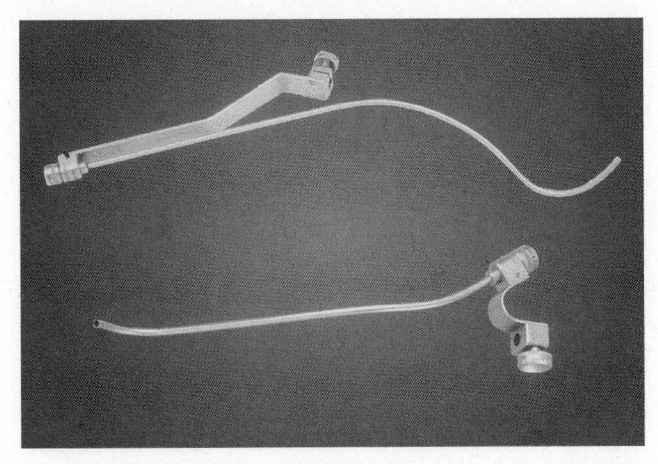

Figure 14.10 Multifunctional stylets with screw clamps. The adult version is at the top. The pediatric version is at the bottom. Note the end of the lumen through which a wire can be inserted. (Courtesy of Circon ACMI, Stanford, CT, a division of Circon Corp.)

3. **Advantages**
   a. The Bullard laryngoscope is especially useful in patients who are difficult to intubate, including those in whom head and neck movement is limited or undesirable; those with limited mouth opening, poor dentition, pharyngeal or laryngeal pathology, or facial fractures; and those who are morbidly obese. It has proved useful in children with Treacher Collins and Pierre-Robin syndromes. It causes less cervical spine movement than conventional rigid laryngoscopy. Compared with flexible fiber-optic intubation, the use of the Bullard laryngoscope is quicker. It may provide better laryngeal views than a video laryngoscope or a rigid laryngoscope blade.
   b. Additional advantages of using the Bullard scope include rapid intubation, low risk of failed intubation or trauma to lips and teeth, and less discomfort in the awake patient than direct laryngoscopy. It is less susceptible to problems with secretions and is more rugged than a flexible fiberscope. While there is a learning curve, this laryngoscope can be used quickly and efficiently. A skilled assistant is not needed to perform a jaw thrust or to hold an airway in place. It requires a mouth opening of only 7 mm. Later versions are fully immersible for cleaning. A video camera can be attached to the eyepiece.
4. **Disadvantages**
   a. Using the Bullard scope requires experience and skills. The equipment is somewhat expensive. Cleaning is somewhat difficult. Intubation may take slightly longer than with a rigid laryngoscope. It cannot be used by an anesthesia provider who has limited use of the left arm.
   b. Using a tracheal tube longer than 7.5 mm may cause the stylet to be displaced posteriorly, which may make intubation more difficult. Certain tracheal tubes (e.g., the metallic laser tube) (Chapter 15) will not fit over the stylet. Double-lumen tubes will not fit the stylets. In these cases, another tube can be inserted by using the Bullard laryngoscope and a tube exchanger can be used to insert the desired tube.
   c. There are reported cases in which the blade extender was accidentally dislodged because it was not securely attached. It is too large to be aspirated if this occurs.

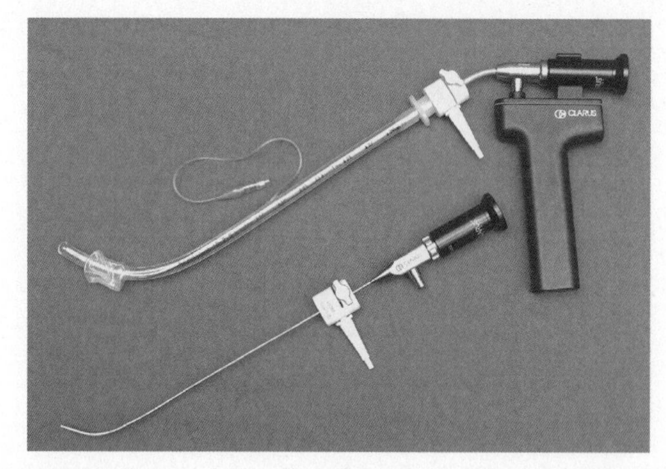

Figure 14.11 Shikani optical stylet. Both the adult and pediatric stylets can be attached to the same handle. Note the tube stop and connection for oxygen tubing. The stylet can be bent at the tip.

IV. Optical Intubating Stylets

A number of devices combine fiber-optic imaging with a stylet. They are referred to as optical intubating stylets, optical stylets, intubating fiber-optic stylets, stylet laryngoscopes, or visual scopes. They include the Shikani optical stylet, Levitan FPS, StyletScope, Airway Rifl, Intubaid Flex, and the Bonfils stylet laryngoscope (Figs. 14.11 to 14.13). Pediatric versions of most of these are available.

A. Description

These devices are used by looking through the eyepiece or they can be connected to a video transmission system so that the intubation can be observed on a monitor. Some have a port for oxygen insufflation, drug administration, or suction. Some are battery operated, others require a separate light source, and some can be used either way. Some can be used with the fiber-optic handle for a rigid blade. Not all stylet laryngoscopes allow the stylet curvature to be changed.

B. Techniques of Use

1. Prior to intubation, an antifogging agent is placed on the lens or the stylet is warmed in water or saline. The blade can be warmed using a convective warming device (Chapter 24). It should be inserted into the tracheal tube without its

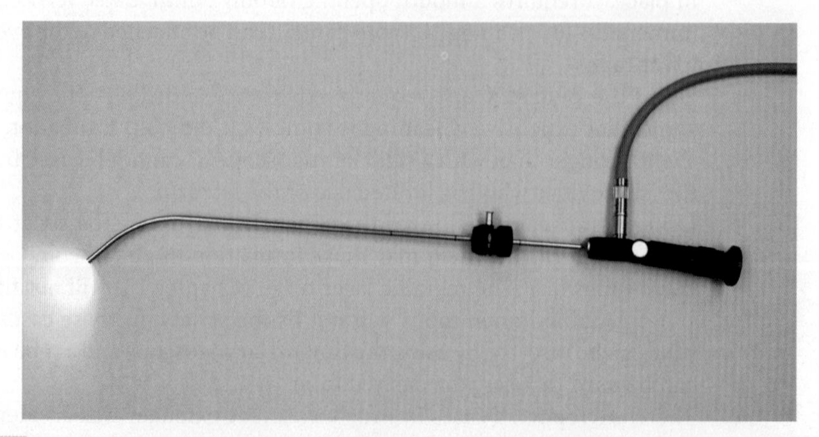

Figure 14.12 Bonfils stylet laryngoscope. The stylet is nonmalleable. It has a 40-degree distal curve. Note the slide adapter for stabilizing the tracheal tube. The adapter has a connector to administer oxygen during intubation. This device can be used with batteries or a separate fiber-optic light source.

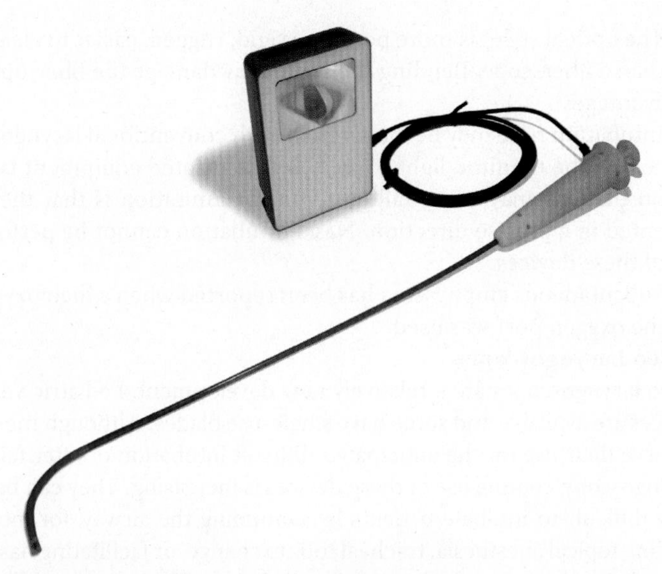

Figure 14.13 Intubaid Flex. The device is single use. The tip is flexible to 90 degrees. (Photograph courtesy of EZC Medical, LLC., San Francisco, CA.)

tip protruding and then fixed to the tube. With a pediatric tracheal tube, it may be necessary to remove the connector.

2. To intubate, the patient is placed in the neutral position or with a pillow under the head. If secretions are present, they should be removed before proceeding further. Some clinicians recommend that a rigid laryngoscope or jaw thrust be used to lift the epiglottis and enlarge the retropharyngeal space. It may also be helpful to grasp the tongue and pull it out of the mouth. The handle is held in the right hand and the stylet is inserted into the mouth in the midline and advanced into the hypopharynx just beyond the tip of the epiglottis. The stylet is then advanced under direct vision through the vocal cords. For some patients, it may be necessary to apply external pressure on the larynx. If secretions are a problem, insufflating oxygen may improve the view. If orientation is lost, the scope should be withdrawn until orientation is reestablished. It may be necessary to remove the stylet and change the curvature, if possible.
3. When an intratracheal position is achieved, the stylet is removed by rotating the handle toward the patient's chest. It should not be pulled straight out.
4. A retromolar approach is sometimes used. The scope is inserted between the cheek and the molars on the patient's right side, with the end of the scope pointing toward the midline.
5. An optical stylet can be used through a Fastrach intubating laryngeal mask airway (ILMA) (Chapter 13). It can also be used as a light wand.

C. Advantages

1. Optical stylets are relatively easy to use for routine and difficult intubations, although skill will be required to achieve and maintain proficiency. Intubation with these devices may be successful after failed direct laryngoscopy. Since the vocal cords are visualized, esophageal intubation should be very uncommon. The incidence of sore throat, increased heart rate, and cervical spine movement are less than with conventional laryngoscopy. The risks of dental trauma and soft tissue damage will be reduced if a conventional laryngoscope is not used in conjunction with the optical stylet.

2. The optical stylet is more portable, rigid, rugged, easier to clean, and less costly than a fiberscope. Bending the stylet may damage the fiber-optic fibers.

D. Disadvantages

1. Intubation time may be longer than with conventional laryngoscopy. The initial cost of the monitor, light source, and associated equipment is high. Secretions on the lens may cause failure. A major limitation is that they cannot be oriented in a precise direction. Nasal intubation cannot be performed with some of these devices.
2. Subcutaneous emphysema has been reported when a high oxygen flow through the oxygen port was used.

V. Rigid Video Laryngoscopes

Rigid video laryngoscopes are a relatively new development. Pediatric versions of some of these devices are available and some have single-use blades. Although most anesthesia providers reserve their use for the anticipated difficult intubation or after failed intubation by direct laryngoscopy, routine use of these devices is increasing. They can be used to evaluate potentially difficult-to-intubate patients by examining the airway, for intubation in awake patients using topical anesthesia, tracheal tube exchange, or facilitating nasotracheal intubation by visualizing the tracheal tube entering the larynx. They can be combined with another device such as a flexible endoscope or video stylet for managing the difficult airway.

A. Description

1. Rigid video laryngoscopes are shown in **Figures 14.14** to **14.16.** There is a rigid curved blade with camera optics built into the blade. The rigid oral portion

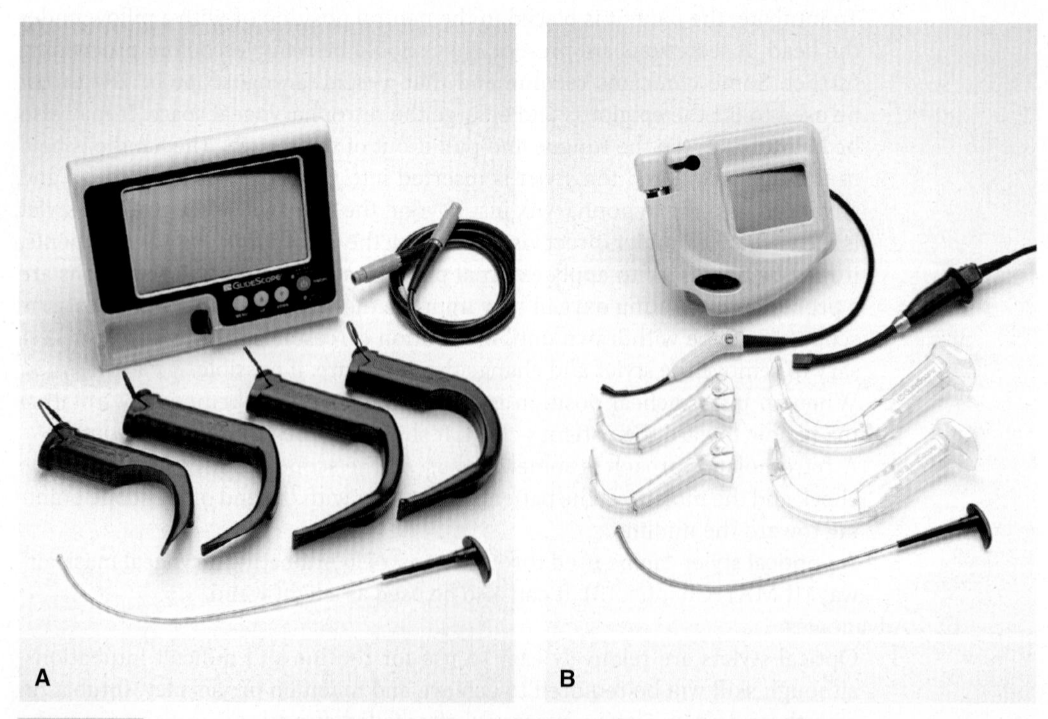

Figure 14.14 **A:** GlideScope GLV reusable laryngoscope. This video laryngoscope has an integral camera and an anti-fogging mechanism. The blade is angulated to 60 degrees and available in several sizes. Note the special stylet for the tracheal tube. (Photograph courtesy of Verathon Medical.) **B:** The GlideScope is also available in the Ranger single-use system. The system has a reusable baton (both pediatric and adult) and plastic outer disposable sheath. The tracheal tube stylet is also shown. (Photograph courtesy of Verathon Medical, Bothwell, WA.)

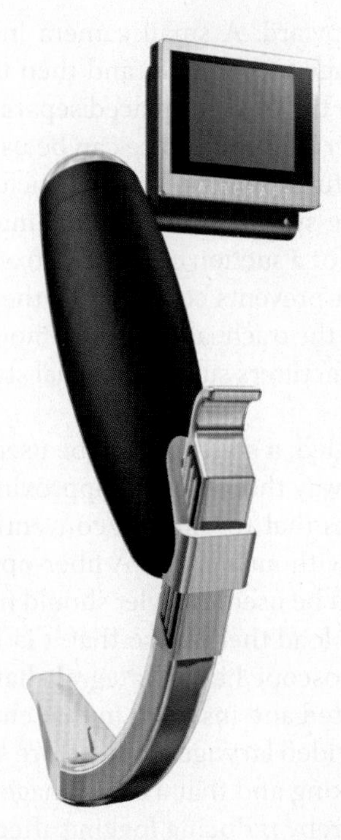

Figure 14.15 McGrath video laryngoscope. It has an adjustable curved blade that is available in different sizes. A miniature camera is located at the blade tip. The blade operates on a single AA battery, making it fully portable. The blade tip is single use. The image is transferred to the attached flat panel, which can be filtered or turned for better viewing. (Photograph courtesy of LMA North America, San Diego, CA.)

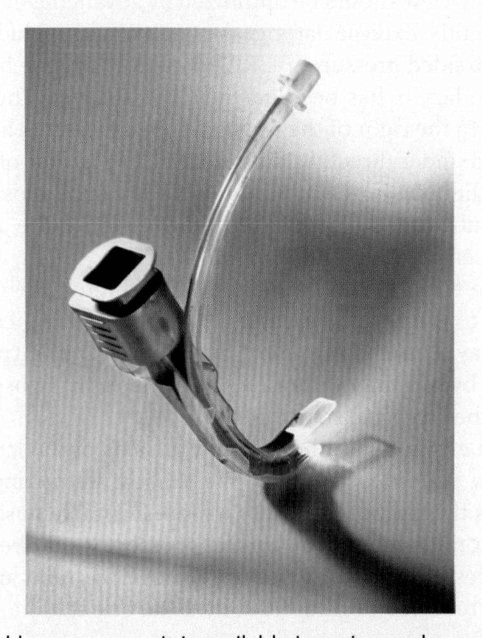

Figure 14.16 Airtraq optical laryngoscope. It is available in various color-coded sizes as well as nasotracheal and double-lumen tube configurations. The blade is disposable. A guiding channel holds the tracheal tube and directs it toward the vocal cords. There is a built-in anti-fog system. A clip-on video system accessory for viewing and recording on an external monitor or personal computer is available.

may be angled upward. A small camera in the blade or a fiber-optic bundle transmits the image to a camera and then to a monitor screen, which may be either attached to the blade or placed separately. The light source may be in the handle, or an external light source can be used.

2. Various other features may be present, including a built-in anti-fog system, an onscreen targeting system that lights the intended path for the tracheal tube, a separate channel for a suction catheter or oxygen insufflation, a disposable transparent sheath that prevents contact with the patient, and an integral channel to contain and guide the tracheal tube. Pole-mounted and portable models are available. Some manufacturers supply a special stylet for use with the laryngoscope.

B. Techniques of Use

1. If the blade is angled, a stylet should be used in the tracheal tube and the tube shaped in such a way that its curve approximates that of the convex side of the blade. With blades that resemble a conventional curved blade, it is often possible to intubate without a stylet. A fiber-optic endoscope with a tracheal tube mounted on it can be used. A stylet should not be used with nasal intubation. It may be helpful to load the tube so that it is 180 degrees from its usual orientation. If the laryngoscope has an integral channel for the tracheal tube, the tube should be lubricated and installed in that channel.
2. Turning ON the video laryngoscope before starting induction will confirm that the device is working and that a clear image can be obtained. It also allows the lens to warm, thereby reducing fogging after it is inserted into the airway.
3. The blade should be inserted in the midline under direct vision and rotated around the tongue until the tip is out of view. The operator should then look at the monitor and advance the blade until the epiglottis is identified. The blade tip may be inserted above or under the epiglottis, lifting it out of the way.
4. The glottic view should be optimized by advancing or withdrawing the laryngoscope slightly. External laryngeal manipulation, including the backward upward and right-sided pressure (BURP) maneuver, may be helpful.
5. Once the larynx has been adequately visualized, the tracheal tube should be inserted to the right of the laryngoscope unless it is inserted into the blade and advanced under direct vision until the tip goes out of view. If there is difficulty placing the tube in the mouth, the blade can be moved slightly to the left. For nasal intubation, the tube should be inserted in the usual manner until the tip can be seen on the monitor.
6. Once the tube tip can be seen on the monitor, the user should direct the tip anterior to the arytenoid cartilages and then advance it off the stylet and into the airway. Uncertainty about the trajectory of a tracheal tube can often be rectified by carefully withdrawing the video laryngoscope to provide a broader view of the laryngeal structures.
7. If the tube is not well aligned with the axis of the larynx, it may be helpful to withdraw the video laryngoscope slightly. Retracting the stylet slightly often advances the tracheal tube into a more favorable position. Forceps can be used to deflect the tube into the correct position. It may be helpful to rotate the tube 90 degrees counterclockwise, or remove the tube and reload it on the stylet with the tube 180 degrees from its usual orientation.

C. Advantages

1. The image is larger and brighter than with a conventional direct laryngoscope. A number of reports show that video laryngoscopes have a better success rate than conventional rigid laryngoscopes, especially in patients who would be

considered difficult to intubate, such as obese patients and even with relatively inexperienced trainees.

2. Because a video laryngoscope does not require the oral, pharyngeal, and tracheal axes to be aligned, less tissue compression, external force, and neck movement are required. They may reduce trauma to the larynx by allowing the user to see what is happening as the tube tip approaches the laryngeal inlet. Their use may result in less dental injury and postintubation sore throat as well as less elevation of blood pressure and heart rate.
3. Because the technique is similar to a traditional laryngoscope, the learning curve is fairly rapid. It may require less operator skill than a conventional rigid laryngoscope. Positioning the monitor over the patient's chest allows the user to move and observe on one axis.
4. The operator and assistant can coordinate their movements because each sees the same image on the monitor. The assistant can more effectively aid in obtaining and maintaining the best possible laryngeal view.
5. The ability to project the image seen through the laryngoscope makes it a good teaching tool, allowing the supervisor to monitor the intubation process more effectively. Video capture permits playback and analysis under less stressful conditions. New users prefer video laryngoscope to direct laryngoscope and learn it more quickly.
6. The video laryngoscope allows the anesthesia provider to maintain a longer distance from the patient during intubation. This could make it useful in patients who have infectious diseases.
7. Recording the intubation can be useful in demonstrating that the intubation is performed properly and is not responsible for a postoperative complication.

D. Disadvantages

1. Video laryngoscopes are more costly and may require more time than conventional laryngoscopes.
2. Airway lacerations have been reported with video laryngoscopes. This may be due to the insertion of the blade or tube without looking directly into the patient's mouth. It is easy to get into the habit of looking only at the monitor and this should be avoided.
3. Some video laryngoscopes require a large video system, making them unsuitable for use outside a healthcare facility.
4. While the video laryngoscope blades are designed to fit most patients properly, patients with anatomical features outside the norm may present a problem for some devices.
5. A video laryngoscope cannot be introduced through the nose or tracheostomy. It cannot be used to position a bronchial blocker or double-lumen tube or perform pulmonary toilet.

VI. Teeth Protectors

A tooth protector (mouth guard, mouth protector, dentguard) (Fig. 14.17) is placed over the upper teeth to protect them from the laryngoscope blade. It may also prevent the blade from getting caught between the teeth. Using a protector does not guarantee safety from dental trauma. Although it will prevent direct trauma to the teeth surface, it cannot prevent transmission of pressure to the roots.

VII. Complications of Laryngoscopy

A. Dental Injury

1. Damage to teeth, gums, or dental prostheses is the most frequent anesthesia-related insurance claim. In addition to cosmetic disfigurement and discomfort,

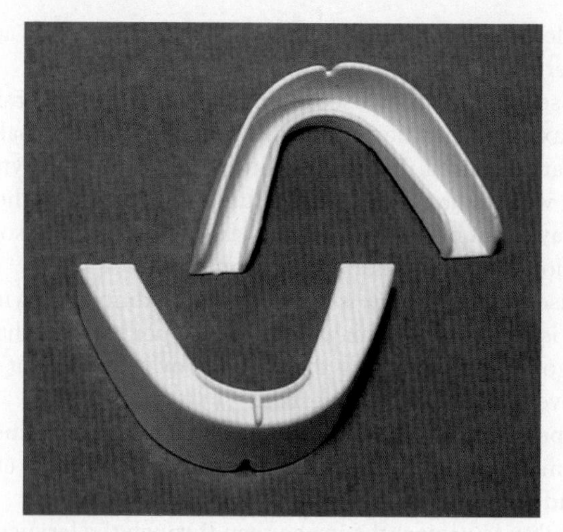

Figure 14.17 Tooth protectors. (Courtesy of Sun Med., Largo, FL.)

there may be pulmonary complications if the dislodged tooth or fragment is aspirated. Profuse bleeding may result.

2. A tooth or prosthetic device may be chipped, broken, loosened, or avulsed. This is usually caused by using the teeth as a fulcrum for the laryngoscope while elevating the epiglottis. The teeth most likely to be damaged are those that have been restored or weakened through periodontal disease, but sound teeth may also be affected. The upper incisors are most frequently involved. Dental implants appear to be less vulnerable to injury.
3. Patients' teeth should be carefully assessed preoperatively to identify possible problems. Inquiry should be made concerning vulnerable dental repair work or loose or carious teeth. Anatomical conditions in the mouth and pharynx that may cause difficulty should be noted. The patient should be advised beforehand if there is likely to be a problem. In patients 4 to 11 years old, the deciduous teeth may be easily dislodged. If such teeth are loose, removal before or during anesthesia may be indicated.

CLINICAL MOMENT A suture may be placed around a loose tooth to capture it if it is dislodged. This can also prevent it from becoming lost in the airway.

4. When there is a gap between the upper front teeth, a portion of a tracheal tube or other device may be used to bridge the gap, or a tooth protector may be used. Keeping a partial upper denture in place may prevent the laryngoscope from slipping into gaps between teeth.
5. If a tooth, fragment, or dental appliance is dislodged, foreign body aspiration is a major concern. An immediate search should be conducted, starting with an examination of the oral cavity and the area surrounding the patient's head. Chest and neck radiographs must be taken if the fragment is not recovered.
6. Various types of tooth damage may occur. These require different treatments. A qualified dentist or oral surgeon should be consulted. If a tooth is avulsed,

immediate replacement in its original position and stabilization will increase the chances of successful reimplantation.

CLINICAL MOMENT If a patient has bad or loose teeth, it may be a good idea to use a fiberscope, an indirect fiber-optic laryngoscope, or a stylet laryngoscope if the clinician has experience with these devices.

B. Damage to Other Structures
   1. Reported injuries to the upper airway include abrasions, hematomas, and lacerations of the lips, tongue, palate, pharynx, hypopharynx, larynx, and esophagus. A common occurrence is rolling the upper or lower lip between the teeth and the laryngoscope blade as the blade is inserted. Osteomyelitis of the mandible has been reported. The lingual and/or hypoglossal nerve may be injured. Arytenoid subluxation may occur. Anterior temporomandibular joint (TMJ) dislocation may occur. Patients with TMJ derangements often state that their problem began following general anesthesia.
   2. Palatopharyngeal wall perforation has been reported with a rigid video laryngoscope.
   3. If a high flow of oxygen is insufflated through a laryngoscopic channel during intubation, there is the possibility that subcutaneous emphysema can result from gas entering the tissues through small tears in the mucosa. Gastric rupture has been reported because of oxygen insufflation through a fiber-optic bronchoscope during a difficult intubation.
   4. There is a significant increase in the rate of airway-related complications with repeated attempts.

C. Cervical Spinal Cord Injury
   1. Aggressive head positioning during intubation, especially head or neck extension, has the potential to cause damage in the patient with an unstable cervical spine. There are case reports of neurologic deterioration after intubation, although the contribution of laryngoscopy to these injuries remains debatable and the overall risk appears to be low. The most appropriate technique for performing tracheal intubation in patients with cervical spine injury continues to be debated. A cervical collar should be not be relied on to prevent damage.

CLINICAL MOMENT When intubating a patient in whom neck motion may be a problem, it is a good idea to have a neurosurgeon present to supervise the extent of neck motion that occurs.

   2. Conventional laryngoscopes require the greatest neck motion during laryngoscopy. Manual in-line immobilization has been thought to reduce spinal movement and the likelihood of secondary injury. This is controversial. Some authors think that manual in-line stabilization causes pressure from the blade of the laryngoscope to be transmitted to the cervical spine. Intubation during in-line stabilization is easier with a rigid video laryngoscope.
   3. Stylet and indirect video laryngoscopes as well as the Bullard laryngoscope have been shown to require less neck motion than conventional laryngoscopes.

D. Shock or Burn

If a laryngoscope light that is left ON contacts the patient, a burn injury may result. A short circuit can result in rapid heating of the handle and blade.

E. Swallowing or Aspirating a Foreign Body

Cases have been reported in which the bulb or other part of a laryngoscope was aspirated or swallowed. It is important to make every effort to find these foreign bodies. If they cannot be found in the oral cavity or around the patient's head, radiographs of the chest and neck should be taken. Part of a tumor may be dislodged into the airway and become implanted.

F. Laryngoscope Malfunction

1. The most common malfunction of a laryngoscope is light failure. This may be the result from a defective power source, lamp, or socket; incorrect assembly; or poor contact between the blade and the handle. Fiber-optic laryngoscopes are more reliable because the useful life of a halogen lamp is longer than an ordinary light bulb, and the lamp is usually in the handle rather than in the blade. Various parts of the blade and the handle may break. Misassembly may result in failure.
2. A preuse check will detect most malfunctions. An extra handle and a blade should always be immediately available. Neglecting to observe these precautions could spell disaster, especially during a rapid sequence induction.

G. Circulatory Changes

Laryngoscopy may result in significant increases in blood pressure and heart rate, although these changes are less than those associated with tracheal intubation.

H. Disease Transmission

The risk of transmission of an infection, particularly Creutzfeldt-Jakob disease, via laryngoscopes is unknown but should be a matter of concern to anesthesia providers. Using a disposable blade cover or a disposable laryngoscope blade should avoid this problem.

SUGGESTED READINGS

Arino JJ, Velasco JM, Gasco C, Lopez-Timoneda F. Straight blades improve visualization of the larynx while curved blades increase ease of intubation: a comparison of the Macintosh, Miller, McCoy, Belscope and Lee-Fiberview blades. Can J Anaesth 2003;50:501–506.

Berry JM. Conventional (laryngoscopic) orotracheal and nasotracheal intubation (single lumen tube). In: Hagberg CA, ed. Benumof's Airway Management: Principles and Practice. Second edition. St Louis, MO: Mosby, 2007: 379–392.

Crosby ET. Airway management in adults after cervical spine trauma. Anesthesiology 2006;104:1293–1318.

Dorsch J, Dorsch S. Laryngoscopes. In: Understanding Anesthesia Equipment. Fifth edition. Philadelphia: Wolters Kluwer/Lippincott Williams & Wilkins, 2008:530–560.

Hagberg CA. Current concepts in the management of the difficult airway. Orlando, FL: American Society of Anesthesiologists, 2008. ASA Refresher Course No. 222.

Hagberg CA, Benumof JL. The American Society of Anesthesiologists' management of the difficult airway algorithm and explanation—analysis of the algorithm. In: Hagberg CA, ed. Benumof's Airway Management: Principles and Practice. Second edition. St. Louis, MO: Mosby, 2007:236–251.

Kuczkowski K, Reisner LS, Benumof JL. Airway problems and new solutions for the obstetric patient. J Clin Anesth 2003;15:552–563.

Law JA, Hagberg CA. The evolution of upper airway retraction: new and old laryngoscope blades. In: Hagberg CA, ed. Benumof's Airway Management: Principles and Practice. Second edition. St. Louis, MO: Mosby, 2007: 532–575.

Mihai R, Blair E, Kay H, Cook TM. Review article. A quantitative review and meta-analysis of performance of non-standard laryngoscopes and rigid fiberoptic intubation aids. Anaesthesia 2008;63:745–760.

Newland MC, Ellis SJ, Peters KR, Simonson JA, et. Al. Dental injury associated with anesthesia: a report of 161,687 anesthetics given over 14 years. J Clin Anesth 2007;19:339–345.

Owen H, Waddell-Smith I. Dental trauma associated with anaesthesia. Anaesth Intensive Care 2000;28:133–145.
Rassam S, Wilkes AR, Hall JE, Mecklenburgh S. A comparison of 20 laryngoscope blades using an intubating manikin: visual analogue scores and forces exerted during laryngoscopy. Anaesthesia 2005;60:384–394.
Walker RM, Ellwood J. The management of difficult intubation in children. Pediatr Anesth 2009;19(suppl 1):77–87.
Warner ME, Benenfield SM, Warner MA, Schroeder DR, Maxson PM. Perianesthetic dental injuries. Frequency, outcomes, and risk factors. Anesthesiology 1999;90:1302–1305.
Wheeler M, Ovassapian A. Fiberoptic endoscopy-aided technique. In: Hagberg CA, ed. Benumof's Airway Management: Principles and Practice. Second edition. St Louis, MO: Mosby, 2007:399–438.

15 Tracheal Tubes and Associated Equipment

THE TRACHEAL (ENDOTRACHEAL, INTRATRACHEAL) TUBE is a device that is inserted through the larynx into the trachea to convey gases and vapors between the breathing system and the lungs. It may also be inserted through a tracheostoma as a temporary measure.

I. General Principles

A. Resistance and Work of Breathing

A tracheal tube places a mechanical burden on the spontaneously breathing patient. It adds resistance and is usually a more important factor in determining the work of breathing than the breathing system. This is particularly significant in pediatric patients. Several factors help to determine the resistance to gas flow imposed by a tracheal tube. The internal diameter is the most important. Decreasing tube length lowers resistance but not significantly. Sharp curves and kinking increase resistance.

B. Dead Space

The tracheal tube and connector constitute mechanical dead space. Because the volume of a tracheal tube and its connector is usually less than that of the natural passages, dead space is normally reduced by intubation. In pediatric patients, however, long tubes and connectors may increase the dead space. Special low-volume pediatric connectors are available.

II. Tracheal Tube System

A. Tube

1. Materials

a. Red rubber tubes are still available. These can be cleaned, sterilized, and reused multiple times. They are not transparent, can become hardened and sticky with age, have poor resistance to kinking, can become clogged by dried secretions more easily than plastic tubes, and do not soften appreciably at body temperature. Latex allergy is another possible problem (see Chapter 11). They usually have high-pressure cuffs.

b. Polyvinyl chloride (PVC) is the substance most widely used in disposable tracheal tubes. It is relatively inexpensive and is compatible with tissues. Tubes made from PVC are less likely to kink than rubber tubes. Their transparency permits observation of moisture and other materials in the lumen. They soften at body temperature, so they tend to conform to the patient's upper airway. Prior to use, a PVC tube may be cooled to make it more firm during intubation or warmed to facilitate placement over a fiberscope. A PVC tube has a smooth surface that facilitates passage of a suction catheter or bronchoscope. Most PVC tubes available today have low-pressure cuffs.

c. Silicone is used in some tracheal tubes. Although more expensive than PVC, silicone tubes are soft and can be sterilized and reused.

d. Polyurethane has been used for tracheal tube cuffs in recent years. Studies indicate that a tube with a polyurethane cuff may be more effective in preventing early postoperative pneumonia than one with a PVC cuff.

2. Tube Design

a. A typical tracheal tube is shown in **Figure 15.1.** The machine end receives the connector and projects from the patient. It may be possible to shorten the tube at this end. The patient (tracheal) end (tip) is inserted into the trachea. It usually has a slanted portion called the bevel. Most commonly, the bevel opening faces to the left on viewing the tube from its concave aspect.

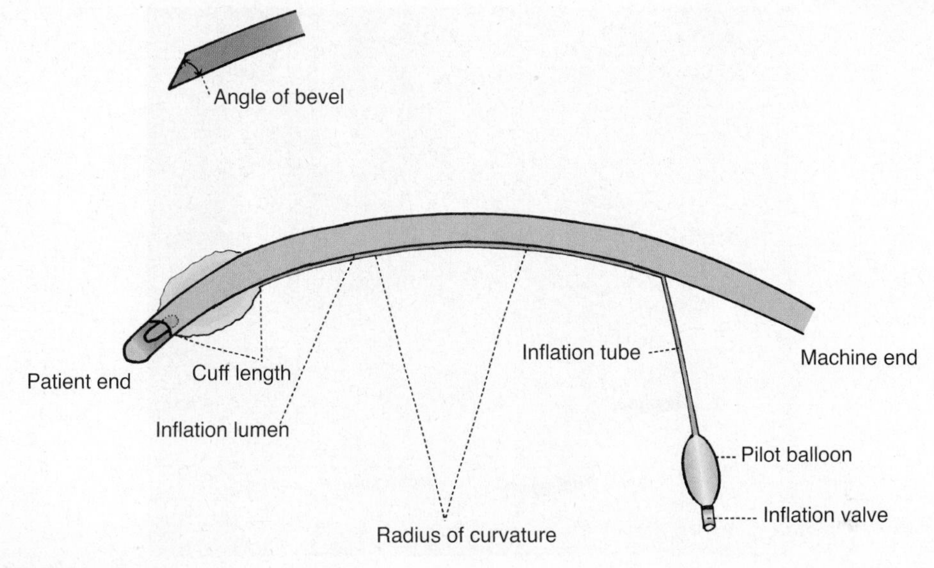

Figure 15.1 Cuffed Murphy tracheal tube.

This is because the tube is usually introduced from the right, and it is easier to visualize the larynx with the bevel facing to the left.

b. The design or orientation at the patient end is important when the tube is advanced over a fiberscope or a catheter is introduced. Insertion is easier if the bevel faces backward, or the tip is specially designed to minimize the distance between the scope and the leading edge of the tube. A hemispherical bevel reduces nasal morbidity during nasotracheal intubation. During nasal intubation, turning the tracheal tube so that the bevel faces up may avoid impinging the tip beside the right vocal cord or on the epiglottis.

c. **Figure 15.1** shows a hole through the tube wall on the side opposite the bevel. This is known as a Murphy eye, and a tube with this feature is called a Murphy eye or a side hole. The purpose of the eye is to provide an alternate pathway for gas flow if the bevel becomes occluded. A forceps, tube changer, or fiberscope may inadvertently advance through a Murphy eye and become caught. Using a tube with a Murphy eye may reduce trauma during nasal intubation. A theoretical disadvantage of the Murphy eye is that secretions may accumulate in it. Some tubes have an additional eye above the bevel. This may provide an additional measure of safety if the tube accidentally advances into a mainstem bronchus.

d. Tracheal tubes lacking the Murphy eye are known as Magill or Magill-type tubes. If a Murphy eye is not present, the cuff can be placed closer to the tip, which may decrease the risk of inadvertent bronchial intubation. When used for nasotracheal intubation, a Magill-type tube causes less trauma.

3. **Special Tubes**

a. Cole Tube

The Cole tube is shown in **Figure 15.2.** It is uncuffed. The patient end has a smaller diameter than the rest of the shaft. This provides some protection against inadvertent bronchial intubation. Cole tubes are sized according to the internal diameter of the tracheal portion. The tube should not be inserted far enough for the shoulder to contact the larynx, because this

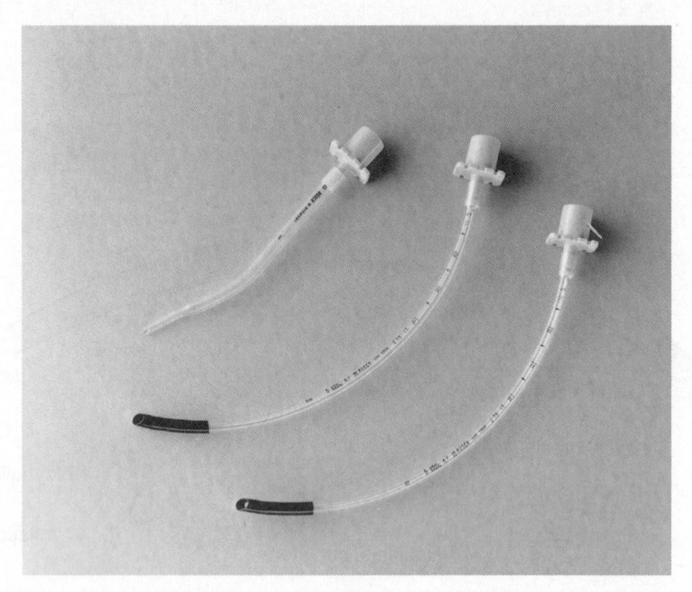

Figure 15.2 Uncuffed pediatric tracheal tubes. The **top** tube is a Cole tube, which is sized by the French scale, according to the intratracheal portion. The **middle** tube is a Magill tube, while the **bottom** tube has a Murphy eye. The dark color is the part of the tube that the manufacturer recommends be below the vocal cords. (Courtesy of Rusch, Inc., Research Triangle Park, NC.)

could result in damage. The resistance offered by the Cole tube is less than that of a comparable tube with a constant lumen. A disadvantage is that it cannot be inserted through the nose.

CLINICAL MOMENT The Cole tube is not suitable for long-term ventilation because if it moves further into the trachea, the wider portion can dilate the larynx.

b. Preformed Tubes

1) Some tracheal tubes are preformed to facilitate surgery about the head and neck. One of these is the Ring-Adair-Elwin (RAE) tube (**Fig. 15.3**), which has a preformed bend that may be temporarily straightened during insertion. The external portion of the oral version is bent at an acute angle so that when in place, it rests on the patient's chin. The nasal version has a curve that is opposite to that of the oral tube so that when in place, the tube is over the patient's forehead. This helps to reduce pressure on the nares. The oral tubes are shorter than the nasal ones. Uncuffed RAE tubes are shorter than cuffed RAE tubes. As the diameter increases, the length and distance from the tip to the curve also increase. In the majority of cases, there is a mark at the teeth or nares, intended to indicate that the tube is satisfactorily positioned in the trachea if the proper size tube for that patient is selected. Unfortunately, the length from the angle to the tube tip varies with similar tubes from different manufacturers.

CLINICAL MOMENT The mark on an RAE tube to be placed at the teeth or nares is only a guide and should not be used as the sole criterion for judging correct tube position.

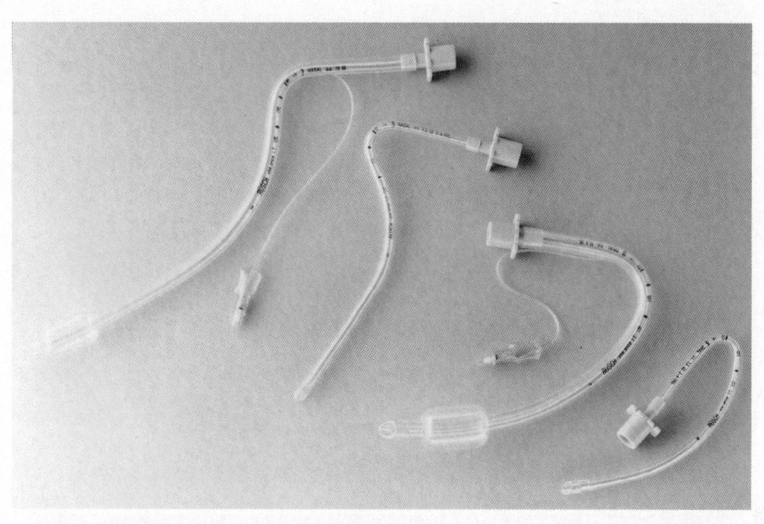

Figure 15.3 Preformed tubes. At **left** are two nasal tubes, one cuffed and one uncuffed; at **right** are two oral tubes. (Courtesy of Rusch, Inc.)

2) Preformed tubes are easy to secure and may reduce the risk of unintended extubation. The curve allows the connection to the breathing system to be placed away from the surgical field during surgery around the head without using special connectors. The long length may make them useful for insertion through a supraglottic airway device (Chapter 13). The nasal tube may be useful for oral intubation in patients who are in the prone position or who are undergoing otolaryngology procedures.
3) A disadvantage of preformed tubes is that it is difficult to pass a suction catheter through them. In critical situations, suctioning can be accomplished by cutting the tube at the curvature and then reinserting the connector into the cut end. These tubes offer more resistance than comparably sized conventional tubes. Since they are designed to fit the average patient, a tube may be either too long or too short for a given patient. When selecting tube size, reference to height and weight may be more useful than the reference to age in years. The user should always be alert to the possibility that bronchial intubation or accidental extubation could occur.

c. Spiral Embedded Tubes
1) The spiral embedded (flexometallic, armored, reinforced, anode) tube has a reinforcing wire covered internally and externally by PVC or silicone (**Fig. 15.4**). The spiral may not extend into the patient and tracheal ends. The connector is frequently bonded to the tube. They usually do not have a Murphy eye.
2) Spiral embedded tubes are especially useful in situations in which the tube is likely to be bent or compressed, as in head, neck, or tracheal surgery. Many clinicians use them for patients in the prone position. The portion of the tube outside the patient can be angled away from the surgical field without kinking. This makes it useful for the patient with a tracheostomy, submental intubation, or retromolar positioning. A spiral embedded tube may pass more easily over a fiberscope than a conventional tube.

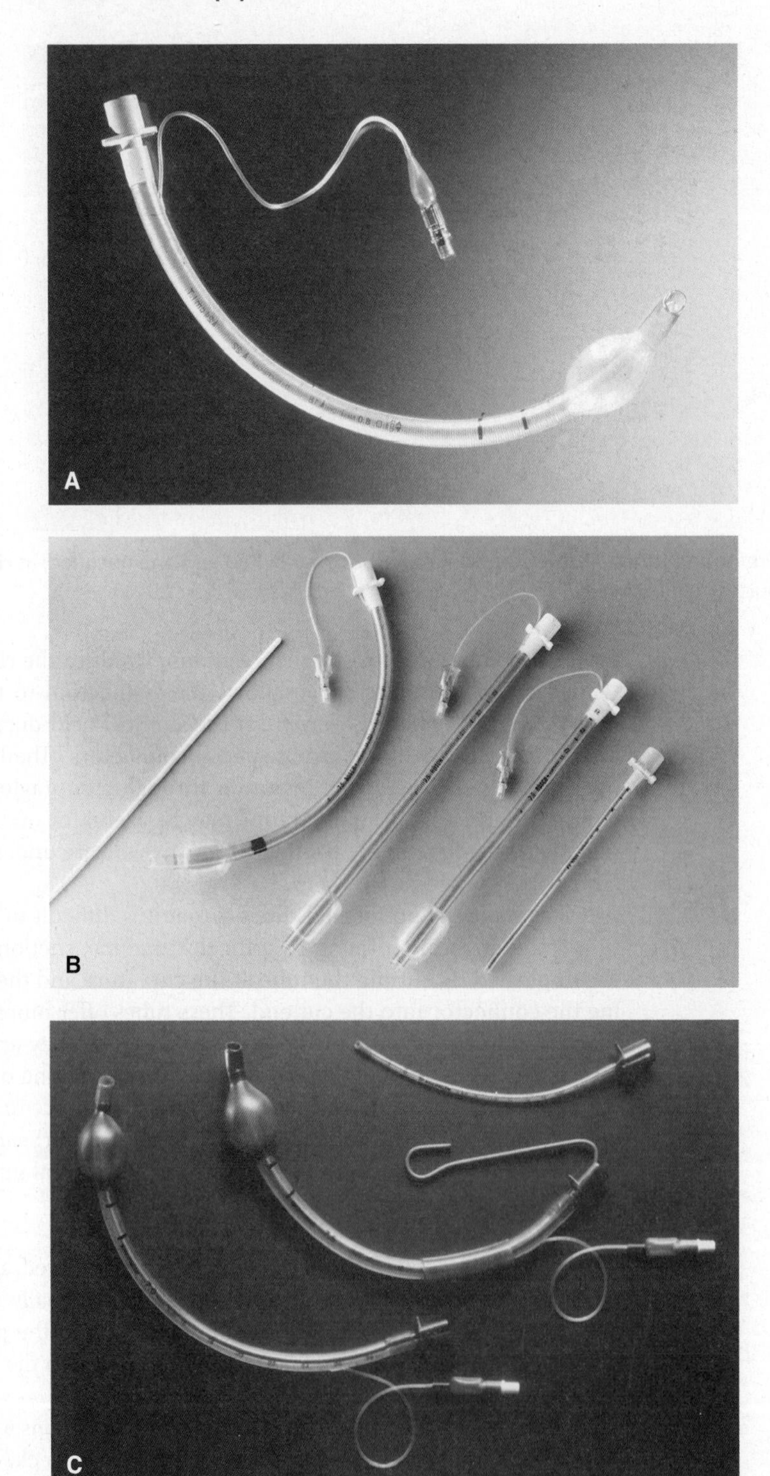

Figure 15.4 Spiral embedded tracheal tubes. **A:** Note the reference marks near the patient end of the tube to aid in positioning with respect to the vocal cords. (Courtesy of Mallinkrodt Medical, Inc., Hazelwood, MO.) **B:** Note that the tube on the **left** has a single reference mark. (Courtesy of Rusch, Inc.) **C:** The **middle** tube has a reinforcing covering over the bite area. Note again the referencing marks. (Courtesy of Kendall Healthcare Products Co., now part of Covidien, Mansfield, MA.)

3) There are a number of problems with spiral embedded tubes. A forceps and/or a stylet will often be needed for intubation. The tube may rotate on the stylet during insertion. It is difficult and sometimes impossible to pass the tube through the nose. Because of the spiral, these tubes cannot be shortened. The elastic recoil force may increase the risk of unintentional extubation. They are difficult to insert through supra-glottic airway devices. Reusable spiral embedded tubes that have been resterilized have a high incidence of problems. For this reason, reuse is not recommended. Even single-use tubes may develop problems. If the patent bites the tube, it can be severed or permanently deformed. A bite block between the molar teeth, not an oral airway, should be used to prevent this. Some spiral embedded tubes have an external reinforced covering over the bite portion (**Fig. 15.4C**). Kinking from compression between a retractor and the teeth has been reported. The absence of a Murphy eye may result in obstruction if the bevel abuts the tracheal wall.

CLINICAL MOMENT While a purported benefit of these tubes is that they do not kink or obstruct, kinking can occur above the spirals and obstruction can occur if the patient forcibly bites on the tube.

d. Laryngectomy Tube

The laryngectomy tube has a "J" configuration near the patient end (**Fig. 15.5, left**). It is designed to be inserted into a tracheostoma. This allows the part of the tube external to the patient to be directed away from the surgical field. The tip may be short and without a bevel to avoid bronchial intubation.

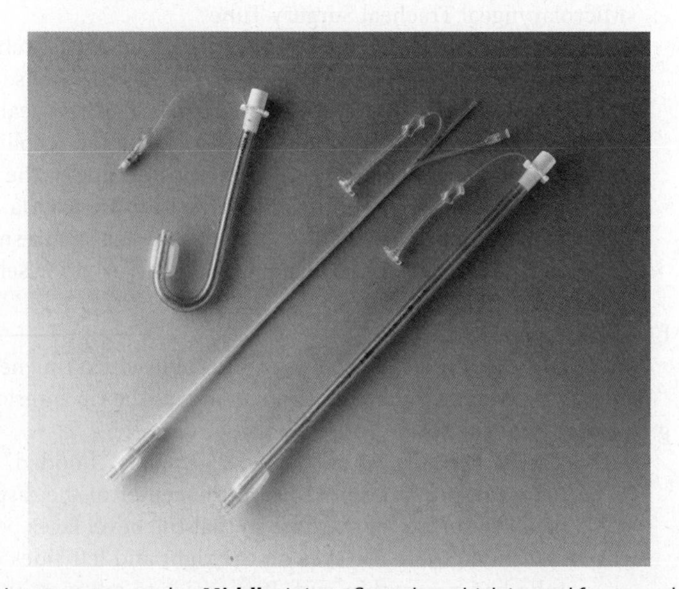

Figure 15.5 Left: Laryngectomy tube. **Middle:** Injectoflex tube, which is used for procedures on the larynx. The tube has an embedded metal spiral. The insufflation lumen and cuff inflation tube are combined in one sheath with the malleable introducer. **Right:** Spiral embedded tube. (Courtesy of Rusch, Inc.)

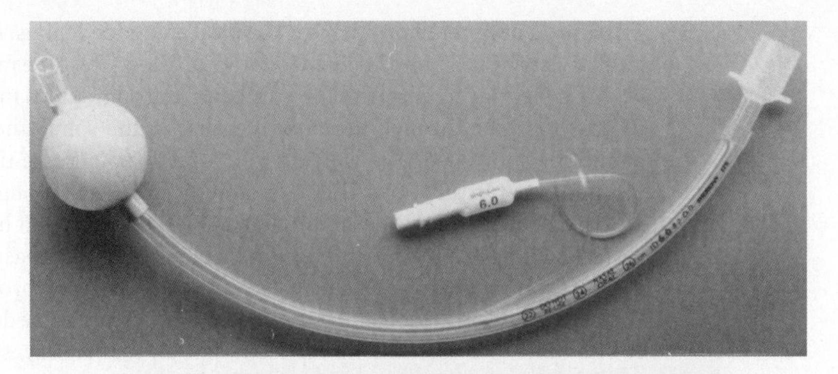

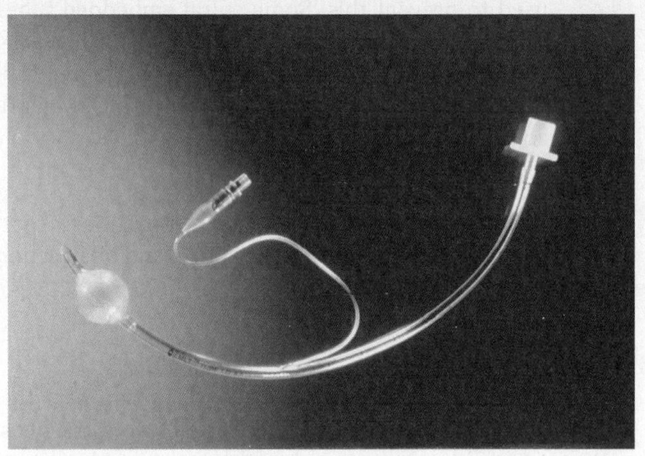

Figure 15.6 Tubes for microlaryngeal tracheal surgery. **Top:** The cuff on this tube is colored yellow for greater visibility. (Courtesy of Sheridan Catheter Corp., now part of Covidien, Mansfield, MA.) **Bottom:** Similar tube with an uncolored cuff.

e. Microlaryngeal Tracheal Surgery Tube
   The microlaryngeal tracheal surgery (LTS or MLT) tube (**Fig. 15.6**) is designed for microlaryngeal surgery or for patients whose airway has been narrowed to such an extent that a normal sized tracheal tube cannot be inserted. It has a small diameter to provide better visibility and access to the surgical site and a large cuff to center the tube in the trachea. Its longer length allows it to be used for intubation through a supraglottic airway device. Possible problems with a tube having such a small bore include increased resistance and occlusion. It can be used for selective bronchial intubation (Chapter 16).
f. Tip Control Tube
   A tip control tube (**Fig. 15.7**) has a pull cable with a ring near the end of the breathing system. Pulling on the ring moves the tip anteriorly.
g. Parker Flex-Tip Tube
   1) The Parker Flex-Tip tube (**Fig. 15.8**) has a "hooded," curved, flexible, tapered tip that points toward the center of the distal lumen on the concave surface of the tube so that the bevel faces posteriorly during insertion. There are eyes on the right and left sides of the tube. This tube has a very thin cuff. It is easier to advance over an intubating catheter or flexible endoscope than a conventional tube. It is also less likely to impinge on the right vocal cord than a tube with the bevel on

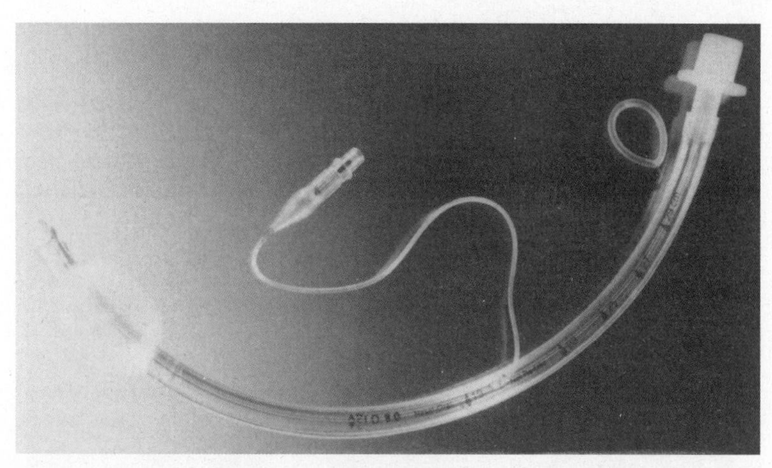

Figure 15.7 Endotrol tracheal tube. The ring is attached to the tip by a cablelike mechanism that allows the tip to be maneuvered. (Courtesy of Mallinckrodt Anesthesiology Division, Mallinckrodt Medical, Inc.)

the side. The tube is available in a variety of shapes with and without a cuff. It may be useful with an intubating laryngeal mask or other supraglottic device or when using a Bullard laryngoscope, flexible endoscope, video laryngoscope, or stylet laryngoscope.

2) The Parker tube tip can fold back and cause obstruction in a patient with subglottic stenosis.

h. Tubes with Extra Lumen(s)

Tubes with one or more separate lumens terminating near the tip are available (**Fig. 15.9**). They are useful for respiratory gas sampling, suctioning, airway pressure monitoring, fluid and drug injection, and jet ventilation. A number of problems are associated with these tubes. Secretions, blood, or moisture can obstruct the extra lumen. The sampling tube must be securely stabilized to minimize tension on the tube.

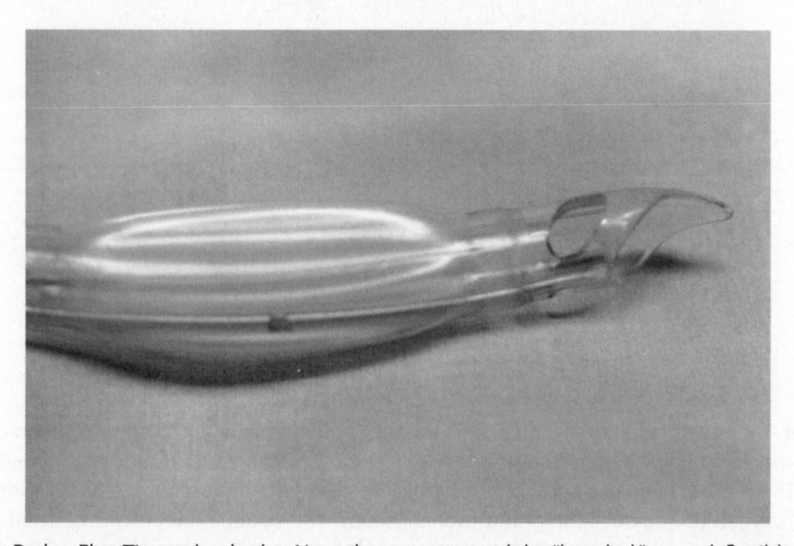

Figure 15.8 Parker Flex-Tip tracheal tube. Note the two eyes and the "hooded," curved, flexible, tapered tip that points toward the center of the distal lumen on the concave surface of the tube so that the bevel faces posteriorly during insertion.

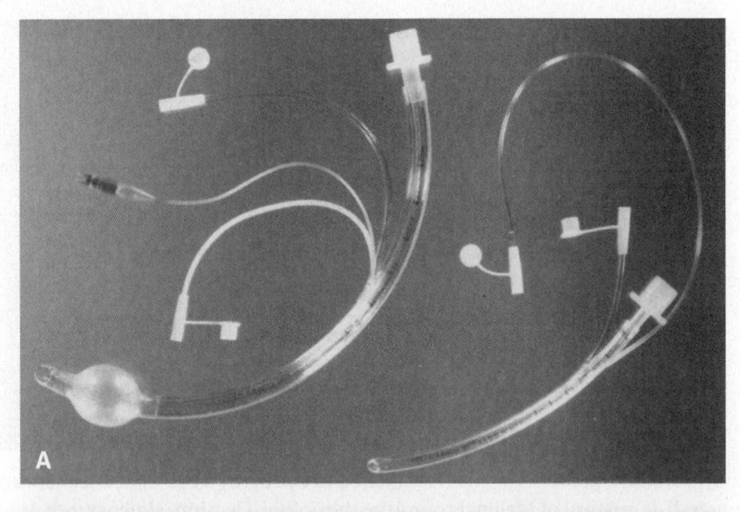

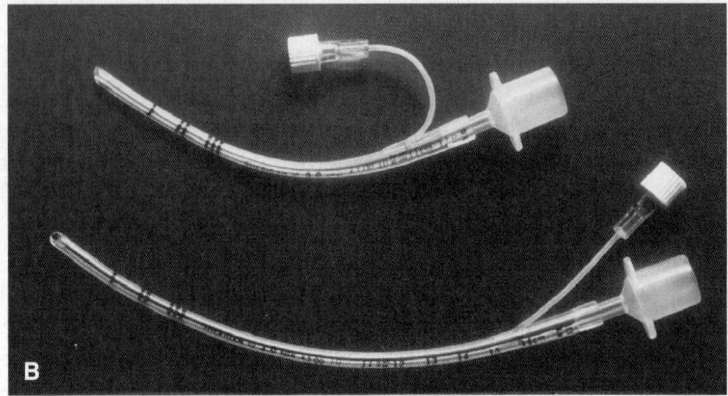

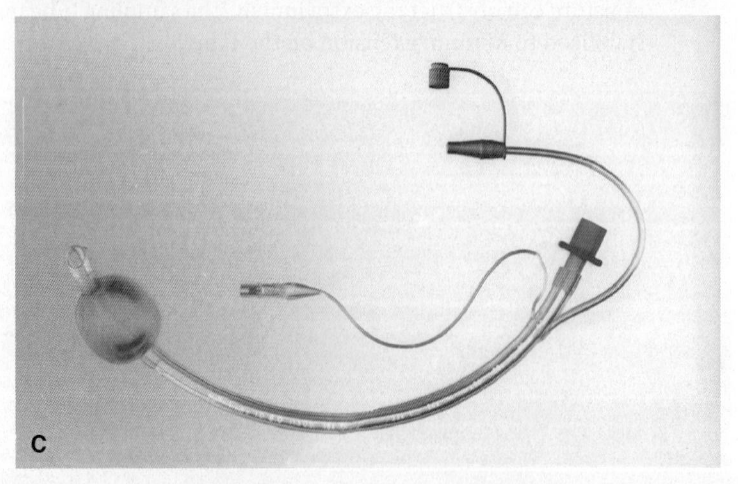

Figure 15.9 Tubes with additional lumen(s). These tubes have a main lumen for ventilation of the patient and one or more additional lumens for monitoring, irrigation, pressure monitoring, suctioning, and/or ventilation. **A:** These tubes have two additional lumens. The clear lumen is used for jet ventilation and administration of oxygen during suctioning and bronchoscopy. The opaque lumen can be used for irrigation and sampling of gases from the trachea. (Courtesy of Mallinckrodt Anesthesiology Division, Mallinckrodt Medical, Inc.) **B:** Pediatric tubes with monitoring lumens. (Courtesy of Kendall Healthcare Products Co.) **C:** Tube with lumen designed for subglottic suctioning. (Courtesy of Mallinkrodt Medical, Inc.)

CLINICAL MOMENT When a tube with an extra lumen is connected to a gas sampling line, moisture may be carried to the gas monitor and cause it to malfunction (see Chapter 17).

i. Laser-Resistant Tubes

A number of tracheal tubes have been designed for laser surgery (**Figs. 15.10** to **15.14**). It is important to understand that these tubes are laser resistant but may catch fire if the laser strength is too great or the laser application too long. Lasers and fires are discussed in more detail in Chapter 25.

CLINICAL MOMENT If a laser-resistant tube is used with a laser other than that for which it was designed, it can catch fire. Always confirm that the type of tube to be used is appropriate for the laser being used and be prepared for a fire in the airway.

CLINICAL MOMENT Even when a tracheal tube is marked as laser-resistant, the cuff is still vulnerable. Methylene blue is sometimes put into a fluid-filled cuff to alert the surgeon that the cuff has been hit. Some surgeons object to the methylene blue because it colors the tissues, making surgery difficult.

CLINICAL MOMENT Laser-resistant tubes are usually not resistant to other heat sources such as an electrocautery or the electrosurgery tip.

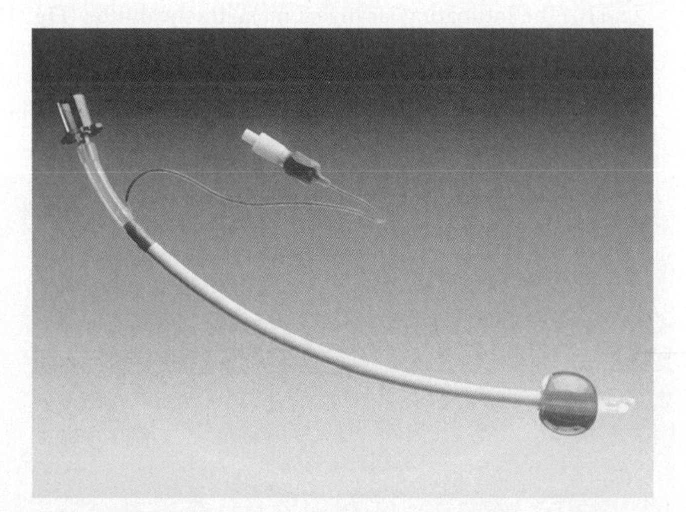

Figure 15.10 Laser-Shield II tracheal tube. It is made from silicone with an inner aluminum wrap and an outer Teflon coating. It is designed for use with CO_2 and potassium-titanyl-phosphate (KTP) lasers. The cuff is not laser-resistant. It contains methylene blue crystals and should be inflated with water or saline. There is 1 cm of unprotected silicone tubing above the cuff. The part of the tube distal to the cuff is also unprotected. Cottonoids for wrapping around the cuff are supplied with each tube. These must be moistened and kept moist during the procedure. (Courtesy of Xomed-Trease Jacksonville, FL.)

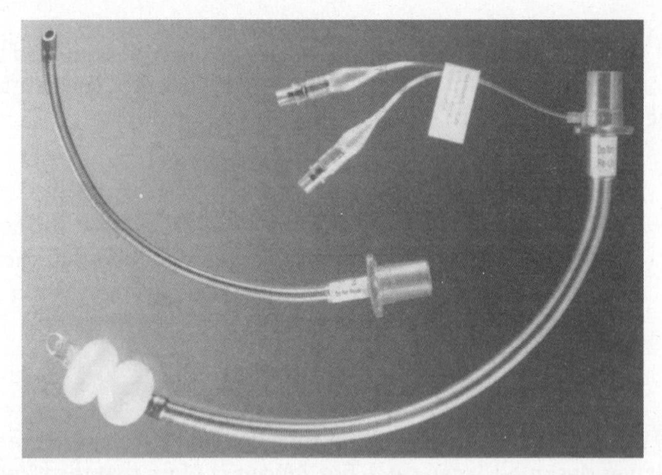

Figure 15.11 Laser-Flex tracheal tubes. The tube is stainless steel with a smooth plastic surface and a matte finish. It has a PVC tip with a Murphy eye. It is designed for use with CO_2 and KTP lasers. The wall of the tube is thicker than that of most other tubes. The adult tube has two cuffs. The distal cuff can be used if the proximal one is damaged. The cuffs should be filled with saline colored with methylene blue. Blood on the outside of the tube renders it less resistant to combustion. The cuff and tip are vulnerable to all lasers. (Courtesy of Mallinckrodt Medical, Inc.)

CLINICAL MOMENT Some laser-resistant tubes are difficult to place in the trachea when intubation is difficult. If the trachea can be intubated with a conventional tube, it may be possible to replace this tube with the laser-resistant tube by using an airway exchange catheter (AEC).

j. Intubating Laryngeal Mask Tracheal Tube and Tube Stabilizer
   1) The intubating laryngeal mask tracheal tube (**Fig. 15.15**) is designed to be inserted through the intubating laryngeal mask (Chapter 13) but can be purchased separately. It is a straight, wire-reinforced silicone tube with a tapered patient end, blunt tip, short bevel, and Murphy

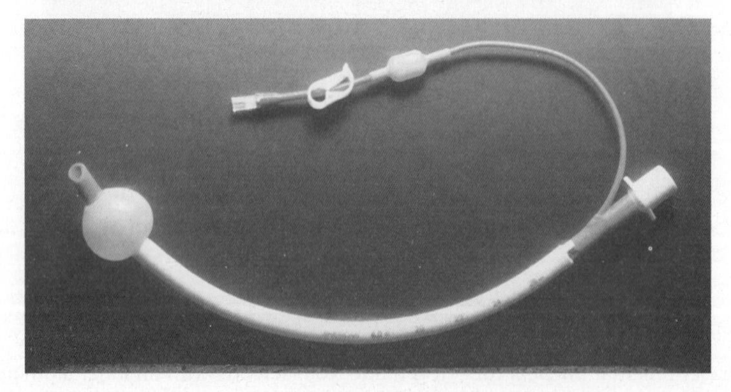

Figure 15.12 Sheridan Laser tracheal tube. The tube is red rubber wrapped with copper foil tape. This is overwrapped with water-absorbent fabric that should be saturated with water or saline prior to use. There is a copper band at the cuff-tube junction. Radiopaque pledgets that are designed to be moistened and placed above the cuff are provided with each tube. It is designed for use with a CO_2 or KTP laser. (Courtesy of Kendall Healthcare Products Co.)

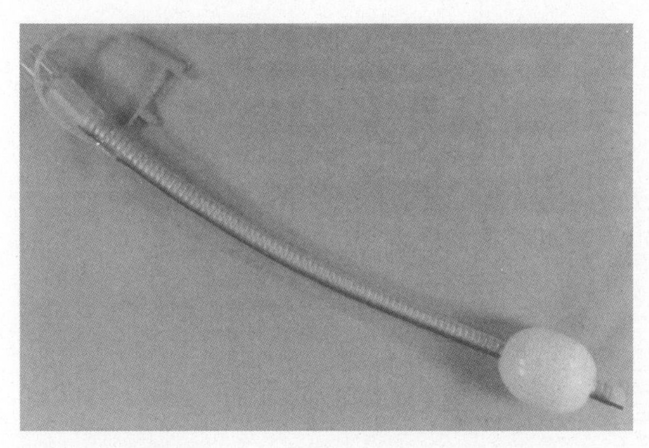

Figure 15.13 Bivona Fome-Cuf laser tube. It has an aluminum and silicone spiral with a silicone covering. The self-inflating cuff consists of a polyurethane foam sponge with a silicone envelope. The cuff must be deflated before intubation or extubation. The cuff should be filled with saline during use. The cuff retains its shape and keeps a seal when it is punctured but it can no longer be deflated. The inflation tube runs along the exterior of the tube and is colored black. It should be positioned away from where the laser with be used. This tube is for use with the CO_2 laser.

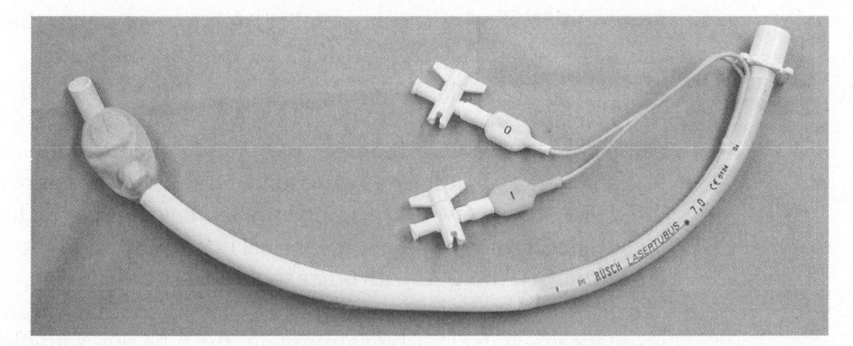

Figure 15.14 Laser tubes. If the outer cuff is perforated by the laser beam, the trachea will still be sealed by the inner cuff. The manufacturer recommends that the inner cuff be filled with air and the outer cuff with water or saline. The shaft above the cuff is covered by a corrugated silver foil which is covered by a Merocel sponge that should be moistened before use. This tube is recommended for use with argon, NdYAG and CO_2 lasers.

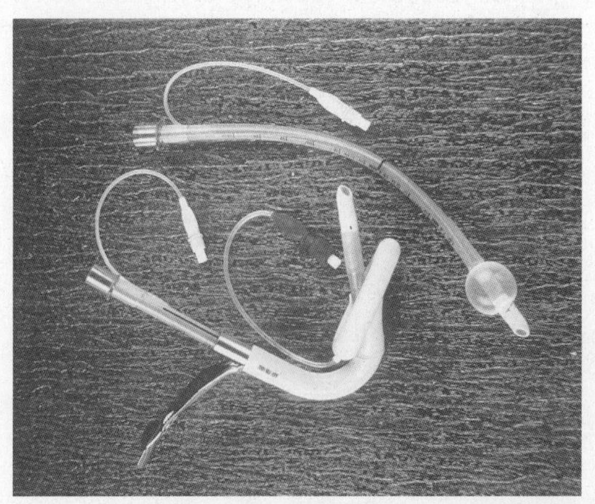

Figure 15.15 ILM-ETT. The *black circle* near the middle of the tube will be at the end of the connector when the tip of the tube is at the entrance to the bowl of the mask. (Courtesy of LMA North America, San Diego, CA.)

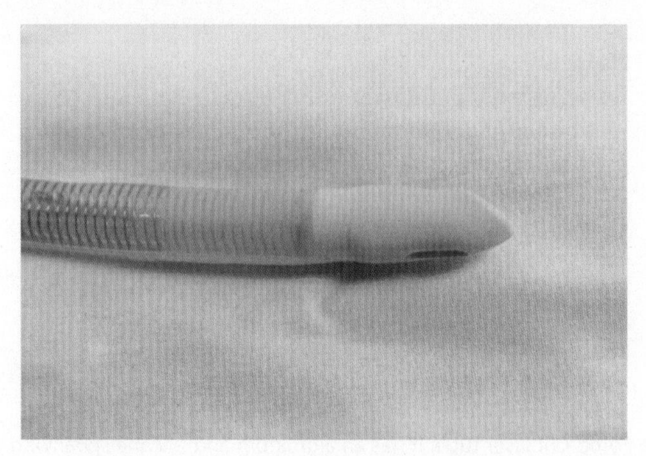

Figure 15.16 Tip of ILM-ETT. Note how the high-pressure cuff situated just above the colored tip lies flat against the tube.

eye. It has a low-volume, high-pressure cuff (**Fig. 15.16**). It is reusable and can be autoclaved. It is available in sizes 6, 6.5, 7, 7.5, and 8. A single-use tube has a low-pressure cuff.

2) **Figure 15.17** shows the tube stabilizer. It is used to steady the tube so it will not be dislocated while the LMA is being removed.
3) The intubating laryngeal mask tracheal tube has been found to be easier to advance over a fiberscope than a conventional tube during oral and nasal intubation. It has been used for submental intubation and tracheal resection and reconstruction after the tip was removed.
4) Problems reported with the intubating laryngeal mask tracheal tube include eccentric cuff inflation, internal deformities, and the tip folding during insertion. As with other spiral wire-reinforced tubes, biting can deform the spirals or cause a leak. When exposed to the magnetic resonance imaging (MRI) environment, the tube poses no direct risk to the patient or other personnel, but the MRI image quality near the tube may be compromised.

CLINICAL MOMENT The reusable intubating laryngeal mask tracheal tube has a low-volume, high-pressure cuff and is not suitable for prolonged ventilation.

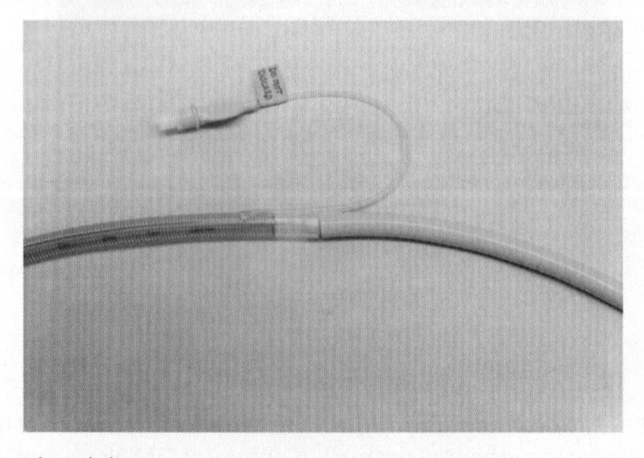

Figure 15.17 ILM-ETT with stabilizer.

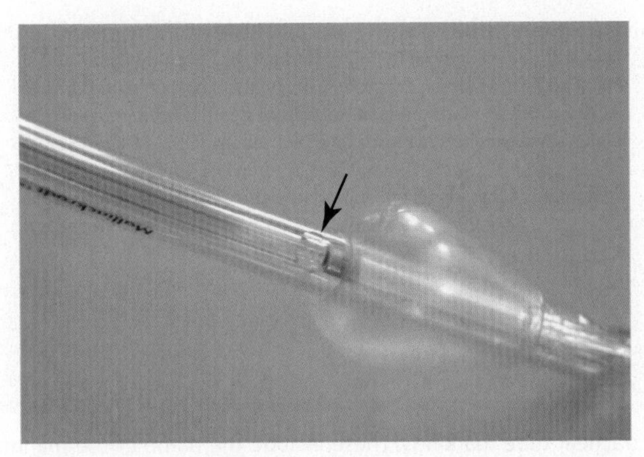

Figure 15.18 Hi-Lo Evac tube. The hole just above the cuff is connected to a channel through which secretions can be aspirated. Note the shape of the cuff, which is designed to reduce the incidence of folds and channels through which secretions can leak.

k. Hi-Lo Evac Tube

The Hi-Lo Evac tube (**Fig. 15.18**) incorporates an evacuation channel that can be used to clear secretions between the vocal cords and the cuff. Results were mixed when this tube was used to prevent or delay development of pneumonia. The lumen may become blocked by secretions or by prolapsed tracheal mucosa. Damage to the tracheal mucosa near the suction port has been reported.

4. **Tube Markings**
   a. Typical tracheal tube markings, shown in **Figures 15.19** and **15.20,** are situated on the beveled side of the tube above the cuff. The following are required:
      1) The word *oral, nasal,* or *oral/nasal.*
      2) The tube size in internal diameter (ID) in millimeters marked on the tube and sometimes also on the pilot balloon.
      3) The outside diameter (OD) for size 6 and smaller tubes.

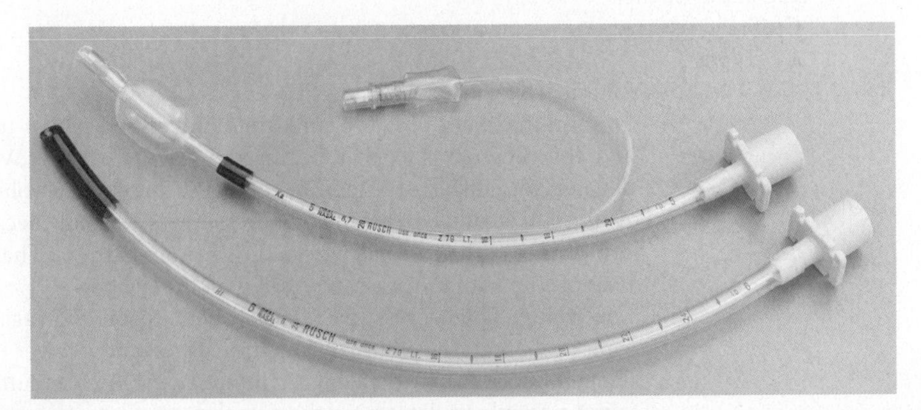

Figure 15.19 Typical tracheal tube markings. The dark marking at the patient end of the bottom tube and the mark above the cuff on the top tube are to aid in proper placement with respect to the vocal cords. The internal and external diameters as well as the size in French scale are shown. For example, on the **top** tube, the internal diameter is 5.0, the external diameter is 6.7, and the French scale size is 20. Z-79 and IT both indicate that the tube material has passed the tissue toxicity test. Length from the patient tip is marked in centimeters. (Photograph courtesy of Rusch, Inc.)

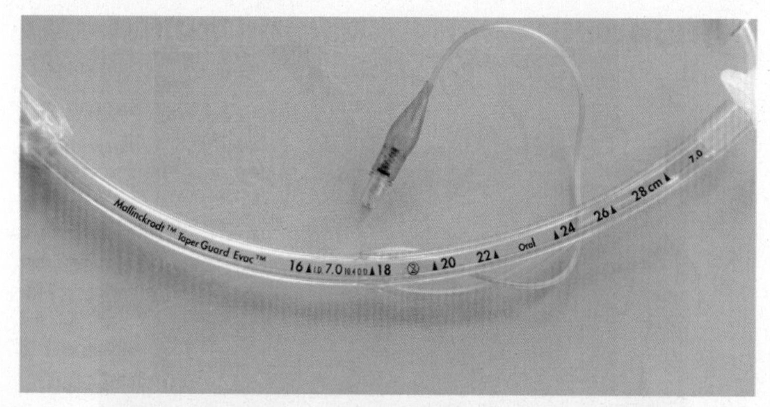

Figure 15.20 Typical tracheal tube markings. These include the name of the manufacturer and type of tube. The internal and external diameters are between the 16- and 18-cm depth marks. Between the 18- and 20-cm marks is a circle with an X through it, indicating that the tube should not be reused. The tube size may also be on the tube near the connector and/or on the pilot balloon.

4) The name or trademark of the manufacturer or supplier.
5) Graduated markings showing the distance in centimeters from the patient end.
6) A cautionary such as "Do not reuse" or "Single use only" if the tube is disposable.
7) A radiopaque marker at the patient end or along the full length.

b. Some tubes have markings (guide marks) to help to position the tube with respect to the vocal cords (**Figs. 15.2, 15.4,** and **15.19**). The design and location of these markings vary.

B. Cuff Systems

A cuff system consists of the cuff plus an inflation tube, pilot balloon, and inflation valve (**Fig. 15.1**). An inflation lumen in the tube wall may also be present. The purpose of the cuff system is to provide a seal between the tube and the tracheal wall to prevent pharyngeal contents from passing into the trachea and ensure that no gas leaks past the cuff during positive pressure ventilation. The cuff also serves to center the tube in the trachea.

1. **Cuff**

a. Types

1) Low-Volume, High-Pressure Cuffs

(i) Low-volume, high-pressure cuffs are found on red rubber tubes and the reusable silicone tube for the LMA-Fastrach. When deflated, the cuff hugs the tube, resulting in a low residual volume. As the cuff is inflated, the inflating pressure rises rapidly because compliance of the cuff wall is low. The pressure in the cuff has no relationship with the pressure exerted on the trachea.

(ii) Low-volume, high-pressure cuffs offer better protection against aspiration, better visibility during intubation, and a lower incidence of sore throat than high-volume, low-pressure cuffs. It is not possible to determine the pressure on the trachea when these cuffs are inflated. When used for a prolonged period of time, ischemic damage to the tracheal mucosa is likely to occur. For prolonged intubation, a tube with one of these cuffs should be replaced with a tube with a high-volume, low-pressure cuff.

CLINICAL MOMENT When a difficult intubation is undertaken and forceps are needed to guide the tube through the vocal cords, a low-volume, high-pressure cuff is less likely to be damaged by the forceps.

2) High-Volume, Low-Pressure Cuffs

(i) High-volume, low-pressure cuffs are most frequently used today. The cuff has a high residual volume and a high compliance. As the cuff is inflated, the pressure rises only slightly until it forms a seal with the tracheal wall. The thin compliant wall can achieve a seal without stretching the tracheal wall. The cuff contacts a wider surface on the tracheal wall than does the low-volume cuff. If inflation continues past the point of sealing, the pressure will increase and the trachea will become distorted (see **Fig. 15.21**).

CLINICAL MOMENT Once the cuff contacts the tracheal wall, the pressure rises rapidly. It is important to inflate only to the point of creating a seal. Measuring intracuff pressure is highly recommended.

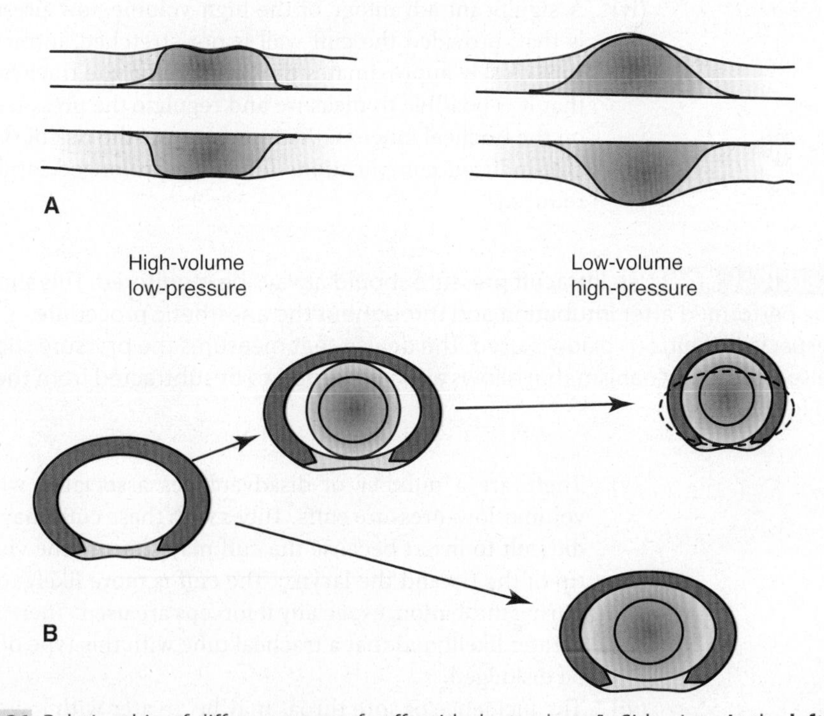

Figure 15.21 Relationship of different types of cuffs with the trachea. **A:** Side view. At the **left,** the high-volume, low-pressure cuff has a large area of contact with the trachea. The cuff adapts itself to the irregular tracheal wall. At the **right,** the low-volume, high-pressure cuff has a small area of contact with the trachea. It distends the trachea and distorts it to a circular shape. **B:** Cross-sectional view. At the **left** is the normal trachea. At the **top,** the low-volume, high-pressure cuff distorts the trachea and makes the tracheal contour the same as the shape of the cuff. At the **bottom,** the soft high-volume, low-pressure cuff conforms to the normal tracheal lumen.

(ii) Intracuff pressure varies during the ventilatory cycle. During spontaneous breathing, airway pressure becomes negative and cuff pressure decreases during inspiration. Positive pressure occurs during exhalation.

(iii) With controlled ventilation, when airway pressure exceeds intracuff pressure, positive pressure is applied to the lower cuff face. If the cuff wall is pliable, the cuff will be distorted into the shape of a cone. The gas in the cuff will be compressed until intracuff pressure equals airway pressure. A leak will develop if the tracheal diameter is greater than the cuff diameter. At that point, more gas must be added to the cuff to abolish the leak. Unfortunately, this additional cuff inflation will elevate the baseline cuff pressure. During exhalation, the intracuff pressure will decrease until its resting pressure is reached. It is desirable that the cuff circumference at residual volume be at least equal to the tracheal circumference. If the cuff is smaller, it must be stretched beyond its residual volume to create a seal. At this point, it will act like a high-pressure cuff. On the other hand, if the residual cuff diameter is much greater than the tracheal diameter, cuff infolding may occur, with the possibility of aspiration along the folds.

(iv) A significant advantage of the high-volume, low-pressure cuff is that, provided the cuff wall is not stretched, intracuff pressure closely approximates the pressure on the tracheal wall so that it is possible to measure and regulate the pressure exerted on the tracheal mucosa. With proper use, the risk of significant cuff-induced complications following prolonged intubation is reduced.

CLINICAL MOMENT Intracuff pressure should always be monitored. This should be performed after intubation and throughout the anesthetic procedure, especially if nitrous oxide is used. The device that measures the pressure should also have a mechanism that allows air to be added to or subtracted from the cuff (**Fig. 15.22**).

(v) There are a number of disadvantages associated with high-volume, low-pressure cuffs. Tubes with these cuffs may be more difficult to insert because the cuff may obscure the view of the tip of the tip and the larynx. The cuff is more likely to be torn during intubation, especially if forceps are used. There may be a greater likelihood that a tracheal tube with this type of cuff will be dislodged.

(vi) The incidence of sore throat may be greater with low-pressure cuffs than with high-pressure cuffs, unless the cuff is specially designed so that the area of tracheal contact is small.

(vii) A major drawback of high-volume, low-pressure cuffs is that they may not prevent fluid from leaking into the lower airway even at high cuff pressures. Fluid leakage is increased with spontaneous respiration and is reduced with continuous positive

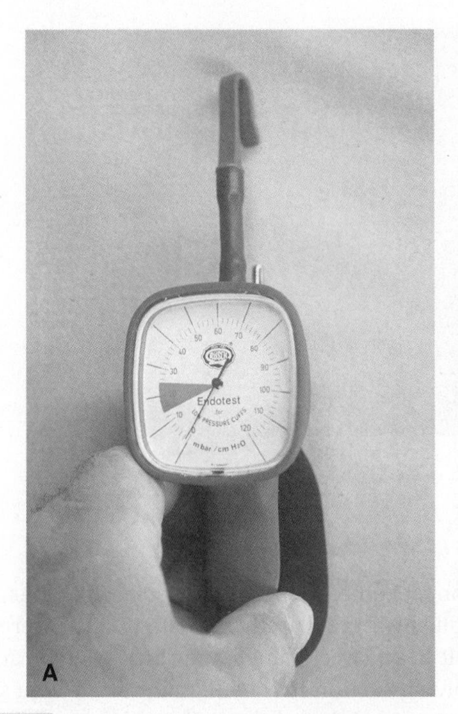

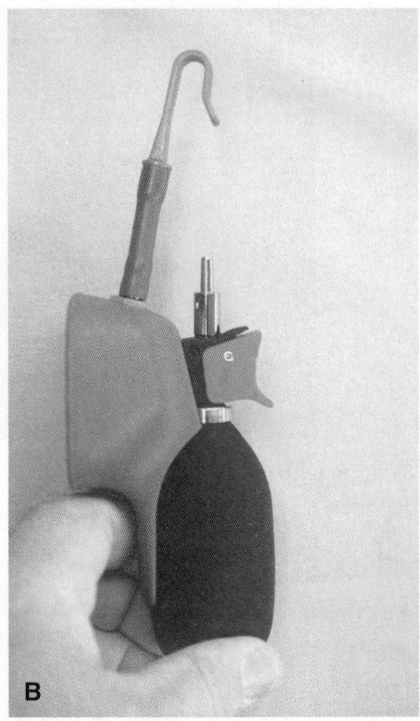

Figure 15.22 Device to measure intracuff pressure. **A:** Front view. **B:** Side view showing the valve used to reduce the pressure. (Courtesy of Rusch, Inc.)

airway pressure, positive end-expiratory pressure (PEEP), and pressure-supported ventilation. Intermittent positive-pressure ventilation adds some protection. Lubrication with a water-soluble gel will reduce fluid leak for a limited period of time.

(viii) It is relatively easy to pass devices such as esophageal stethoscopes, temperature probes, and enteric tubes around low-pressure cuffs.

(ix) Another problem with low-pressure cuffs is the belief that simply using this type of cuff will prevent high pressures from being exerted on the tracheal wall. Any cuff can be overfilled or the volume and pressure can increase during use, resulting in high-intracuff and tracheal wall pressures. In fact, tracheal injury can occur even when these cuffs are used properly.

CLINICAL MOMENT When nitrous oxide is used, it will diffuse into the cuff. This added volume will increase the pressure on the tracheal mucosa. Continuously monitoring cuff pressure will allow the clinician to relieve excess pressure when needed.

3) Microthin Cuffs

The microthin cuff is a high-volume, low-pressure cuff with a very thin wall that allows the channels to self-seal, preventing liquid from entering the trachea. These cuffs have been shown to cause lower pressure on the tracheal wall and a better seal than conventional cuffs (1, 2).

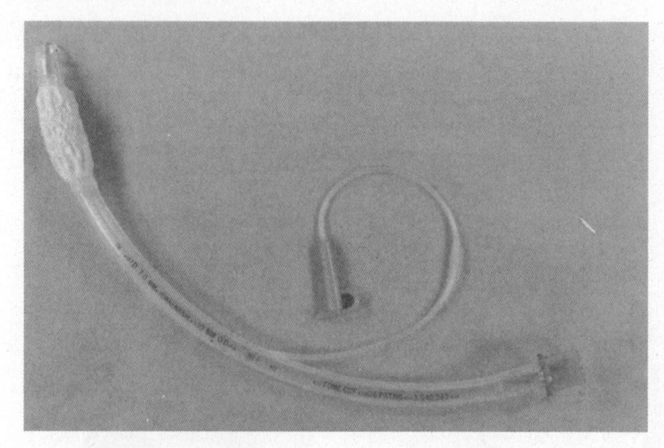

Figure 15.23 Tube with deflated foam cuff.

4) Foam Cuffs
   (i) The foam (sponge, Fome, Kamen-Wilkinson) cuff (**Figs. 15.13** and **15.23**) is filled with polyurethane foam that is covered with a thin sheath. It has a large diameter, residual volume, and surface area. Applying suction to the inflation tube with a syringe causes the foam to shrink and the cuff to contract. When the negative pressure is released, the foam and the cuff expand.
   (ii) The tube is supplied with a T-piece to fit between the connector and the breathing system (**Fig. 15.24**). When the inflation tube is connected to this T-piece, the pressure inside the cuff follows proximal airway pressure during the ventilatory cycle.
   (iii) When in place in the trachea, the volume that the foam expands determines the pressure exerted laterally on the tracheal wall. The more the foam expands, the lower the pressure. Thus, the pressure on the tracheal wall depends on the relationship between the cuff diameter at residual volume and the tracheal diameter. If too large a tracheal tube is used, the cuff:tracheal wall pressure ratio will be high. If too small a cuff is used, there will be no seal. The risk of fluid leaking past the cuff is similar to that with most high-volume, low-pressure cuffs.

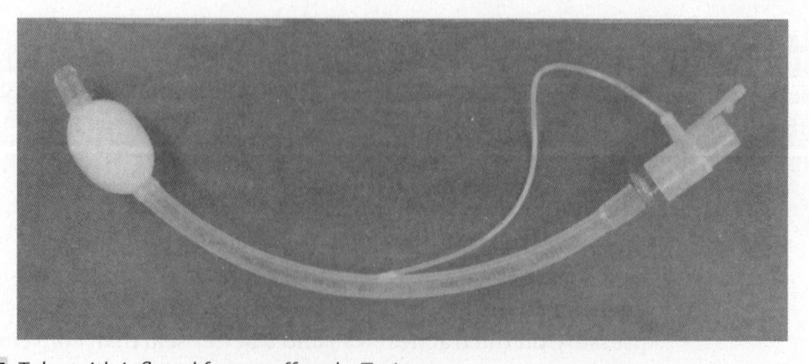

Figure 15.24 Tube with inflated foam cuff and a T-piece.

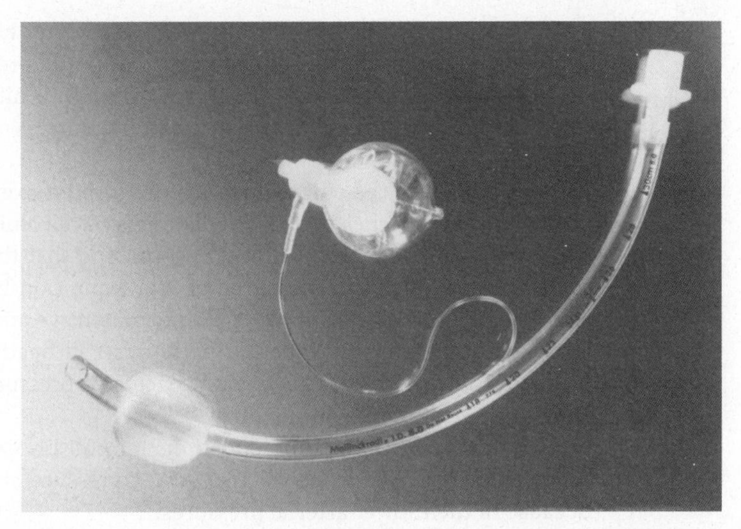

Figure 15.25 Lanz pressure-regulating valve. The pilot balloon is confined inside a transparent plastic sheath. There is a pressure-regulating valve between the pilot balloon and the cuff. Air should be injected into the cuff until the pilot balloon is stretched, but it should be smaller than the confining sheath.

(iv) Anesthetic agent can diffuse into the cuff but will not cause an increase in pressure. It is not possible to monitor cuff pressure with this device. It can provide a seal at a low tracheal wall pressure, provided the relationship between the diameter of the cuff and that of the tracheal tube is optimal.

(v) Before extubation, the cuff should be collapsed by aspirating the residual air and then clamping the inflation tube.

5) Lanz Cuff System

(i) The Lanz pressure-regulating valve (McGinnis balloon system) consists of a very compliant latex pilot balloon inside a transparent plastic sheath with an automatic pressure-regulating valve between the balloon and the cuff (**Fig. 15.25**). The pilot balloon has three parts: an indicator for cuff inflation, an external reservoir for the cuff, and a pressure-limiting device.

(ii) The Lanz valve permits a rapid gas flow from the balloon to the cuff but only a slow flow from the cuff to the balloon. This prevents gas from being squeezed back into the balloon when the airway pressure rises rapidly, so there is no gas leak around the cuff during positive-pressure ventilation. It also prevents increases in cuff volume and pressure caused by nitrous oxide and other gases diffusing into the cuff.

(iii) As air is injected into the Lanz cuff, the cuff and the balloon are inflated in parallel. When the balloon has a stretched appearance, a pressure of approximately 26 to 33 cm H_2O will be present in the cuff. As injection continues, the pilot balloon fills preferentially. The intraballoon pressure remains constant and will not increase until it strikes the confining sheath. Should the trachea expand, air will slowly flow from the balloon into the cuff. The pressure-regulating valve protects against rapid loss of cuff volume into the balloon during inspiration.

(iv) The pressure-regulating valve of the Lanz cuff has been found to be effective in keeping lateral tracheal wall pressure low and preventing increases in cuff pressure due to nitrous oxide. It eliminates the need to measure cuff pressure.

b. Cuff Pressure

1) It is desirable that the cuff seal the airway without exerting so much pressure on the trachea that its circulation is compromised or the tracheal wall is dilated. Most authors recommend that the pressure on the lateral tracheal wall measured at end expiration be between 20 and 30 cm H_2O (18 to 25 mm Hg) in normotensive adults. A patient who requires high peak inflation pressures will need a higher cuff pressure to prevent leaks (minimum occlusive pressure), increasing the risk of ischemic tracheal injury.
2) For children, no firm recommendations for cuff pressure have been reported, but it seems logical that lower pressure should be used because of their lower arterial pressures.
3) A number of techniques have been advanced to determine the proper cuff inflation volume and by extension the proper cuff pressure. These include allowing a minimal leak, injecting a certain amount of air into the cuff, injecting enough volume to minimally occlude a leak, and palpating the pilot balloon.

CLINICAL MOMENT Many anesthesia providers inject air into the cuff with little regard for how much pressure is needed to achieve a seal. When the intracuff pressure is measured, the pressure is often quite high. Pressure increases during nitrous oxide anesthesia administration cannot be detected without measuring the pressure. It is recommended that every anesthesia location have a means for measuring cuff pressure and that it be used with each patient.

4) If a cuff is inflated with air, the intracuff pressure and cuff volume will rise when nitrous oxide is administered. The increase varies directly with nitrous oxide partial pressure, permeability of the cuff wall, and time. When nitrous oxide administration is discontinued, the pressure in the cuff decreases.

CLINICAL MOMENT If the tracheal tube is to remain in place after surgery is finished and nitrous oxide is used, the cuff should be evacuated and filled with air. When nitrous oxide diffuses out, the cuff volume will decrease and a leak may result in the postoperative period. Four hours may be needed to stabilize cuff pressure after using nitrous oxide.

5) There are a number of reasons beside nitrous oxide diffusion for cuff pressure variation. Cuff pressures are lower during hypothermic bypass. Increases in cuff pressure may result from pressure from nearby surgical procedures, higher altitude, oxygen diffusion into the cuff, and changes in head position away from the neutral position. Cuff pressure will also be affected by coughing, straining, and changing muscle tone. Foam-filled cuffs do not exhibit these fluctuations.

c. Ways to Limit Cuff Pressure

1) Cuff pressure can be measured continuously or at frequent intervals and altered by inflating or deflating the cuff as needed. This is the only way to provide adequate protection from both aspiration and tracheal ischemia. Measurement is easy, and cuff pressure monitors are relatively inexpensive. Pressures higher or lower than recommended are common when cuff pressure is not monitored.
2) The cuff can be filled with a gas mixture containing oxygen and nitrous oxide or nitrous oxide alone. This is awkward to perform. A cuff inflated with nitrous oxide will lose volume and may allow a leak when nitrous oxide administration is discontinued or during extracorporeal circulation.
3) The cuff can be filled with water or saline. This results in a more stable pressure. Adjusting cuff pressure is more difficult than when air is used. It may also be difficult to remove the tube quickly when the cuff is filled with liquid.

CLINICAL MOMENT Fluid-filled cuffs cannot be deflated rapidly. This could be a disadvantage if a fire occurs.

4) Specialized balloon systems such as the Lanz pressure-regulating valve (see earlier discussion) and various other devices for controlling cuff pressure have been developed. A cuff designed to reduce nitrous oxide diffusion, a cuff with a high compliance, or a cuff with a large, thin-walled pilot balloon can be used.

CLINICAL MOMENT Assessing cuff pressure by manual palpation or pinching the pilot balloon is inaccurate, as is using a minimal leak volume, minimal occlusive volume, or a predetermined volume to inflate the cuff.

2. **Inflation System**

The tracheal tube inflation system (**Fig. 15.1**) consists of an external inflation tube with a lumen that terminates inside the cuff. There is a pilot balloon in the inflation tube or near the inflation valve. The inflation valve is the point where air or liquid is introduced into the cuff. The valve is opened when a syringe is attached and closes automatically when it is removed.

C. Tracheal Tube Connector

The connector of the tracheal tube links the tracheal tube to the breathing system. The tube end varies with the tube size, whereas the breathing system end has a 15-mm male end. The connector may be straight or curved. Flexible connectors or flexible extenders may also be used.

CLINICAL MOMENT The connector on a new tracheal tube is commonly only partially inserted into the tube. When the tube is to be used, the connector should be removed and the tracheal end moistened with alcohol so as to slide into the tube more easily. This makes a strong bond between the tube and the connector.

CLINICAL MOMENT Using a connector longer than the one supplied with the tube will increase the dead space. The same is true if extenders are added between the tracheal tube and the Y-piece. This may not be significant for adult patients but the added dead space can cause problems with small patients.

III. Using the Tracheal Tube

A. Tube Choice

1. Cuffed versus Uncuffed

a. Cuffed tubes are routinely used for adult patients. Cuffed tubes for children are also available (**Fig. 15.19**) and their use has become common. Studies indicate that the use of cuffed tubes in children is not associated with an increased risk of complications.

b. Advantages of cuffed tubes include improved monitoring accuracy for end-tidal gases, tidal volume, compliance, and oxygen consumption; decreased aspiration risk; ability to use high inflation pressures or PEEP, and low fresh gas flows; less operating room (OR) pollution; decreased risk of fire; and fewer tube changes.

c. Drawbacks of using a cuffed tube in children include the need to choose a slightly smaller tube (which makes suctioning more difficult and tube obstruction more likely and increases resistance and the work of breathing); the risk of injury to the vocal cords; a reduced margin of safety (the need to avoid the cuff impinging on the glottis yet avoid bronchial intubation) and possible trauma to the tracheal mucosa or mucosal ischemia caused by cuff overinflation. Cuff pressure measurement is especially important for pediatric patients because a small air addition causes a considerable pressure increase.

2. Size

a. Smaller tubes are easier to insert and require less reshaping force to adapt to the patient's airway but are associated with higher resistance, difficulty passing a fiberscope or suction catheter, and increased risk of occlusion and kinking. Larger tubes are associated with less risk of occlusion and less resistance but a higher incidence of trauma and postoperative sore throat. Larger tubes are more difficult to insert.

b. Because no system for choosing the correct size tube is foolproof, the user should always have tubes that are both larger and smaller than the tube chosen readily available. A smaller tube should be used when a difficult intubation is anticipated.

c. When using cuffed tubes, the cuff circumference should equal that of the tracheal lumen. If the tube is too small, a high cuff pressure will be needed to achieve a seal, increasing pressure on the mucosa. If the cuff is too large, it will have folds when inflated. Aspiration may occur along these folds.

d. One study found that the ideal tube in the average adult is a 7.5-mm ID tube for females and an 8.5-mm ID tube for males. However, there is great variation in the sizes and shapes of tracheas in adults.

e. Choosing the correct tracheal tube size in children remains a major challenge. Age is recognized as the most reliable indicator. **Table 15.1** shows some recommendations. There are many other formulae and guidelines, but they should be regarded only as rough estimates. A child with Down syndrome has a smaller trachea, so a tracheal tube at least two sizes smaller

Table 15.1 Some Recommendations for Tube Size in Children

Patient Age (years)	Uncuffed	Cuffed
Premature	2.5–3	
Birth to <0.5	3.5–4	3.0
0.5 to <1.0	3.5–4	3.0–3.5
1.0 to <1.5	4–4.5	3.5
1.5 to <2.0	4–4.5	3.5–4
2.0 to <3.0	4.5	3.5–4
3.0 to <4.0	4.5–5	4–4.5
4.0 to <5.0	5.0	4–4.5

than usual may be needed. Premature babies have relatively elastic laryngeal structures that may allow a large tube to be inserted, but this may result in injury to the posterior part of the glottis.

f. When uncuffed tubes are used in children, the size should be large enough to provide effective ventilation but not so large as to cause pressure on the mucosa. This is commonly achieved by allowing a leak between the tube and the tracheal wall at peak airway pressures (commonly 15 to 25 cm H_2O). Many factors influence the leak pressure, and these should be borne in mind when performing the leak test. Measuring the leak when the child's head is turned to one side or when the child is not paralyzed increases the pressure required to cause the leak.

CLINICAL MOMENT When selecting a tracheal tube based on the internal diameter, it is important to realize that the outer diameter will vary between tubes of the same internal diameter from different manufacturers.

B. Checking the Tube

1. Before insertion, the tube should be examined for defects such as splitting, holes, and missing sections. The tube should be checked for patency. With transparent tubes, simple observation will suffice. With other tubes, the user should look into both ends and/or insert a stylet.
2. The cuff, if present, should be inflated and the syringe removed to check for leaks in the inflation valve. The cuff should be inspected to make certain that it inflates evenly and does not cause the tube lumen to be reduced. It should remain inflated for at least 1 minute to detect a slow leak.
3. If the tube has a sponge cuff, all the air should be aspirated. The inflation tube should then be closed or clamped. The cuff should remain collapsed. If it fills and there is a leak, then the tube should be discarded.

C. Preparing the Tube

After the sterile wrapping is opened, the tube should be handled only at the connector end. The connector should be lubricated with alcohol and inserted as far as possible. Using sterile water-soluble lubricant jelly on a high-volume, low-pressure cuff may decrease the aspiration risk by filling in the folds. For oral intubation, only the cuff should be lubricated. If nasal intubation is planned, lubricant should be applied along the entire tube.

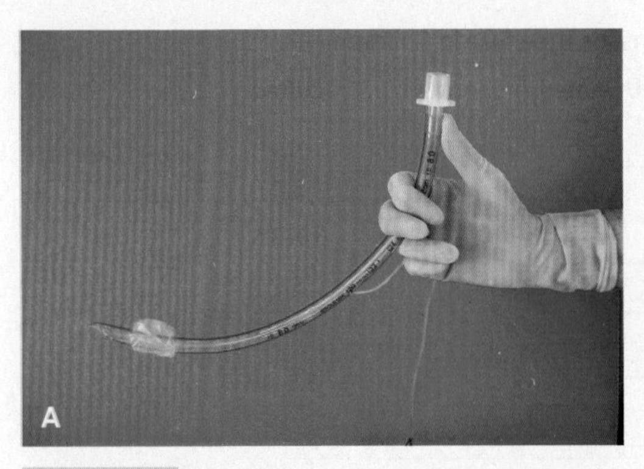

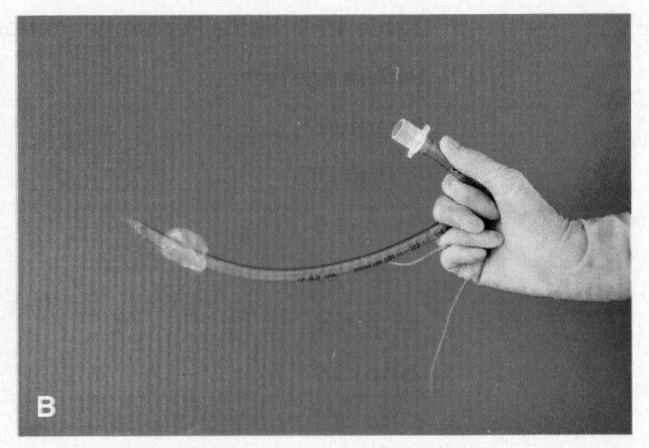

Figure 15.26 **A:** The tracheal tube is gripped as shown in the picture with the thumb on the shaft near the connector and two fingers around the tube. **B:** Pushing forward with the thumb will cause the tip to move forward.

D. Inserting the Tube

1. **Techniques**

a. Oral Intubation

1) Oral intubation is generally preferred for general anesthesia and in emergencies because it can be performed more quickly and easily and allows a wider and shorter tube to be used than with nasal intubation. Disadvantages include the possibility of oropharyngeal complications. The patient with an oral tube has difficulty swallowing. Obstruction from biting can occur with oral intubation.

2) Insertion of the tube is usually easy once the vocal cords are exposed. The tube should be introduced into the right corner of the mouth and directed toward the glottis with the bevel parallel to the vocal cords. If there is cord movement, the tube should be inserted during maximum abduction. Gripping the tube as shown in **Figure 15.26** may facilitate anterior movement at the patient end during insertion.

3) A blind oral technique is performed with the head flat. A stylet with a bend is inserted into the tracheal tube. The intubator should apply pressure on the cricoid cartilage with one hand while the tracheal tube is introduced into the mouth with the other, following the curve of the tube. The tube is advanced until the intubator feels the tip or feels the tube advance into the trachea. It may be necessary to manipulate the larynx to the right or left in order to advance the tube into the trachea. A tube with tip control (**Fig. 15.7**) may be useful in blind oral intubations. If the patient is breathing spontaneously, blind intubation may be performed by capnography to obtain the optimal CO_2 waveform or by hearing or feeling spontaneous breathing.

4) A bite block, rolled gauze, or oral airway should be placed between the teeth to prevent the patient from biting the tube and occluding the lumen.

b. Nasal Intubation

1) The nasal route is commonly used for surgical procedures involving the oral cavity, oropharynx, or face where an oral tube would hinder the surgeon's access. Other indications may include a fractured mandible, movement limitation at the temporomandibular joints, a neck

injury or cervical spine disease, intraoral pathology, and intolerance to direct laryngoscopy.

2) Intubation by the nasal route has many advantages. Securing the tube is easier. The nasal route eliminates the possibility that the tube will be occluded by biting. Nasal intubation may cause less cervical spine movement than oral intubation.
3) Disadvantages include using a smaller tube, which will result in increased resistance and difficulty suctioning or performing endoscopy. Intubation usually takes longer. Severe bleeding may occur. Nasal intubation has been shown to result in a higher incidence of bacteremia, sinusitis, and otitis.
4) Contraindications to nasotracheal intubation include anticoagulation, coagulopathy, and any nasal or paranasal pathology (including polyps, abscesses, foreign bodies, or epiglottitis). A fracture at the base of the skull is usually considered a contraindication to nasotracheal intubation, although it has been safely used in this situation. Traumatic brain injury with cerebrospinal fluid leakage is also considered a contraindication.
5) A tracheal tube one size smaller than would be considered optimal for oral intubation is preferable to minimize trauma. It should be thoroughly lubricated along its entire length with a sterile, water-soluble lubricant. The cuff should be fully deflated.
6) If possible, a fiberscope should be passed through the nostrils to determine the presence of abnormalities. Clinical tests such as estimating the air flow rate by palpation when the contralateral nostril is occluded or asking the patient to assess airflow through the nostrils do not correlate with nasal abnormalities. Inserting progressively larger, lubricated nasal airways will test nostril patency and dilate it. Other methods to decrease trauma include applying a vasoconstrictor; using a Magill tube or a tube with a hemispherical bevel; thermosoftening the tube; passing the tube through a nasal airway; using an intraluminal balloon; slipping the end of a catheter or gloved finger over the tracheal tube tip; and inserting the tube over a bougie, stylet, fiberscope, stethoscope, gastric tube, or catheter passed through the nose.
7) When the tube is inserted, the bevel opening should face laterally. It should be advanced along the floor of the nose while slightly lifting the nose tip. The tube should be tilted cephalad over the patient's face as it is passed posteriorly until it contacts the posterior pharyngeal wall. From this point, the natural curve of the tube and the anterior body of the cervical spine will usually direct it anteriorly. Only gentle pressure should be used. If excessive resistance is encountered, the other nostril or a smaller tube should be tried.
8) Sometimes, the tube will impact the posterior pharyngeal wall and resist attempts to advance it farther. The tube should be pulled back a short distance and the patient's head extended to facilitate passage beyond this point. If the tube is turned so that the tip is posterior, it may be easier to advance it into the trachea. It may be useful to withdraw the tube and place a stylet with an acute bend in the distal 1.5 cm into the tube. The tube is inserted until the tip passes the posterior nasopharynx and then the stylet is withdrawn. Passage beyond the

epiglottis may be facilitated if the tube is rotated so that the bevel is facing up.

9) After the tube is in the pharynx, the larynx is exposed by using a rigid laryngoscope. If the tube impinges on the anterior commissure, it should be twisted while applying gentle downward pressure. The position of the larynx relative to the tube tip may be altered by flexing or extending the neck and/or applying external pressure on the larynx. If these manipulations do not align the tube and laryngeal opening, forceps can be used to grasp the tip and direct it through the vocal cords.

CLINICAL MOMENT The cuff should not be grasped using forceps because it may be damaged. This is especially important when using high-volume, low-pressure cuffs.

CLINICAL MOMENT Adding 10 to 15 mL of air to the tracheal tube cuff may cause the tip to align itself with the vocal cords. The tube tip is then advanced until the cuff contacts the vocal cords, at which point the cuff is deflated and the tube is inserted into the trachea.

10) If the tip passes through the vocal cords and then encounters resistance, it is likely that the tube curve is directing the tip into the anterior wall of the larynx. Withdrawing the tube slightly and flexing the neck will usually allow the tube to advance into the trachea. Other techniques include rotating the tube 180 degrees, passing a suction catheter or bougie through the tube into the larynx as a guide, and inserting a stylet with an anterior bend near the tip.

11) A blind technique may be useful when direct laryngoscopy or fiber-optic intubation would be difficult. There are instances in which blind nasal intubation may prove life saving, making the technique worth learning.

CLINICAL MOMENT Blind nasal intubation may start bleeding and ruin the chance to view the larynx through a fiberscope. A wire-reinforced or warmed standard tracheal tube may facilitate intubation with a fiberscope.

12) Blind nasal intubation may be performed under general or local anesthesia. A vasoconstrictor is usually used to prevent bleeding. A tracheal tube with directional tip control may improve the success rate. The patient is placed in the classical intubating position with the neck flexed and the head extended. After the tube is inserted through the nostril, it is advanced blindly. If the patient is breathing spontaneously, breath sounds can be heard as the tip approaches the larynx. When the sounds are at maximal intensity, the tube is gently but swiftly advanced during inspiration. If the sounds suddenly cease but the patient continues to breathe, the tube has entered the esophagus.

13) End-tidal CO_2 can be used as a guide to blind intubation. If CO_2 is no longer detected, the tube has entered the esophagus.
14) If the patient is not breathing, certain landmarks on the front of the neck (hyoid bone, notch of the thyroid cartilage, and the cricoid cartilage) can be observed. As the tube moves anteriorly, the tip will move these landmarks. The object is to move the tip to the midline at the thyroid angle, where it should enter the larynx. If the tip is above the thyroid cartilage, flexing the head will move the tip caudally. If the tip is below the thyroid cartilage, neck extension will move it cephalad. If the tip is lateral, then the tube should be withdrawn and twisted to direct it toward the midline. If the tube tip passes the laryngeal inlet but impinges on the anterior trachea, cervical flexion or rotating the tube 180 degrees may allow it to pass into the trachea.

c. Insertion Depth
1) Bronchial intubation and accidental extubation are common in spite of formulae and guidelines for tracheal tube insertion depth. These guidelines should be regarded only as a starting point because there is great variation in tracheal length.
2) In adults, the tube should be inserted until the cuff is 2.25 to 2.50 cm below the vocal cords. For uncuffed tubes, the tube tip should be inserted not more than 1 cm past the cords in children younger than 6 months; not more than 2 cm past the cords for patients up to 1 years of age; and 3 to 4 cm past the cords in older patients.
3) Some manufacturers place a mark above the cuff and recommend that the tube is advanced until this mark lies at the vocal cords (**Fig. 15.19**). There are variations in this type of marking and their position on the tube.
4) In adult patients of average size, securing the tube at the anterior incisors at 22 to 23 cm in men and 21 cm in women has been shown to be a reasonable starting point for tube placement. For nasal intubations, 5 cm should be added to these lengths for positioning at the nares.

E. Checking Tube Position

After the tube has been inserted, its position should be checked to be certain that it is in the tracheobronchial tree and that it is neither too deep nor too shallow. Methods to detect bronchial or esophageal intubation are discussed later in this chapter. After correct placement is confirmed, the portion external to the patient may be shortened to prevent kinking.

F. Inflating the Cuff

1. **Low-Volume, High-Pressure Cuff**

A high-pressure cuff should be inflated with the minimal amount of gas that will cause it to seal against the trachea at peak inspiratory pressure and prevent aspiration. Listening with the unaided ear will often miss small leaks. These can be detected by palpating or auscultating the pretracheal area. Inflating the cuff until the pilot balloon is tense and/or inflating beyond seal will result in unnecessarily high cuff volume and pressure. Intracuff pressure cannot be used to indicate the pressure on the trachea.

2. **Low-Pressure, High-Volume Cuff**

a. A low-pressure, high-volume cuff should be inflated to a pressure of 20 to 34 cm H_2O at end expiration in adults. A lower pressure should be used in children. The pressure should be measured (**Fig. 15.22**) and adjusted approximately 10 minutes after the tube has been inserted. This delay is necessary to allow the cuff material to soften at body temperature and for the patient to become settled. The volume necessary for occlusion will vary with muscle tone. Not measuring the pressure usually results in a pressure well above that recommended.

b. After the cuff pressure has been adjusted, check to make certain that there is no leak at peak airway pressure. A leak can be detected by measuring the difference between inhaled and exhaled volumes, hearing a noise with a stethoscope or detecting CO_2 in the upper airway.

CLINICAL MOMENT Cuff pressure should be measured and adjusted frequently. Changes in muscle tone in the trachea and gas diffusion across the cuff may result in large changes in pressure. Peak inspiratory pressure may also change, so frequent checks for leaks should also be performed.

c. When a tracheal tube with a Lanz pressure-regulating valve is used, the cuff should be inflated until a seal is achieved during peak inspiration. The pilot balloon should be distended but to a lesser extent than the confining sheath.

3. **Sponge Cuff**
   a. After intubation, the inflation tube should be opened to atmosphere and the cuff allowed to fill with air. The amount of air in the cuff should be determined by withdrawing the air with a syringe. The ability to remove 2 to 3 mL from the smallest cuff or 5 to 6 mL or more from the largest cuff usually signifies that the cuff:tracheal wall pressure ratio will allow adequate mucosal perfusion. If little or no air can be aspirated, the cuff may be too large.
   b. If a leak is present after the cuff has been allowed to expand, wrinkles in the cuff may be present and may be straightened out by injecting 2 or 3 mL of air into the cuff and then allowing it to deflate. If the leak persists, a larger tube may be needed.

G. Securing the Tube

1. Adhesive tape is most commonly used to maintain the tube in the desired position. A variety of taping methods have been used. The part of the tube to which the tape is to be applied should be thoroughly dried. Tapes do not adhere to all tracheal tubes equally well, so it is advisable to test available tapes in order to determine which works best for the chosen tube.
2. Many patients have beards or mustaches, making it difficult to attach the tape. For patients with sufficiently long mustache, it can be taped to the tracheal tube. Because hair is an insecure medium for fixing a tube, a close-fitting skullcap, elastic net, or a towel taped around the head may be used to provide a structure to attach the tape or ties (**Fig. 15.27**). Another method is to use double-sided tape to attach an elastic strap.
3. Some patients have cutaneous responses to adhesive tape. Fragile skin is commonly associated with prematurity, long-term steroid treatment, zinc deficiency, amyloidosis, epidermolysis bullosa, and cosmetic skin exfoliant use. In such cases, other means such as a tie around the patient's head should be used to anchor the tube.
4. Special devices (tube holders, fixation devices) for securing tracheal tubes without using adhesives or ties are available commercially. A tube holder may be combined with a bite block and/or a nasogastric tube holder.

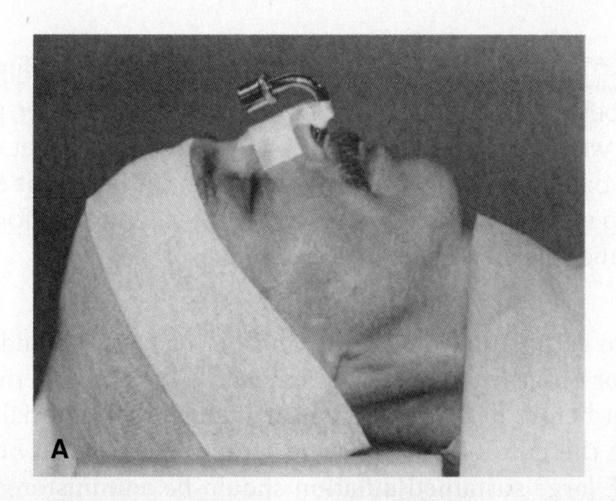

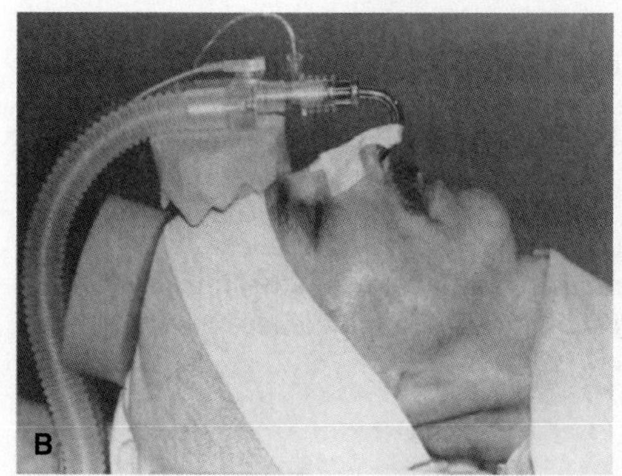

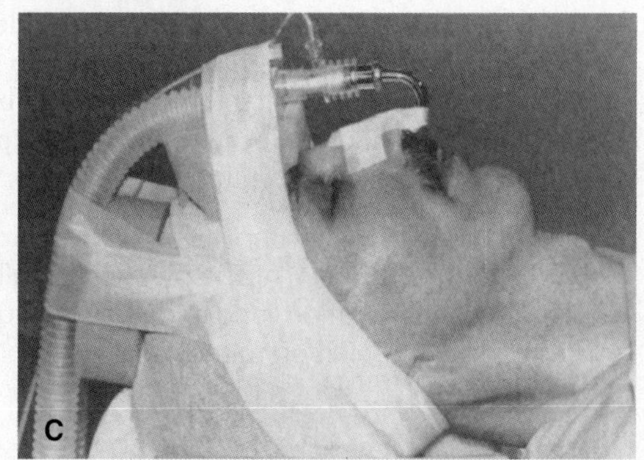

Figure 15.27 Method of securing a nasotracheal tube. **A:** A skullcap is placed around the head. An acute-angle connector is used and taped so that it does not exert pressure on the nasal ala. **B:** Foam padding is used to keep the breathing system from exerting pull on the tracheal tube. **C:** Tape is added to keep the breathing system firmly in place.

5. Craniofacial procedures and burns or other conditions in which adhesive tape is not acceptable may be managed by securing the tracheal tube to a stable tooth, the tongue, mandible, maxilla, or the nasal septum by using a wire or suture.
6. Nasal preformed and other tubes and breathing systems that run over the top of the head present a particular problem. Backward pull on the breathing system will cause the tube to put pressure on the cartilage and skin at the tip of the nose. This may cause necrosis that is difficult to repair. One method to secure the tube is shown in **Figure 15.27.**

H. Removing the Tube

1. The oral airway or bite block should remain in place until after extubation to prevent the patient from biting the tube during emergence from anesthesia. Spraying lidocaine down the tracheal tube or inflating the cuff with lidocaine will attenuate the airway and circulatory reactions during emergence from anesthesia and extubation, as will intravenous lidocaine. Respiratory and cardiovascular complications that are commonly associated with extubation can be decreased by inserting a supraglottic airway device (Chapter 13) before or just after the tracheal tube is removed.

CLINICAL MOMENT Extubating a patient in whom it may be difficult to reestablish an airway is best carried out in a staged or "reversible" manner, permitting reintubation while administrating oxygen by insufflation or jet ventilation when the airway is being secured. An airway exchange catheter that can be connected to the breathing system or another oxygen source can be used for this purpose. In the very small patient, a guide wire may be used.

2. Before extubation, the mouth and the pharynx should be suctioned and the tape or other fixation means removed. Withdrawing the tube until resistance is met before deflating the cuff may push the material that has accumulated above the cuff into the pharynx, from where it can be removed by suctioning. A large sustained inflation should be administered through the tracheal tube. Alternately, the adjustable pressure-limiting (APL) valve can be closed and airway pressure allowed to rise to 5 to 10 cm H_2O. While the lung is near total capacity, the cuff should be deflated and the tube removed. If a syringe cannot be located, the tip of a pen can be inserted into the valve assembly to deflate the cuff.

CLINICAL MOMENT The practice of pulling the pilot balloon and the inflation valve from the inflation tube to deflate the cuff should be discouraged because this can cause the inflation tube to seal.

CLINICAL MOMENT Suction should not be applied to the tracheal tube during extubation because this can deflate the lung and result in oxygen desaturation.

CLINICAL MOMENT If the tracheal tube cannot be easily removed, the inflation tube should be checked for obstruction, especially at the point where tape is used to hold the tube in place. If the surgery involves the mouth, neck, or thorax, a suture may be placed through or around the tube. If the tube is forcibly removed in this circumstance, the surgical site may be disrupted. If there is a possibility that the tube has been fixed in the airway, consult the surgeon before tube removal.

I. Using Open but Unused Tubes

Many clinicians feel that it is necessary to open one or more tubes of different sizes. This raises the question as to whether it is safe to store these tubes for use on another day. Studies indicate that tracheal tubes can be safely used up to 14 days after being opened if the tip is kept in its original wrapper. If a lubricant was used, it may dry out and form flakes, so the tube should be discarded.

IV. Perioperative Complications

A. Failure of the Tube to Pass into the Trachea over an Intubating Device

It is sometimes difficult to pass (railroad) a tracheal tube over a fiberscope, bougie, or AEC and through the glottic opening. When using a flexible endoscope, this can often be prevented by using the largest scope that fits easily inside the tracheal tube and keeping the fiberscope in the midline. A tube with a tip designed to minimize the distance between the fiberscope and the leading edge of the tube may pass more easily than a standard tube. A spiral embedded tube may pass more easily over a fiberscope than a tube with a preformed curve. Warming and thereby softening a standard tracheal tube may facilitate its passage. The tube may pass more easily if it is reverse loaded (upside down from its natural curvature) or with the bevel facing posteriorly.

CLINICAL MOMENT The tube tip may impinge on laryngeal structures. If this occurs, then the tube should be withdrawn a short distance, rotated counterclockwise 90 degrees, and finally advanced. This will overcome the obstruction in most cases.

B. Trauma

1. Reported injuries to the larynx include hematomas, contusions, lacerations, puncture wounds, cord avulsions, and fractures. Arytenoid cartilage dislocation may also occur.
2. With nasotracheal intubation, nasal mucosa abrasion or laceration is common. The nasal septum may be dislocated or perforated. Fragments of adenoid tissue, nasal polyps, or turbinates may be dislodged. Blood clots from epistaxis may enter the trachea and block a bronchus. Softening by prewarming has been shown to decrease trauma.
3. Cases of tracheal, bronchial, pharyngeal, nasal, hypopharyngeal, pyriform sinus, esophageal, and laryngeal perforation have been reported, sometimes with fatal consequences.

CLINICAL MOMENT When using a stylet in the tracheal tube to facilitate intubation, ensure that the stylet tip does not protrude from the end of the tracheal tube or through the Murphy eye. If the stylet protrudes through the Murphy eye, it may be difficult or impossible to remove.

4. The best way to avoid trauma is never to use more than a gentle pressure. Methods to decrease trauma to the nose are discussed in the nasal intubation section.

C. Esophageal Intubation

Esophageal intubation can occur even with an experienced anesthesia provider. Recognition and prompt correction are necessary to prevent dire consequences. In most patients, recognizing esophageal intubation is not difficult. Sometimes, the signs so closely resemble tracheal placement that they can deceive even a careful and experienced individual. In many of the reported cases of esophageal intubation, one or more of the following tests were performed but were misleading.

1. **Direct Visualization**

   Directly visualizing the tube passage between the vocal cords is one of the most reliable methods. Unfortunately, the glottis often cannot be seen well. Even if the tube is visualized between the cords, it may slip out as the laryngoscope or stylet is removed or the tube is secured.

2. **Reservoir Bag Compliance or Movement**

   Normal reservoir bag compliance and refilling with manual ventilation is an unreliable method to determine correct tracheal tube placement. It may be more reliable if performed with no fresh gas flow. A related test is observing reservoir bag movement in time with the patient's spontaneous respiratory efforts. However, tidal volumes have been noted with the tube in the esophagus. This method is not useful if the patient has received muscle relaxants.

3. **Chest Wall Motion**
   Some anesthesia providers rely on visual and/or manual evidence of chest wall movement during ventilation. Unfortunately, chest wall movement simulating lung ventilation can occur with the tube in the esophagus, especially in patients whose respiration is primarily abdominal. Chest wall movement may be difficult to assess in the obese patient or the patient with large breasts. Low lung or chest wall compliance may result in little chest movement, even when the tube is in the trachea. Listening through the open end of the tracheal tube while the sternum is abruptly depressed can also be misleading.
4. **Auscultation**
   a. Auscultation should be performed in the high region of each midaxillary area and not just the anterior chest region. The sound quality is important. A gurgling sound (death rattle) suggests esophageal placement. This test is not always reliable. Auscultating the upper abdomen as well as the lungs may increase reliability, although these sounds may be confused with breath sounds that are often heard in the epigastric area in thin individuals and pediatric patients.
   b. Auscultation can also be helpful if the stethoscope is placed on the neck at the cricoid cartilage level. If the tracheal tube is then moved upward and downward, the sound of the tube moving over tracheal rings may be heard.
   c. Another method to determine tracheal tube location is breathing system auscultation. A stethoscope is attached to an adaptor in the breathing system adjacent to the tracheal tube. If the tube is in the trachea, loud breath sounds can be heard. If the tube is in the esophagus, squeaks or flatus-like sounds may be heard. This test is also not totally reliable.
5. **Epigastric Distention**
   The abdomen can be observed for gastric distention. Unfortunately, the abdomen does not always distend with intermittent gastric inflation. Gastric distention could also result from mask ventilation before intubation is attempted. If there is a hiatal hernia or intrathoracic gastrointestinal contents, abdominal distention may not occur with esophageal intubation. The presence of a nasogastric tube may make gastric filling difficult to distinguish from normal abdominal movements during ventilation.
6. **Oxygenation**
   Good patient color and satisfactory pulse oximeter readings have been advocated as a means to confirm tracheal tube placement. Unfortunately, with preoxygenation, hypoxemia may be delayed for a few minutes after esophageal intubation. A later onset of hypoxemia may occur from other causes beside esophageal intubation and must be ruled out. By that time, esophageal intubation may not be suspected. If oxygen saturation improves after intubation and ventilation, it is likely that the tube is in the tracheobronchial tree.
7. **Palpation**
   During intubation, a washboard-like sensation can often be felt by the individual who manipulates the larynx or tube or applies cricoid pressure as the tube passes over the tracheal rings. After tube placement, maneuvers such as

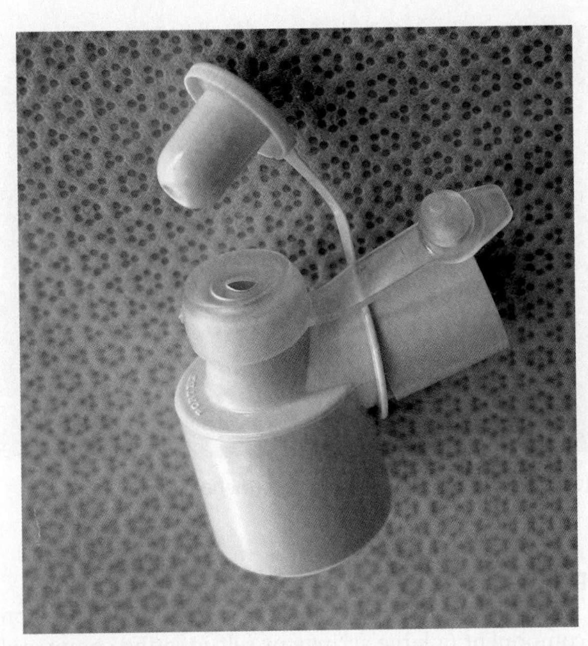

Figure 15.28 Adaptor to allow a fiberscope or other device (such as an AEC) to be inserted without interrupting ventilation.

inflating and deflating the cuff rapidly, squeezing the pilot balloon, or moving the tube in and out may be felt when the neck is palpated at the suprasternal notch. The "roll test" involves gentle backward pressure on the cricoid cartilage and simultaneous side-to-side displacement of the cartilage in an attempt to detect a tracheal tube lying behind in the esophagus. None of these tests is reliable.

8. **Fiberscopic View**
   The tracheal rings can be visualized with a fiberscope or an optical stylet. A special adaptor (**Fig. 15.28**) with a port allows ventilation while the examination is carried out. This is a reliable method but requires special instrumentation, skill, and time. If the tube tip hangs up on the anterior commissure, it may be possible to visualize the trachea, even though the tube is not in the trachea.
9. **Intentional Bronchial Intubation**
   The tracheal tube may be intentionally advanced into a mainstem bronchus. The chest is then auscultated during positive-pressure ventilation. If breath sounds can be heard on only one side, bronchial intubation has been achieved. With esophageal intubation, the breath sounds are either equal bilaterally or equally diminished or absent on both sides of the chest.
10. **Pressure- and Flow-Volume Loops**
    Pressure- and flow-volume loops are discussed in Chapter 18. If the tracheal tube is in the esophagus, the loops will not have their characteristic shapes. The loop will probably be open, indicating that some gas went into the patient's stomach but failed to return to the breathing system during exhalation. Although it will not detect all esophageal intubations, this test has a high likelihood of success.

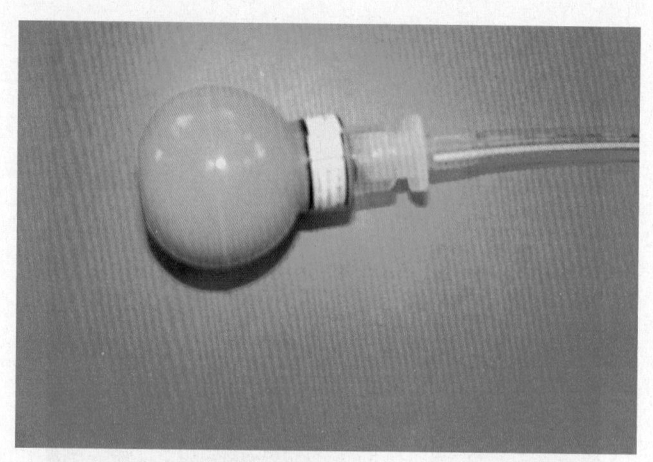

Figure 15.29 Esophageal detector device attached to a tracheal tube.

11. **Esophageal Detector Device**
    a. The esophageal detector device (EDD) (**Fig. 15.29**) consists of an aspirating component (a large syringe or self-inflating compressible bulb) attached to the tracheal tube with an adaptor. First, gas is forced though the tracheal tube by pushing the syringe plunger or by squeezing the bulb. The plunger is then withdrawn, or the compressed bulb is released. If the tube is in the trachea and an airtight seal has been achieved, gas will aspirate from the patient's lungs without resistance. If the tube is in the esophagus, apposition of the esophageal walls around the tube tip will occlude the lumen and cause a negative pressure or resistance. As a confirmatory test, the device can be used to inject a bolus of air into the tube while listening over the epigastrium. This test will also detect a blocked tracheal tube. The EDD should be used immediately after tube placement, before delivering the first breath.
    b. Most studies show that the EDD has a high degree of accuracy in identifying esophageal intubation even with inexperienced users, but one study indicated poor sensitivity. The presence of a nasogastric tube or tracheal tube cuff deflation does not limit its efficacy. Its accuracy is not affected by a lack of pulmonary perfusion. It is faster than most other methods. This device may be more accurate than exhaled CO_2 in the cardiac arrest patient. This device is unreliable in patients younger than 1 year.
    c. It is possible to get a false-negative result with the EDD when the tube is in the trachea but the bulb expands too slowly or not at all. Some investigators found that there were fewer false-negative results if 10 seconds were allowed for reinflation. The bulb will not reexpand rapidly in patients with decreased expiratory reserve volume (e.g., morbidly obese or pregnant patients; patients with bronchospastic disease; tracheomalacia; pulmonary edema; bronchial intubation; and upper or lower airway obstruction). A high number of false-positive and false-negative results were found in patients having cesarean delivery. The incidence of false-negative results is reduced if the bulb is compressed after connection to the tracheal tube. Another cause of a false-negative result is the tube bevel resting against the tracheal wall. If the tracheal tube tip is above the cords, a false-negative result can be obtained.

d. False-positive results with the EDD have been reported in patients in whom the tracheal tube was not in the trachea but the device suggested otherwise. These are often associated with an incompetent gastroesophageal junction (obesity, pregnancy) or gastric inflation.

12. **Exhaled Carbon Dioxide Monitoring**

a. Carbon dioxide monitoring is discussed in detail in Chapter 17. Although not foolproof, this is generally considered the most reliable method to detect esophageal intubation. The American Society of Anesthesiologists Standards for Basic Anesthetic Monitoring and the American Association of Nurse Anesthetists require that when a tracheal tube is inserted, its correct position must be verified by identifying CO_2 in the exhaled gas. It has been found to be reliable in circumstances in which the EDD was unreliable.

b. Carbon dioxide may not be detected despite correct placement because of severe bronchospasm, cardiac arrest, no pulmonary blood flow (from problems such as pulmonary embolism), or a one-way obstruction in the tracheal tube. The EDD may be a more reliable device in these circumstances. Carbon dioxide may be detected when the tube tip is above the vocal cords.

c. There are some circumstances in which CO_2 may be detected if the tube is in the esophagus. Exhaled gases may have been forced into the stomach during mask ventilation before intubation. Carbon dioxide can be in the stomach either as a by-product of antacids that have reacted with gastric acid or from ingested carbonated beverages. In these cases, the end-tidal CO_2 will be low and the capnogram (Chapter 17) will have an abnormal and irregular configuration. Carbon dioxide levels will rapidly diminish with repeated ventilation.

D. Inadvertent Bronchial Intubation

1. **General**

a. Bronchial placement can lead to atelectasis in the nonventilated lung. The lung that is ventilated may become hyperinflated, leading to barotrauma and hypotension. If the tip impinges on the carina, persistent coughing and bucking may occur.

b. Bronchial intubation is a relatively common problem. It occurs more frequently with emergency intubations and in pediatric and female patients. Proper positioning can be especially difficult in pediatric patients. Preformed tubes may be more likely than standard tubes to cause bronchial intubation, especially in children.

c. Bronchial intubation can occur after correct initial placement. A tracheal tube may descend into a bronchus from the weight of the attachments, suctioning, neck or head movement, or patient repositioning. The tube will usually move caudally with neck or head flexion, mouth opening, or a change in position from erect to recumbent. The distance from the cords to the carina is decreased during laparoscopy and with the Trendelenburg position. Manipulating an instrument introduced into the mouth, such as a transesophageal echocardiography probe, gastroscope, or tongue depressor, can result in tracheal tube movement.

CLINICAL MOMENT It is important that correct tube position is confirmed after the patient's position has been altered or the head and neck has been moved. A tube originally, properly placed in the trachea may have entered a mainstem bronchus.

2. **Detection**

A number of techniques and tests have been recommended to avoid or detect bronchial intubation. These should be performed just after intubation and at intervals during an anesthetic procedure, especially after the patient is repositioned or the head and neck are moved.

a. Lung Auscultation

Auscultation for bronchial intubation should be performed bilaterally in the midaxillary areas. Auscultation may be misleading, as breath sounds can be transmitted to the opposite side of the chest in the presence of bronchial intubation, unless the tube is wedged firmly in a bronchus. A Murphy eye may reduce the reliability of chest auscultation to detect bronchial intubation.

b. Chest Radiograph

Chest X-rays are reliable but time-consuming and expensive. The tracheal tube has a radiopaque marker at the patient end or along the full length of the tube. In adults, the tube tip should be 3, 5, or 7 cm above the carina, with the neck flexed, neutral, or extended. The tip should lie over the second to fourth thoracic vertebrae or at the clavicle level with the head in the neutral position. In neonates, infants, and young children, the tip should be 2 cm above the carina, with the neck in the neutral position. In children approaching 5 to 6 years of age, this distance should be increased to 3 cm.

c. Tube Position at the Lips/Nostril

1) In adults, it has been recommended that oral tubes be positioned at the 21-cm mark on the tube at the teeth (or upper anterior edge of the gums in edentulous patients) in normal sized women and 22 to 23 cm in normal-size men. For nasal intubation, 5 cm needs to be added to these lengths for positioning at the nostril. Studies show that this is a better method of preventing bronchial intubation than chest auscultation. It will, however, result in bronchial intubation in some patients.
2) There is a correlation between airway length and body height. For patients whose body lengths lie outside the normal range, the tube can be placed alongside the patient's face and neck. The tube tip is aligned to the suprasternal notch, and the tube's machine end is aligned to conform to the position of a nasal or oral tracheal tube. The point on the tube at which the tube intersects with the teeth or gums (oral intubation) or the nares (nasal intubation) is noted and then the tube is secured at that point.
3) The margin of safety in children is less than in adults. While using special formulas may decrease the incidence of bronchial intubation, they are based on averages and should not be considered totally reliable. A number of formulas have been developed, including the following:
4) Oral Intubation
   (i) Length in centimeters = (age/2) + 12.
   (ii) Length in centimeters = (weight in kilograms/5) + 12.
   (iii) Length in centimeters = (height in centimeters/10) + 5.
   (iv) Rule of 7-8-9: Infants weighing 1 kg are intubated to a depth of 7 cm, 2-kg infants to a depth of 8 cm, and 3-kg infants to a depth of 9 cm.

5) Nasotracheal Intubation
   (i) $L = (S \times 3) + 2$, where L is the length in centimeters and S is the ID of the tube in millimeters.
   (ii) Multiplying the crown-heel length by 0.21.
   (iii) For total tube length, 0.16 × height in centimeters + 4.5 cm and then leave 2 cm of the tube outside the nostril of an infant and 3 cm outside for an older child.

d. Placing the Cuff Just below the Vocal Cords
Placing the cuff only a few centimeters below the vocal cords should prevent bronchial intubation in adults.

e. Guide Marks on the Tracheal Tube
Many tubes have lines or rings to help to position the tube with respect to the vocal cords (**Figs. 15.2** and **15.4**), whereas the distal portion of some pediatric tubes are colored (**Fig. 15.19**). Guide (depth) marks vary in their position relative to the cuff and tube tip. These guide marks have been shown not to be consistently accurate enough to avoid bronchial intubation.

f. Fiberscopic Observation through the Tube
Passing a fiberscope through the tube is equal in accuracy and faster than a chest X-ray for determining tube position in both adults and pediatric patients and is more accurate than auscultation. The ready availability of fiberscopes in most OR suites makes this a practical method for checking the tube position. Head and neck movement during the examination may cause the tube to move.

g. Monitoring Exhaled Carbon Dioxide
Monitoring exhaled CO_2 is not a reliable means to detect bronchial intubation, as either increased or decreased end-tidal CO_2 may be seen.

h. Pressure- and Flow-Volume Loops
Pressure–volume loops (Chapter 18) can often be used to detect bronchial intubation. The pressure–volume loop will show decreased compliance when the tracheal tube enters a mainstem bronchus. As the tube is withdrawn, there will be a marked sudden improvement in compliance as the tube leaves the bronchus. If peak inflation pressure is monitored while delivering a constant tidal volume, bronchial intubation will cause an increase in peak inflation pressure.

CLINICAL MOMENT Pressure- and flow-volume loops may be used to determine proper tracheal tube placement. After the tube is inserted below the vocal cords, reference loops are recorded. The tube is then advanced into a bronchus. When there is a sharp reduction in tidal volume or compliance, the tube tip is in the bronchus. It is then withdrawn until the loops return to normal.

i. Other
Decreased oxygen saturation measured by pulse oximetry (Spo_2) or transcutaneous oxygen is often seen with bronchial intubation. Desaturation will not always be seen, even with massive atelectasis. If the patient is receiving a high oxygen concentration, the oxygen saturation may not fall.

3. **Treatment**
   When a tracheal tube is assumed to be in a bronchus, the cuff should be deflated and the tube gently withdrawn, the cuff reinflated, and the position rechecked. If reintubation would be difficult, consideration should be given to advancing a fiberscope or AEC (see the following text) into the tube before withdrawing it. If extubation occurs, the tracheal tube can be quickly reinserted.

E. Swallowed Tracheal Tube
There are a number of case reports of a tracheal tube being lost in the esophagus, often during newborn resuscitation or in an adult following emergency intubation. Using a connector that fits firmly into the tube can prevent this complication. The tube should be long enough so that it protrudes from the mouth when correctly placed and firmly secured. Tape should be attached to the tube rather than the connector. If this complication occurs, the tube may not need to be removed immediately unless it interferes with ventilation.

CLINICAL MOMENT Bonding between the connector and the tube will be increased if the connector is wiped with alcohol before being inserted into the tube.

F. Foreign Body Aspiration
1. During intubation, a variety of materials can be aspirated into the trachea. The tracheal tube may dislodge fragments of tissue from the oral or nasal cavity, pharynx, or larynx.
2. A portion of a cuff or the tube shaft, including the punched out area from the Murphy eye still in situ, may remain in the airway. A tracheal tube can separate from its connector and slip below the cords. This is most likely to occur with shortened and pediatric tracheal tubes.
3. Other foreign bodies that have been found in tracheal tubes include cottonoids or pieces of aluminum used to protect the cuff or shaft from a laser beam, the distal portion of a tracheal tube, a cap liner from a tube of anesthetic ointment, teeth, and parts of spray devices and a laryngoscope.
4. Careful equipment inspection before use will help to avoid foreign body aspiration. The connector should fit firmly in the tracheal tube, and the tape or securing device should be attached to the tube and not the connector. When a cuff leaks, it should be carefully examined for missing portions after it is removed from the patient.
5. Foreign body aspiration should be suspected whenever obstructive signs or symptoms appear. The patient's airway should be searched immediately and should include bronchoscopy if the foreign body is not discovered above the larynx. If the foreign body is above the cuff, it might be possible to blow it out of the trachea by deflating the cuff while forcibly compressing the reservoir bag in the breathing system.

CLINICAL MOMENT If there are any teeth that are loose and likely to become dislodged, a suture should be tied around them before induction so that they can be easily retrieved if they are dislodged.

G. Leaks

1. A leak may make it difficult to maintain adequate ventilation, fail to protect against aspiration, and make oral surgery difficult. During insertion, the cuff, inflation tube, or the tube itself may be torn by a tooth, turbinate, implant, laryngoscope blade, forceps, or stylet. A problem with the inflation system may make it impossible to inflate the cuff. A defect in the tube or eccentric cuff inflation can cause a leak. The cuff may be located above the vocal cords, which could result in a leak despite a large amount of air being injected into the cuff.

CLINICAL MOMENT If there is a leak with the pilot balloon inflated, the cuff may be resting above the vocal cords.

2. The cuff can develop a leak while the tube is in place. Applying local anesthetic spray has been associated with cuff leaks. The cuff or other parts of the tube may be damaged during internal jugular or subclavian vein cannulation or during percutaneous dilatational tracheostomy or other nearby procedures. A laser beam can perforate the cuff. A tube may be damaged by biting.

CLINICAL MOMENT If a leak becomes evident after a gastric tube or other device has been placed, the device may have passed into the trachea alongside the tracheal tube instead of passing into the esophagus.

3. When a leak is present, laryngoscopy should be performed, if possible. If the cuff is above the vocal cords, it should be deflated and the tube advanced before the cuff is reinflated. Consideration should be given to using a tube changer or fiberscope during this procedure, especially if intubation was difficult.
4. If the problem is in the inflation system, it may be possible to repair the damage, or bypass the leak by inserting a stopcock, small catheter, or needle into the line below the defect. It may be possible to seal a cut in the tube itself by using glue. Approximating the cut edges and circumferential packing may be helpful.

CLINICAL MOMENT If the cuff is leaking, pharyngeal packing or placing a supraglottic device over the tube may help to control the leak. The fresh gas flow can be increased to overcome the loss of gas. Injecting a mixture of lidocaine and saline or a saline infusion into the cuff may be helpful. In some cases, it may be necessary to change the tube.

CLINICAL MOMENT When a damaged tube is removed, it should be carefully examined to make certain there are no missing portions.

CLINICAL MOMENT If the cuff develops a small leak and the tube cannot be easily changed, air can be added to the cuff by using a syringe pump.

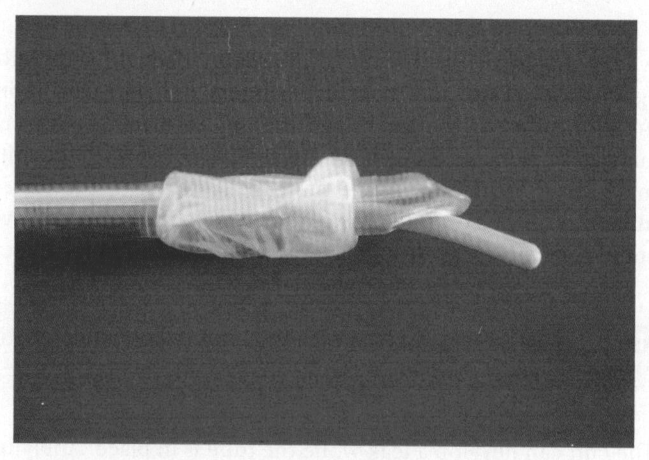

Figure 15.30 The tube changer has become caught in the Murphy eye.

H. Device Trapped inside the Tracheal Tube

Whenever any device is placed through a tracheal tube, there is a risk that it could become entrapped in the tube. Anything passed down the tracheal tube such as a suction catheter, tube exchanger, or fiberscope can pass through a Murphy eye and become caught (**Fig. 15.30**).

CLINICAL MOMENT In most cases, the best course of action when something is caught in a tracheal tube is to replace the tube.

I. Tracheal Tube Fires

Fires in tracheal tubes have a high likelihood of causing serious harm. They are discussed in Chapter 25.

J. Tracheal Tube Obstruction

One reason for inserting a tracheal tube is to provide a patent airway. Unfortunately, the tube itself may become the cause of obstruction. This is especially a problem with infants and children. Obstruction can be partial or complete. Inspiration may be unimpeded while resistance to exhalation is increased or vice versa.

1. **Causes**

a. Biting

Unless protection in the form of a bite block or oral airway is provided, the patient may bite and obstruct the tube. Many of the reported cases involve spiral embedded tubes that were permanently deformed after the bite was released (**Fig. 15.31**).

b. Kinking

Kinking is a frequent cause of tracheal tube obstruction. Spiral embedded tubes have been used to overcome this problem, but kinking can still occur at the breathing system end if the connector is not inside the spirals. Kinking sometimes occurs when the patient's head position is changed, especially when the neck is flexed. Another site prone to kinking is where the inflation tube exits the tracheal tube wall. It can also occur when a tube is moved from one side of the mouth to the other. Some tubes may kink after they become warmed and softened in the pharynx. Kinking can be caused by other equipment, such as a retractor, in the mouth. A manufacturing defect can also cause obstruction.

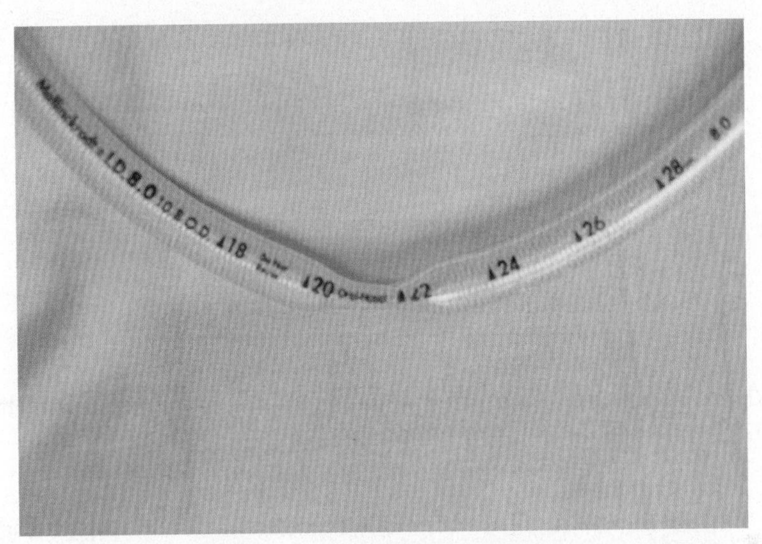

Figure 15.31 Spiral embedded tube permanently deformed by patient biting down on it.

CLINICAL MOMENT If there is a sudden increase in breathing system pressure or a change in the pressure–volume loop, tracheal tube kinking should be suspected. A digital examination may be required to determine the kink location.

CLINICAL MOMENT If a tracheal tube kinks in the mouth and cannot easily be changed, it may be possible to insert an intubating airway around the tube to relieve the kink.

c. Material in the Tube Lumen
A tracheal tube may be obstructed by dried secretions, blood, pus, adenoid tissue after a nasotracheal intubation, tumor, or other tissue. Lubricant that is used to help put the connector into the tube may dry and form a film. A variety of foreign bodies have been found in tracheal tubes, including a tooth, foam rubber from a mask, an inflation valve, a cleaning brush, an adaptor from an intravenous set, an intravenous needle, a stopcock from a stylet, a cork, a glass ampoule, pieces of plastic, part of a nasogastric tube, an oral medication tablet, a smaller tracheal tube, part of a paper towel, part of a sampling tube, caps from syringes, and dead organisms. Part of a stylet or stylet cover can be detached and remain in the lumen.

d. Spiral Embedded Tube Occlusion
Most spiral embedded tubes do not have a Murphy eye. Anything that blocks the bevel can cause obstruction. In some spiral embedded tubes, the part of the tube distal to the cuff has no spirals. This part may become soft and easily occluded. Reusing spiral embedded tubes predisposes to problems. Even single-use tubes may have air bubbles in the wall that enlarge with exposure to nitrous oxide and cause obstruction.

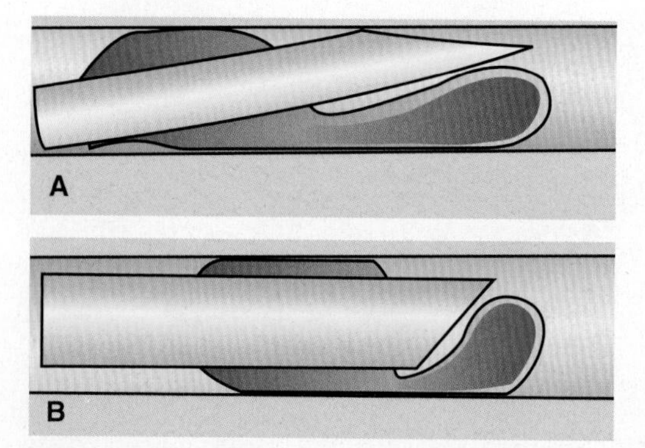

Figure 15.32 Causes of tracheal tube obstruction. **A:** The bevel is pushed against the wall of the trachea by an eccentrically inflated cuff. **B:** The cuff has ballooned over the end of the tube.

e. Cuff Problems
If the cuff herniates or inflates eccentrically, it may displace the bevel from the center of the trachea (**Fig. 15.32**). Eccentric cuff expansion from diffused anesthetic gases can cause it to expand in one direction and cause the bevel to impinge against the tracheal wall (**Figs. 15.32A** and **15.33**). An inflated cuff may balloon over the tube tip (**Fig. 15.32**). Inflating the cuff may compress the tube lumen (**Fig. 15.34**). Obstruction from these causes may not occur until sometime after initial cuff inflation.

CLINICAL MOMENT Deflating the cuff may relieve tracheal tube obstruction.

f. External Compression or Displacement
The trachea may be displaced by the aorta. The thyroid gland may cause the bevel to lie against the tracheal wall or compress the tube. A nasogastric tube or suction catheter knotted around the tube or a nearby surgical retractor can cause compression. External tracheal tube compression has been reported in association with Ludwig's angina, Forestier's disease, and "saber-sheath" trachea. Bony fragments from a LeFort fracture can cause

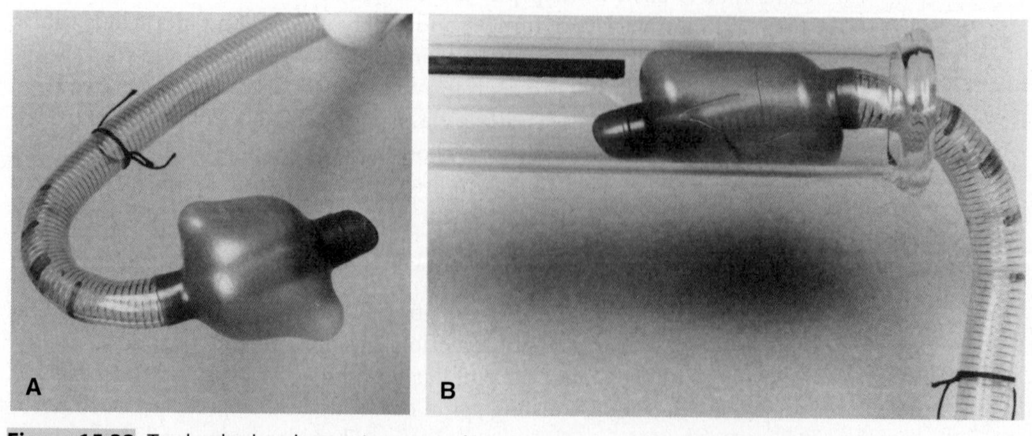

Figure 15.33 Tracheal tube obstruction secondary to eccentric cuff inflation. **A:** The cuff as removed from the patient. **B:** When placed in a glass tube, the inflated cuff pushes the bevel toward the wall of the tube.

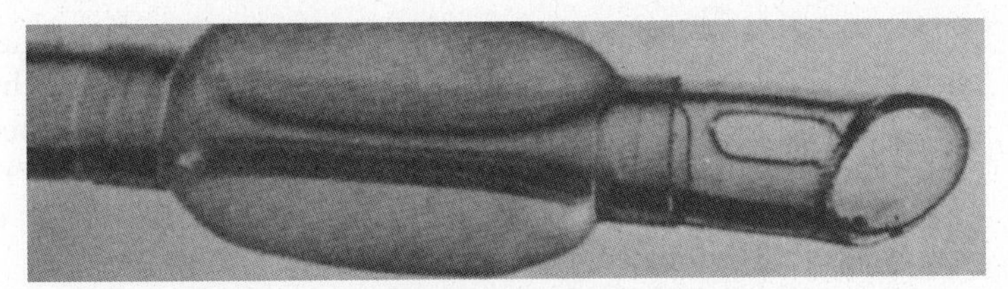

Figure 15.34 Reduction in tube lumen by cuff. Inflation of the cuff causes narrowing of the tube lumen.

external tube compression. Compression may not occur until the tracheal tube has warmed and softened.

g. Defective Connector

If the connector is defective or damaged, it can partially or completely obstruct the lumen. To avoid problems when reinserting the connector after shortening the tracheal tube, the tube should be cut diagonally. The connector should be lubricated slightly with alcohol, brought into the longitudinal axis of the tube, and then gently slid into the tube.

h. Change in Body Position

A shift in body position may cause the tracheal tube to become obstructed. When the tube orifice faces in one direction and the head is turned to the other, the orifice may face the tracheal wall.

2. **Prevention**

a. Prevention of tracheal tube obstruction starts with tube choice. Transparent tubes facilitate identification of material or objects blocking the lumen. Using a Murphy tube may avoid obstruction in some cases. A spiral embedded tube may be useful if an operation involves turning the head or other maneuvers that may cause kinking. Solutions or lubricants that can form a film barrier should be prevented from entering the tube lumen.

b. The tracheal tube should be examined carefully before use and the lumen patency verified. Foreign bodies and other obstructions inside the lumen can be detected by inserting a stylet. The cuff should be examined to make certain that it is securely attached and inflates symmetrically. The lumen should not be reduced when the cuff is inflated. If the tube has a soft flexible tip, a stylet should be used during insertion. After insertion, the cuff should be inflated as described earlier in this chapter. Cuff pressure should be readjusted frequently, especially if nitrous oxide is used. When an X-ray is taken, the orifice position and cuff configuration should be examined.

CLINICAL MOMENT Once inserted, the tube should not be withdrawn while the cuff is inflated, because this may cause the cuff to balloon over the end of the tube.

c. Placing a bite block securely between the molar teeth and maintaining an adequate level of anesthesia will prevent biting on the tube.

3. **Diagnosis and Treatment**

a. Partial tracheal tube obstruction may present as a decrease in compliance or expiratory flow, high inspiratory pressures, an increase in the difference between peak and plateau airway pressures with volume-controlled ventilation, reduced tidal volume during pressure-controlled ventilation, or wheezing. Pressure–volume loops (Chapter 18) are very helpful in diagnosing an obstruction. Paradoxical chest movements may be seen in spontaneously breathing patients. The capnograph (Chapter 17) may show an increased slope in phase III and a larger α angle. Relying on the anesthesia provider's "educated hand" is not reliable.

b. Passing a fiberscope down the tube may facilitate diagnosis. Altering the patient's head position or cuff deflation may relieve the obstruction. The tube can be checked for kinking either by examining manually with a gloved finger or visually with a laryngoscope or bronchoscope. Passing a suction catheter or stylet down the tube may be helpful.

c. Digital pressure at the site of the kink may relieve the obstruction. A kink in a small tube can sometimes be remedied by placing a larger tube over the kinked tube. If a large tube kinks, it may be possible to pass a smaller tube through it. A hemostat applied at 90 degrees to the occlusion may relieve obstruction caused by biting.

d. Equipment placed between the breathing system and the tracheal tube may be the source of the obstruction. These components should be considered in the differential diagnosis of obstruction, especially if they are added after the initial equipment check or just before the obstruction was detected.

K. Aspirating Fluid from above the Cuff

Although it is generally assumed that a tracheal tube will prevent foreign material from entering the lungs, aspiration can occur around the cuff. In one study of long-term intubation, secretions leaking around the tracheal tube cuff were the most important risk for developing pneumonia in the first 8 days of intubation. Use of a polyurethane cuffed tracheal tube may prevent early postoperative pneumonia by decreasing aspiration of contaminated upper airway secretions.

1. **Low-Pressure Cuffs**

Low cuff pressure (below 20 mm Hg) is associated with an increased risk of pneumonia in patients with long-term intubation. Many low-pressure cuffs wrinkle despite proper inflation and allow fluid to pass along the folds. Infolding can be decreased by increasing the pressure in the cuff, using a thin-walled cuff, and using a tube in which cuff diameter at residual volume approximates the internal tracheal diameter. Applying lubricant jelly to the cuff may fill in the folds and prevent aspiration. When nitrous oxide administration is discontinued, there will be an outflow of that gas from the cuff. This can cause the cuff to lose volume and decrease the seal. Using a tube with a polyurethane cuff may prevent fluid aspiration.

2. **Spontaneous Ventilation**

During spontaneous ventilation, there will be negative pressure in the airway during inspiration. In addition, the trachea tends to dilate during spontaneous inspiration. With thin-walled cuffs, the negative airway pressure will be transmitted to the cuff. If the negative pressure exceeds the leak pressure around the tube, blood or secretions may be drawn into the trachea. Intermittent positive pressure, PEEP, and pressure-supported ventilation will lower the incidence of aspiration but not totally prevent it.

3. **Fluid and Blood Accumulation above the Cuff**

a. Suctioning to maintain a clear oropharynx will decrease the fluid pressure above the cuff. If the patient is in a head-up position, the hydrostatic pressure exerted by the fluid will be higher than if the patient is supine or in a slightly head-down position. It has been suggested that the cuff be placed just below the vocal cords to reduce the volume of fluid that cannot be removed by suctioning, but in this position, head movement may cause the tube to move upward, causing the cuff to exert pressure on the cords and increasing the risk of inadvertent extubation. Furthermore, a cuff placed just below the cords may compress nerve endings against the thyroid cartilage, resulting in vocal cord paralysis.

CLINICAL MOMENT Blood from the pharynx can flow through the vocal cords and accumulate above the cuff. If sufficient time elapses, the blood clot can form a sheath above the cuff and between the tube and the tracheal wall. During extubation, this sheath may fall into the trachea or a bronchus, causing complete or partial obstruction. If any surgery occurs above the cuff, a gauze packing should be applied around the tube to collect any blood that could drain beneath the vocal cords.

b. A tracheal tube that incorporates a dedicated suction lumen and channel above the cuff can be used to clear secretions above the cuff. Using this tube may reduce the incidence of ventilator-associated pneumonia during long-term intubation.
c. Aspiration can occur on extubation. Pharyngeal suction may not remove all of the fluid above the tube, and it can find its way into the lungs when the tube is removed.

CLINICAL MOMENT Recommendations to avoid aspiration during extubation include withdrawing the inflated cuff until it impinges on the lower surface of the vocal cords, placing the patient in a head-down and lateral position before cuff deflation, and deflating the cuff while positive airway pressure is applied to blow material collected above the cuff into the pharynx, from where it can be removed by suctioning.

L. Other Equipment Entering the Trachea

A tracheal tube keeps the glottis open, making it easier to pass other equipment into the tracheobronchial tree. Items entering the trachea include gastric tubes, esophageal stethoscopes, temperature probes, and electrocardiogram (ECG) leads.

M. Scan Artifacts

Artifacts may be seen on a computed tomographic (CT) scan when radiopaque markers are present on a tracheal tube. Tubes without these markers are available and should be used for this application. The metallic spring in the tracheal tube inflation device can form an artifact on an MRI scan. Repositioning the spring away from the patient will usually solve the problem. Wire-reinforced tracheal tubes will cause image distortion when used in an MRI unit. Nylon-reinforced tubes are recommended for this application.

N. Unintended Extubation

1. Accidental (spontaneous) tracheal tube extubation is at best a nuisance and at worst a life-threatening emergency. It occurs more commonly in smaller patients and in patients with burns.
2. Neck extension or lateral head rotation can cause cephalad tube movement. This movement is increased with nasal intubation. The prone position or upper-airway swelling can cause the tube to move cephalad.

3. Removing a gastric tube entwined around the tracheal tube can cause accidental extubation.
4. Inadvertent extubation can occur when the cuff is positioned between or just below the cords. If the cuff is distended as a result of overinflation or nitrous oxide diffusion, it may herniate and push the tube upward. This may result in a leak. A common response is to inject more air into the cuff. If the cuff is at or just above the vocal cords, this may cause the tube to move farther out of the trachea.

CLINICAL MOMENT Removing an adhesive surgical drape that is positioned over the tracheal tube may result in unintended tube removal. This can be avoided by placing a nonstick cover over all tracheal tube parts that come into contact with the adhesive drape.

5. Antidisconnect devices may increase the risk of inadvertent extubation. It may be preferable for the connection between the tube and the breathing system to give way under strain than to cause the tube to be pulled out.
6. To prevent inadvertent extubation, the tube should be positioned with the tip in the middle third of the trachea and the neck in a neutral position. A cuff that requires frequent inflation may be situated between the vocal cords. The tube should be well secured. If the securing tape becomes wet, it should be replaced. Care should be taken to avoid extubation whenever the patient is positioned. Using an RAE tube may decrease the incidence of accidental extubation.

CLINICAL MOMENT If unplanned extubation occurs in the lateral or prone position, using a supraglottic device (Chapter 13) may be a better option than attempting tracheal intubation.

O. Infection

A high incidence of sinusitis and otitis during and following nasotracheal intubation has been reported. During long-term intubation, the rates of nosocomial sinusitis and pneumonia do not differ significantly between oral and nasal intubation. The incidence of bacteremia after oral or nasal intubation is approximately the same.

P. Difficult Extubation

1. A difficult extubation is a rare but dangerous problem. A common cause is failure to deflate the cuff. This may be caused by inflation tube obstruction. If the obstruction is distal to the pilot balloon, the balloon will offer no clue that the cuff has not deflated. Heat from a laser or a drill may melt the inflating tube or the patient may bite it, causing it to occlude. Some users pull the pilot balloon and inflation valve from the inflation tube to deflate the cuff. This can cause the inflation tube to seal. The connector may occlude the inflation tube if it fits below the point where the inflation tube leaves the tracheal tube wall. A retaining bandage may kink the inflation tube. The inflating tube may become entangled with a nasogastric tube or turbinate. A fold or flange in the cuff may impede extubation. Edema in the larynx may make extubation difficult. With a sponge cuff, deflation will be difficult if the inflation tube is cut or detached.

CLINICAL MOMENT If the tracheal or inflation tube is transfixed to adjacent tissues, extubation will not be possible. This problem occurs with surgical procedures near the tube. Forcibly removing the tube may cause tissue disruption and possibly lead to fatal consequences. Consult the surgeon to determine whether a suture or staple could be in the tracheal or inflating tube.

2. When it is impossible to deflate the cuff, a cut in the inflation tube may relieve the pressure in the cuff. It may be possible to insert a syringe and a needle into the stump of the pilot tube and deflate the cuff. If the cuff still remains inflated, the tube should be pulled out until the cuff is close to the undersurface of the vocal cords. A needle can then be inserted through the cricothyroid membrane, puncturing the cuff. Alternately, the tube can be withdrawn so that the cuff is seen below the cords and punctured from above with a sharp object. Removal may be aided by relaxing the vocal cords and/or tube rotation. If the tube is surgically fixed to adjacent tissues, surgical reexploration will probably be required.

Q. Emergence Phenomena

Undesirable phenomena during emergence and extubation include coughing, bucking, restlessness, increases in blood pressure, tachycardia, and increases in intraocular pressure. The incidence of most of these problems can be decreased by filling the tracheal tube cuff with a lidocaine solution. The addition of sodium bicarbonate increases the diffusion rate of lidocaine into the trachea. Spraying the trachea with lidocaine before intubation will decrease coughing on emergence from anesthesia of less than 2 hours' duration.

CLINICAL MOMENT If it is important that emergence phenomena not occur, a supraglottic device can be inserted and the tracheal tube removed while the patient is still deeply anesthetized.

R. Postoperative Sore Throat

Sore throat is a common postoperative complaint. It is more common in females, following operations involving the head and neck, when larger tubes are used, and when the patient is in the prone position. Cuff design may be a contributing factor. Limiting intracuff pressure may decrease the incidence. The incidence of sore throat is high with the sponge cuff.

S. Hoarseness

Hoarseness is commonly seen after intubation. Its incidence may be decreased by using tubes with low-pressure cuffs, smaller tubes, and lubrication with lidocaine jelly. Hoarseness increases with difficult or prolonged intubation but not with increased intracuff pressure. Hoarseness that is persistent or that develops later in the postoperative period should be investigated.

T. Neurologic Injuries

Trigeminal, lingual, buccal, and hypoglossal nerve palsies have been reported following short-term intubation. Mental nerve neuropraxia has been reported after an oral RAE tube was used.

U. Upper-Airway Edema

1. Edema may occur anywhere along the tube's path including the tongue, uvula, epiglottis, aryepiglottic folds, ventricular folds, vocal cords, and the retroarytenoid

and subglottic spaces. The mouth floor can swell due to sialadenitis from a submandibular duct obstructed by a tracheal tube.

2. Laryngeal edema (postintubation croup or inflammation, acute edematous stenosis, stridor, subglottic edema) encroaches on the airway lumen, especially in the young child in whom a mild degree of edema may produce a significant reduction in the internal cross-sectional area. Because the cricoid cartilage completely surrounds the subglottic region, swollen tissues may not expand externally at this location.
3. Laryngeal edema has a peak incidence between 1 and 4 years of age. The presence or absence of a leak or the history of a recent respiratory infection does not correlate with the incidence of croup. It is more common in women than in men. It is most commonly seen after surgery involving the head and neck and with longer surgical procedures.
4. Edema may manifest itself any time during the first 48 hours after extubation. Usually, the first signs are evident 1 to 2 hours postoperatively. In its mildest form, there is hoarseness or croupy cough. In the most severe cases, respiratory obstruction will occur. Decompensation can be rapid.
5. Preventing laryngeal edema begins with avoiding irritating stimuli. If there is an upper respiratory infection, using a face mask or supraglottic airway should be strongly considered. Tubes, sprays, and lubricants that are used on the tubes should be sterile. Intubation should be atraumatic, and adequate anesthetic depth and/or good muscle relaxation should be maintained to prevent tube movement. Head movement should be kept to a minimum.

V. Vocal Cord Dysfunction

Vocal cord paralysis and paresis have been reported after tracheal intubation despite the intubation being atraumatic and the site of surgery remote from the head and neck. Most cases resolve spontaneously, usually within days or weeks. Factors associated with vocal cord dysfunction include hypertension or diabetes, intubation greater than 6 hours, and age 50 years and above. Positioning the tube with the cuff just below the cords and high cuff pressure may increase the incidence of this problem. Because a tube moves cephalad with head or neck extension, the cuff may become positioned in the subglottic region when the patient remains in this position for a long time.

W. Ulcerations

Ulcerations (erosions) in the larynx and the trachea are common, even when a tube has been in place only a short time. The incidence and severity increase with the duration of intubation. Ulcers vary from superficial lesions involving only the mucosa to deep lesions in which the underlying cartilage is exposed. The end result will depend on the location and severity of the ulcer, as well as other factors such as infection that affect the healing process. If the ulcer is superficial, regeneration to normal epithelium occurs relatively quickly. When the damage is deeper, regeneration follows the same pattern as that for superficial damage but is more protracted. If the ulcer is very deep, scar tissue may form. Uvular necrosis following intubation has been reported.

X. Vocal Cord Granuloma

1. The incidence of vocal cord granuloma following intubation (intubation or postanesthesia granuloma) is reported to be between 1 in 800 and 1 in 20,000. Most occur in adults. They are more common in women. A number of possible etiologies have been proposed, including trauma, infection, too large a tracheal tube, excessive cuff pressure, duration of intubation, and the tube position.

2. Symptoms associated with vocal cord granuloma include persistent hoarseness, intermittent voice loss, pain or discomfort in the throat, a feeling of fullness or tension in the throat, chronic cough, hemoptysis, and pain extending to the ear. Occasionally, respiratory obstruction is seen. Symptoms may start after extubation or may not develop for as long as several months. Some cases are symptomless.
3. Persistent hoarseness after intubation warrants laryngeal examination. If the examination reveals ulceration over the vocal processes, strict voice rest to allow healing to take place may prevent granuloma development.

Y. Latex Allergy

While most tracheal tubes are made of PVC, some regular and some laser tubes are made of latex-containing rubber. A careful history and proper precautions should be taken when these tubes are used. Latex allergy is discussed in Chapter 11.

Z. Gastric Tube Knotted around the Tracheal Tube

A gastric tube may form a knot around the tracheal tube. Tandem movement of both the nasogastric tube and the tracheal tube should suggest this problem. Options for dealing with this include cutting the knot under direct vision, leaving the knotted tube in place until tracheal extubation is performed, and performing reintubation.

AA. Macroglossia

Macroglossia can be a serious problem resulting in airway obstruction after extubation. Patients in the prone position, especially for prolonged periods, usually have edema in the dependent facial structures. Macroglossia has also been reported in patients in the sitting position. Hemorrhage into the tongue can occur in an anticoagulated patient.

BB. Tracheal Stenosis

Tracheal stenosis following brief intubation has been reported. This problem is more common with long-term intubation.

CC. Cuff Inflated with Medication or Fluid

Cases have been reported in which a syringe or intravenous catheter was erroneously connected to the cuff inflation system and medication or fluid was then injected.

DD. Tube or Cuff Failure

There may be tube or cuff system defects that could cause the cuff to deflate or make inflation difficult.

V. Airway Management Adjuncts

A. Stylets

A stylet (introducer, guide, or intubating or malleable stylet) is designed to fit inside a tracheal tube but not extend beyond its tip. It is used to change the tracheal tube shape to facilitate intubation. It is also useful to check tracheal tube patency. A stylet should always be immediately available when intubation is performed. Many anesthesia providers routinely use a stylet, whereas others reserve its use for difficult intubations.

1. **Description**

A stylet is made of a material that can be bent into the desired shape. Some have a plastic coating to make them easier to insert and remove from the tracheal tube. There should be a means to prevent the stylet from going beyond the tracheal tube tip (**Fig. 15.35**). This could be a stopcock attached to the tube or simply a bend in the stylet. Pediatric stylets are available.

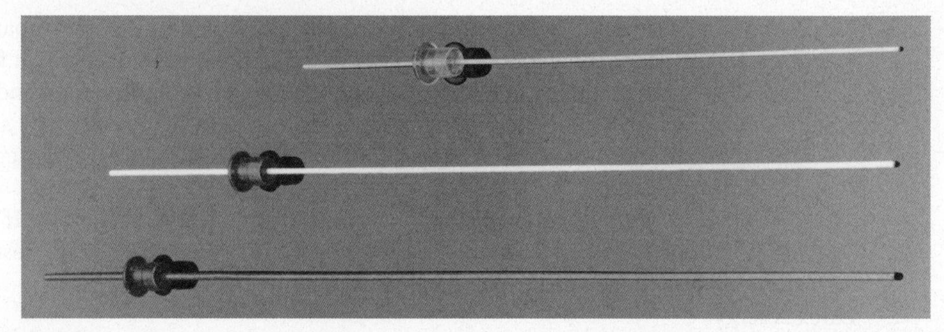

Figure 15.35 Malleable stylets with adjustable stops. The stop fits into the tracheal tube and prevents the stylet from protruding beyond the distal tip of the tube. (Courtesy of Rusch, Inc.)

2. **Use**
   a. Unless the stylet has a nonstick coating, a thin film of water-soluble lubricant should be spread over its entire length before insertion. The stylet should be inserted into the tube until the distal end is near the bevel and fixed so that it cannot advance further. Occasionally, the patient's airway may require extending the stylet tip beyond the bevel of the tracheal tube, but this is best avoided if possible.
   b. The tube with the stylet inserted should then be bent to the desired shape. For routine intubations, a straight or slightly curved configuration is usually the best option. When dealing with an anterior larynx, a "hockey stick" configuration, with the patient end of the tube bent anteriorly at an angle of 70 degrees to 80 degrees, is most commonly used. Bending the tube at the midpoint to the right or left may result in a better view of the larynx.
   c. The tracheal tube is held so that the thumb rests on the connector. The larynx is exposed and the tracheal tube is inserted. In most cases, unimpeded passage is achieved by introducing the unit through the right side of the mouth while pointing the tracheal tube tip toward the larynx and simultaneously supinating the hand 30 degrees to 40 degrees from the vertical position. Adjustments to the entry angle are easily made by moving the connector and/or supinating or pronating the hand. The thumb is used to advance the tracheal tube. When the distal part of the tube is believed to have passed the vocal cords, the stylet should be carefully withdrawn from the tube. Counterpressure on the tube in the opposite direction from the pull on the stylet may be necessary to prevent the tracheal tube from being removed. As the stylet is withdrawn, the tube tip typically moves anteriorly. If this anterior movement is timed with passage under the epiglottis, it may help to direct the tube through an anteriorly positioned glottis.
3. **Problems**
   a. Using a stylet may be associated with trauma to the airway or esophagus. The risk is increased if the stylet tip protrudes from the patient end of the tube. If the tube is advanced into the airway with the stylet bent at an acute angle, the tube tip may be forced into the anterior larynx.
   b. Part of the stylet may be sheared off. The stylet may damage the tracheal tube. The inflation tube can become entangled in the stylet. The tracheal tube may not advance over the stylet after intubation.

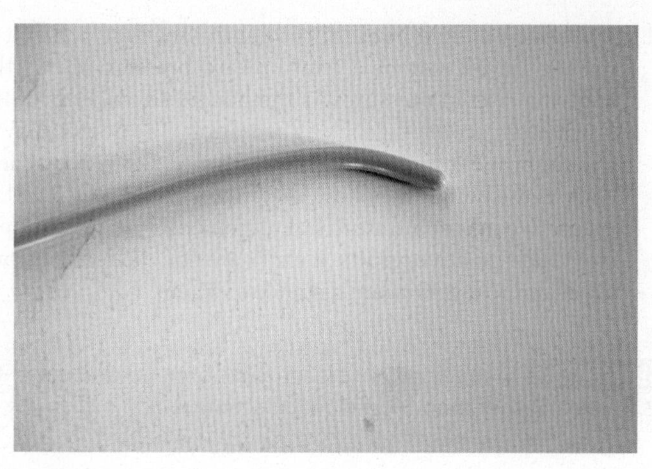

Figure 15.36 Tip of bougie.

B. Bougies

1. **Description**

a. The classic bougie (intubating or intubation catheter or introducer, guide, introducer, or stylet; Eschmann tracheal introducer) is fabricated from a braided polyester base with resin coating. Some are hollow except at the ends, but the ends may be cut away so that it can be passed over a smaller guide wire or used to monitor CO_2. Placing twisted wires in the hollow lumen allows the bougie to be shaped. Single-use bougies are available. Some bougies have length markings.

b. One end may be angled (**Fig. 15.36**). Either end can be placed into the tracheal tube to facilitate passage of the device through the laryngeal inlet. A bougie with a straight tip may be useful for tracheal tube exchange but is less advantageous than an airway exchange catheter.

CLINICAL MOMENT It is important to have bougies of various diameters available.

2. **Techniques of Use**

a. Before use, the bougie should be carefully inspected for fractures and tested for rigidity. It should be well lubricated with a water-soluble lubricant. It can be placed first in the tracheal tube with the tip protruding, or it can be advanced into the glottis and the tracheal tube then advanced over it.

b. A bougie can be blindly placed in the trachea or with the aid of a rigid laryngoscope, a rigid video laryngoscope, a flexible endoscope, or a supraglottic airway device. It is better to preposition the bougie in the laryngeal mask so that it exits through the middle between the bars rather than pass it blindly.

c. If the tip is angled, it should be introduced pointing anteriorly. If the tip becomes stuck at the anterior commissure, it should be rotated 180 degrees and then advanced. If the airway curvature is extreme, the tip can be directed even more anteriorly by lifting it with forceps. Applying cricoid pressure during tracheal tube insertion may prevent the tube from impinging on the anterior commissure during rotation.

d. The bougie should be advanced gently. The first sign that the tip is traversing the larynx may be a faint upward pressure felt by the person who is applying cricoid pressure. As the bougie advances over the tracheal rings, it will often produce a clicking sensation. The bougie may rotate as it enters a main bronchus and may come to a stop when it reaches a smaller bronchus. If the bougie is hollow, the proximal end may be attached to a capnograph to confirm intratracheal placement. Pharyngeal tip placement could yield false-positive results. If clicks are not elicited, the bougie can be gently advanced to a maximum distance of 45 cm.

CLINICAL MOMENT In the lightly anesthetized, nonparalyzed patient, coughing suggests tracheal rather than esophageal placement.

e. During nasal intubation, the bougie is advanced through the nostril and into the larynx. It is then visualized with a laryngoscope. The bougie is directed toward the vocal cords under direct vision. When the tip is inside the laryngeal inlet, the bougie is rotated so that the tip points posteriorly. It will usually then advance into the trachea. In the patient with a limited mouth opening, it may be possible to blindly pass the bougie through a nostril and into the trachea.

f. Once the bougie is believed to be in the trachea, the tracheal tube is gently advanced (railroaded) over the bougie by a rotary motion. A tracheal tube that is designed to minimize the gap between the leading edge of the tube and the intubation catheter may facilitate insertion. Intubation may be facilitated by leaving the laryngoscope in the mouth, a jaw thrust, or rotating the tracheal tube counterclockwise 90 degrees. A second technique is to preinsert the bougie into the tracheal tube so that its tip protrudes approximately 5 cm beyond the tube tip. This may save a few seconds but may make steering the tip to the left or right more difficult.

3. **Evaluation**

a. As an aid to the difficult intubation, the bougie may be superior to a stylet. It may be the first item that should be tried when tracheal intubation is not successful.

b. A bougie may be especially useful in the patient with a severely compromised upper airway, anterior larynx, or limited mouth opening. If glottic exposure is impossible, the bougie may be inserted blindly toward the laryngeal inlet and advanced until resistance is encountered. The tracheal tube is then threaded over the bougie.

c. Using a bougie may result in airway trauma. The force exerted by the tip is increased when the bougie is held near the tip. The bougie tip may become detached and the outer layer may become fractured. The bougie can be a source of contamination.

C. Airway Exchange Catheters

1. **Description**

a. AECs are shown in **Figures 15.37** and **15.38.** An AEC is more flexible and longer than a bougie. Some have an angular tip. Some have a stiffening cannula. Depth markings that are large, circumferential, and bold are helpful as they allow an estimation of how far the catheter has been inserted.

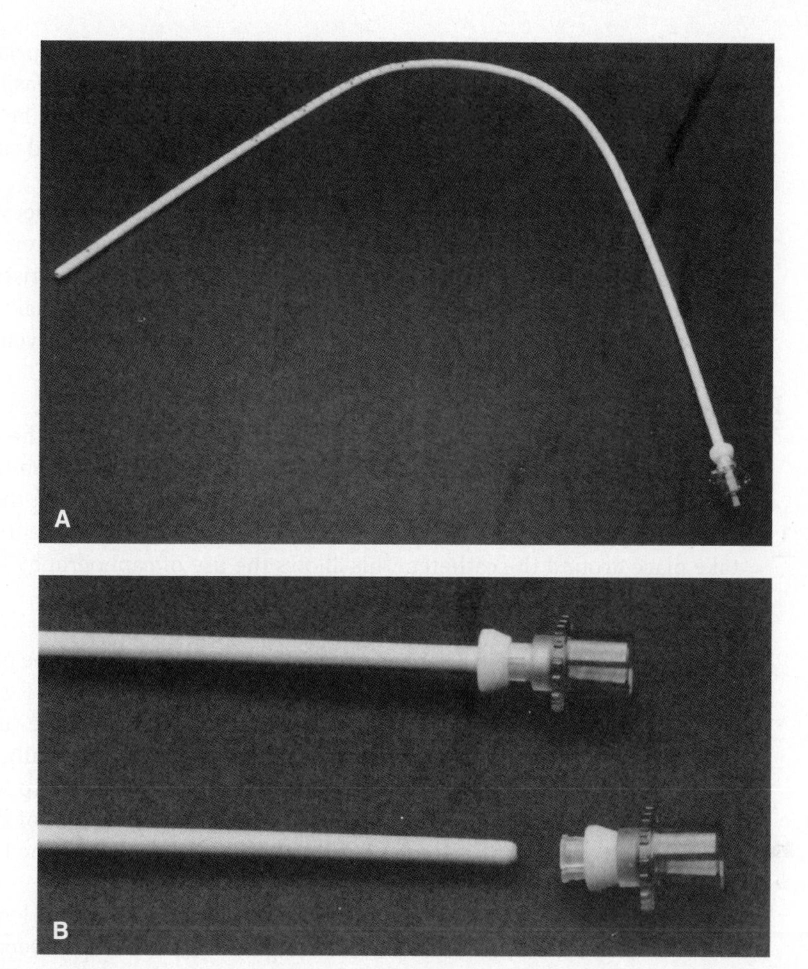

Figure 15.37 **A:** Airway exchange catheter. Note the marks showing the distance from the tip to the holes near the tip. **B:** The proximal connections allow administration of oxygen, jet ventilation, connection to a CO_2 analyzer, or suctioning. (Courtesy of Cook Critical Care, a division of Cook, Inc., Gloomington, IN.)

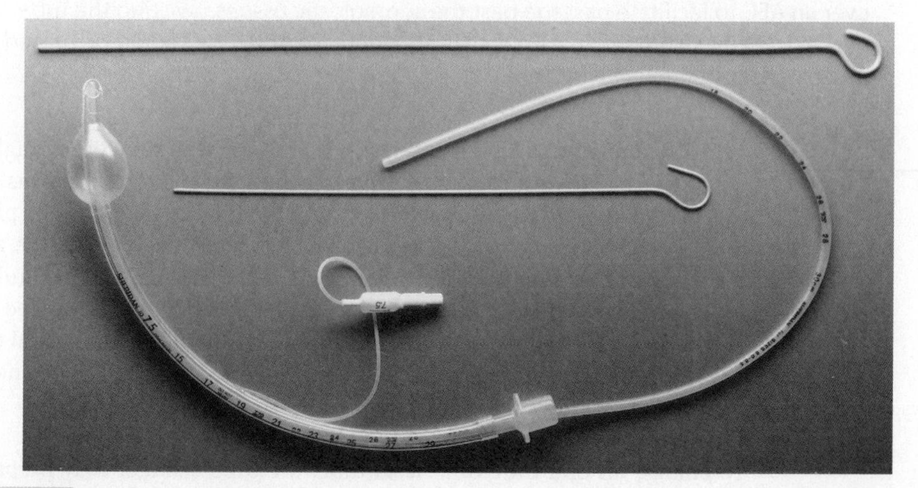

Figure 15.38 Tube changer in place. (Photograph courtesy of Kendall Healthcare Products, Inc.)

b. AECs in various sizes are available. The choice of an appropriately sized AEC can be vital. The best chance of a tracheal tube passing easily over the catheter into the trachea occurs when the catheter and the tracheal tube are close in size. The AEC may be labeled with the recommended size tube to be used with it.

c. Hollow devices allow oxygen administration by insufflation or jet ventilation and CO_2 measurement. Adaptors for these purposes are often furnished with the AEC. Jet ventilation through an AEC can provide satisfactory gas exchange in most cases. The length and small ID make manual ventilation with a resuscitation bag impractical. An AEC can be used for ventilation in children with tracheal stenosis.

2. **Uses**

A silicone spray or water-soluble lubricant should be applied to the outside of the AEC before use. Oxygen insufflation can be achieved by connecting the exchange catheter to an oxygen flowmeter. If the AEC is passed through the self-sealing diaphragm on a bronchoscopy adaptor (**Fig. 15.28**), ventilation can take place around the catheter. This allows the use of capnography to confirm tracheal placement location without removing the catheter.

a. Tracheal Tube or Supraglottic Device Exchange

1) This technique has been used to exchange a tracheal tube placed submentally with a nasotracheal tube, a double-lumen tube for a conventional single-lumen tube, or a Univent tube for a single-lumen tube and to replace a tracheostomy tube. An AEC is especially useful for exchanging a tracheal tube in a patient who is difficult to intubate.

2) The length of the AEC must be more than double that of the tube. It should be stiff enough so that it will not kink as the tube is removed or reinserted.

3) The marking on the catheter should be matched with the length markings on the tube to avoid advancing the AEC too deeply. Deep insertion increases the risk of perforation and barotrauma with jet ventilation. The AEC should never be inserted if resistance is encountered.

CLINICAL MOMENT A laryngoscope should be used when passing a tracheal tube over an AEC to facilitate passage past the supraglottic tissues. Twisting the tube may aid its advancement. If resistance is encountered, the tube should be turned 90 degrees counterclockwise.

4) The lubricated AEC is inserted into the tracheal tube or supraglottic device and advanced until it has reached the end of the tube as indicated by depth markings. Alternately, the tube changer may be placed alongside the tube. The tube changer is held steady while the existing tube or supraglottic device is withdrawn. A new tracheal tube or supraglottic device is then threaded over the AEC and advanced until it is at the proper depth. Proper placement should be confirmed using CO_2 monitoring, an EDD, or a flexible endoscope. The tube changer is then withdrawn.

b. Changing a Tracheal Tube from Oral to Nasal

To change an oral tube to a nasal tube, the tube changer may be passed through the oral tube along with a tracheal tube through the nose into the pharynx. The oral tube is removed, leaving the tube changer in the trachea. The nasal tube is inserted into the trachea next to the exchange catheter.

c. Changing a Tracheal Tube from Nasal to Oral
In one technique, a tube changer is placed orally alongside the tracheal tube (using a direct laryngoscope or a flexible endoscope). Alternately, a fiberscope loaded with a tracheal tube can be placed alongside the tracheal tube. A tube changer is passed through the nasal tube, which is then withdrawn into the pharynx. A tracheal tube is advanced over the first tube changer (or the fiberscope) until it is in the trachea. The nasal tube and the tube exchanger are then removed. If it is not possible to advance the oral tube, the nasal tube can be passed back into the trachea over the tube changer.

d. Intubation
The AEC can be used similarly to a bougie to facilitate intubation with a single-lumen or double-lumen tube or a supraglottic airway device. A guide wire may be inserted into the trachea and the tube changer then inserted over the guide wire. A supraglottic airway device can be used to place the catheter, although the success rate is not high with blind insertion.

e. Extubation
   1) Despite established extubation criteria, it is often difficult to reliably predict subsequent respiratory distress. An extubation trial (staged extubation) should be considered, especially for a patient who might be difficult to reintubate. The AEC is inserted into the tracheal tube, which is then removed. Placement in the tracheobronchial tube should be confirmed. The catheter forms a bridge that allows reintubation, administration of supplemental oxygen, ventilation, or end-tidal CO_2 measurement from the trachea. If the patient requires reintubation, this can be accomplished more easily and dependably with the AEC in place. Using an AEC might be cost saving by demonstrating that the patient will tolerate extubation earlier.
   2) While tracheostomy is being performed, the AEC may be useful to reestablish an airway if a problem occurs and may guide the surgeon to the tracheal lumen.

3. **Complications**
   a. Airway perforation has been reported as a complication of an AEC. The risk of perforation is related to the insertion depth. The exchange catheter should never be inserted if resistance is encountered. Gastric perforation can occur if the AEC enters the stomach.
   b. Using jet ventilation through the AEC may result in barotrauma. Using standard ventilation through a 15-mm connector is less dangerous, so jet ventilation should be used only if standard ventilation fails to provide adequate gas exchange. The risk of barotrauma with jet ventilation may be decreased by lowering the gas pressure, using a short inspiratory time, providing a long exhalation time, selecting a properly sized exchange catheter, and keeping the AEC tip above the carina. If incomplete chest deflation occurs, jet ventilation should be discontinued.
   c. There are other complications associated with the AEC. The tracheal tube may fail to pass over the AEC. Part of the catheter may break off and be aspirated. The exchange catheter may be inadvertently removed. The replacement tracheal tube may not end up in the trachea. The channel in the exchange catheter may become occluded by secretions, incorrectly implying esophageal

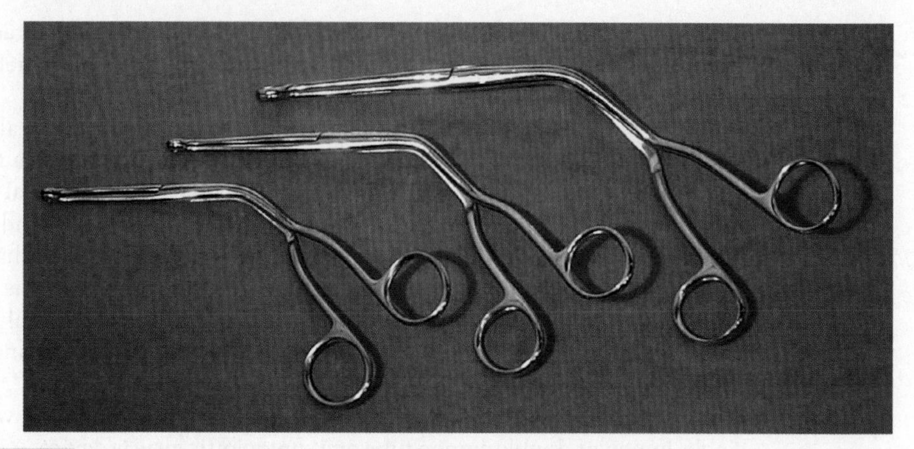

Figure 15.39 Magill's forceps. (Photograph courtesy of Sun Med., Largo, FL.)

placement. The catheter may dislodge a mucous plug, causing airway obstruction. The catheter may exit through a side hole (Murphy eye) in the tracheal tube. The catheter may shear. If the catheter is large relative to the internal diameter of the tracheal tube, it will increase the work of breathing. If the AEC kinks, it may not be possible to pass a tracheal tube over it.

VI. Forceps

Forceps can be used to direct a tracheal tube into the larynx or a gastric tube or other device into the esophagus. It may also be used to insert or remove pharyngeal packing and to remove foreign bodies from the upper airway or esophagus. Forceps should be immediately available whenever intubation is performed.

A. Description

A popular type is Magill's forceps (**Fig. 15.39**). These are designed so that when the grasping ends are at the axis of the tracheal tube, the handle is to the right. When the larynx is exposed, most of the forceps is out of the line of sight. Modifications of Magill's forceps and other devices have been described.

B. Problems

The tracheal tube cuff may become damaged, especially when forceps are used with high-volume, low-pressure cuffs. The tube should not be grasped at the cuff. Another way to avoid cuff damage is to smooth the ridges on the forceps. The forceps may cause damage to the airway mucosa. Another problem is that one arm of the forceps may become lodged in a Murphy eye. A forceps may also break.

REFERENCES

1. Dullenkopf A, Gerber A, Weiss M. Fluid leakage past tracheal tube cuffs: evaluation of the new Microcuff endotracheal tube. Intensive Care Med. 2003:1849–1853.
2. Dullenkopf A, Schmitz A, Gerber AC, Weiss M. Tracheal sealing characteristics of pediatric cuffed tracheal tubes. Ped Anesth. 2004;14:825–830.

SUGGESTED READINGS

Berry JM. Conventional (laryngoscopic) orotracheal and nasotracheal intubation (single lumen tube). In: Hagberg C, ed. Benumof's Airway Management. Second edition. Philadelphia: Mosby, 2007:379–392.

Coffin SE, Klompas M, Classen D, Arias KM. Strategies to prevent ventilator-associated pneumonia in acute care hospitals. Infect Contr Hosp Epidemiol 2008;29(suppl 1):S31–S40.

Cook TM, Seller C, Gupta K, et al. Non-conventional uses of the Aintree intubating catheter in management of the difficult airway. Anaesthesia 2007;62:169–174.

Cooper RM. Extubation and changing endotracheal tubes. In Hagberg C, ed. Benumof's Airway Management. Second edition. Philadelphia: Mosby, 2007:1146–1180.

Dorsch J, Dorsch S. Tracheal tubes and associated equipment. In: Understanding Anesthesia Equipment. Fifth edition. Philadelphia: Wolters Kluwer/Lippincott Williams & Wilkins, 2008:561–632.

Dullenkopf A, Gerber A, Weiss M. Fluid leakage past tracheal tube cuffs: evaluation of the new Microcuff endotracheal tube. Intensive Care Med 2003;29(10):1849–1853.

Dullenkopf A, Schmitz A, Gerber AC, Weiss M. Tracheal sealing characteristics of pediatric cuffed tracheal tubes. Pediatr Anesth 2004;14:825–830.

Givol N, Gershtansky Y, Halamish-Shani, T, et al. Perianesthetic dental injuries: analysis of incident reports. J Clin Anesth 2004;16:173–176.

Hagberg CA, Georgi R, Krier C. Complications of managing the airway. In: Hagberg C, ed. Benumof's Airway Management. Second edition. Philadelphia: Mosby, 2007:1181–1216.

Hagberg CA. Current concepts in the management of the difficult airway. Orlando, FL: American Society of Anesthesiologists, 2008. ASA Refresher Course No. 222.

Hall CEJ, Shutt LE. Nasotracheal intubation for head and neck surgery. Anaesthesia 2003;58:249–256.

Henderson JJ, Popat MT, Latto IP, Pearce AC. Difficult Airway Society guidelines for management of the unanticipated difficult intubation. Anaesthesia 2004;59:675–694.

Ho, AM-H, Aun CST, Karmakar. The margin of safety associated with the use of cuffed paediatric tubes. Anaesthesia 2002;57:169–182.

Latto IP, Stacey M, Mecklenburgh J, Vaughan RS. Survey of the use of the gum elastic bougie in clinical practice. Anaesthesia 2002;57:379–384.

McHardy FE, Chung F. Postoperative sore throat: cause, prevention and treatment. Anaesthesia 1999;54:444–453.

Mort TC. Continuous airway access for the difficult extubation: the efficacy of the airway exchange catheter. Anesth Analg 2007;105:1357–1362.

Newth CJL, Rachman B, Patel N, et al. Cuffed versus uncuffed endotracheal tubes in pediatric intensive care. J Pediatr 2004;144:333–337.

Ramez Salem M, Baraka A. Confirmation of tracheal intubation. In: Hagberg C, ed. Benumof's Airway Management. Second edition. Philadelphia: Mosby, 2007:697–727.

Szekely SM, Webb RK, Williamson JA, Russell WJ. Problems related to the endotracheal tube: an analysis of 2000 incident reports. Anaesth Intensive Care 1993;21:611–616.

Weber T, Salvi N, Orliaguet G, Wolf A. Cuffed vs non-cuffed endotracheal tubes for pediatric anesthesia. Pediatr Anesth 2009;19(suppl):46–54.

16 Double-Lumen Tracheobronchial Tubes, Bronchial Tubes, and Bronchial Blocking Devices

I. Indications for Lung Isolation

A. Double-lumen tracheobronchial tubes (double-lumen tubes, DLTs) and bronchial blocking devices (bronchial blockers) are lung isolation devices used to provide better operating conditions and reduced trauma during thoracic surgical procedures and prevent infected material from one lung from contaminating the other. When hemorrhage occurs in one lung, an isolation device allows the unaffected lung to be ventilated.

B. A bronchopleural or bronchocutaneous fistula may have such a low resistance to gas flow that most of the tidal volume passes through it, making it impossible to adequately ventilate the other lung. Large cysts or bullae may rupture under positive pressure, making it mandatory that they be excluded from ventilation. Another indication for lung separation is for ventilation when lungs have markedly different compliance or airway resistance such as occurs following single lung transplantation or unilateral injury.

C. Other indications for one-lung ventilation include bronchiectasis, lung transplantation, minimally invasive cardiac surgery, thoracic aneurysm procedures, tracheobronchial obstruction, tracheoesophageal fistula, video thoracoscopy, esophagogastrectomy, chest wall and thoracic vascular procedures, patent ductus arteriosus ligation, plural striping or biopsy, coarctation of the aorta correction, and lung, lobe, or segmental resection.

II. Anatomical Considerations

The right mainstem bronchus is shorter, straighter, and has a larger diameter than the left. It takes off from the trachea at an angle of 25 degrees in adults while the left mainstem bronchus diverges at a 45-degree angle. These angles are slightly larger in children. The right upper lobe bronchus takeoff is very close to the origin of the right mainstem bronchus. These anatomical features mean that it is usually easier to intubate the right mainstem bronchus than the left, but it is very difficult to place a tube in the right mainstem bronchus without obstructing the upper lobe orifice.

III. Double-Lumen Tubes

The DLT is the device most commonly used to provide lung isolation.

A. Description

1. A DLT is essentially two single-lumen tubes bonded together and designated as right- or left-sided, depending on which mainstem bronchus the tube is designed to be placed into. The distal bronchial portion is angled to fit into the appropriate mainstem bronchus.
2. The bronchial cuff for right-sided tubes varies in shape, depending on the manufacturer. Some right-sided tubes have a slanted cuff and a slot in the bronchial tube (**Fig. 16.1**) to ventilate the right upper lobe. Some right-sided DLTs have two bronchial cuffs with an opening in between (**Figs. 16.2B** and **16.3**). The resting volume and compliance of bronchial cuffs varies among different DLT sizes and brands. Most manufacturers color the bronchial cuff blue. They also use blue markings on the pilot balloon and/or the inflation device for the bronchial cuff.
3. A few DLTs have a carinal hook (**Figs. 16.4** and **16.5**) to aid in proper placement and minimize tube movement after placement. Potential problems with carinal hooks include increased difficulty during intubation, trauma to the airway, tube malposition because of the hook, and interference with bronchial closure during pneumonectomy. The hook can break off and become lost in the bronchial tree.

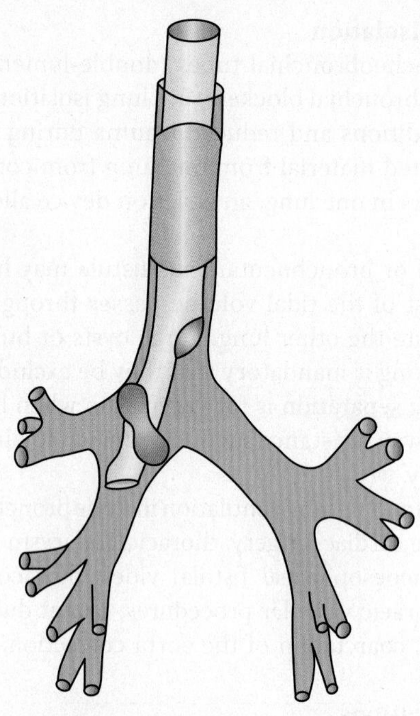

Figure 16.1 Broncho-Cath right double-lumen tube. The bronchial cuff has the shape of an S or a slanted doughnut, with the edge of the cuff nearest the right upper lobe bronchus closer to the trachea than the part of the cuff touching the medial bronchial wall. A slot in the tube beyond the cuff corresponds to the opening of the right upper lobe bronchus. Newer versions have no bevel on the bronchial segment.

4. Most manufacturers place a radiopaque marker at the patient end of the tracheal cuff or at the end of the tracheal lumen. Other marks may be placed above and/or below the bronchial cuff. Some have a radiopaque line running the tube length.
5. Disposable DLTs are supplied in sterile packages, which include a stylet, connectors, and a suction catheter(s) (**Fig. 16.4**). A means to supply continuous positive airway pressure (CPAP) may be included with the tube or can be purchased separately.

B. Sizing

Adult DLTs commonly come in sizes 35, 37, 39, and 41 Fr. The French scale is the external diameter of the tracheal segment times three. Some manufacturers also provide 26, 28, and 32 Fr tubes for younger patients. Unfortunately, the French gauge markings are of limited value in determining the most important measurement—the diameter of the bronchial segment. There are major variations among manufacturers in the bronchial segment dimensions for tubes that are the same nominal size and even among tubes that are the same size from the same manufacturer.

C. Margin of Safety

The margin of safety for a DLT is the tracheobronchial tree length between the most distal and proximal acceptable positions for the bronchial tube. The margin of safety will depend on the length of the lumen into which the cuff is placed and the length of the cuff and tip. If the cuff is short or the mainstem bronchus long, the margin of safety will be greater. Because there is significant variation among manufacturers and different sized DLTs, each tube must be matched to the patient to ensure an adequate margin of safety.

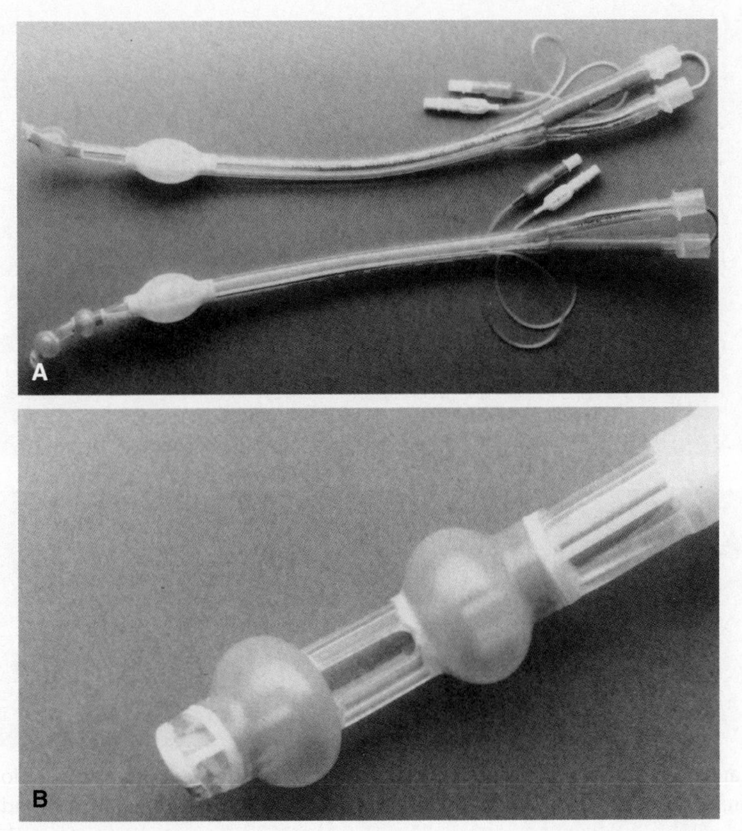

Figure 16.2 Sher-I-Bronch double-lumen tubes. **A:** Left-sided tube (*top*). Right-sided tube (*bottom*). **B:** Close-up of right bronchial segment, showing opening to the right upper lobe. (Courtesy of Sheridan, Inc., now part of Covidien, Mansfield, MA.)

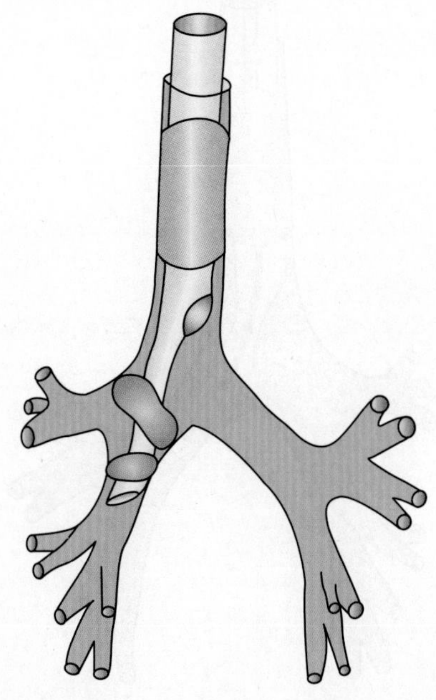

Figure 16.3 Sher-I-Bronch right double-lumen tube. Note the two cuffs proximal and distal to the opening to the right upper lobe.

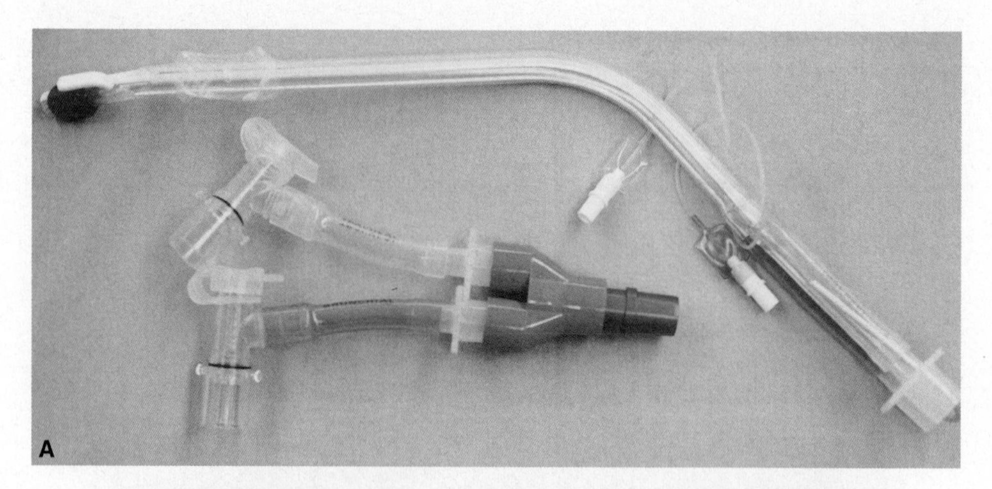

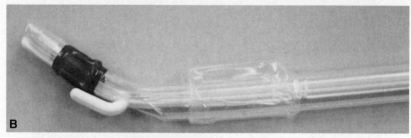

Figure 16.4 Carlens double-lumen tube. **A:** The connector has ports for fiberscope insertion or suctioning and areas where a clamp can be applied to occlude gas flow. **B:** Note the carinal hook and the blue bronchial cuff.

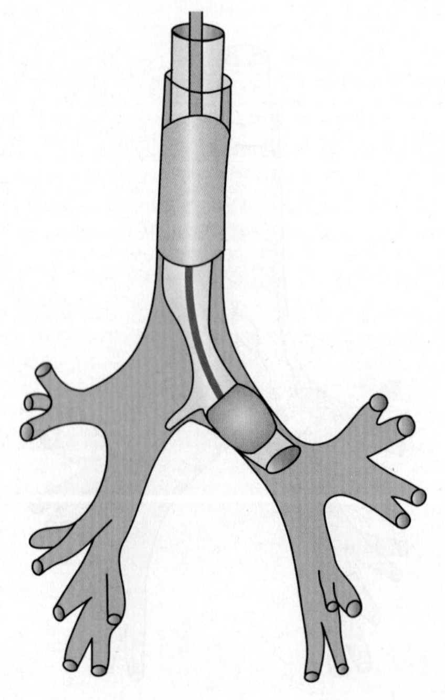

Figure 16.5 Carlens tube in place.

1. **Left-Sided Tubes**
   a. The outermost acceptable position for a left DLT is when the bronchial cuff is just below the carina. If the tube were higher, the bronchial cuff could obstruct the trachea and/or the contralateral (right) mainstem bronchus. The most acceptable distal position is when the bronchial segment tip is at the proximal edge of the upper lobe bronchial orifice. More distal insertion would obstruct the upper lobe bronchus.
   b. The average left bronchus length from the carina to the upper lobe bronchus takeoff is 5.6 cm. This leaves a relatively small margin for placement, because there could be up to 3.5 cm of movement with neck flexion and extension.
2. **Right-Sided Tubes**
   The margin of safety is defined differently for right-sided tubes and is considerably less than for left-sided tubes. A right-sided DLT is acceptably positioned if the right upper lobe ventilation opening is aligned with the right upper lobe orifice. Thus, the margin of safety is the length of the ventilation opening minus the diameter of the orifice.

D. Use

1. **Tube Choice**
   a. Right versus Left
      1) One study showed that right- and left-sided DLTs are associated with the same incidence and severity of hypoxemia, hypercapnia, and high airway pressures (1).
      2) When surgery is performed on the right lung, a left-sided DLT should be used. Because the margin of safety in positioning a right-sided DLT is very small, some prefer to use a left-sided DLT whenever possible for left lung surgery. During left pneumonectomy, immediately before the left mainstem bronchus is clamped, the DLT can be pulled from the bronchus and used for ventilating the right lung without being placed in the right mainstem bronchus. A disadvantage of this technique is the risk of blood and secretions moving from the operative (left) bronchus to the nonoperative (right) bronchus. Other possible problems include the tube becoming dislodged or inadvertently sutured in place.
      3) A right DLT should be used when it is important to avoid manipulation/intubation of the left main bronchus (e.g., an exophytic lesion), when the left main bronchus is narrowed or so cephalad that the bronchial lumen will not enter the left mainstem bronchus, left lung transplantation, a left mainstem bronchial stent in place or when there is tracheobronchial disruption on the left.
   b. Size
      1) A DLT that is too small may fail to provide lung isolation or may require bronchial cuff volumes and pressures that could produce mucosal ischemia or bronchial rupture. Using too small a DLT can result in the tube advancing too far into the bronchus, a high level of auto positive end-expiratory pressure (PEEP), or barotrauma. An undersized tube may be more likely to become displaced. Ventilation and suctioning are more difficult with a small tube.
      2) Using a large DLT will result in less resistance to gas flow, facilitate suctioning and passing a fiberscope, and reduce the risk of advancing

Table 16.1 Sizes of Double-Lumen Tubes for Children

Age (years)	Double-Lumen Tube (French)
8–10	26
10–12	26–28
12–14	32
14–16	35

From Hammer GB, Fitzmaurice BG, Brodsky JB. Methods for single-lung ventilation in pediatric patients. Anesth Analg 1999;89:1426–1429.

the DLT too far into the bronchus but may result in trauma. Inability to insert a DLT through the larynx or past the carina or intrinsic or extrinsic obstruction in the mainstem bronchus to be intubated may necessitate using a smaller tube.

3) A tube is oversized if the bronchial lumen will not fit into the bronchus or there is no air leak with the bronchial cuff deflated. It is too small if the bronchial cuff inflation volume is greater than the resting cuff volume. Not more than 3 mL of air in the bronchial cuff should be required to create a seal.
4) Suggested sizes for DLTs in children are shown in **Table 16.1.**
5) While it has been advocated that the largest tube that can safely fit that bronchus should be selected, using a smaller tube does not result in more complications (2). The size of the mainstem bronchus may be determined by measuring its width on a chest radiograph or computed tomographic scan. Unfortunately, it is not possible to accurately measure bronchial width on many radiographs.

2. **Preparing the Double-Lumen Tube**

The tracheal and bronchial cuffs should be inflated and checked for leaks and symmetrical cuff inflation, making certain that each inflation tube is associated with the proper cuff. The cuffs and the stylet should be lubricated with a water-soluble gel and the stylet placed inside the bronchial lumen, making certain that it does not extend beyond the tip.

3. **Insertion**

a. The DLT is advanced through the larynx with the angled tip directed anteriorly. After the bronchial cuff has passed the cords, the tube is turned 90 degrees so that the bronchial portion points toward the appropriate bronchus. If the tube is to be placed in the left mainstem bronchus, the head and neck should be rotated to the right before rotating and advancing the tube. Leaving the stylet in place for the entire intubation procedure rather than removing it once the bronchial cuff has passed the vocal cords may result in more rapid and accurate placement. Some clinicians recommend that the stylet be removed after the tube passes the vocal cords to prevent trauma.

b. A DLT is most accurately placed by inserting a fiberscope into the bronchial lumen and directing it into the appropriate bronchus under direct vision. This ensures that the correct bronchus is intubated on the first attempt and avoids inserting the tube too deeply or the tube becoming kinked in the upper lobe bronchus. Concurrent direct laryngoscopy may be required to elevate the supraglottic tissues to facilitate passing the DLT through the glottic opening.

c. Insertion of the bronchial portion into the mainstem bronchus can be performed blindly. This method may be useful where rapid lung isolation or collapse is necessary. In some cases (e.g., bronchorrhea, bleeding), blind placement may succeed whereas the fiber-optic technique does not. With blind insertion, the correct insertion depth may be difficult to determine. In adults, there is a correlation between the ideal left DLT insertion depth and patient height but not weight or age. The ideal insertion depth can be estimated from the chest radiograph. Advancing the tube with the bronchial cuff partially inflated until an increase in resistance is felt (or only one side of the chest moves and compliance is reduced) may prevent inserting the tube too deeply. The bronchial cuff is then deflated and the tube advanced a distance equal to the length of the bronchial cuff plus 1 to 1.5 cm.

d. Since the DLT usually moves upward with positioning, some clinicians recommend that the tube should initially be inserted more deeply than would be the ideal position, but the risk of trauma may be greater if the tube is intentionally placed too deep.

4. **Cuff Inflation**

a. Once the tip is thought to be in a mainstem bronchus, the tracheal cuff should be inflated in a manner similar to that on a tracheal tube. It is more difficult to inflate the bronchial cuff correctly. An overinflated bronchial cuff is more likely to herniate into the trachea, cause the carina to be pushed toward the opposite side, or result in bronchial segment lumen narrowing. Inflating the bronchial cuff beyond its resting volume may result in dangerously high pressure.

b. The bronchial cuff should be inflated with small incremental volumes until an airtight seal is just achieved. The total volume should be less than 3 mL. One technique is to immerse the proximal tracheal lumen in water during ventilation via the bronchial lumen. The bronchial cuff is inflated until no bubbles are seen escaping during positive-pressure inspiration (**Fig. 16.6**). Variations include connecting a balloon or a capnograph to the tracheal lumen.

5. **Confirming Position**

Confirming proper tube position is essential because the tube may not perform properly if incorrectly positioned. Tube position should be checked after insertion, after the patient is repositioned, and before beginning one-lung ventilation, because these tubes often move. The most frequent DLT movement is during lateral decubitus positioning. While movement is usually outward, distal migration may also occur. DLT position should be confirmed whenever there is evidence of malfunction.

CLINICAL MOMENT Always check tube position after the patient is repositioned. The DLT can become displaced when the patient is turned. Moving the head can cause the tube to move deeper or out of the mainstem bronchus.

a. Auscultatory Techniques

1) Unfortunately, auscultation detects DLT malposition only part of the time because breath sounds can be transmitted from one region of the lung to adjacent areas. Studies have shown that a significant percentage of DLTs thought to be positioned satisfactorily by auscultation were inappropriately positioned on subsequent fiber-optic

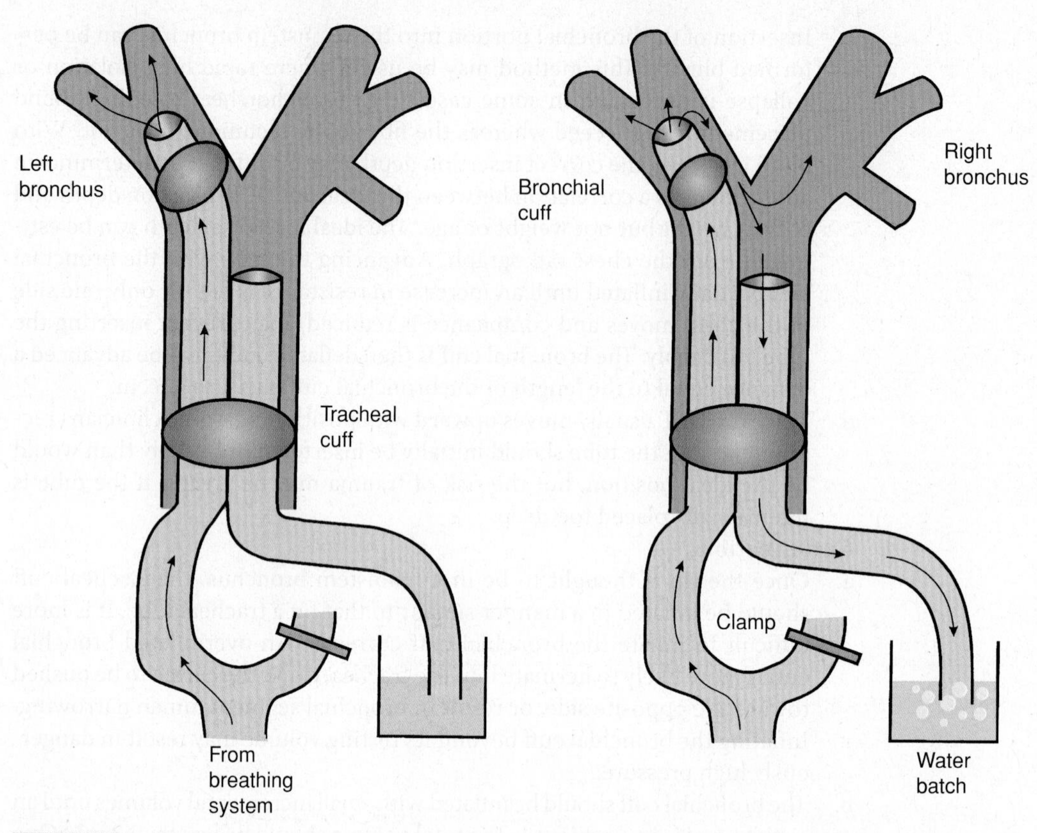

Figure 16.6 Inflating the bronchial cuff. With the tracheal cuff inflated, the bronchial cuff is slowly inflated. **Right:** A bronchial cuff leak is indicated by bubbles when the end of the tracheal lumen is placed under water. **Left:** With a seal, no bubbles appear.

examination. Another problem is that once the patient is prepped and draped, the chest is no longer available for auscultation.

2) For left-sided tubes when only the tracheal cuff is inflated and the tracheal lumen connected to the breathing system, both lungs should be auscultated in the axillary regions and upper lung fields to detect differences. The bronchial cuff should then be inflated and both lumens connected to the breathing system. Auscultation should then be repeated and breath sounds heard over both lungs.

3) To determine if a left-sided bronchial tube is correctly placed, the attachment between the breathing system and the tracheal lumen should be occluded and the tracheal lumen opened to atmosphere. Breath sounds should be heard only over the left lung. If breath sounds are heard bilaterally, the tube is too high in the trachea. Both cuffs should be deflated and the tube advanced. If breath sounds are heard only over the right lung, the bronchial segment is in the wrong bronchus. If this is the case, both cuffs should deflated, the tube withdrawn until its tip is above the carina, rotated, and then advanced. These steps should be repeated.

4) To further check for correct left bronchial tube placement, the attachment between the breathing system and the bronchial lumen should

be clamped and the patient ventilated through the tracheal lumen. The bronchial lumen should be opened to atmosphere. Breath sounds should be heard only over the right lung. If there is marked resistance to ventilation, the tube is either too far into the left bronchus or not deep enough. The position can be determined by deflating the bronchial cuff while continuing to ventilate through the tracheal lumen with the bronchial lumen clamped. If the tip is too deep in the left bronchus, breath sounds will be heard only on the left side. If the tube is not deep enough in the bronchus, breath sounds will be present bilaterally. The tracheal cuff also should be deflated and, depending on where breath sounds were heard, the tube pulled back or advanced. Both cuffs should be reinflated and the auscultatory sequence repeated.

5) Right-sided DLT auscultation is similar to that of a left-sided tube. It is especially important to confirm right upper lobe ventilation.

b. Flexible Endoscopic Techniques

1) Flexible endoscopy is the most accurate method for determining DLT position. Many recommend that it be the standard of care. There is general agreement that fiber-optic endoscopy is always needed for right-sided DLTs. Fiber-optic methods may not work in the presence of blood or secretions. An advantage is that it can be used to remove blood or secretions. It can also be used after the patient is prepared and draped.

2) Left-sided DLT position can be confirmed by placing the fiberscope in the tracheal lumen through the open end or through a port in the connector that is specially designed for this purpose (**Fig. 16.4A**). As the fiberscope is advanced, the carina should come into view. The top surface of the blue bronchial cuff should be seen below the carina in the mainstem bronchus. The bronchial cuff should neither herniate over the carina nor the carina be pushed to the side. An unobstructed view of the nonintubated mainstem bronchus should be obtained.

3) After the location has been checked through the tracheal lumen, the fiberscope should then be advanced through the bronchial lumen to check for narrowing in the lumen at the level of the cuff and an unobstructed view of the distal bronchial tree.

4) Looking down a right-sided tube tracheal lumen, the clinician should see the upper surface of the bronchial cuff below the carina in the right mainstem bronchus. The fiberscope is then placed in the bronchial lumen. The right middle lower lobe bronchial carina should be seen below the end of the tube. The endoscopist should be able to look into the right upper lobe orifice by flexing the tip of the fiberscope superiorly.

5) Once correct tube position is confirmed, the tube should be secured in place. During positioning, the tube should be held at the incisors and the head immobilized in a neutral or slightly flexed position to prevent the tube from migrating.

6. **Intraoperative Care**

The bronchial cuff should be kept deflated (unless the lung needs to be isolated to prevent spread of blood or infection) until the lung needs to be collapsed. Lung collapse will be most rapid if lung separation is initiated at end expiration. Suction is of limited utility because the gas trapped in the lung is distal to collapsible airways. If despite best efforts complete lung separation cannot be accomplished and gas is introduced into the ipsilateral lung with each breath, then continuous suction may be helpful to evacuate the gas as it enters the lung. Bronchial cuff pressure should be monitored and adjusted to the minimum necessary to achieve an airtight seal.

7. **Replacing a Double-Lumen Tube with a Single-Lumen Tube**
   a. If mechanical ventilation needs to be continued at the conclusion of a case in which a DLT was used, it is usually desirable to replace the DLT with a standard tracheal tube. Personnel who are caring for the patient in the postoperative period are not always familiar with a DLT. Suctioning through a DLT can be difficult. After pneumonectomy, when all of the patient's ventilation is conducted through one lumen, the small lumen may make it difficult for the patient to breathe spontaneously. Pressure support ventilation (Chapter 6) can be used to decrease the work of breathing during spontaneous ventilation if the DLT cannot be replaced.
   b. In most cases, the DLT is removed and a single-lumen tube is inserted in its place. If the patient is difficult to intubate or circumstances make visualizing the larynx difficult, other techniques should be considered. One would be to insert a long airway exchange catheter into the tracheal lumen before the DLT is removed. After the DLT has been removed, the single-lumen tube is then advanced over the catheter. Oxygen insufflation via the catheter will reduce the incidence of hypoxemia.

CLINICAL MOMENT If an airway exchange catheter is used when replacing a DLT with a single-lumen tube, it should be at least twice as long as the DLT to avoid it being pulled from the trachea.

IV. Bronchial Blocking Devices

A. Indications and Use

1. Indications for bronchial blockers are similar to those for a DLT, with the exception of independent lung ventilation. They are often employed when the use of a DLT is not possible or advisable (nasal intubation, small patient, difficult intubation, the patient with a tracheostomy, subglottic stenosis, thick and excessive secretions, or need for continued postoperative intubation). A blocker may be especially useful for providing lung separation in a patient with a single-lumen tracheal tube already in place. Another indication may be the patient on anticoagulants, since placing a blocker is usually less traumatic than inserting a DLT. A blocker may allow a larger fiber-optic endoscope to be used and provide better suctioning than a DLT.
2. A blocker can be used to block a lung segment rather than the entire lung. This cannot be done with a DLT. A blocker may be used to sequentially block different parts of the lung.
3. A blocker may be used to achieve lung isolation in the patient with an improperly positioned double-lumen or bronchial tube or if both lungs require sequential blockage. The blocker can be shifted to the opposite lung when needed. If one blocker does not provide complete one-lung isolation, a second blocker may be used.
4. There is no need to change the tube at the end of the operation if postoperative mechanical ventilation is needed when a bronchial blocker is used.

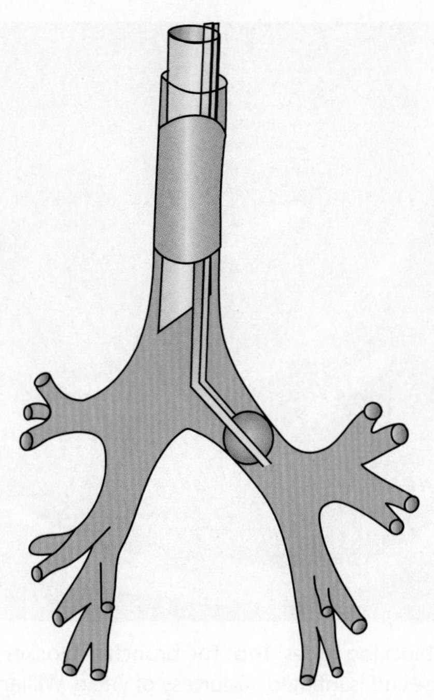

Figure 16.7 Univent bronchial blocker. The cuffed tracheal tube has a small lumen along its concave side, which contains a tubular cuffed bronchial blocker. The blocker can be advanced into a mainstem bronchus or smaller airway.

B. Devices

1. **Univent Bronchial Blocking Tube**
   a. The Univent blocker (**Figs. 16.7** and **16.8**) fits into a special tracheal tube that has a channel to accommodate it. The blocker is hollow and semirigid with a cuff at the end. It can be retracted into the tracheal tube during intubation. It is curved to facilitate being directed into a mainstem bronchus. A fiberscope or guide wire is used to guide the blocker into the bronchus. The cuff is then inflated. The channel through the cuff allows the lung to be deflated.
   b. The Univent blocker can provide lung isolation equivalent to a DLT. The Univent blocker may be easier to insert than a DLT. CPAP, oxygen, jet ventilation, or suction can be applied to the channel in the blocker. If jet ventilation is used, the cuff must be deflated. Problems include the fixed shape and inability to soften when warmed. Bronchial perforation has been reported with its use.
2. **Arndt Bronchial Blocker**
   a. The Arndt bronchial blocker is designed for a patient with a standard tracheal tube in place. It consists of a blocking catheter and a special airway adaptor. The catheter has a high-volume, low-pressure balloon that has either an elliptical or a spherical shape. A flexible nylon wire passes through the proximal end of the catheter, extends to the patient end, and then exits as a small loop (**Fig. 16.9**). The loop size may be increased or decreased by advancing or retracting the wire assembly. The multiport adaptor (**Fig. 16.9**) allows simultaneous introduction of a bronchoscope and the blocker while maintaining mechanical ventilation.

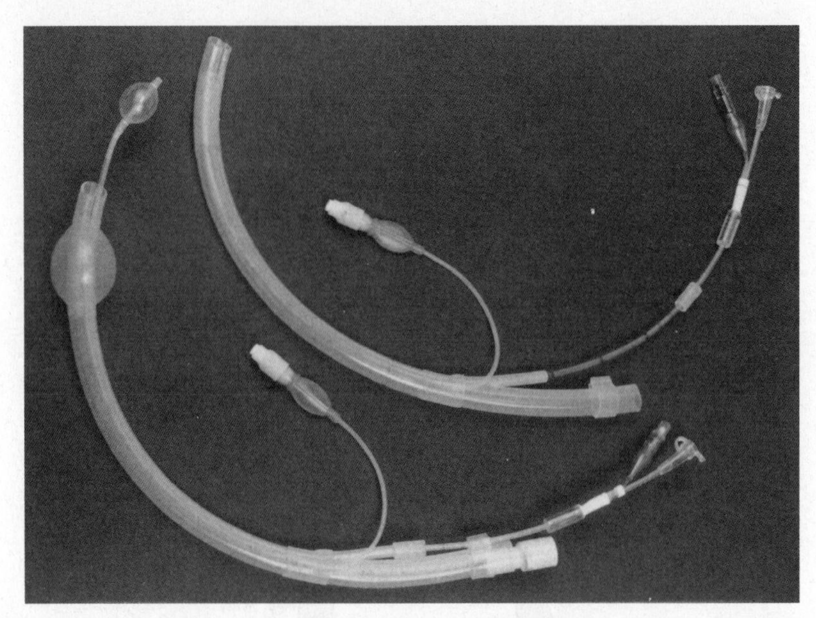

Figure 16.8 Univent bronchial blocking tubes. **Top:** The bronchial blocker is retracted. **Bottom:** The bronchial blocker is advanced, and the cuff is inflated. (Courtesy of Vitaid, Williamsville, NY.)

b. The wire in the blocker lumen is used in either of two ways. When the loop is cinched tightly around the tip of the fiberscope, the fiberscope carries the blocker to its desired location. Alternately, the fiberscope can be passed through the loop so that it provides a track for the blocker to pass through after the fiberscope is in the bronchus.

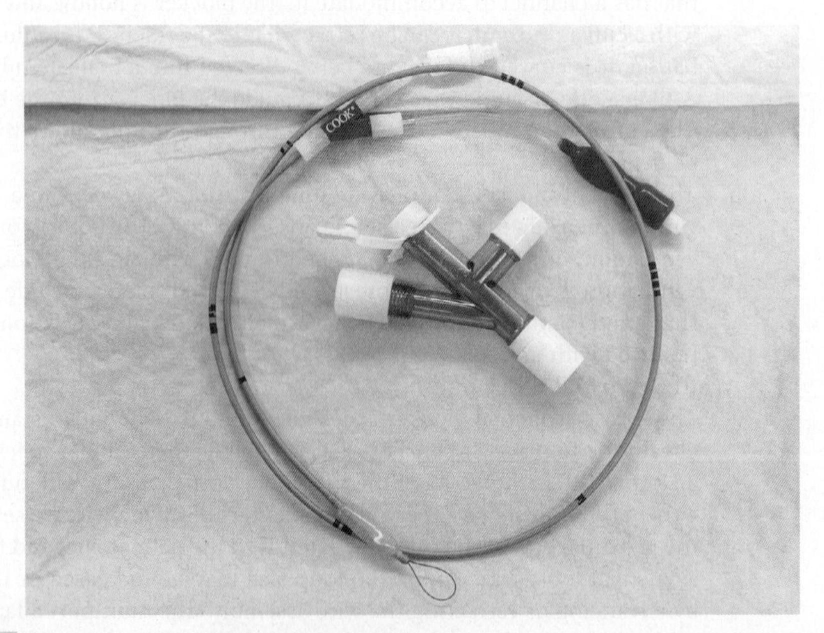

Figure 16.9 Arndt bronchial blocker with multiport adaptor. The wire loop can be cinched around the tip of the fiberscope, or the fiberscope is passed through the loop. The adaptor has ports for attachment to the tracheal tube and the breathing system, for introducing the blocker, and for a fiberscope.

c. When placing the blocker, it may be advisable to advance the blocker approximately 1 cm beyond the optimal position when the patient is in the supine position, in order to avoid dislodging the blocker into the trachea when the patient is placed in the lateral decubitus position. The balloon is then inflated under direct vision so that it fills the entire bronchial lumen but does not herniate into the trachea. Following placement, the balloon may be deflated until one-lung ventilation is required. Lung collapse can be expedited by applying suction to the blocker channel.

d. The Arndt bronchial blocker has been used to provide single-lung ventilation in young children. If the wire is removed, the lumen can be used for suctioning, administering oxygen, or providing CPAP. A disadvantage is that once the wire loop is removed, it cannot be reinserted to allow the blocker to be repositioned. Placement requires the availability of fiber-optic equipment.

e. If the wire is not removed after the blocker has been properly placed, it can be inadvertently cut or stapled into place during surgery.

3. **Cohen Tip-Deflecting Bronchial Blocker**

a. The Cohen tip-deflecting bronchial blocker (**Fig. 16.10**) has a 9-Fr external diameter and a central lumen with a 1.6-mm diameter. The high-volume, low-pressure blue balloon at the tip has a spherical shape. The average inflation volume is 5 to 8 mL. There are side holes between the tip and the balloon to evacuate gas from the distal lung or insufflate oxygen. A proximal control wheel that can be operated with the thumb and the forefinger is used to adjust tip deflection. The catheter has depth markings and an indicator arrow that shows the direction in which the tip deflects.

b. In most cases, the blocker and a fiberscope are inserted through an appropriately sized tracheal tube. The blocker can also be placed outside the tracheal tube and guided into place with a fiberscope placed through the tracheal tube. A multiport airway adaptor such as the Arndt bronchial blocker is attached to the breathing system end of the tracheal tube. Alternatively, a standard swivel adaptor can be used for insertion. An assistant with a video-flexible fiber-optic scope may be necessary because it may require two hands to manipulate the blocker into position, one to deflect the tip and the other to rotate and advance the catheter.

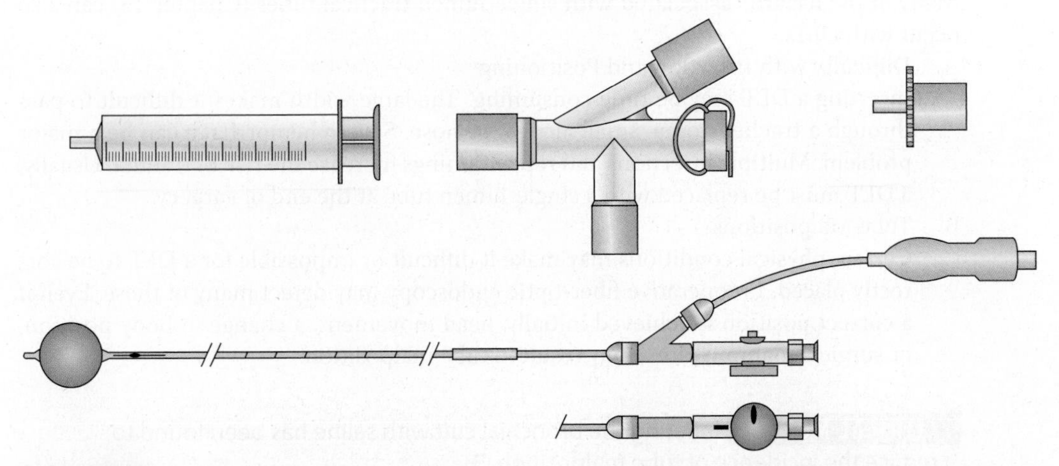

Figure 16.10 Cohen tip-deflecting bronchial blocker. The proximal control wheel is used to adjust tip deflection. An arrow on the wheel indicates the direction to which the tip deflects. (Courtesy of Cook Critical Care, Bloomington, IN.)

4. **Embolectomy Catheter**
   a. An embolectomy (Fogarty) catheter can be used as a bronchial or segmental blocker. This is readily available in most operating suites where vascular surgery is performed. It comes with a stylet in place. It is possible to place a curvature in the distal tip to facilitate guiding the catheter into the target bronchus. The occlusion balloon has a low-volume, high-pressure cuff. It comes in a variety of sizes. Adult bronchi can be blocked with 7-Fr catheters, whereas 2- to 5-Fr catheters are suitable for segmental or pediatric bronchial blockade.
   b. An embolectomy catheter may be placed before or after intubation with a single-lumen tracheal or tracheostomy tube and can be passed either through or alongside the tube. An alternative method is to insert the catheter through a hole made on the side of the tracheal tube.
   c. If the patient is already intubated, the catheter may be passed through a fiber-optic endoscope adaptor. An endoscope is passed down the tracheal tube, and the embolectomy catheter is guided into the appropriate bronchus under direct vision.
   d. An embolectomy catheter can be passed through a single-lumen tracheal tube in an already intubated patient, and there is no need for reintubation if postoperative mechanical ventilation is needed. It may be useful in pediatric patients, the patient with a tracheostoma, or for nasal intubation. A Fogarty catheter is relatively thin for a given balloon volume when compared with other bronchial blockers and thus will allow larger tracheal tubes to be used, especially in pediatric patients in whom they are placed side by side in the trachea.
   e. A significant disadvantage is the lack of a hollow center. Suctioning, differential ventilation, oxygen insufflation, or applying CPAP to the blocked lung is not possible. Lung collapse takes longer and may not be as complete as with a DLT or a blocker with a hollow lumen. The obstructed lung segment cannot be reexpanded until the blocker is removed. Another disadvantage is that it is made of latex, so it cannot be used in the patient with potential latex allergy (Chapter 11). Most of these devices have low-volume, high-pressure cuffs and can damage the airway, although the pressure may be less than that exerted by the cuff on a DLT.

V. **Hazards Associated with Double-Lumen Tubes and Blockers**

Many of the hazards associated with single-lumen tracheal tubes (Chapter 15) can also occur with DLTs.

A. Difficulty with Insertion and Positioning

Inserting a DLT may be time consuming. The large width makes it difficult to pass through a tracheostoma, small airway, or nose. Severe hemorrhage can be a major problem. Multiple insertions and repositionings increase the risk of trauma. Usually, a DLT must be replaced with a single-lumen tube at the end of surgery.

B. Tube Malpositions

Certain physical conditions may make it difficult or impossible for a DLT to be correctly placed. Preoperative fiber-optic endoscopy may detect many of these. Even if a correct position is achieved initially, head movement, a change in body position, or surgical manipulations may result in tube malposition.

CLINICAL MOMENT Inflating the bronchial cuff with saline has been found to reduce the incidence of tube malposition (3).

CLINICAL MOMENT If DLT malposition is suspected, a fiberscope can be used to define the problem and provide a means of correction.

1. **Consequences**
   a. An obstruction in the unventilated lumen can prevent the unventilated lung from deflating. If the lung cannot be collapsed, operating time will be increased and the surgical result may be compromised.
   b. If the bronchial cuff is not below the carina, it may obstruct the trachea and mainstem bronchus. With right-sided tubes, the port needed to ventilate the right upper lobe may be misaligned, causing obstruction. If the bronchial cuff on a left-sided DLT is too deep, it may obstruct the left upper lobe bronchus.
   c. Gas trapping can result from a one-way valve effect. This can lead to cardiorespiratory embarrassment and/or lung damage.
   d. If the airway to a bronchopleural fistula cannot be isolated from the normal lung, barotrauma may develop with positive-pressure ventilation. The air leak through the fistula may be so large that ventilation of the normal lung is compromised.
   e. An incompletely protected dependent lung may be flooded with blood or secretions.
2. **Possible Malpositions**
   a. In some cases, the bronchial portion will enter the opposite lung. This is usually easy to detect and correct by fiber-optic endoscopy. In some cases, it may be best to leave the bronchial lumen in the operative bronchus and isolate the operative lung by clamping the bronchial limb and using the tracheal lumen for ventilation. This may be appropriate for surgery on the right lung but not for surgery on the left lung, since the right upper lobe bronchus would almost certainly be occluded.
   b. It may be possible for the surgeon to assist in correctly placing the DLT once the chest is open. If it is determined that the tube is in the wrong bronchus, both cuffs are deflated and the tube is withdrawn into the trachea. The surgeon then compresses the bronchus, and the anesthesia provider advances the tube into the correct side. The cuffs are then reinflated.
   c. If a left-sided DLT is inserted too deeply, the upper lobe may be obstructed. The problem may be that the tube is too small. A high peak airway pressure during one-lung ventilation should suggest this malposition.
   d. If the DLT is not sufficiently advanced into the bronchus, the bronchial cuff may protrude into the trachea. The need to inject more than 3 mL of air into the bronchial cuff to achieve a seal should alert the user that the tube may be malpositioned. The bronchial segment may slip out of the bronchus, especially during changes in the patient's position. In many cases, no untoward sequelae will occur. However, there may be gas flow obstruction to the other lung and inability to isolate the surgical lung.
   e. The bronchial lumen tip may be above the carina because of a tracheal lesion that prevents the tube from being advanced farther. With this malposition, there will be unsatisfactory lung deflation and failure to separate the lungs.
   f. DLT malposition with respect to the upper lobe bronchus is particularly a problem with right-sided tubes. The result of such a malposition is usually hypoxemia and unsatisfactory upper lobe deflation.

g. The inflated bronchial cuff can cause the bronchial lumen tip to face the bronchial wall, producing a one-way valve obstruction that allows lung inflation but not deflation.

C. Hypoxemia

1. In many instances, hypoxemia during one-lung ventilation is at least partly the result of a malpositioned DLT. For this reason, whenever hypoxemia occurs, tube position should be reassessed and adjusted if necessary. Even with correct positioning, hypoxemia can result from continuous blood flow through the unventilated lung (shunting) after one-lung ventilation has begun.
2. Another cause of hypoxemia is the presence of a tracheal bronchus arising from the lateral tracheal wall. In some of these cases, a bronchial blocker may be a better choice than a DLT for one-lung ventilation.
3. If hypoxemia is a problem despite proper tube position, CPAP can be applied to the nondependent lung by using the oxygen flow from a separate source. Some DLT manufacturers include a CPAP device with each DLT, or they may be purchased separately (**Fig. 16.11**).

CLINICAL MOMENT A Mapleson D system can be used to provide CPAP. The pressure can be adjusted using the adjustable pressure-limiting valve and oxygen from the courtesy flowmeter.

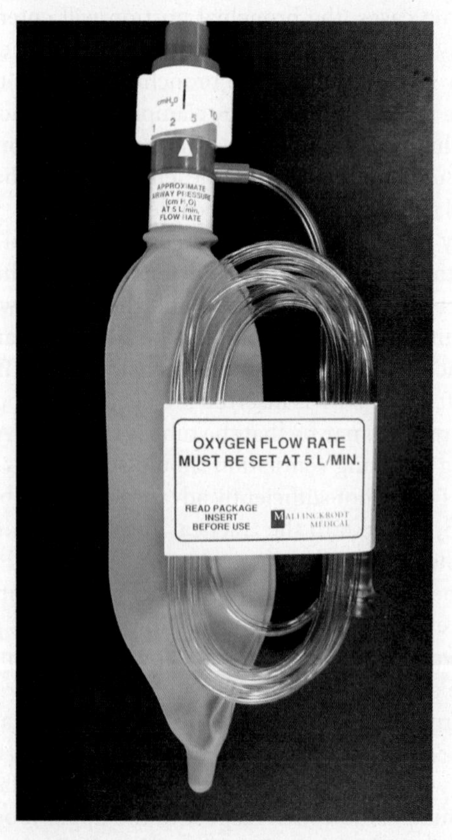
OXYGEN FLOW RATE
MUST BE SET AT 5 L/MIN.
READ PACKAGE INSERT BEFORE USE

Figure 16.11 Device for applying continuous positive airway pressure to a nonventilated lung. The adjustable valve supplies pressures from 1 to 10 cm H_2O.

4. Other measures to improve oxygenation include dependent lung PEEP, occasional ventilation of the nondependent lung (one breath every 5 to 10 minutes), oxygen insufflation to the nonventilated lung, and clamping the pulmonary artery before clamping the bronchus.

D. Obstructed Ventilation

Many cases of obstruction are the result of a malpositioned tube. Inflating the bronchial cuff can cause bronchial lumen narrowing or may cause the carina to be displaced laterally, causing the other mainstem bronchus to be narrowed. A defective tube or connector may cause obstruction. The bronchial lumen can become twisted. An endoluminal tumor can cause obstruction.

E. Trauma

1. Hoarseness, sore throat, and vocal cord injuries are common complications with DLTs. These problems are less frequent when a bronchial blocking device is used.
2. Trauma to the respiratory tract can occur whenever intubation with a DLT is performed. Tears in the trachea and mainstem bronchus have been reported. The arytenoid cartilage can become dislocated. The incidence of bronchial injuries is comparable between DLTs and blockers, but minor airway injuries are more common with DLTs.
3. Tube size is a factor. Large tubes have been involved more often in injury than smaller ones. A tube that is too small and requires excessive cuff inflation may cause ischemic injury.
4. Measures to reduce airway trauma include removing the stylet after the tube tip has passed the vocal cords, avoiding cuff overinflation, deflating the tracheal and bronchial cuffs when repositioning the patient or the tube, and not advancing the tube when resistance is encountered. Some bronchial cuffs can provide one-lung isolation with significantly lower pressures than others. It has been recommended that the bronchial cuff be kept deflated until needed. This may not be wise if there is a bronchial tumor, because necrotic tumor may migrate into the other lung.

F. Tube Problems

Tracheal or bronchial cuff rupture can occur. This most commonly results from contact between the tube and the teeth or laryngoscope during insertion. Proposed methods to avoid this include using a retractable protective sheath, a lubricated Penrose drain, and lubricated teeth guards and increasing the DLT bronchial portion curve with the stylet. Movement during repositioning may also cause cuff rupture.

There may be manufacturing defects that result in a blocked lumen. These are not easy to determine in tubes that are not opaque.

G. Surgical Complications

The bronchial cuff may be punctured by the surgeon. A suture or staple may be placed in or through the DLT. The surgical procedure may result in a tight stenosis, which could entrap the bronchial segment.

CLINICAL MOMENT When the surgical site is near a DLT, there is the possibility that a suture could be placed in the tube wall. If it is difficult to remove the tube, stop and consult the surgeon since forcible tube removal could disrupt the surgical site with fatal consequences.

H. Failure to Seal
Failure to prevent fluids from passing the bronchial cuff could result from malposition or improper cuff inflation. Neither an airtight bronchial seal nor a cuff pressure of 25 cm H_2O guarantees protection against aspiration. Lubricating the cuff with a gel may reduce the risk that fluid will leak past the cuff.

I. Difficult Extubation
Difficulty removing a DLT may be due to anatomical abnormalities, surgical fixation, or entanglement with other surgical or anesthetic hardware.

J. Excessive Cuff Pressure
It is important to remember that cuffs on DLTs and blockers can be overinflated and exert excessive pressure on the tracheal or bronchial mucosa.

REFERENCES

1. Ehrenfeld JM, Walsh JL, Sandberg WS. Right- and left-sided Mallinckrodt double-lumen tubes have identical clinical performance. Anesth Analg 2008;106:1847–1852.
2. Amar D, Desiderio DP, Heerdt PM, Kolker AC, Zhang H, Thaler HT. Practice patterns in choice of left double-lumen tube size for thoracic surgery. Anesth Analg 2008;106:379–383.
3. Suzuki M, Haraguchi S, Kitamura A, et al. Inflation of the distal cuff by saline reduces the incidence of malposition of the bronchial tube during lung separation in patients receiving nitrous oxide. J Cardiothorac Vasc Anesth 2007;21:838–842.

SUGGESTED READINGS

Brodsky JB, Lemmens HJM. Left double-lumen tubes: clinical experience with 1,170 patients. J Cardiothorac Vasc Anesth 2003;17:289–298.

Campos JH. Current techniques for perioperative lung isolation in adults. Anesthesiology 2002;97:1295–1301.

Campos JH. An update on bronchial blockers during lung separation techniques in adults. Anesth Analg 2003;97:1266–1274.

Campos JH. Which devices should be considered the best for lung isolation: double-lumen endotracheal tube versus bronchial blockers. Curr Opin Anesthesiol 2007;20:27–31.

Cohen E. New Developments in Thoracic Anesthesia. Orlando, FL: American Society of Anesthesiologists, 2008. ASA Refresher Course No. 326.

Conacher ID, Velasquez H, Morrice DJ. Airway rupture from double-lumen tubes. J Cardiothorac Vasc Anesth 1999;13:322–329.

Dorsch J, Dorsch S. Lung isolation devices. In: Understanding Anesthesia Equipment. Fifth edition. Philadelphia: Wolters Kluwer/Lippincott Williams & Wilkins, 2008:633–660.

Hammer GB. Single-lung ventilation in infants and children. Pediatr Anesth 2004;14:98–102.

Klafta JM. Strategies for Success in One-Lung Anesthesia. Orlando, FL: American Society of Anesthesiologists, 2008. ASA Refresher Course No. 309.

Sheinbaum R, Hammer GB, Benumof JL. Separation of the two lungs (double-lumen tubes, bronchial blockers and endobronchial single-lumen tubes). In: Hagberg CA, ed. Benumof's Airway Management. Second edition. St Louis, MO: Elsevier, 2007:576–593.

V Monitoring Devices

17 Gas Monitoring

RELIABLE, AFFORDABLE, AND USER-FRIENDLY MONITORS for respired gases are now available and may be either added to or integrated into the anesthesia machine (**Fig. 17.1**).

I. Definitions

A. *Delay time* (transit time, response time, transport delay, time delay, lag time) is the time to achieve 10% of a step change in reading at the gas monitor.

B. *Rise time* (response time) is the time required for a change from 10% to 90% of the total change in a gas value with a change in concentration at the sampling site.

C. The *sensor* (measuring head or chamber) is the part of a respiratory gas monitor that is sensitive to the gas being measured.

D. A *nondiverting* (mainstream, direct probe) *monitor* measures the gas concentration at the sampling site.

E. A *diverting* (sidestream, withdrawal, sampling, aspirating) *monitor* transports gas from the sampling site through a sampling tube to the sensor, which is remote from the sampling site.

F. The *sampling* (sensing) *site* is the location from which gas is diverted for measurement in a diverting monitor or the location of the sensor in a nondiverting monitor.

G. The *sampling tube* (inlet line, sample line) is the conduit for transferring gas from the sampling site to the sensor in a diverting gas monitor.

H. The *partial pressure of a gas* is the pressure that a gas in a gas mixture would exert if it alone occupied the volume of the mixture at the same temperature.

I. The *volumes percent* (%, v/v, vol %) of a gas is the volume of a gas in a mixture, expressed as a percentage of the total volume.

II. Monitor Types

There are two general types of gas monitors: diverting (sidestream) and nondiverting (mainstream). These terms refer to the measurement site and not to the technology being used.

A. Nondiverting

A nondiverting gas monitor (**Fig. 17.2**) measures the gas concentration by using a sensor located directly in the gas stream. Only oxygen and carbon dioxide (CO_2) are

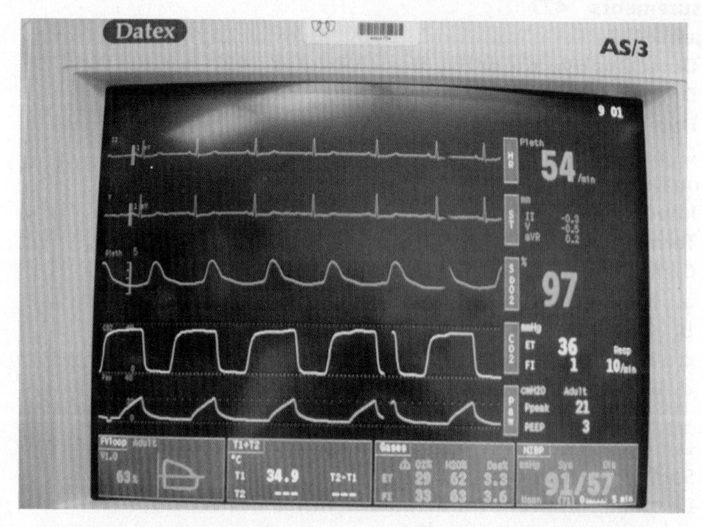

Figure 17.1 Multipurpose monitor. Most gas monitors are now part of a physiologic monitor that includes other monitors such as electrocardiograph, blood pressure, pulse oximetry, and the like. A gas monitor may also be part of the anesthesia machine. Newer anesthesia machines have one or more screens to display monitored functions, and the gas concentrations and waveforms may also be displayed.

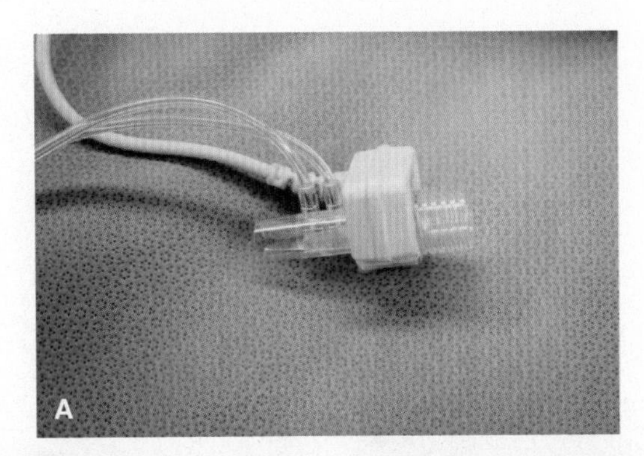

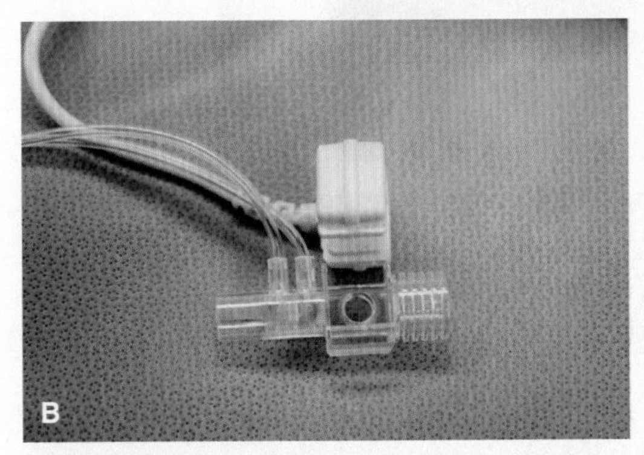

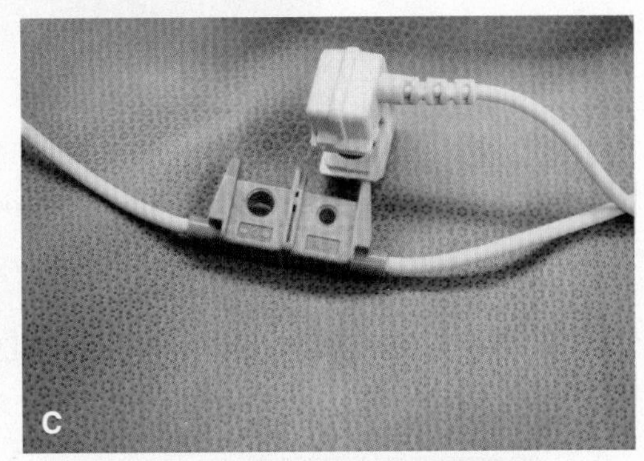

Figure 17.2 Nondiverting gas monitor. **A:** The sensor is in position over the cuvette, which is placed between the patient and the breathing system. The two clear tubings to the left are for spirometry loops (Chapter 18). **B:** The sensor is separated from the cuvette, which contains the window through which the infrared light passes. **C:** Calibration cells. For convenience, they are attached to the cable to the sensor. During calibration, the sensor is placed over each cell in sequence.

being measured by nondiverting monitors at this time. Carbon dioxide is measured by infrared (IR) technology, with the sensor located between the breathing system and the patient. A mainstream oxygen sensor uses electrochemical technology and is usually placed in the inspiratory limb of the breathing system. If the technology is fast enough to measure both inspired and exhaled oxygen, it can be placed between the patient and the breathing system.

B. Diverting

1. **Operation**

a. A diverting monitor uses a pump to aspirate gas from the sampling site through a tube to the sensor that is located in the main unit. Keeping the sampling tube as short as possible will decrease the delay time and result in more satisfactory waveforms.

b. To avoid water or particulate contamination in the monitor, a number of devices have been used. These include traps (**Fig. 17.3**) (which must be emptied periodically), filters and hydrophobic membranes (which must be changed periodically), and special tubing that allows water to diffuse through its walls. Most diverting capnometers are accurate at the respiratory rates normally encountered in clinical practice (20 to 40 breaths per minute). Accuracy decreases with increasing respiratory rate and longer sampling lines.

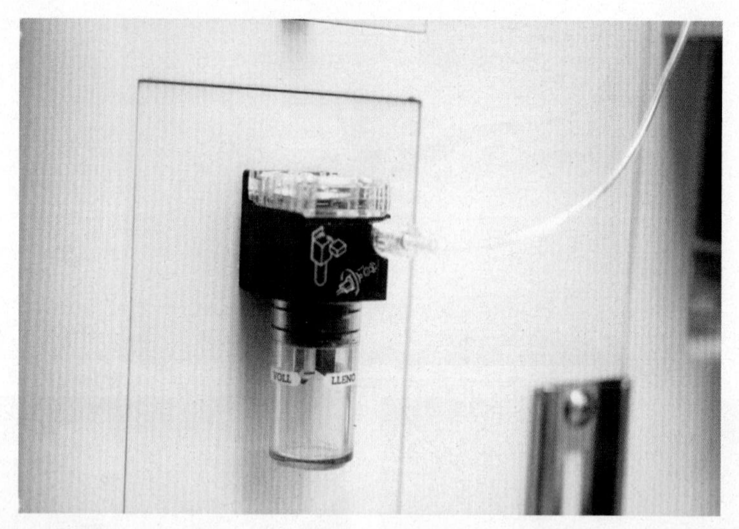

Figure 17.3 Water trap. This should be emptied periodically to prevent water from entering the monitor.

CLINICAL MOMENT If the water trap is located beneath a vaporizer, the plastic that makes up the trap can be damaged if contacted by a liquid anesthetic agent.

CLINICAL MOMENT Many clinicians use a heat and moisture exchanger (HME) (Chapter 9) at the patient port in the breathing system. If the gas monitor line is attached to the breathing system side of the HME, the end-tidal CO_2 value measured will be lower than that measured on the patient side. A disadvantage of attaching the sample line on the patient side of the HME is water and bacterial/viral contamination of the sample line and then the monitor.

2. **Devices**
   a. Face Masks, Tracheal Tubes, and Supraglottic Airway Devices
      1) To measure both inspired and exhaled gases, the sampling site must be between the patient and the breathing system. Most disposable breathing systems and HMEs have built-in sample ports. A sample line can be attached to other breathing system components (**Fig. 17.4**).
      2) When respiratory gases are measured at a facemask, there is a relatively large dead space compared with a tracheal tube. This may result in slightly lower end-tidal carbon dioxide values.
      3) Some tracheal tubes incorporate a sampling lumen that extends to the patient end of the tube (Chapter 15). This provides measurements that more closely approximate alveolar values, especially in small patients and with the Mapleson breathing systems (Chapter 5) in which the fresh gas can mix with exhaled gases.

CLINICAL MOMENT When a tracheal tube with a sampling lumen is used, more moisture will be drawn into the sample line. This can increase resistance in the sample line and possibly damage the monitor if not removed.

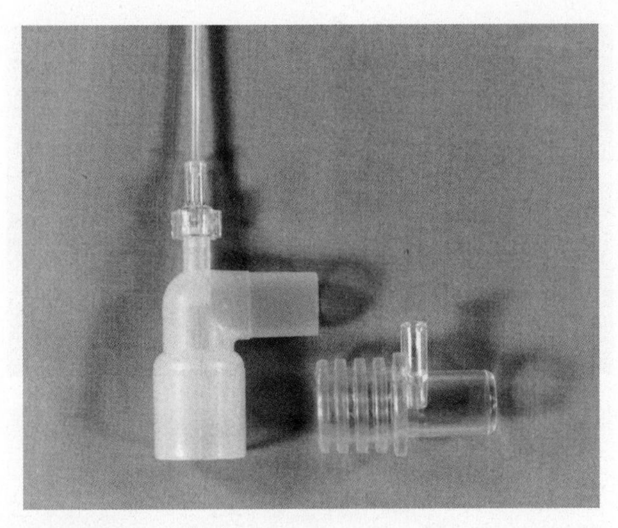

Figure 17.4 Ports for gas sampling in breathing system components.

b. Oxygen Supplementation Devices
   1) Nasal cannulae with a connection for a sample line to measure carbon dioxide are available in several configurations (**Figs. 17.5** and **17.6**). Mouth breathing, airway obstruction, and oxygen delivery through the ipsilateral nasal cannula can affect the accuracy of the readings.
   2) A plastic oxygen mask may be fitted with a sampling port (**Fig. 17.7**). Alternatively, the sampling tube may be connected to the mask outlet, inserted through a vent hole or a slit in the mask, or slipped under the mask and attached near the nostrils. A sampling catheter can also be attached to the upper lip or placed in the patient's nares or the lumen of an oral or nasopharyngeal airway under the mask. In this configuration, air or oxygen will also enter the sample line, lowering the exhaled CO_2 and anesthetic gas values.

CLINICAL MOMENT Loosely fitting masks and nasal cannulae that deliver oxygen do not provide accurate end-tidal carbon dioxide readings because oxygen and air will dilute the sample. This does not mean that it is not useful to measure carbon dioxide when using these devices. The presence of exhaled carbon dioxide provides assurance that the patient is breathing.

c. Other

The end of a sampling line can be placed in front of or inside the patient's nostril or a nasopharyngeal airway. If the patient is a mouth breather, the sample line can be placed in front of the mouth or in the nasopharynx or hypopharynx. A bite block can be modified to accommodate a sampling line. A sampling line can be placed over or in a tracheostoma. Optimal placement should be determined by the CO_2 waveform. Mucosal irritation, catheter blockage, and mechanical interference sometimes cause problems. As with the loosely fitting masks and nasal cannula, the end-tidal CO_2 readings will not be accurate with these monitoring methods.

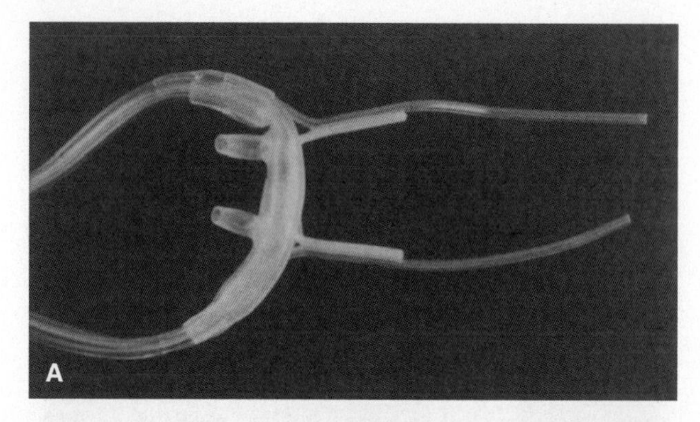

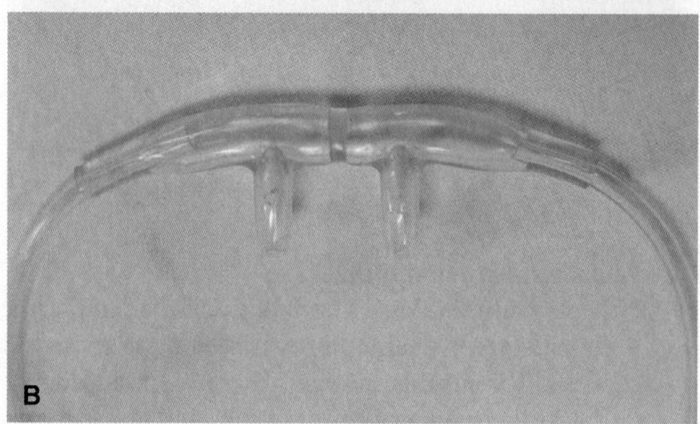

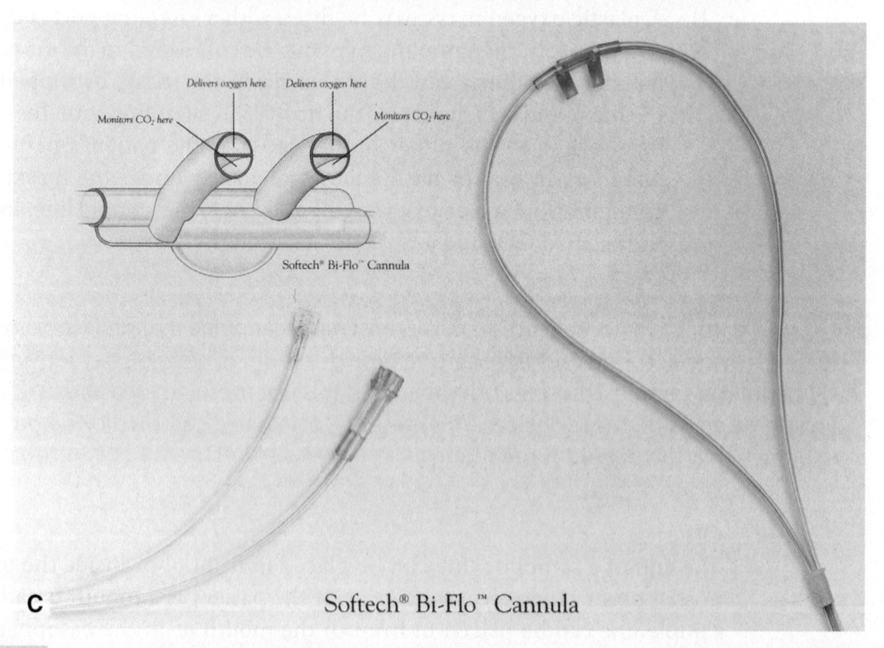

Figure 17.5 Devices for simultaneous administration of oxygen and gas sampling. **A:** This device is designed for patients who are predominantly mouth breathers. The longer oral sampling prongs can be cut and shaped to suit individual patients. (Courtesy of Biochem International, Inc., Waukesha, MI.) **B:** One prong is used for the administration of oxygen and one for gas sampling. There is a septum between the two prongs. **C:** With this device, the two prongs are divided so that oxygen is delivered and gas is sampled through each prong.

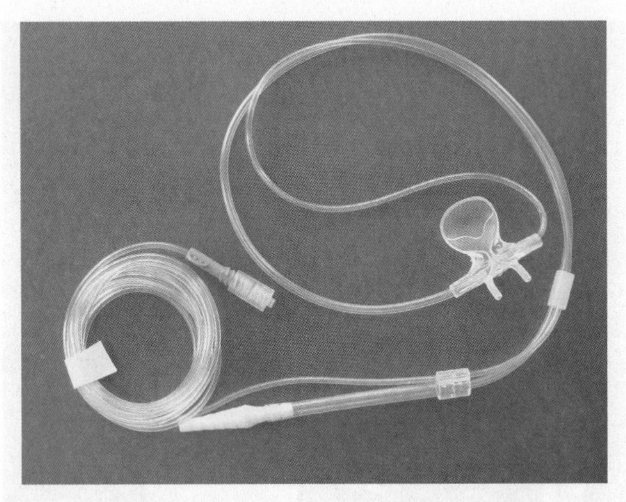

Figure 17.6 This device is used for CO_2 sampling in nonintubated patients who are exhaling either by mouth or by nose.

III. **Technology**

A. Infrared Analysis

IR analysis is the technology most often used to measure carbon dioxide, nitrous oxide, and volatile anesthetic agents.

1. **Technology**

a. IR analyzers are based on the principle that gases with two or more dissimilar atoms in the molecule (nitrous oxide, CO_2, and the halogenated agents) have specific and unique IR absorption spectra. Since the amount of IR rays absorbed is proportional to the concentration of the absorbing molecules, the concentration can be determined by comparing the IR absorbance in the sample with that of a known standard. The nonpolar molecules of argon, nitrogen, helium, xenon, and oxygen do not absorb IR rays and cannot be measured using this technology.

b. Most investigators believe that these monitors are sufficiently accurate for clinical purposes, although they tend to underestimate the inspired level and overestimate end-tidal values at high respiratory rates.

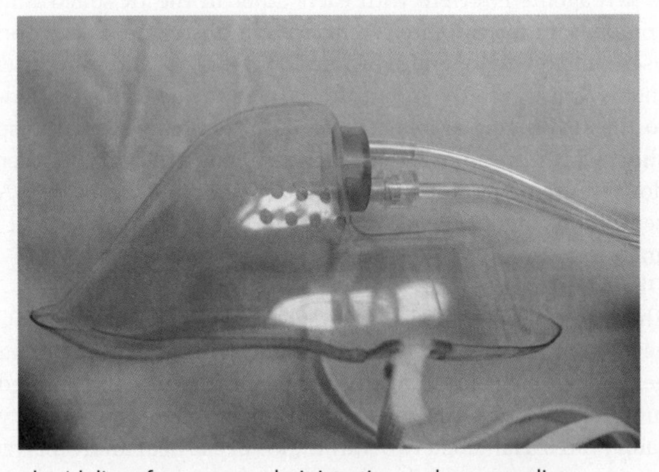

Figure 17.7 Face mask with lines for oxygen administration and gas sampling.

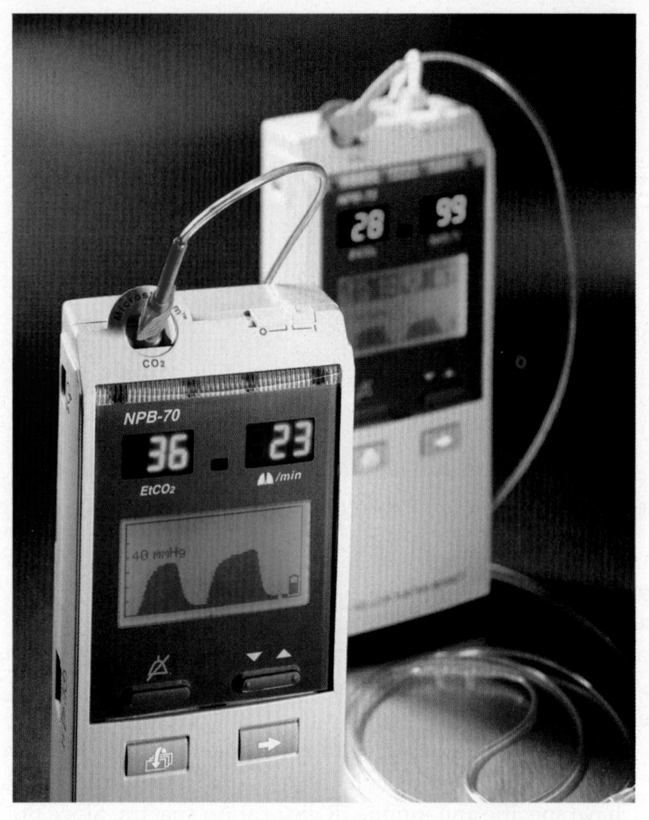

Figure 17.8 Microstream infrared analyzer. Small handheld device. (Photograph courtesy of Oridion Medical, Needham, MA.)

2. **Advantages of Infrared Analysis**
   There are many advantages to using IR monitors. These include the ability to measure nitrous oxide, carbon dioxide, and volatile anesthetic agents. They can discriminate between volatile agents and detect mixtures of these agents. When agents interfere with each other in the IR spectrum, the monitor can compensate for the interference. Some instruments are portable and can be used outside the operating room for transport and other uses (**Fig. 17.8**). Gas that is drawn into the monitor can be returned to the breathing system or sent to the scavenging system. These monitors have a quick response time and a short warm-up time. Agent analyzers may indicate that there is agent breakdown (but do not detect carbon monoxide) (see Chapter 5). Argon or low concentrations of nitric oxide do not interfere with volatile agent monitoring by IR analyzers.
3. **Disadvantages**
   There are a number of disadvantages to using IR technology. Oxygen and nitrogen cannot be measured. There is interference from other gases, such as oxygen in high concentrations, although this can be compensated for by most new monitors. Water vapor can absorb IR light. There is inaccuracy with rapid respiratory rates. Handheld two-way radios in use near an IR analyzer may cause CO_2 readings to be increased.

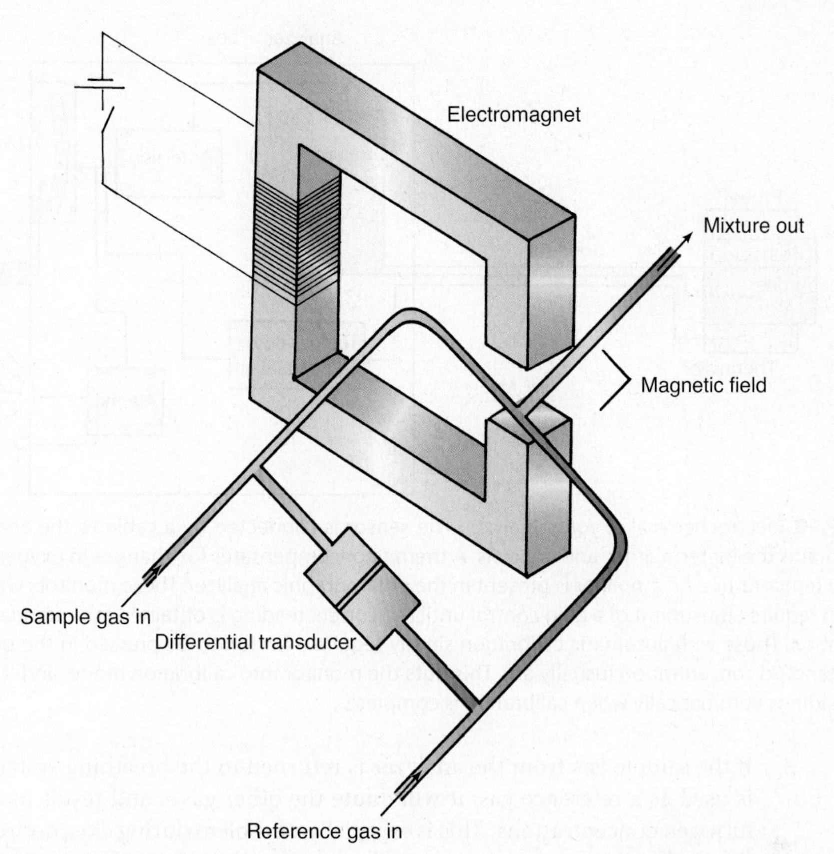

Figure 17.9 Paramagnetic oxygen analyzer. A reference gas of known or no oxygen content and the gas whose oxygen level is to be measured are pumped through the analyzer and converge into a tube at the outlet. The two gas paths are joined at their midpoints by a differential pressure or flow sensor. The magnet is switched on and off at a rapid rate. Because the reference and sample gases have different oxygen levels, the pressures in the paths will differ. The pressure difference is detected by the sensor.

B. Paramagnetic Oxygen Analysis

1. When introduced into a magnetic field, some substances locate themselves in the strongest portion of that field. These substances are termed *paramagnetic*. Oxygen is the only paramagnetic gas that is important in anesthesia. When a gas that contains oxygen is passed through a switched magnetic field, the gas will expand and contract, causing a pressure wave that is proportional to the oxygen partial pressure.
2. A paramagnetic oxygen analyzer is shown diagrammatically in **Figure 17.9**. Reference and sample gases are pumped through the analyzer. The two gas paths are joined by a differential pressure or flow sensor. If the sample and reference gases have different oxygen partial pressures, the magnet will detect the difference. This difference is converted into an electrical signal that is displayed as oxygen partial pressure or volumes percent. The short rise time allows both inspired and end-tidal oxygen levels to be measured even at rapid respiratory rates. Many monitors combine IR analysis of CO_2, volatile anesthetic agents, and nitrous oxide with paramagnetic oxygen analysis by using the same diverted gas (**Fig. 17.1**). This allows most gases of interest to be measured using a single monitor.

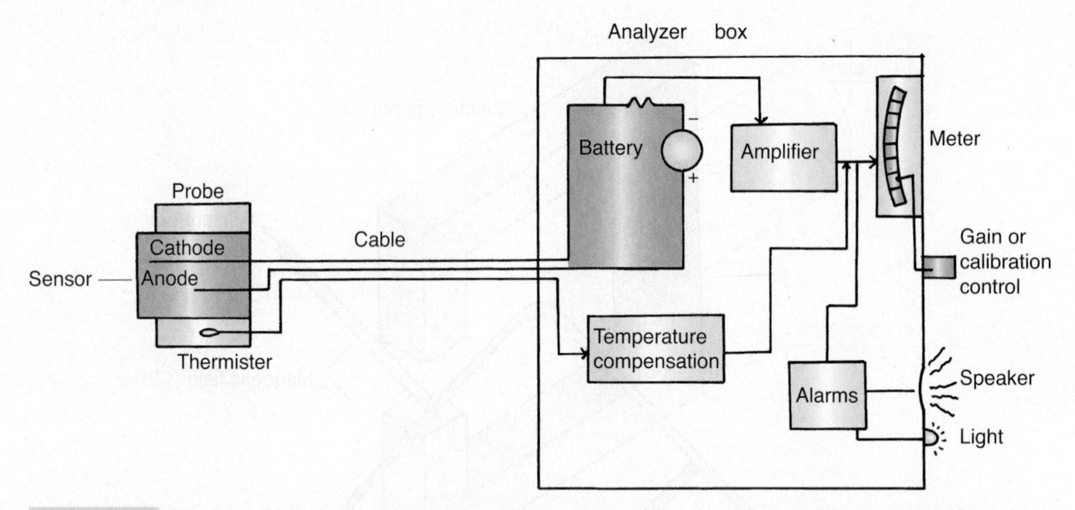

Figure 17.10 Electrochemical oxygen analyzer. The sensor is connected by a cable to the analyzer box, which contains the meter, alarms, and controls. A thermistor compensates for changes in oxygen diffusion caused by temperature. An amplifier is present in the polarographic analyzer. Those monitors with manual calibration require adjustment of a gain control until the correct reading is obtained for a standard oxygen concentration. Those with automatic calibration simply require a button to be pressed in the presence of a gas of standard concentration (usually air). This puts the monitor into calibration mode, and it returns to normal readings automatically when calibration is complete.

3. If the sample gas from the analyzer is returned to the breathing system and air is used as a reference gas, it will dilute the other gases and result in increased nitrogen concentrations. This is especially a problem during closed-circuit anesthesia. If oxygen is used as the reference gas, the accumulation of nitrogen is significantly reduced.

C. Electrochemical Oxygen Analysis

An electrochemical oxygen analyzer consists of a sensor, which is exposed to the gas being analyzed, and the analyzer box, which contains the electronic circuitry, display, and alarms (**Fig. 17.10**). The sensor contains a cathode and an anode surrounded by electrolyte. The gel is held in place by a membrane that is nonpermeable to ions, proteins, and other such materials yet is permeable to oxygen. The membrane should not be touched, because dirt and grease reduce its usable area.

In most cases, the sensor is placed in the inspiratory limb of the breathing system. Most of these analyzers respond slowly to changes in oxygen pressure, so they cannot be used to measure end-tidal concentrations. Some newer monitors can analyze oxygen quickly enough to measure inspired and exhaled concentrations.

CLINICAL MOMENT The life of an electrochemical analyzer sensor is measured in percent hours. This means that the higher the oxygen concentration that it is exposed to, the shorter the sensor life. The life of an electrochemical oxygen analyzer sensor can be prolonged by removing it from the breathing system and exposing it to air when not in use (**Fig. 17.11**).

1. **Use**

a. Calibration

Unless the monitor is self-calibrating, calibration should be performed daily before use and at least every 8 hours after that. Some instruments remind

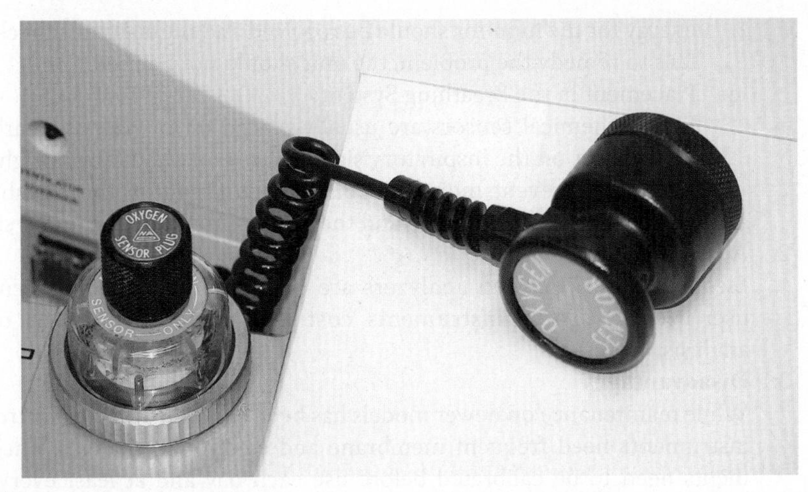

Figure 17.11 The life of a galvanic (fuel cell) electrochemical oxygen analyzer can be prolonged by leaving it exposed to room air when not in use.

the user when calibration is needed and will not give a reading until calibration is performed (**Fig. 17.12**). The calibration can be checked by exposing the sensor to room air and verifying that it indicates approximately 21% oxygen.

b. Checking the Alarms

The sensor should be exposed to room air and the low oxygen alarm limit set above 21%. The visual signal should flash, and the audible signal sound. If the unit has a high oxygen alarm, the setting for that should be moved below 21%. Both the visual and audible signals should be activated. If the visual signal fails or the audible signal is weak, the batteries supplying

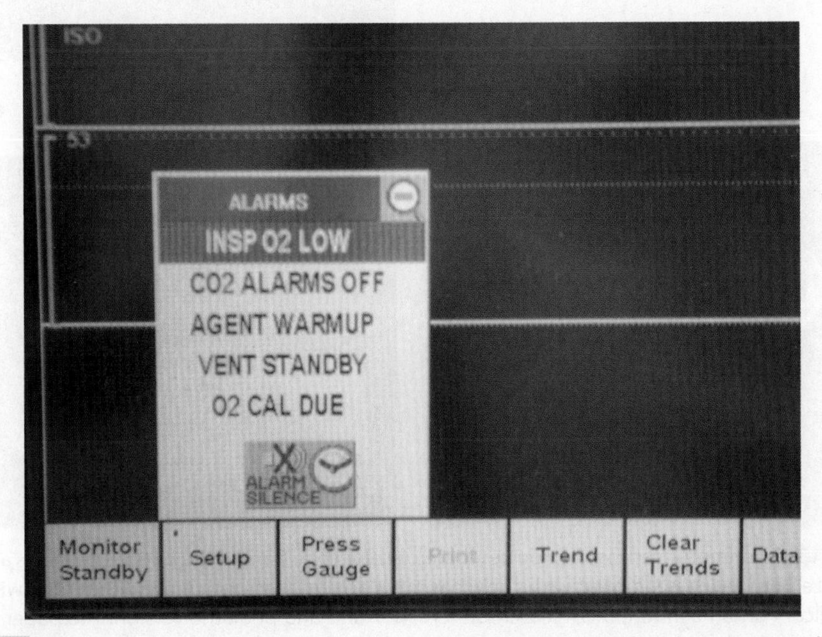

Figure 17.12 The display on the anesthesia machine provides a reminder that the oxygen analyzer needs to be calibrated.

energy for the monitor should be replaced and the alarms rechecked. If this fails to remedy the problem, the unit should not be used.

c. Placement in the Breathing System

Electrochemical sensors are usually placed on or near the carbon dioxide canister on the inspiratory side. The sensor should be upright or tilted slightly to prevent moisture from accumulating on the membrane. The junction between the cable and the sensor should not be under strain.

2. **Advantages**

Electrochemical oxygen analyzers are compact, dependable, accurate, and user-friendly. These instruments cost less than other means of oxygen analysis.

3. **Disadvantages**

While maintenance on newer models has been simplified, some electrochemical instruments need frequent membrane and electrolyte changes. These instruments need to be calibrated before use each day and at least every 8 hours. Instruments that are not an integral part of and powered by the anesthesia machine need to be turned on by the user.

D. Chemical Carbon Dioxide Detection

1. **Technology**

A chemical (colorimetric) detector (**Fig. 17.13**) consists of a pH-sensitive indicator enclosed in a housing unit. When the indicator is exposed to carbonic acid that is formed as a product of the reaction between CO_2 and water, it becomes more acidic and changes color. During inspiration, the color returns to its resting state unless it is used with a breathing system that allows rebreathing. The inlet and outlet ports are 15 mm, so the device can be placed between the patient

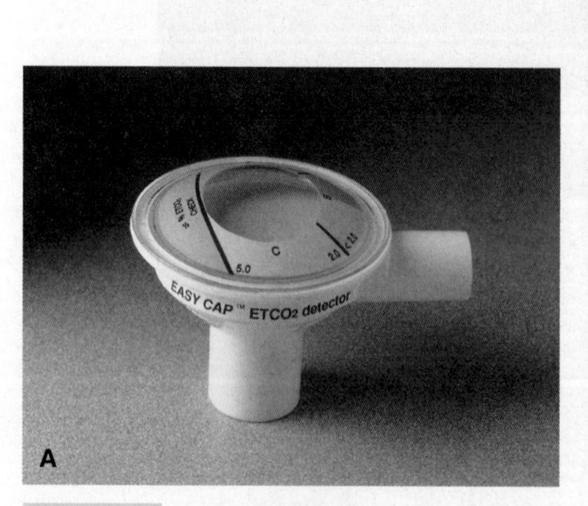

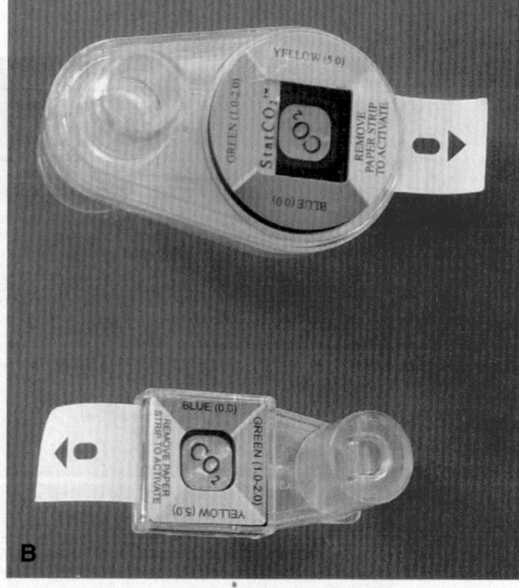

Figure 17.13 Colorimetric carbon dioxide detectors. A color code around the outside provides a reference. **A:** Adult size. The device is supplied with caps that must be removed before use. (Reprinted with permission of Nellcor Puritan Bennett, Inc., Pleasanton, CA.) **B:** Adult and pediatric version. The paper strip must be removed to use the device.

and the breathing system or resuscitation bag. Pediatric versions are available (**Fig. 17.13B**).

2. **Advantages**

Chemical carbon dioxide detectors are small, portable, easy to use, and not affected by nitrous oxide and other anesthetics or carbon monoxide. They do not depend on external power sources and can therefore be used in remote locations. They are low in cost. These devices accurately detect esophageal intubation if carbon dioxide is present in exhaled gases. Flow resistance is minimal. Since they are disposable, they need not be cleaned and cannot transmit infection.

3. **Disadvantages**

Six breaths are recommended to determine tracheal tube location. False-negative results may be observed with very low tidal volumes and low end-tidal carbon dioxide concentrations. Drugs instilled into the trachea or gastric contents may disable the device. The color may be difficult to determine in low light or with low end-tidal carbon dioxide levels. These devices are semiquantitative and cannot give accurate measurements for carbon dioxide.

CLINICAL MOMENT If stomach acid is regurgitated into the colorimetric device, the color change may indicate that carbon dioxide is present. The color change may be permanent.

CLINICAL MOMENT False-positive results may occur if there is carbon dioxide in the stomach and the tracheal tube is in the esophagus.

IV. Gas Measurements

A. Oxygen

The standards for basic anesthesia monitoring of the American Society of Anesthesiologists (ASA) and American Association of Nurse Anesthetists state that the concentration of oxygen in the breathing system shall be measured by an oxygen analyzer with a low oxygen concentration alarm. There are a number of important reasons to monitor oxygen.

1. **Detecting Hypoxic or Hyperoxic Mixtures**
   a. The first line of defense against hypoxemia is to avoid a hypoxic inspired gas mixture. An oxygen monitor provides an earlier warning of inadequate oxygen than pulse oximetry. Hypoxia is discussed in Chapter 10.
   b. Oxygen analysis can also help to prevent problems resulting from hyperoxygenation, such as patient movement during surgery, awareness, damage to the lungs and eyes, and fires. Fires are discussed in detail in Chapter 25.
2. **Detecting Disconnections and Leaks**

An oxygen monitor can detect disconnections in the breathing system. However, oxygen monitoring cannot be depended on for this purpose. Whether or not the oxygen level falls at the point being monitored depends on several factors, including the type of breathing system in use, position of the sensor, site of disconnection, alarm set points, whether the patient is breathing spontaneously or ventilation is controlled, and the type of ventilator in use. A disconnected tube to an oxygen mask may be detected by using a diverting oxygen analyzer. Disconnections are discussed in Chapter 10.

3. **Detecting Hypoventilation**

Normally, the difference between inspired and expired oxygen is 4% to 5%. A difference of more than 5% after a steady state has been reached is a sensitive indicator of hypoventilation. Hypoventilation is discussed in detail in Chapter 10.

4. **Other**

a. End-tidal oxygen can be used to determine adequate preoxygenation.

b. Knowing the expired oxygen concentration allows the patient's oxygen consumption to be estimated and can aid in diagnosing malignant hyperthermia.

c. End-tidal oxygen has been used to detect air embolism. When a significant amount of air enters the vascular bed, there is an increase in end-tidal oxygen and a decrease in the difference between inspiratory and end-tidal oxygen concentrations.

B. Carbon Dioxide Analysis

1. **Importance**

a. ASA guidelines for basic anesthetic monitoring state that when a tracheal tube or supraglottic airway device is inserted, its correct positioning must be verified by identifying CO_2 in the expired gas. Continual end-tidal CO_2 analysis shall be performed until the device is removed or the patient is transferred to a postoperative care location. In 2005, an audible alarm was added to the monitoring standard. Some states have mandated using CO_2 monitors.

b. Carbon dioxide analysis provides a means for assessing metabolism, circulation, and ventilation and can detect many equipment- and patient-related problems that other monitors either fail to detect or detect so slowly that patient safety may be compromised. A closed claims analysis found that capnography plus pulse oximetry could potentially prevent 93% of avoidable anesthetic mishaps. Carbon dioxide monitoring detects acute complete airway obstruction, apnea, and extubation more rapidly than pulse oximetry or vital sign monitoring.

2. **Terminology**

Capnometry is the measurement of CO_2 in a gas mixture, and a *capnometer* is the device that performs the measurement and displays the readings in numerical form. *Capnography* is the recording of CO_2 concentration versus time, and a *capnograph* is the machine that generates the waveform. The *capnogram* is the actual waveform.

3. **Clinical Significance of Capnometry**

Carbon dioxide is produced in the body tissues, conveyed by the circulatory system to the lungs, excreted by the lungs, and removed by the breathing system. Therefore, changes in respired CO_2 may reflect alterations in metabolism, circulation, respiration, or the breathing system. **Tables 17.1** to **17.4** list some causes of changes in CO_2 levels.

a. Metabolism

1) Monitoring CO_2 elimination gives an indication of the patient's metabolic rate. An increase or decrease in end-tidal CO_2 (P_{ETCO_2}) level is a reliable indicator of metabolism only in mechanically ventilated subjects. In spontaneously breathing patients, end-tidal carbon dioxide may not increase with increased metabolism because the patient may compensate for the increased CO_2 by hyperventilating.

Table 17.1 Capnography and Capnometry with Altered Carbon Dioxide Production[a]

	Waveform on Capnograph	End-Tidal Carbon Dioxide	Inspiratory Carbon Dioxide	End-Tidal to Arterial Gradient
Absorption of CO_2 from peritoneal cavity	Normal	↑	0	Normal
Injection of sodium bicarbonate	Normal	↑	0	Normal
Pain, anxiety, shivering	Normal	↑	0	Normal
Increased muscle tone (due to muscle relaxant reversal)	Normal	↑	0	Normal
Convulsions	Normal	↑	0	Normal
Hyperthermia	Normal	↑	0	Normal
Hypothermia	Normal	↓	0	Normal
Increased depth of anesthesia (in relation to surgical stimulus)	Normal	↓	0	Normal
Use of muscle relaxants	May see curare cleft	↓	0	Normal
Increased transport of CO_2 to the lungs (restoration of peripheral circulation after it has been impaired, e.g., after release of a tourniquet)	Normal	↑	0	Normal

[a]Normal end-tidal CO_2 is 38 torr (5%). Inspired CO_2 is normally 0. The arterial to end-tidal gradient is normally less than 5 torr.

2) **Table 17.1** lists some metabolic causes of increased or decreased CO_2 excretion. Increased exhaled CO_2 can result from CO_2 used to inflate the peritoneal cavity during laparoscopy, the pleural cavity during thoracoscopy, and a joint during arthroscopy or to increase visualization for endoscopic vein harvest.

CLINICAL MOMENT Malignant hyperthermia is a hypermetabolic state with a massive increase in CO_2 production that occurs early, before the temperature rises. Detecting this syndrome in the early stages is one of the most important reasons for routinely monitoring CO_2. Capnometry can be used to monitor the treatment effectiveness.

Table 17.2 Capnographic and Capnometric Alterations as a Result of Circulatory Changes

	Waveform on Capnograph	End-Tidal Carbon Dioxide	Inspiratory Carbon Dioxide	End-Tidal to Arterial Gradient
Decreased transport of CO_2 to the lungs (impaired peripheral circulation)	Normal	↓	0	Normal
Decreased transport of CO_2 through the lungs (pulmonary embolus, either air or thrombus; surgical manipulations)	Normal	↓	0	Elevated
Increased patient dead space	Normal	↓	0	Elevated

Table 17.3 Capnometry and Capnography with Respiratory Problems

	Waveform on Capnograph	End-Tidal Carbon Dioxide	Inspiratory Carbon Dioxide	End-Tidal to Alveolar Gradient
Disconnection	Absent		0	
Apneic patient, stopped ventilator	Absent		0	
Hyperventilation	Normal	↓	0	Normal
Hypoventilation, mild to moderate	Normal	↑	0	Normal
Upper airway obstruction	Abnormal[a]	↑	0	Elevated
Rebreathing (e.g., under drapes)	Baseline elevated	↑	↑	Normal
Esophageal intubation	Absent		0	

[a]See Figure 17.22.

b. Circulation

1) **Table 17.2** lists some of the circulatory changes that affect exhaled CO_2. A decrease in end-tidal CO_2 level is seen with a decrease in cardiac output if ventilation remains constant whereas end-tidal CO_2 level increases with increased cardiac output.

Table 17.4 Capnographic and Capnometric Alterations with Equipment

Problem	Waveform on Capnograph	End-Tidal Carbon Dioxide	Inspiratory Carbon Dioxide	End-Tidal to Arterial Gradient
Increased apparatus dead space	Baseline Elevated	↑	↑	Normal
Rebreathing with circle system: faulty or exhausted absorbent, bypassed absorber (may be masked by high fresh gas flow)	Baseline Elevated See Figure 17.14	↑	↑	Normal
Rebreathing with the Mapleson system (inadequate fresh gas flow, misassembly, problem with inner tube of the Bain system)	Baseline Elevated See Figure 17.14	↑	↑	Decreased
Rebreathing due to malfunctioning nonrebreathing valve	Baseline Elevated See Figure 17.14	↑	↑	Decreased
Obstruction to expiration in the breathing system	See Figure 17.22	↑	0	Decreased
Blockage of sampling line	Absent	0	0	
Leakage in sampling line	See Figure 17.24	↓	0	Increased
Low sampling rate with diverting device		↓	↑	Increased
Too high a sampling rate with diverting device		↓	0	Increased
Inadequate seal around tracheal tube	See Figure 17.26	↓	0	Increased

2) In addition to reduced cardiac output, reduced blood flow to the lungs can result from surgical manipulations of the heart or thoracic vessels, dissecting aortic aneurysm, wedging of a pulmonary artery catheter, or pulmonary embolism (thrombus, tumor, gas, fat, marrow, or amniotic fluid). If the embolized gas is CO_2, the end-tidal CO_2 level will initially increase and then decrease. Although not as sensitive as the Doppler system for detecting air embolism, CO_2 monitoring is less subjective, is unaffected by electrosurgery apparatus, and can be used in many cases for which the Doppler apparatus is not applicable. End-tidal CO_2 levels may be used to predict resuscitation outcomes and the resolution of a pulmonary embolus. However, capnometry may not be sufficiently sensitive to detect fat and marrow microemboli.

3) During resuscitation, exhaled CO_2 is a better guide to the effectiveness of resuscitative measures than the electrocardiogram, pulse, or blood pressure. The capnometer is not susceptible to the mechanical artifacts that are associated with chest compression. Resuscitative measures do not need to be interrupted to assess circulation. If high-dose epinephrine or bicarbonate is used, the end-tidal CO_2 level is not a good resuscitation indicator.

CLINICAL MOMENT During situations such as acute blood loss causing reduced cardiac output, it may be difficult to monitor blood pressure. The presence of end-tidal carbon dioxide will confirm that at least some circulation is present. As the situation is corrected, the end-tidal carbon dioxide will increase and may overshoot the preincident levels as carbon dioxide is released from various hypoperfused organs.

CLINICAL MOMENT If there is no blood flow to the lungs (as occurs in cardiac arrest), any residual CO_2 may be washed out of the lungs before intubation is attempted. CO_2 monitoring will not help to determine tracheal tube placement in this situation.

c. Respiration

1) Carbon dioxide monitoring gives information about the rate, frequency, and depth of respiration. It can be used to evaluate the patient's ability to breathe spontaneously as well as the effect of bronchodilator or nitric oxide treatment or altered ventilation parameters. It allows ventilatory control with fewer blood gas determinations. End-tidal analysis is noninvasive, available on a breath-by-breath basis, and not affected by hyperventilation induced by drawing an arterial blood sample.

2) **Table 17.3** lists some respiratory causes of increased and decreased end-tidal CO_2 levels associated with respiration. A capnometer can warn about esophageal intubation, apnea, extubation, disconnection, ventilator malfunction, a change in compliance or resistance, airway obstruction, poor mask fit, a malpositioned supraglottic airway, or a leaking tracheal tube cuff.

CLINICAL MOMENT Monitoring end-tidal CO_2 level is useful for patients undergoing sedation or monitored anesthesia care (MAC) and may provide an earlier warning of a potentially dangerous respiratory pattern than pulse oximetry.

3) A dependable means to determine when a tracheal tube has been placed in the tracheobronchial tree is obviously of great value. Inadvertent esophageal intubation has been a leading cause of death and cerebral damage in the past. A discussion of various ways to detect proper tracheal tube position is given in Chapter 15. Carbon dioxide monitoring is usually considered the most reliable method but has some drawbacks and limitations.

CLINICAL MOMENT If there is mechanical blockage in both mainstem bronchi, there will be no detectable CO_2 in spite of the tracheal tube being present in the trachea. Carbon dioxide may not be detectable in cardiac arrest patients if no circulation has been present.

CLINICAL MOMENT With esophageal intubation, small waveforms may be seen transiently resulting from CO_2 that has entered the stomach during mask ventilation or from carbonated beverages or medications. This could give the impression that the tube is correctly placed in the trachea. Rapidly diminishing concentrations and abnormal waveforms will usually differentiate esophageal from tracheal intubation.

CLINICAL MOMENT While esophageal intubation will likely be detected by monitoring CO_2, there is no guarantee that the tube is present in the trachea. Carbon dioxide can be detected from a tracheal tube positioned above the vocal cords or in a bronchus.

4) A diverting CO_2 monitor can be used to monitor respiratory rate and exhaled CO_2 in unintubated patients who are breathing spontaneously. Apnea, airway obstruction, or oxygen source disconnection may be detected.

CLINICAL MOMENT If the breathing space under the surgical drapes is not adequately ventilated, rebreathing will occur and may be detected by a rising inspired CO_2 level.

CLINICAL MOMENT Carbon dioxide monitoring in combination with pulse oximetry has been found useful in detecting respiratory depression during patient-controlled analgesia and MAC (1, 2).

5) Capnometry can be used to help to determine double-lumen tube position. Correct placement can be verified by examining the waveform from

each lung during clamping and unclamping procedures. This method is less reliable than other methods that are discussed in Chapter 16. During independent lung ventilation, capnography can be used to determine the proper settings for ventilating each lung. Capnography can be used to detect tracheobronchial injury during thoracoscopic procedures.

6) Accidental bronchial intubation may result in a transient fall or rise in the end-tidal CO_2 level. Monitoring CO_2 is not a good method to detect bronchial intubation.

d. Equipment Function

1) A problem with the breathing system can cause an inspired CO_2 level of more than zero. Examples of such problems are listed in **Table 17.4.**

2) Incompetent unidirectional valves are an inherent danger of the circle system. An incompetent expiratory valve allows reverse gas flow that contains CO_2 from the expiratory limb during the inspiratory phase, resulting in an elevated baseline on the capnogram (**Fig. 17.14**). If the inspiratory valve is incompetent, CO_2 will enter the inspiratory limb during exhalation. During the next inspiration, CO_2 will be rebreathed. This will cause the plateau on the capnogram to be lengthened and a decrease in the steepness of the inspiratory downslope (**Fig. 17.15**). An elevated baseline may not be seen. Carbon dioxide analysis can be used to detect a disconnected oxygen tube to a mask during local or regional anesthesia. If the oxygen source becomes detached, there will be a rise in CO_2 level because of rebreathing.

CLINICAL MOMENT If the patient is spontaneously breathing and a disconnection occurs between the breathing system and the sampling site, the disconnection may not be detected by carbon dioxide monitoring.

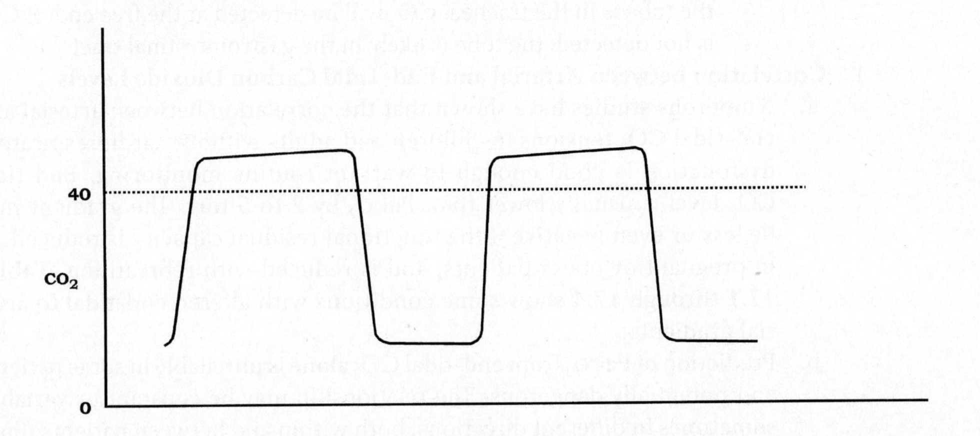

Figure 17.14 Inspired carbon dioxide. The capnogram baseline is normally zero. In this figure, the baseline is elevated and the waveform has a normal shape. This may be caused by an incompetent expiratory valve or exhausted absorbent in the circle system; insufficient fresh gas flow to a Mapleson system; problems with the inner tube of a coaxial (Bain or coaxial circle) system; deliberate addition of CO_2 to the fresh gas; or in some cases, an incompetent inspiratory valve. It may also be the result of rebreathing under drapes in a spontaneously breathing patient who is not intubated.

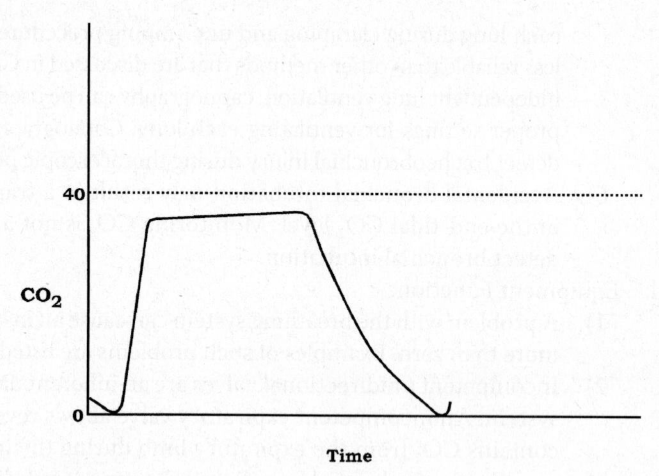

Figure 17.15 Incompetent inspiratory unidirectional valve. The waveform has a prolonged plateau and a slanting inspiratory downstroke. The inspiratory phase is shortened, reflecting the presence of CO_2 in the first inhaled gas. The baseline may or may not reach zero, depending on the fresh gas flow. A similar pattern may be seen with suction applied to a chest tube.

e. Other Uses

1) A diverting capnometer can be used to localize the leak sites in CO_2 insufflation equipment, diagnose a tracheoesophageal or bronchoesophageal fistula, guide blind intubation, determine when the tip of an exchange catheter or fiberscope is in the trachea, or confirm that the needle or catheter is positioned in the trachea during cricothyrotomy or percutaneous dilatational tracheostomy.

2) Carbon dioxide analysis may be used to assess enteric tube position. If the tube is in the trachea, CO_2 will be detected at the free end. If CO_2 is not detected, the tube is likely in the gastrointestinal tract.

4. **Correlation between Arterial and End-Tidal Carbon Dioxide Levels**

a. Numerous studies have shown that the correlation between arterial and end-tidal CO_2 tensions in children and adults without cardiorespiratory dysfunction is good enough to warrant routine monitoring. End-tidal CO_2 level is usually lower than $Paco_2$ by 2 to 5 torr. The gradient may be less or even negative if the functional residual capacity is reduced, as in pregnant or obese patients, and is reduced with rebreathing. **Tables 17.1** through **17.4** show some conditions with altered end-tidal to arterial gradients.

b. Prediction of $Paco_2$ from end-tidal CO_2 alone is unreliable in some patients and potentially dangerous. The relationship may be constant or variable, sometimes in different directions, both within and between patients. End-tidal CO_2 cannot replace $Paco_2$ measurement in the intensive care unit or emergency department, although it is useful for trending or screening.

5. **Sampling Problems**

a. Sampling at the patient end of the tracheal tube or supraglottic airway device results in a closer approximation to arterial CO_2 than sampling at the breathing system end. Placing the gas sampling line on the breathing system side of an HME may avoid water being sucked into the monitor.

Sampling on the breathing system side of the HME may cause erroneous values and a poor waveform.

b. One source of sampling error is a leak at the interface between the patient and the equipment. Poor mask fit, using an uncuffed tracheal tube or a tube with a defective cuff, or a loose connection or leak in the sampling catheter may cause erroneously low end-tidal CO_2 readings. The correlation between arterial and end-tidal CO_2 tensions is better during ventilation with a supraglottic device than with a face mask.

c. With unintubated, spontaneously breathing patients, poor correlation between end-tidal and arterial CO_2 tensions is associated with partial airway obstruction, high respiratory rates, low tidal volumes, oxygen delivery through the ipsilateral nasal cannula or into a plastic face mask, and mouth breathing. Results may be improved by isolating insufflated oxygen from exhaled gases, observing the waveform for normal configuration, and decreasing the oxygen flow rate.

6. **Disturbances in the Ventilation:Perfusion Ratio**

a. When there is ventilation–perfusion mismatching, the relationship between end-tidal and arterial CO_2 tensions is disturbed. Clinical conditions that can alter the volume and/or distribution of pulmonary blood flow include pulmonary embolism, pulmonary artery occlusion, reduced cardiac output, hypovolemia, and certain heart lesions.

b. The end-tidal to arterial CO_2 gradient increases as venous admixture (right to left shunt) occurs. This can be caused by atelectasis, bronchial intubation, or certain heart conditions. The effect is less dramatic than that caused by an increase in dead space, but when the venous admixture is large (as in cyanotic congenital heart disease), its contribution can be considerable.

c. Patients with pulmonary disease have an uneven distribution of ventilation and, to a lesser extent, blood flow. This leads to an increased gradient. Since positive end-expiratory pressure (PEEP) may decrease the gradient, the arterial to end-tidal CO_2 gradient can be a useful tool for optimizing PEEP. Changes in body position, such as the lateral or prone position, may cause an increase in the $Paco_2$/$Petco_2$ gradient.

7. **Capnometer Problems**

a. If there is a leak or break in the sampling line or its connections, air will be added to the sample and the end-tidal CO_2 reading will be lower than the actual value. A partially obstructed sampling catheter can cause the capnogram to be dampened and lead to both falsely high inspired and falsely low end-tidal CO_2 values. An occluded sampling or exhaust line can result in no CO_2 being detected. An internal leak in the analyzer can result in artifactually high values.

b. Other problems that may result in an inaccurate $Petco_2$ reading include increased sampling tube resistance, changes in atmospheric pressure, improper calibration, drift, signal noise, selectivity, pressure effects from the sampling system or patient environment, water vapor, and foreign substances. With some analyzers, air is used for zeroing. If CO_2-containing gas enters the zeroing sample, there will be falsely low CO_2 readings with a normal-looking waveform.

8. **Capnography**

a. All CO_2 monitors today include a waveform (**Fig. 17.16**). Waveforms can be either displayed on an oscilloscope or printed on paper. Slow speeds can be used to show trends. Faster speeds are used for examining individual waveforms. Most monitors provide end-tidal trends.

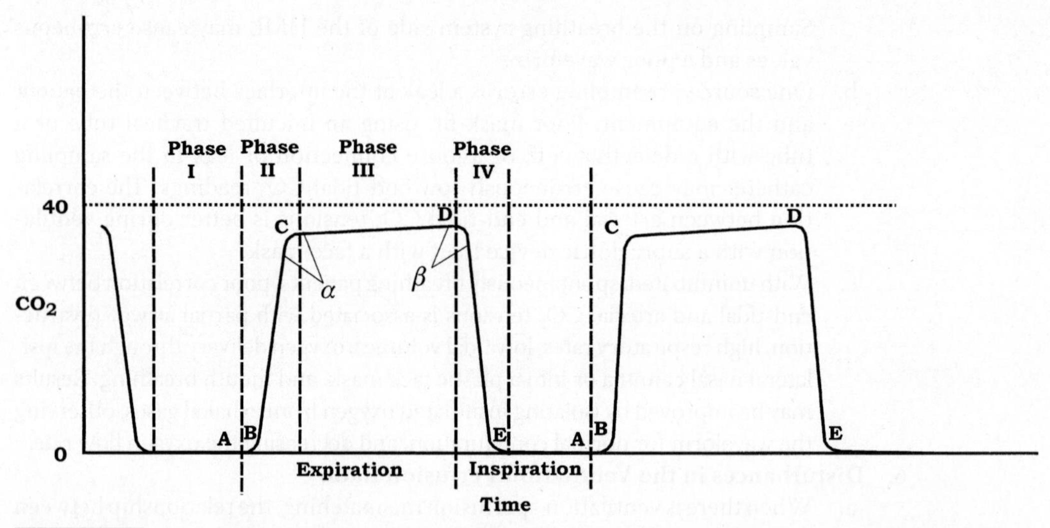

Figure 17.16 The normal waveform. Phase I begins at E and is at zero, since under normal circumstances the inspired gas does not contain CO_2. Phase II (expiratory upstroke) begins at B and continues up to C. This rapid S-shaped upswing represents the transition from dead space gas that does not participate in gas exchange to alveolar gas that contains CO_2. Phase III begins at C and continues to just before D. As gas coming almost entirely from alveoli is exhaled, a plateau is normally seen. If a plateau is not present, the maximum value obtained may not be equivalent to the end-tidal level and the correlation between arterial and end-tidal CO_2 gradients is not likely to be good. The phase III slope is increased by ventilation-perfusion abnormalities in the lung as well as external factors such as a kinked tracheal tube. The last portion of phase III, identified by D, is referred to as the end-tidal point. The CO_2 level here is normally at its maximum. In normal individuals, this is 5% to 5.5%, or 35 to 40 torr.

The angle between phase II and phase III is called the α (takeoff, elevation) angle. Normally, it is between 100 degrees and 110 degrees. It is decreased with obstructive lung disease. The slope of phase III depends on the ventilation-perfusion status of the lung. Airway obstruction and PEEP cause an increased slope and a larger α angle. Other factors that affect the angle are the response time, sweep speed, and respiratory cycle time of the capnometer.

The angle between the end of phase III and the descending limb of the capnogram is called the β angle. Normally, it is approximately 90 degrees. The angle increases with rebreathing. Another possible cause of an increased β angle is a prolonged response time compared with the respiratory cycle time, particularly in children. The angle will be decreased if the phase III slope is increased.

In phase IV, the patient inhales. Normally, CO_2 falls abruptly to zero and remains at zero until the next exhalation.

b. Examining the waveform will often explain readings that appear inaccurate. If the capnometer shows several peaks per breath or does not distinguish breaths that do not have a plateau, the respiratory rate and peak CO_2 readings will be inaccurate.

c. The waveform should be examined systematically for height, frequency, rhythm, baseline, and shape.

d. **Figures 17.14 to 17.30** illustrate various waveforms that may be observed. These waveforms are stylized to illustrate one clinical situation. Often waveforms will represent more than one clinical condition. There is a Web site devoted to capnography (www.capnography.com).

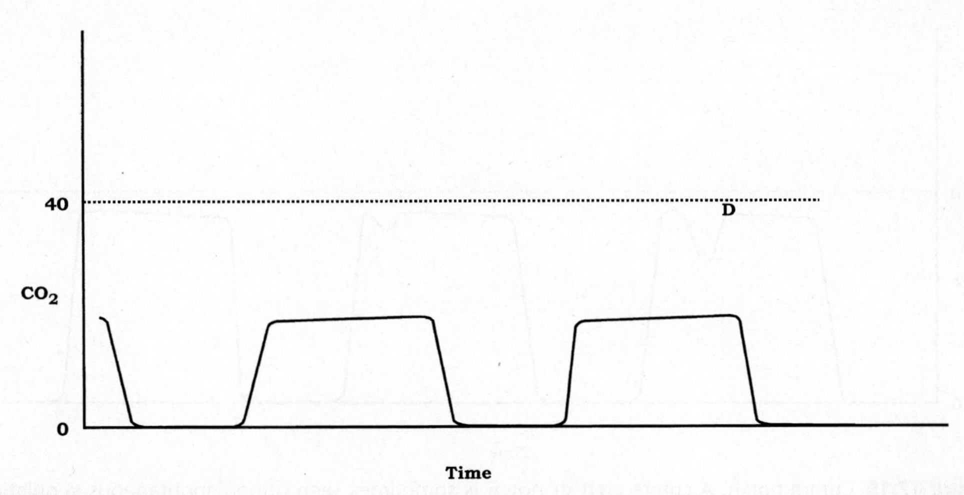

Figure 17.17 Low end-tidal CO_2. The normal value for end-tidal carbon dioxide (40 torr) is illustrated by the dotted line. The waveform illustrated shows a normal configuration but the plateau is well below the normal CO_2 value. This indicates a low end-tidal value. This can occur with hyperventilation or an increase in dead space ventilation.

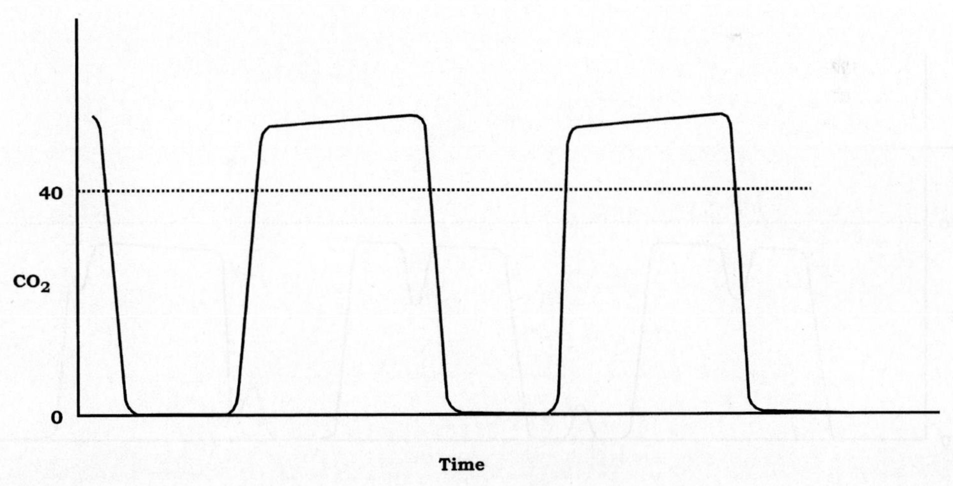

Figure 17.18 Elevated end-tidal CO_2 with good alveolar plateau. The waveform is normal but the plateau is higher than normal. The baseline is zero, which indicates that carbon dioxide is not present in the inspired mixture. This situation can occur if carbon dioxide production increases (such as in malignant hyperthermia) or with hypoventilation. Other causes can be CO_2 being absorbed during laparoscopy, tourniquet release, increased muscle tone (as from muscle relaxant reversal), shivering, or convulsions.

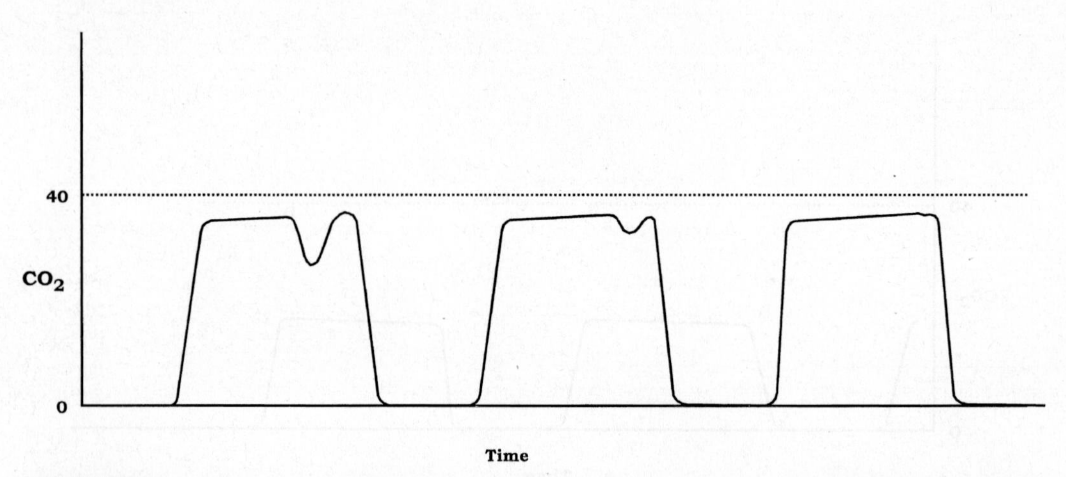

Figure 17.19 Curare notch. A curare cleft or notch is sometimes seen during spontaneous ventilation. The capnogram on the left shows the notch. The cleft is in the last third of the plateau and is thought to be caused by a lack of synchronous action between the intercostal muscles and the diaphragm, most commonly caused by inadequate muscle relaxant reversal. The depth of the cleft is proportional to the degree of remaining muscle paralysis. The position of the cleft is fairly constant on the same patient but is not necessarily present with every breath. As the muscle relaxant is reversed, the curve becomes normal in shape. The notch can also be seen in patients with cervical transverse lesions, flail chest, hiccups, and pneumothorax.

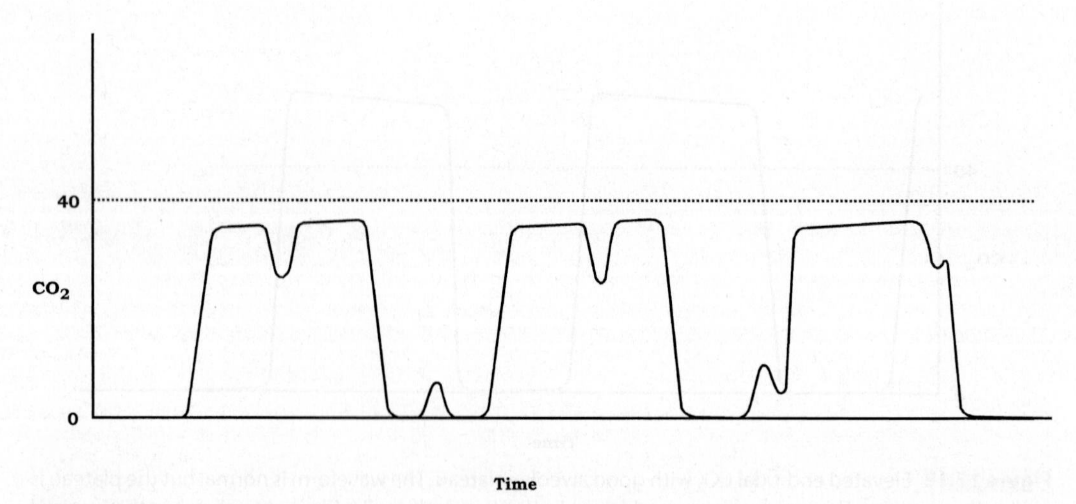

Figure 17.20 Spontaneous respiratory efforts during mechanical ventilation. The capnogram shows small breaths at various places during exhalation and inspiration. Its causes include hypoventilation, inadequate muscle paralysis, severe hypoxia, or the patient waking up. The end-tidal CO_2 may rise slightly because of the increased metabolism of the contracting respiratory muscles. This pattern may also be caused by pressure on the patient's chest or ventilator malfunction.

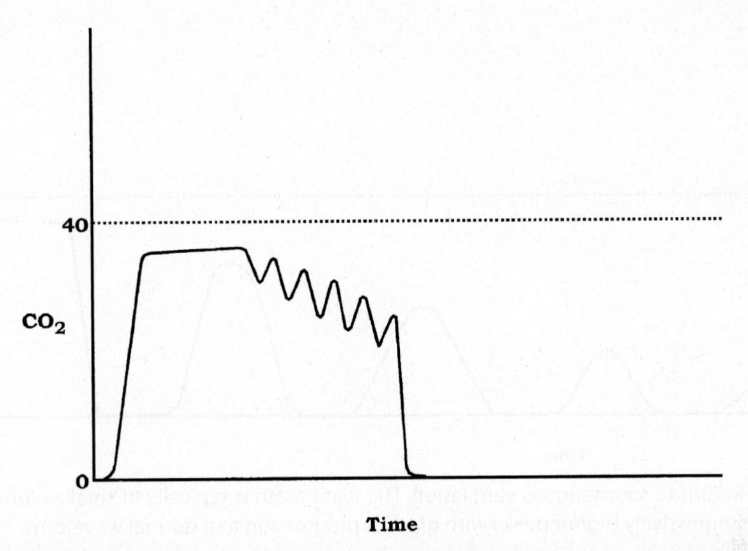

Figure 17.21 Cardiogenic oscillations. These appear as small, regular, toothlike humps at the end of the expiratory phase. They may be single or multiple, and the heights may vary considerably. They are believed to be due to the heart beating against the lungs. A number of factors, including negative intrathoracic pressure, a low respiratory rate, diminished vital capacity:heart size ratio, a low inspiratory:expiratory ratio, low tidal volumes, and muscular relaxation, contribute to their appearance. In many cases, adjusting the ventilator rate, flow, or tidal volume will remove this pattern from the screen. At other times, however, they cannot be eliminated. Cardiogenic oscillations are more common in pediatric patients because of the relative size of the infant's heart and thorax. Capnograms from patients with severe emphysema tend not to register cardiogenic oscillations. Less sophisticated capnometers may count each oscillation as a breath, displaying an erroneously high respiratory rate. Placing the sampling site on the patient side of a heat and moisture exchanger or using low levels of positive end-expiratory pressure may remove the oscillations.

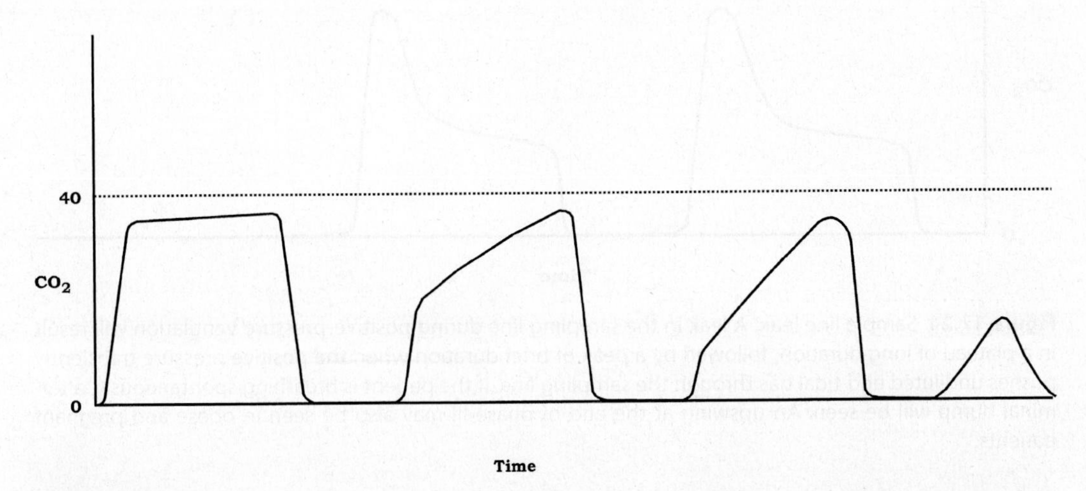

Figure 17.22 Prolonged upstroke. The left curve shows a normal waveform. The other three curves show progressive slanting. As expiration is progressively prolonged, inspiration may start before exhalation is complete so that the end-tidal CO_2 reading but not the actual end–tidal value is decreased. Without the plateau, the end-tidal CO_2 reading will not necessarily be an accurate representation of the actual end-tidal value. This pattern can be caused by obstructed gas flow due to a partially obstructed tracheal tube or obstruction in the patient's airways (chronic obstructive lung disease, bronchospasm, or upper airway obstruction).

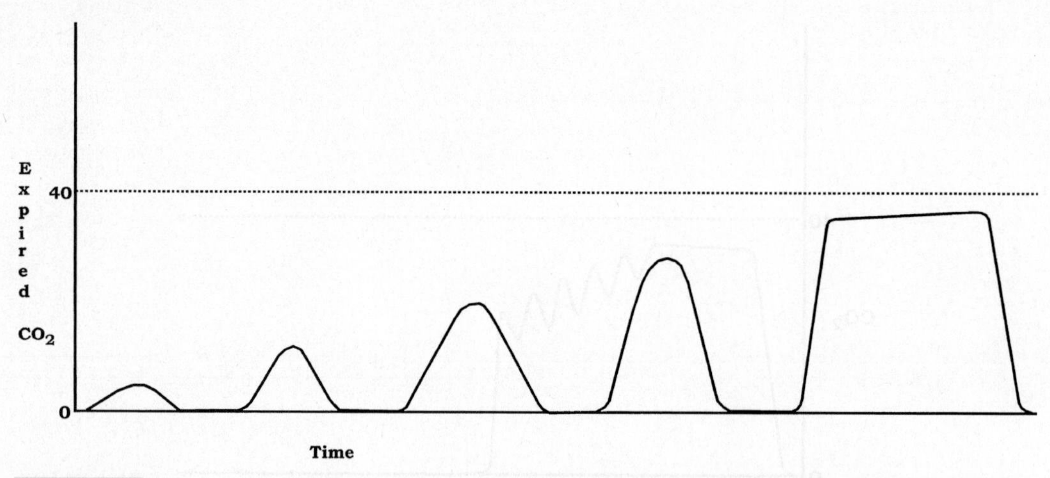

Figure 17.23 Return to spontaneous ventilation. The first breath is typically of small volume. Subsequent breaths show progressively higher peaks with gradual progression to a normal waveform.

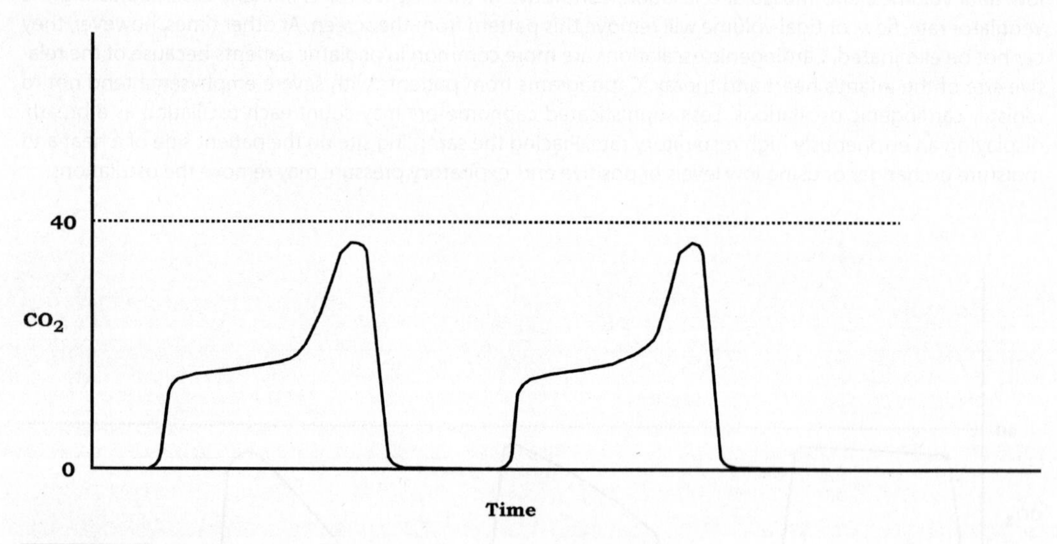

Figure 17.24 Sample line leak. A leak in the sampling line during positive-pressure ventilation will result in a plateau of long duration, followed by a peak of brief duration when the positive pressure transiently pushes undiluted end-tidal gas through the sampling line. If the patient is breathing spontaneously, a terminal hump will be seen. An upswing at the end of phase III may also be seen in obese and pregnant patients.

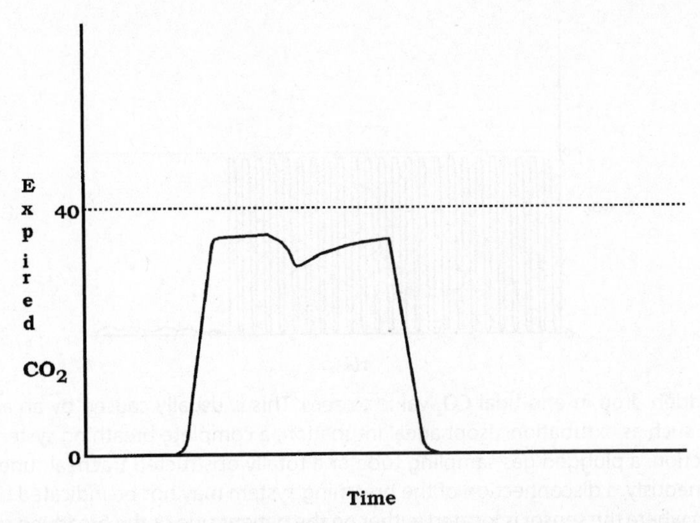

Figure 17.25 Variations between lungs. If the compliance, airway resistance, or ventilation-perfusion ratio in one lung differ substantially from the other lung, a biphasic expiratory plateau may be seen. This type of capnogram has been reported in a patient with severe kyphoscoliosis and following single-lung transplantation.

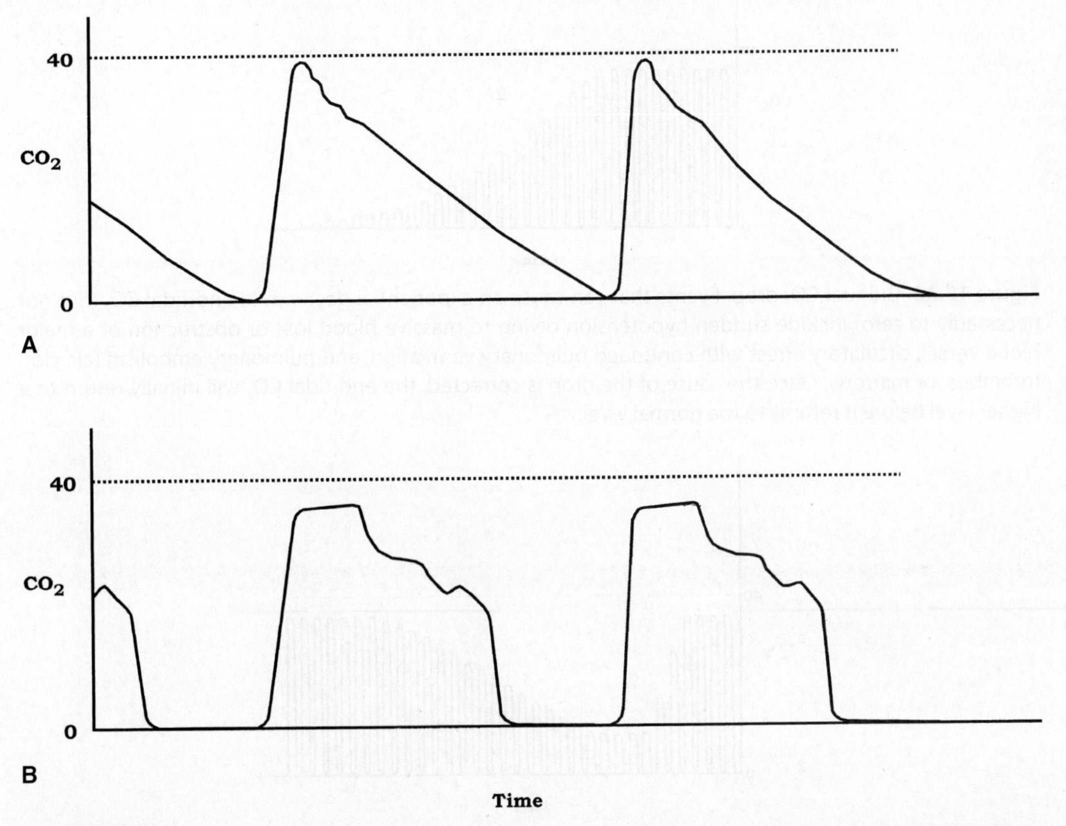

Figure 17.26 Contaminated gas sample. Contamination of the expired gas sample by fresh gas or ambient air may be caused by placing the sampling site too near the fresh gas inlet, a leak, or too high a sampling flow rate. **A:** A large leak is indicated by the progressive decrease in the plateau. **B:** If the contamination is of lesser magnitude, a drop-off occurs at the end of the plateau.

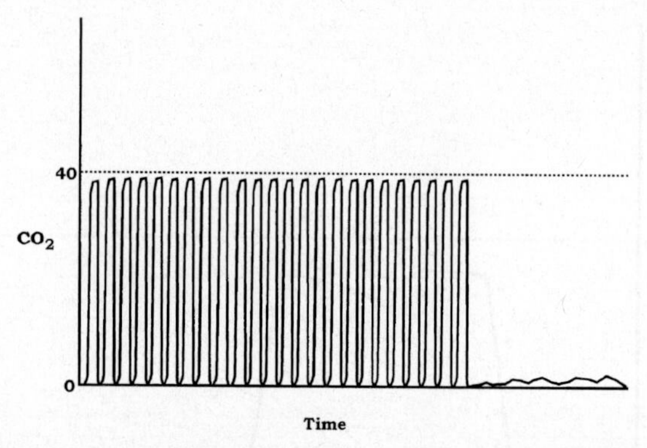

Figure 17.27 Sudden drop in end-tidal CO_2 value to zero. This is usually caused by an acute event relating to the airway, such as extubation, esophageal intubation, a complete breathing system disconnection, ventilator malfunction, a plugged gas sampling tube or a totally obstructed tracheal tube. If the patient is breathing spontaneously, a disconnection of the breathing system may not be indicated by the absence of CO_2 depending on where the sensor is located (either on the patient side or the breathing system side of the disconnection).

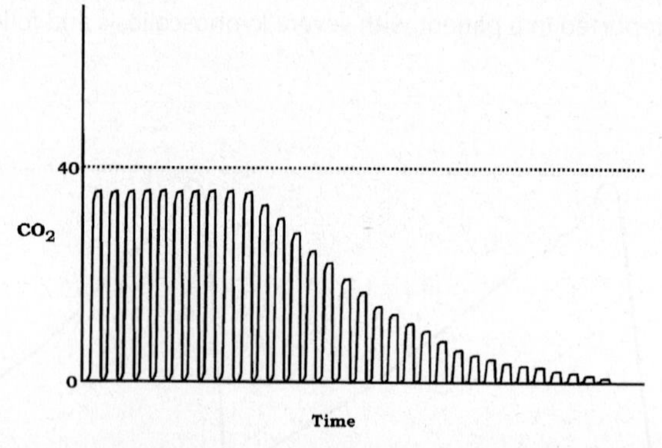

Figure 17.28 Gradual CO_2 drop. Events that can cause an exponential decrease in end-tidal CO_2 (but not necessarily to zero) include sudden hypotension owing to massive blood loss or obstruction of a major blood vessel, circulatory arrest with continued pulmonary ventilation, and pulmonary embolism (air, clot, thrombus, or marrow). Once the cause of the drop is corrected, the end-tidal CO_2 will initially return to a higher level before it returns to the normal level.

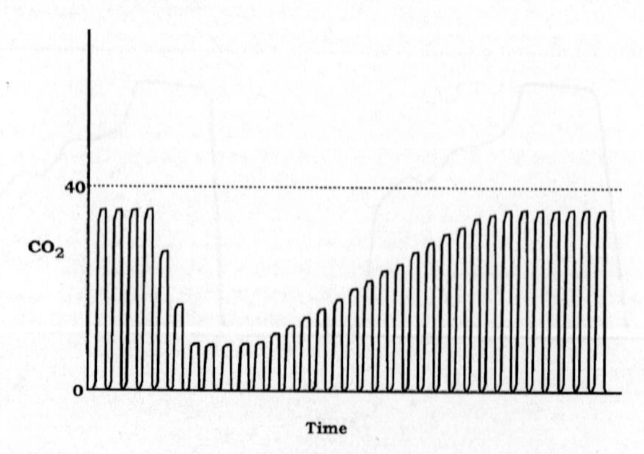

Figure 17.29 Small air embolus with resolution. If air enters the vascular system of the lung, it will obstruct a certain portion of the circulation. If the embolus is large enough, it will cause the end tidal CO_2 to decrease suddenly but not necessarily to zero. Often these emboli resolve quickly and the end-tidal CO_2 returns to normal level.

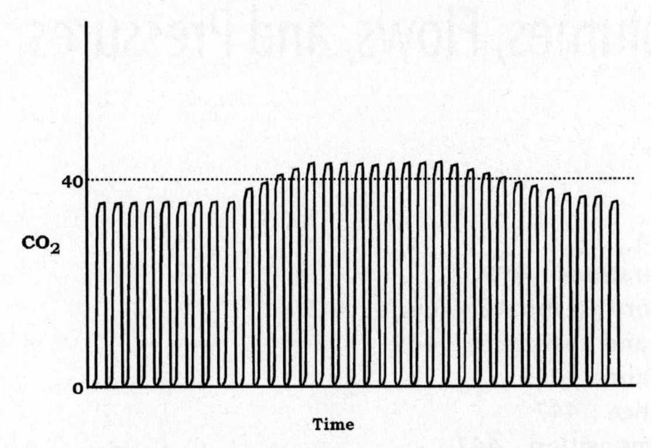

Figure 17.30 Tourniquet release. Releasing a tourniquet or unclamping of a major vessel may result in a sudden increase in end-tidal CO_2 level that gradually returns to normal.

C. Volatile Anesthetic Agents
   1. Measuring concentrations of volatile anesthetic gases is now a common practice. In some countries (but not the United States at the time of this writing), agent monitoring is a standard of care.
   2. An anesthetic agent monitor is usually a part of a multiparameter monitor since the same IR bench monitors both anesthetic agents and carbon dioxide.
   3. An agent monitor is useful for monitoring vaporizer function and determining incorrect contents, providing information on agent uptake and distribution, assessing anesthetic depth, providing information into an electronic record, and detecting disconnections.

D. Nitrous Oxide
   1. Nitrous oxide can be measured directly only by IR technology.
   2. Analysis of nitrous oxide will show whether or not the flowmeters are functioning properly and determine the adequacy of nitrous oxide washout at the end of a case.

REFERENCES

1. Overdyk FJ, Carter R, Maddox RR, et al. Continuous oximetry/capnometry monitoring reveals frequent desaturation and bradypnea during patient-controlled analgesia. Anesth Analg 2007;105:412–418.
2. Soto RG, Fu ES, Vila H Jr, Miguel RV. Capnography accurately detects apnea during monitoring anesthesia care. Anesth Analg 2004;99:379–382.

SUGGESTED READINGS

Barker L, Webb RK, Runciman WB, Van Der Walt JH. The oxygen analyzer: applications and limitations—an analysis of 2000 incident reports. Anaesth Intensive Care 1991;570–574.

Dorsch J, Dorsch S. Gas monitoring. In: Understanding Anesthesia Equipment. Fifth edition. Philadelphia: Wolters Kuluwer/Lippincott Williams & Wilkins, 2008:685–727.

Gravenstein JS, Jaffe MB, Paulus DA, eds. Capnography: Clinical Aspects. Cambridge, MA: Cambridge University Press, 2004.

Tinker JH, Dull DL, Caplan RA, Ward RJ, Cheney FW. Role of monitoring devices in prevention of anesthetic mishaps: a closed claims analysis. Anesthesiology 1989;71:541–546.

18 Airway Volumes, Flows, and Pressures

I. Definitions

A. *Compliance*: Ratio of a change in volume to a change in pressure. It is a measure of distensibility and is usually expressed in milliliters per centimeter of water (mL/cm H_2O). Compliance commonly relates to the lungs and chest wall. Breathing system components, especially breathing tubes and the reservoir bag, also have compliance.

B. *Expiratory Flow Rate*: Rate at which gas is exhaled by the patient expressed as volume per unit of time.

C. *Expiratory Flow Time*: Time between the beginning and end of expiratory flow (**Fig. 18.1**).

D. *Expiratory Pause Time*: Time from the end of expiratory flow to the start of inspiratory flow (**Fig. 18.1**).

E. *Expiratory Phase Time*: Time between the start of expiratory flow and the start of inspiratory flow. It is the sum of the expiratory flow and expiratory pause times (**Fig. 18.1**).

F. *Inspiratory Flow Time*: Period between the beginning and end of inspiratory flow (**Fig. 18.1**).

G. *Inspiratory Pause Time*: The portion of the inspiratory phase time during which the lungs are held inflated at a fixed pressure or volume (i.e., the time of zero flow) (**Fig. 18.1**). It is also called the *inspiratory hold, inflation hold,* and *inspiratory plateau.*

H. *Inspiratory Phase Time*: Time between the start of inspiratory flow and the beginning of expiratory flow (**Fig. 18.1**). It is the sum of the inspiratory flow and inspiratory pause times. The inspiratory pause time:inspiratory phase time (T_{IP}:T_I) may be expressed as a percentage.

I. *Inspiratory:Expiratory Phase Time Ratio (I:E ratio)*: Ratio of the inspiratory phase time to the expiratory phase time. For example, an I:E ratio of 1:2 means that the inspiratory phase time is one third of the ventilatory cycle time.

J. *Inspiratory Flow Rate*: Rate at which gas flows into the patient expressed as volume per unit of time.

K. *Minute Volume*: Sum of all tidal volumes within 1 minute.

L. *Peak Pressure*: Maximum pressure during the inspiratory phase time (**Fig. 18.1**).

M. *Plateau Pressure*: Resting airway pressure during the inspiratory pause. There is usually a lowering of airway pressure from its peak when there is an inspiratory pause (**Fig. 18.1**). This lower pressure is called the *plateau pressure*.

N. *Positive End-Expiratory Pressure (PEEP)*: Positive pressure in the airway at the end of exhalation.

O. *Resistance*: Ratio of the change in driving pressure to the change in flow rate. It is commonly expressed as centimeters of water per liter per second (cm H_2O/L/second).

P. *Tidal Volume*: Volume of gas entering or leaving the patient during the inspiratory or expiratory phase time.

Q. *Ventilatory (Respiratory) Rate or Frequency*: Number of respiratory cycles per unit time, usually per minute.

R. *Work of Breathing*: Energy expended by the patient and/or ventilator to move gas in and out of the lungs. It is expressed as the ratio of work to volume moved, commonly as joules per liter. It includes the work needed to overcome the elastic and flow-resistive forces of both the respiratory system and the apparatus.

II. General Considerations

A. The Ventilatory (Respiratory) Cycle

1. Airway pressure with volume controlled ventilation is shown in **Figure 18.1A.** There is a rise in pressure with no preceding negative pressure. A fast rise to peak pressure suggests that the flow is too high. The peak pressure will increase if tidal volume, inspiratory flow rate, or resistance increases or compliance decreases. A decrease in peak pressure may result from a leak, spontaneous inspiratory effort by the patient, a decrease in resistance, or an increase in compliance.
2. **Figure 18.1B** shows the respiratory cycle with an inspiratory pause. If the pause is long enough, a plateau pressure will be seen. Plateau pressure depends on tidal volume and the total static compliance but is independent of resistance.
3. **Figure 18.1C** shows the effect of fresh gas entering the breathing system during controlled ventilation during inspiration. This occurs when the anesthesia ventilator does not prevent fresh gas from entering the breathing system during inspiration. The inspired volume increases, and the peak pressure falls and then rises.

B. Compliance and Resistance

1. **Compliance**

   a. Compliance measurement may be dynamic or static. Dynamic compliance is calculated by dividing the difference in volume by the difference in pressure at two points during the ventilatory cycle. This is not a true measure of total compliance because the airway pressure includes the pressure needed to overcome resistance.

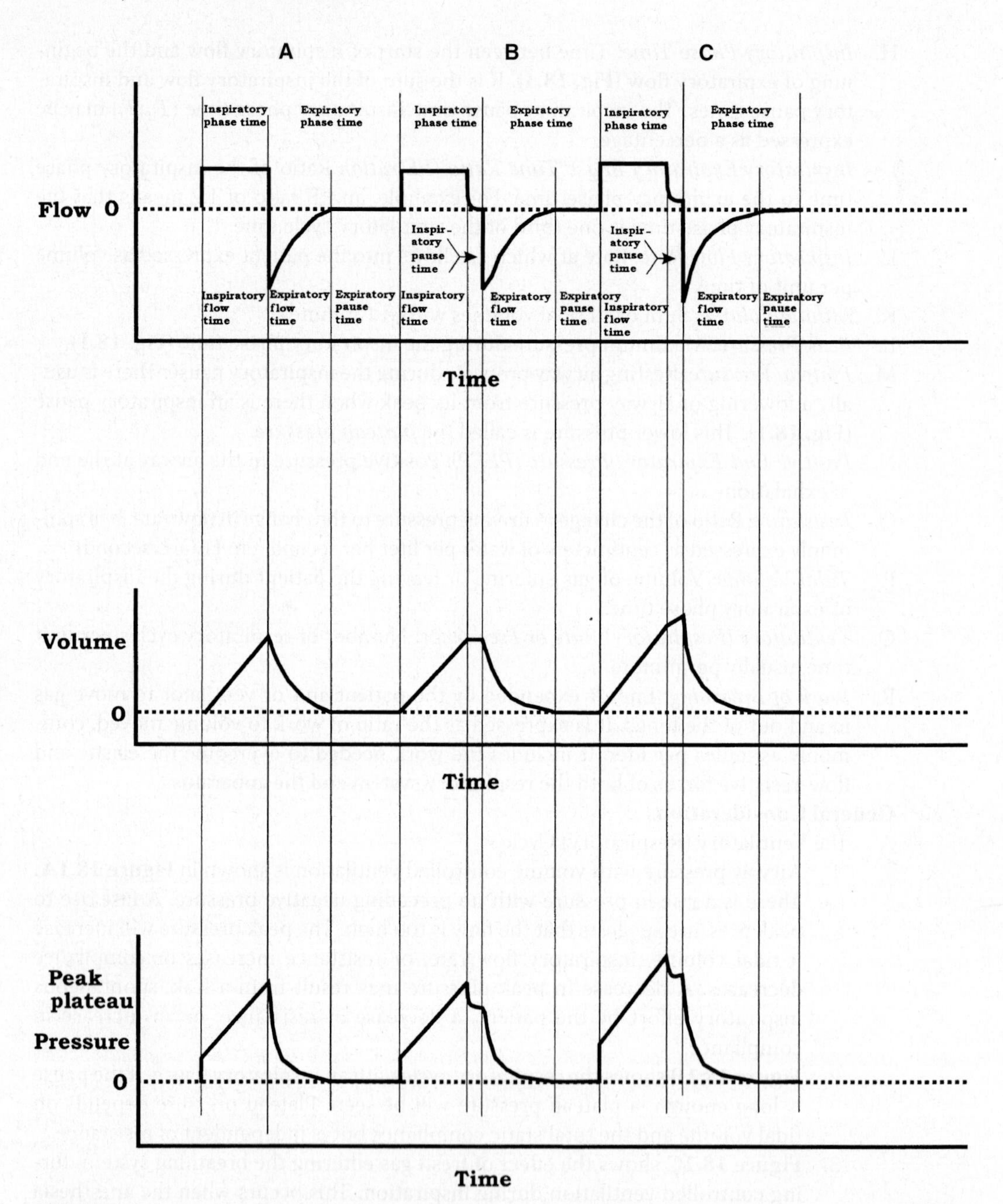

Figure 18.1 Flow, volume, and pressure curves from a ventilator that produces a rectangular inspiratory flow wave. **A:** This represents controlled ventilation with no inspiratory pause. The end-inspiratory pressure will equal the peak pressure. **B:** With an inspiratory pause, there is a decrease from peak pressure to a lower plateau pressure. **C:** This illustrates the effect of continuing fresh gas flow during inspiration. The inspired volume increases, and the peak pressure falls and then rises.

b. Static compliance is calculated by using the end-inspiratory occlusion pressure. Conditions of zero gas flow are achieved by employing an inspiratory hold or occluding the expiratory port long enough to allow airway pressure to reach a constant value. This pressure, commonly termed *plateau pressure*, represents the total respiratory system elastic recoil at end-inflation volume.

$$\text{Static compliance} = \frac{\text{Tidal volume}}{\text{Plateau pressure} - \text{Positive end-expiratory pressure}}$$

c. Total compliance reflects the elastic properties of the lungs, thorax, abdomen, and the breathing system. Using muscle relaxants will increase chest wall and abdominal compliance but will not affect lung compliance, so in paralyzed patients, changes in compliance reflect mainly alterations in lung compliance. In adults, normal total static compliance is 35 to 100 mL/cm H_2O. In children, static compliance is normally greater than 15 mL/cm H_2O.

2. **Resistance**

a. Resistance occurs when gas flows through a tube and energy is lost. This is reflected by decreased pressure. The pressure drop depends on both resistance and flow rate. For a given tidal volume, a higher resistance may be overcome by using a lower flow for a longer time or a higher driving pressure. During controlled ventilation, if there is an increase in airway resistance, the pressure needed to deliver a given tidal volume will increase. This pressure increase can usually be supplied by the ventilator or the person squeezing the reservoir bag. Because exhalation is passive, expiratory flow depends on the elastic and resistive forces in the lungs and the resistance in the airway device (tracheal tube, supraglottic airway) and the breathing system expiratory limb.

b. Total resistance, which may differ during inspiration and exhalation, is determined by the patient's airway, the airway device (tracheal tube or supraglottic device), and the breathing system. Decreased airway caliber from bronchoconstriction, secretions, tumor, edema, a foreign body, or airway closure is associated with increased resistance. Tracheal tube resistance depends primarily on its internal diameter. Partial tube obstruction by secretions, kinking, or other problems will increase resistance. Breathing system resistance is affected by the length and internal diameter of its components and is increased by sharp bends and constrictions.

c. Total airway resistance can be estimated by the difference between peak and plateau pressures, which is normally 2 to 5 cm H_2O. If there is an increase in resistance, a higher peak pressure will be necessary to produce the same flow. Plateau pressure, however, depends only on compliance and will not be affected by resistance. If the inspiratory flow and tidal volume remain constant but resistance increases, there will be a greater difference between the peak and plateau pressures.

3. **Gas Composition**

The composition of the gas being measured will affect the accuracy of flow-measuring devices. Differences in the density and viscosity of gases can induce an error in flow measurement.

III. Respiratory Volume

A. A respirometer (spirometer) is a device that measures the volume of gas passing through a location in a flow pathway during a given period of time.

B. Monitoring respiratory volumes can aid in detecting breathing system obstructions, disconnections, apnea, leaks, ventilator failure, and high or low volumes in spontaneously breathing patients as well as in those whose ventilation is controlled. Some monitors can detect reversed flow that can indicate an incompetent unidirectional valve or a leak. A discrepancy between expired and inspired tidal volume should suggest a leak. A decrease in tidal volume as a result of migration of the tracheal tube into a bronchus may be detected. Although there are other ways of detecting these problems, such as observing chest wall movements, monitoring breath sounds, capnometry, and airway pressure monitoring, using a volume monitor provides additional protection. The American Society of Anesthesiologists strongly encourages monitoring the volume of expired gas.

C. Respiratory volume monitoring may fail to detect some problems. It is possible to have fairly normal flow with esophageal intubation. With airway occlusion, there may be enough flow during exhalation resulting from gas compression within the breathing system during inspiration to prevent the respirometer alarm from being activated.

D. A high-volume alarm may be useful to detect unanticipated increases in tidal volume. This may be due to improper ventilator settings or increased gas flow into the breathing system during inspiration. Increased tidal volume can be caused by a hole in the ventilator bellows, an increased I:E ratio, or fresh gas flow (if there is no fresh gas flow compensation or decoupling).

E. Possible sites for the location of a respirometer are shown in **Figure 18.2.** From the standpoint of accuracy, the most desirable location is between the breathing system and the patient (position C). In this location, readings are not affected by breathing system leaks, expansion of breathing system components, or gas compression. Both inspired and expired volumes can be measured. Placing the sensor at this site will increase the dead space and water condensation may be a problem. This position may result in increased likelihood of damage, disconnection, or tracheal tube kinking.

CLINICAL MOMENT With the respirometer sensor between the patient who is spontaneously breathing and the breathing system, a disconnection between the sensor and the breathing system may not be noticed. There will continue to be a tidal volume. End-tidal carbon dioxide readings will also be present if the sample line is connected to or near the respirometer sensor. This disconnection would not be missed if the gas sample line were attached to the breathing system and the respirometer sensor were on the absorber.

1. A common practice is to locate the respirometer in the exhalation limb upstream or downstream of the unidirectional valve (positions B and A). An advantage of these positions is that if the respirometer can sense a reverse flow, a malfunctioning unidirectional valve can be detected. If a disconnection that prevents exhaled gases from passing down the exhalation tubing occurs, the respirometer will not sense a gas flow and an alarm will be activated. A respirometer in this location will usually read accurately during spontaneous respiration, but during controlled respiration, it will usually give inaccurately high readings. This is due to expansion in components of the breathing system and gas compression. If a ventilator with a hanging bellows is used, a respirometer in this position may still indicate flow when a disconnection occurs.
2. If the respirometer is located downstream of the absorber (position E), the volume of gas measured will be decreased by the amount of carbon dioxide absorbed in the absorber.

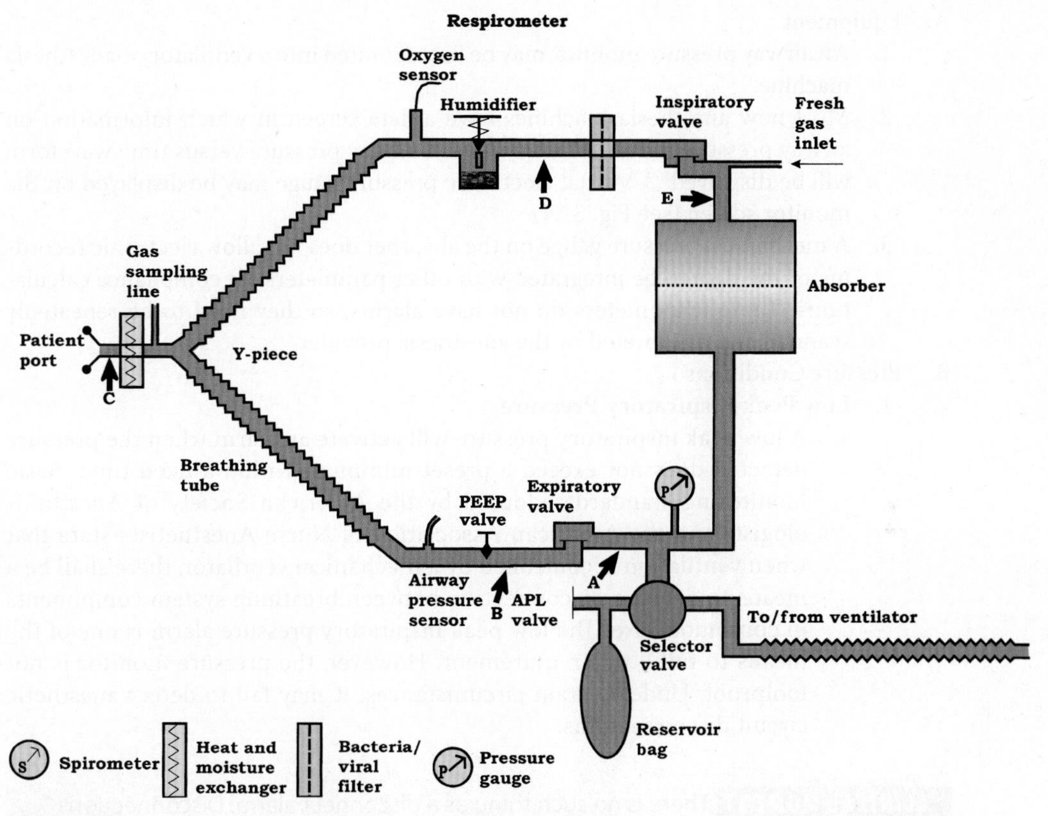

Figure 18.2 Possible sites for a respirometer in the circle system. (See text for details.) PEEP, positive end-expiratory pressure; APL, adjustable pressure limiting.

3. Another possible location for the respirometer is on the inspiratory side of the system (position D). In this location, the respirometer will display erroneously high readings since gas that does not inflate the patient's lungs will also pass through it. During controlled ventilation, a disconnection may not be detected.
4. It is common to locate pressure-flow sensors at both positions B and D. This allows both the inspiratory and exhalation volumes and pressures to be measured. This provides the information to produce a flow-volume or pressure–volume loop. Sensors in both these positions are sometimes used by the anesthesia ventilator to compensate for changes in tidal volume due to fresh gas flow or leaks. Machines with electronic checkouts can determine the component expansion and gas compression in the system with sensors in these positions.

IV. Airway Pressure Monitoring

Continuous airway pressure monitoring is now the norm in both the operating room and critical care areas. High- and low-pressure conditions in the breathing system have been a major cause of anesthesia-related mortality and morbidity. Other parameters such as exhaled carbon dioxide and exhaled volumes may remain relatively normal in the presence of dangerously abnormal airway pressures.

A. Equipment
   1. An airway pressure monitor may be incorporated into a ventilator or anesthesia machine.
   2. Most new anesthesia machines have a data screen in which information on airway pressure is available. Usually, an airway pressure versus time waveform will be displayed. A virtual electronic pressure gauge may be displayed on the monitor screen (see Fig. 5.24).
   3. A mechanical pressure gauge on the absorber does not allow electronic recording or the data to be integrated with other parameters for compliance calculations. These manometers do not have alarms, so they need to be repeatedly scanned and interpreted by the anesthesia provider.

B. Pressure Conditions
   1. **Low Peak Inspiratory Pressure**
      a. A low peak inspiratory pressure will activate an alarm when the pressure detected does not exceed a preset minimum within a fixed time. Basic monitoring standards adopted by the American Society of Anesthesiologists and the American Association of Nurse Anesthetists state that when ventilation is controlled by a mechanical ventilator, there shall be a means to detect a disconnection between breathing system components in continuous use. The low peak inspiratory pressure alarm is one of the means to fulfill this requirement. However, the pressure monitor is not foolproof. Under certain circumstances, it may fail to detect anesthetic circuit disconnections.

CLINICAL MOMENT There is no such thing as a disconnect alarm. Disconnections can be determined by decreased pressure, volume, or flow below a certain minimum or absent expired carbon dioxide. A false-negative alarm situation can occur with any one of these modalities under certain circumstances and often only one or two will activate the alarm when a disconnection occurs.

CLINICAL MOMENT Many clinicians set the low peak inspiratory pressure alarm threshold much lower than the peak pressure to prevent the alarm from being activated. This is a very dangerous practice because partial or complete disconnections can occur but the pressure remains above the low threshold. The low pressure alarm limit should be set only slightly below the peak inspiratory pressure. It should be readjusted for every patient and after every change in ventilation.

      b. Conditions that can cause a low peak pressure include a disconnection or major leak in the breathing system; an obstruction upstream of the pressure sensor; inadequate fresh gas flow (disconnection of the fresh gas line, an internal machine obstruction, or loss of or reduction in pipeline pressure); the bag/ventilator selector valve in the wrong position; a leaking tracheal tube cuff; extubation; a faulty, poorly set, or disconnected ventilator; gas or power supply failure to the ventilator; a malfunctioning scavenging system; increased compliance; and reduced resistance. Low-pressure alarms are of little or no use during spontaneous breathing when the pressure in the system does not rise and fall appreciably.

CLINICAL MOMENT The low-pressure alarm is usually activated when mechanical ventilation commences. During spontaneous or manually controlled ventilation, this alarm is not useful. Other pressure alarms such as continuous, negative, or sustained high pressure are always active.

c. Problems with pressure monitors have been reported. A disconnection or leak may not be detected if the alarm is not switched ON or the threshold is set too low. A false-negative condition may occur if the end-expiratory pressure is above the threshold pressure. Other conditions that may produce a pressure high enough to exceed the threshold when a disconnection occurs include the breathing system connector obstructed by a pillow, sheet, or surgical drape; a high-resistance component such as a heat and moisture exchanger, capnometer cuvette, or humidifier; air entrainment into the breathing system (especially with a ventilator bellows descending during expiration); partial extubation; compression of an empty ventilator bellows; and a Mapleson system with a high resistance. Devices operating on batteries will not alarm if the batteries fail.

CLINICAL MOMENT The low peak inspiratory pressure alarm should always be checked before use. Unfortunately, studies show that this test is often not performed or performed correctly.

2. **Sustained Elevated Pressure**
   a. A sustained (continuous, continuing) pressure monitor activates an alarm if the pressure does not fall below a certain level during part of the respiratory cycle.
   b. Several mechanisms can produce a sustained elevated pressure: accidental oxygen flush valve activation; an obstructed expiratory limb; an improperly adjusted pressure-limiting valve; scavenging system occlusion; a malfunctioning ventilator; or a malfunctioning or incorrectly set PEEP valve.
3. **High Pressure**
   a. A high-pressure alarm is activated if the pressure exceeds a certain limit. On some devices, the threshold is fixed (usually 50 to 80 cm H_2O); on others, it is adjustable. On some machines, the alarm threshold is automatically set a certain amount above the average peak pressure for several previous breaths. Some anesthesia delivery systems are fitted with pressure-limiting valves that vent gas from the breathing system when a high pressure is detected.
   b. Possible causes of high pressure include airway obstruction, reduced compliance, increased resistance, the oxygen flush activated during the inspiratory phase, a punctured ventilator bellows, an occluded or obstructed breathing system expiratory limb, scavenging system malfunction, or the patient coughing or straining.

CLINICAL MOMENT During pressure-controlled ventilation, the inspiratory airway pressure is preset and thus cannot warn that the tracheal tube is becoming occluded.

4. **Subambient Pressure**

A subambient (subatmospheric) pressure alarm is activated when the pressure falls below atmospheric by a predetermined amount. Subatmospheric pressure can be generated by a patient attempting to inhale against a collapsed reservoir bag or increased resistance; a blocked inspiratory limb during the expiratory phase of the ventilator; a malfunctioning scavenging system; suction applied to a tube placed in the tracheobronchial tree or to the working channel of an endoscope passed into the airway; a sidestream gas analyzer; or by a hanging ventilator bellows refilling.

C. Monitoring Site

1. The site of pressure sensing will affect its usefulness. **Figure 18.3** shows possible sites. Ideally, the site should be close to the patient's airway (position C). Pressures during both inspiration and exhalation can be measured at this site. Many disposable breathing systems have a small port at the Y-piece that can serve as the connection site for tubing that transmits the pressure to a monitoring device. Pressure- and flow-volume loops can also be generated from this site. Placement between the patient and the breathing system may present problems with dead space, disconnections, tracheal tube kinking, and water buildup in the pilot line. The line(s) must be connected for every patient.

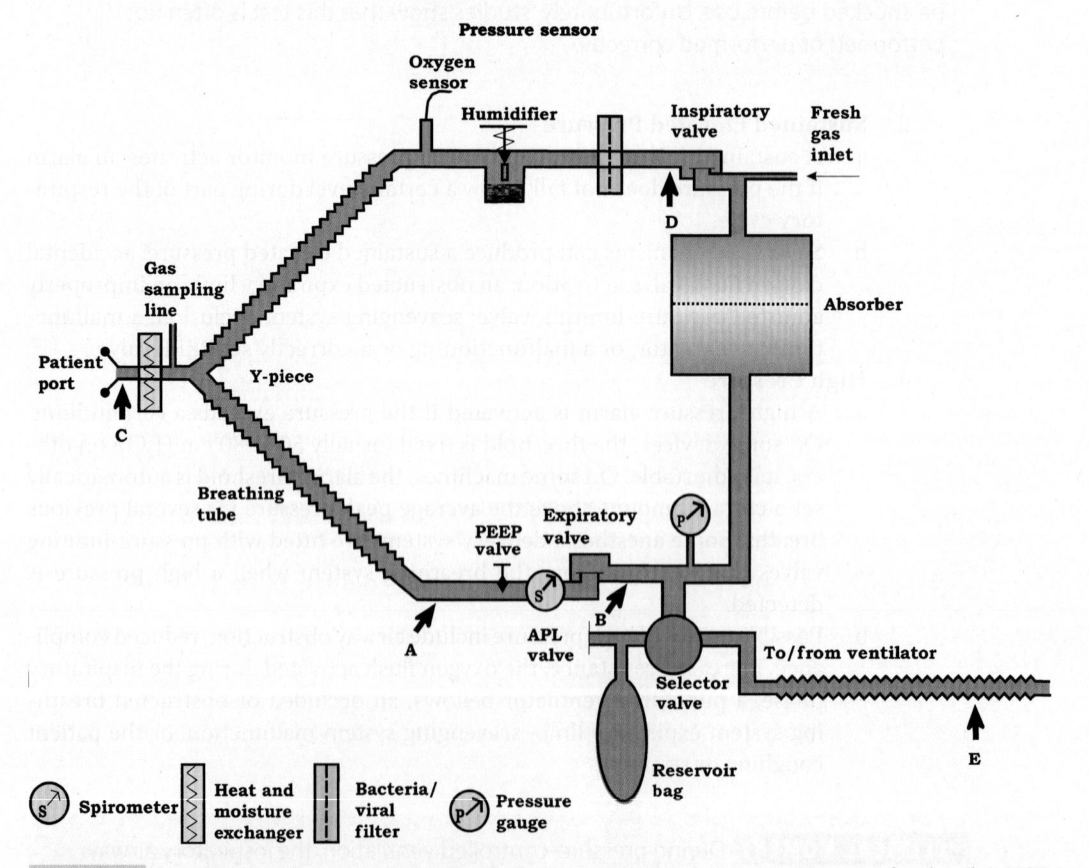

Figure 18.3 Possible sites for monitoring airway pressure in the circle system. (See text for details.) PEEP, positive end-expiratory pressure; APL, adjustable pressure limiting.

2. The more distant the measurement site is from the patient, the less useful it is for estimating airway pressure. Breathing system resistance and compliance, leaks, obstructions, and other mechanical factors may cause the measured pressure to be quite different from the pressure in the patient's airway.
3. Frequently, the monitoring site is in the breathing system (positions A, B, and D). An occlusion in the breathing system will cause a low-pressure state downstream from the obstruction and a high-pressure state upstream of it, so certain types of problems may be missed. If PEEP is used, it will not be indicated on a pressure monitor located at position B. Positions A and D are frequently used to monitor pressure during inspiration and exhalation and to provide pressures for pressure–volume loops.
4. In the past, the sensor was sometimes located in the ventilator (position E). This is unsatisfactory because under certain circumstances, sufficient back pressure to inhibit the low peak inspiratory pressure alarm may be generated at the bellows even when there is a disconnection.

V. Spirometry Loops

A. General Information

1. A loop is a graphic representation of the dynamic relationship between two related variables (pressure and volume or flow and volume) during both inspiration and exhalation. Pressure- and flow-volume loops are available on most later generation anesthesia machines, critical care ventilators, and physiologic monitors.
2. Pressure- and flow-volume loops provide the clinician with real-time information. Many problems (e.g., kinked tracheal tube, disconnection, migration of a tracheal tube into a bronchus) can occur quickly and unexpectedly during a case. Without loops, these problems might not be recognized promptly and corrective action delayed. While many of these problems could be determined by monitoring pressure, volume, and flow individually, loop technology integrates this information into a form that makes changes more likely to be quickly discovered.

B. Illustrative Loops

1. **The Pressure–Volume Loop**
   a. The pressure–volume loop shows volume on the vertical axis and pressure on the horizontal axis (**Fig. 18.4**). With controlled ventilation, the pressure in the breathing system increases during inspiration. At the same time, the inspired volume increases. The tidal volume is the point on the vertical axis that corresponds to the highest point on the loop. The peak pressure is the highest value on the horizontal axis. The shape of the inspiratory phase is determined by the type of ventilation being used. The portion of the loop representing exhalation starts at the point of highest volume and moves downward toward zero.
   b. A line drawn from the zero point through the point of end inspiration during controlled ventilation represents compliance. With good compliance, this line forms a 45-degree angle or less with the volume scale. A loop that becomes more horizontal indicates decreased compliance. The area inside the loop is related to the work of breathing.
2. **The Flow-Volume Loop**
   a. The flow-volume loop (**Fig. 18.5**) has volume on the horizontal axis and flow on the vertical axis. The zero point for volume is to the right on the horizontal axis. Loop generation proceeds in a clockwise direction. During inspiration, flow rate increases (plotted downward). The tidal volume is the

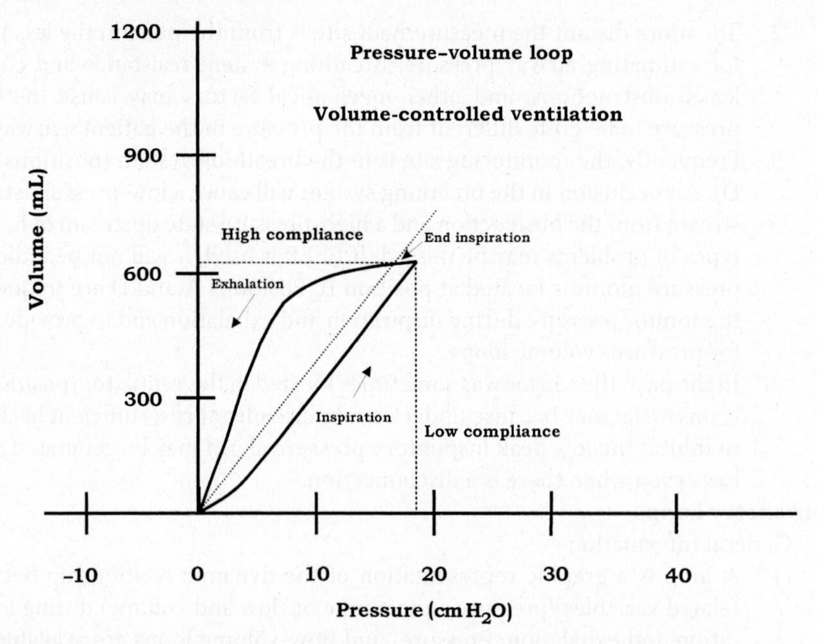

Figure 18.4 Pressure-volume loop. The pressure–volume relationship reflects pulmonary and tracheal tube mechanics. During controlled ventilation, a line drawn from the zero point through the point of end inspiration represents the compliance, which is determined by dividing the tidal volume by the pressure at end inspiration. With good compliance, that line forms an angle of 45 degrees or less with the volume scale. A loop that becomes more horizontal indicates a decrease in compliance.

point where flow returns to zero and the loop crosses the horizontal axis. The shape of this part of the loop depends on the type of respiration (e.g., volume controlled, pressure controlled, manual, or spontaneous).

b. Exhalation is represented by the part of the loop above the horizontal axis. The shape of this portion is determined by the rate of passive lung

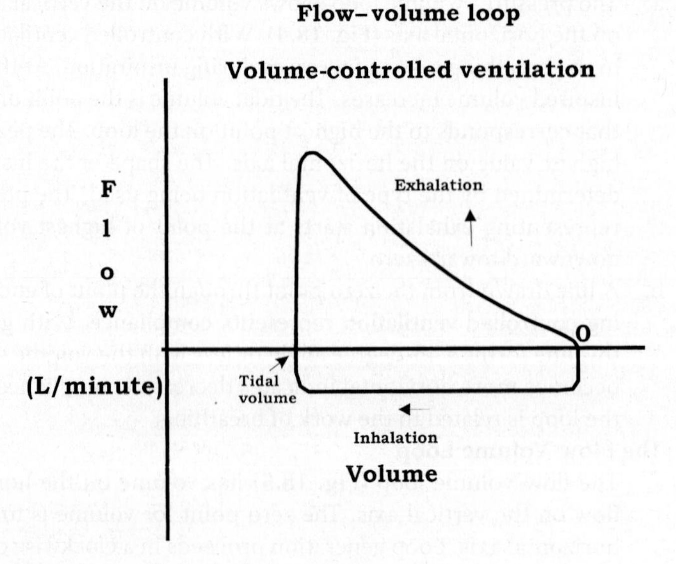

Figure 18.5 Flow-volume loop with controlled ventilation.

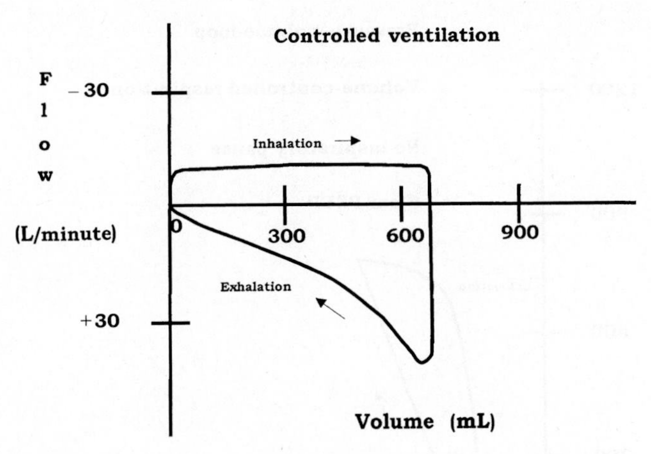

Figure 18.6 Alternative method of displaying a flow-volume loop. (See text for details.)

deflation, which is, in turn, determined by elastic recoil of the lungs and chest wall and by the total flow resistance offered by the bronchial tree, airway device, and the expiratory limb of the breathing system. With a normal loop, the flow rate during exhalation increases rapidly at the beginning, quickly reaches a peak, then slows, and gradually returns to zero.

c. Another way of illustrating a flow-volume loop places the zero point at the junction of the horizontal and vertical axes (**Fig. 18.6**). When this configuration is used, inspiration is usually above the horizontal axis and exhalation below it. Loop generation is clockwise. It has also been represented with the zero point at the junction of the horizontal and vertical axes, inspiration below the horizontal axis and exhalation above it.

C. Representative Loops

Representative loops are shown in **Figures 18.7** to **18.45.** These loops are stylized to illustrate certain aspects of respiratory mechanics. They are based on actual loops as much as possible. The reader should not expect to see an exact reproduction of these loops when monitoring a patient. Clinical conditions and ventilator function are rarely straightforward. There are usually a number of factors that contribute to the loop that is seen on the monitor.

CLINICAL MOMENT Use loops routinely. Gradually you will become familiar with the normal loop and recognize when it is abnormal. Using the examples illustrated in this text, you should be able to interpret changes taking place.

CLINICAL MOMENT Most monitors that present loops have a way to save one or more loops. After the anesthetic has begun and ventilation has stabilized, it is useful to save a set of loops for future comparison. Frequently one of the saved loops can be displayed on the screen along with the active loop. This feature can help to identify changes that occur during the case.

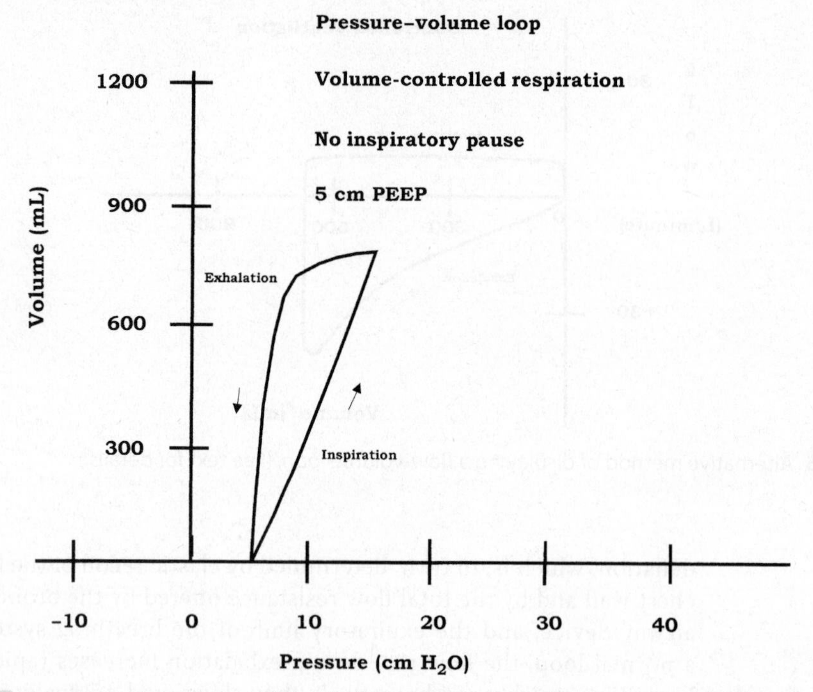

Figure 18.7 Pressure–volume loop with positive end-expiratory pressure (PEEP). With PEEP, the loop starting point is shifted to the right.

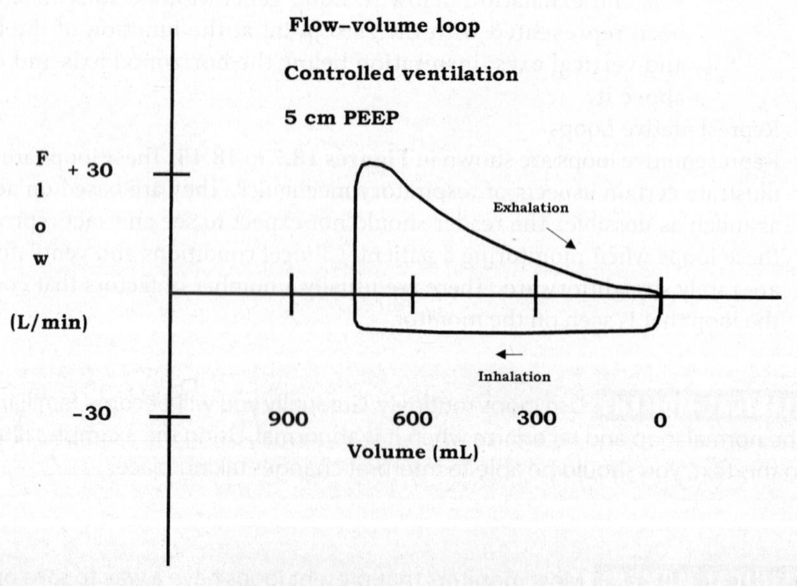

Figure 18.8 Flow-volume loop with positive end-expiratory pressure (PEEP). PEEP will decrease the expiratory driving pressure, causing a lower expiratory flow so the loop will appears flatter during exhalation.

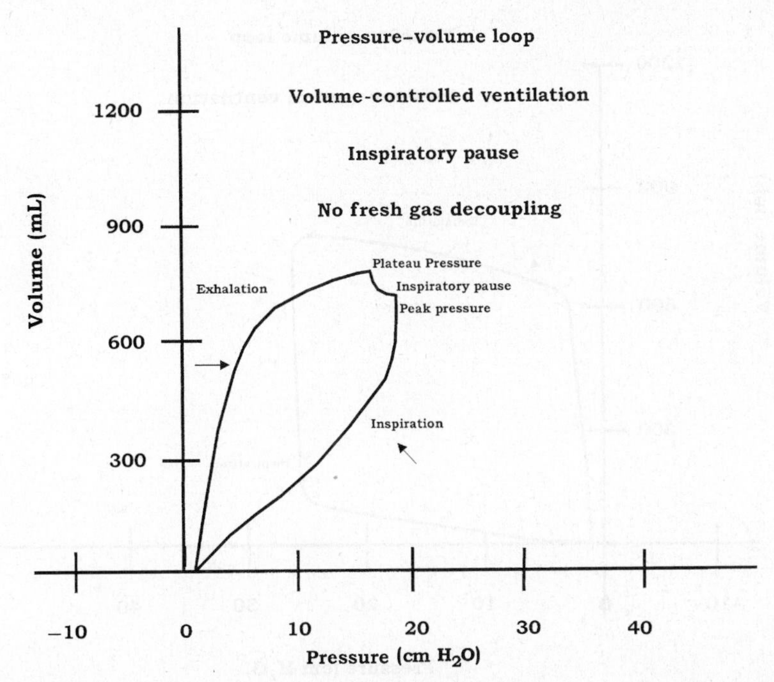

Figure 18.9 Pressure–volume loop with an inspiratory pause. When there is an inspiratory pause with controlled ventilation, it is common for the airway pressure to decline 2 to 5 cm H_2O after the peak pressure is reached. The lower pressure is called the plateau pressure. In this illustration, a ventilator without the ability to exclude fresh gas from the breathing system during inspiration is being used (see fresh gas decoupling in Chapter 6). The additional fresh gas increases the tidal volume.

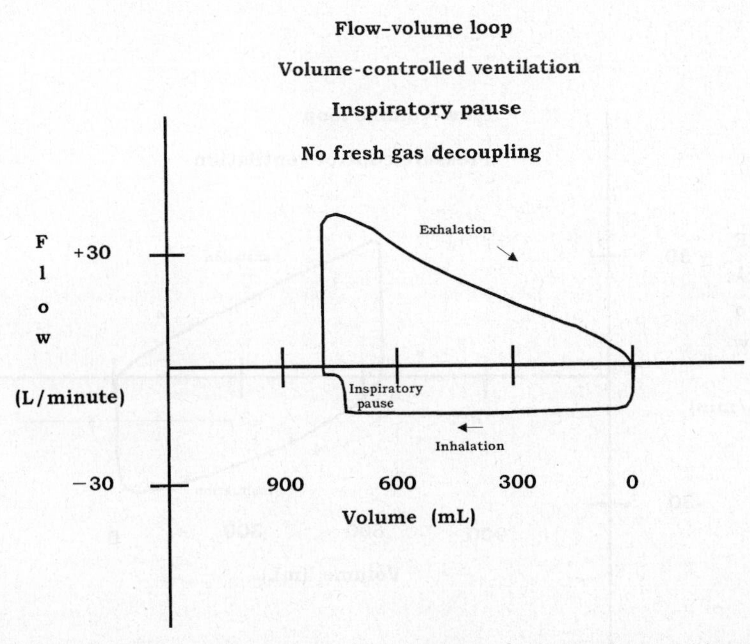

Figure 18.10 Flow-volume loop with an inspiratory pause. There is a drop in flow at end inspiration. During the pause, there is a slight increase in tidal volume during the pause because fresh gas continues to flow into the breathing system (if there is no fresh gas decoupling) (see Chapter 6). This pattern should not be confused with a spontaneous breathing during controlled ventilation. Exhalation is similar to the loop without an inspiratory pause.

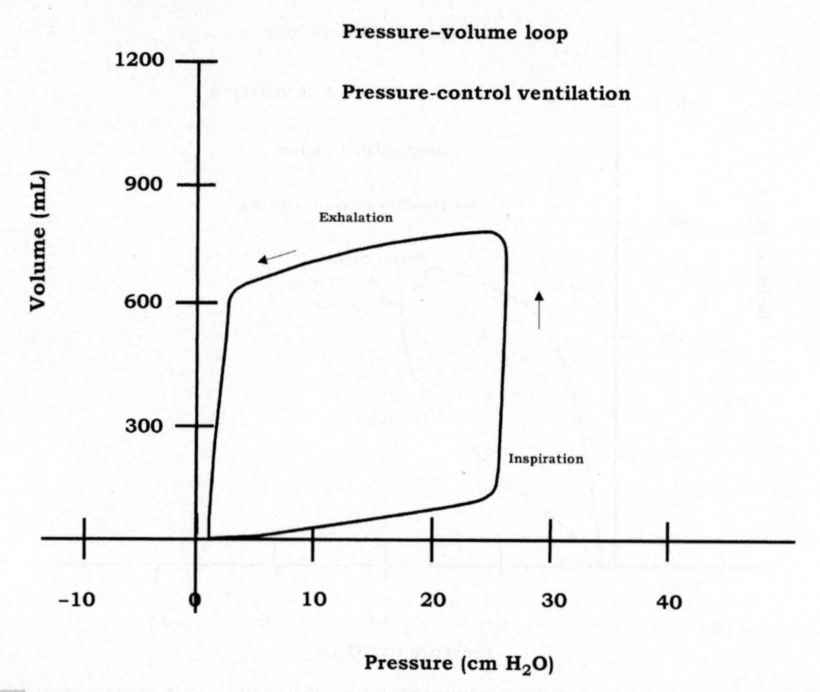

Figure 18.11 Pressure–volume loop with pressure-controlled ventilation. Pressure-controlled ventilation differs from volume-controlled ventilation in that inspiratory flow is not constant. There is a rapid initial increase in pressure to the set pressure. Tidal volume rises slowly at first but after the set pressure is reached, it increases rapidly to its maximum point. This results in a wide loop. The relatively flat beginning of exhalation results from residual pressure, which initially slows exhalation.

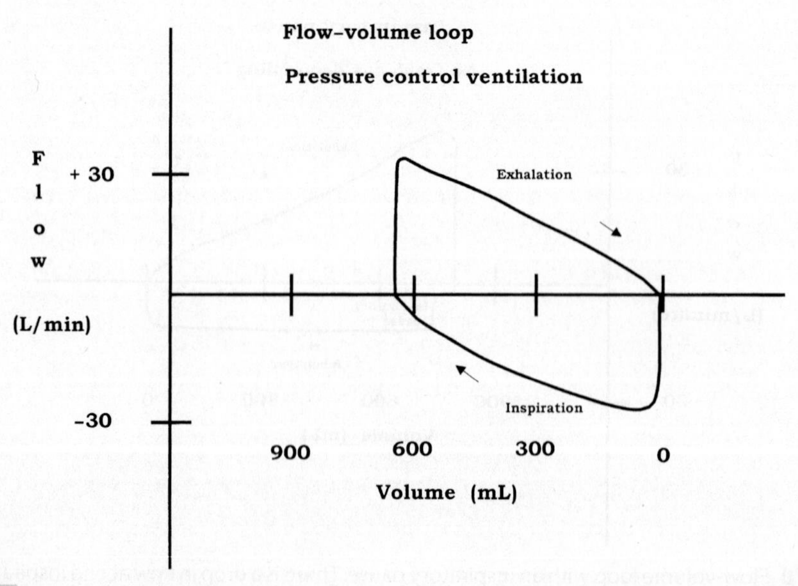

Figure 18.12 Flow-volume loop with pressure-controlled ventilation. Flow is rapid at the beginning of inspiration and then decreases. The exhalation pattern is nearly a mirror image of inspiration in that the flow is initially rapid and then slower as exhalation proceeds.

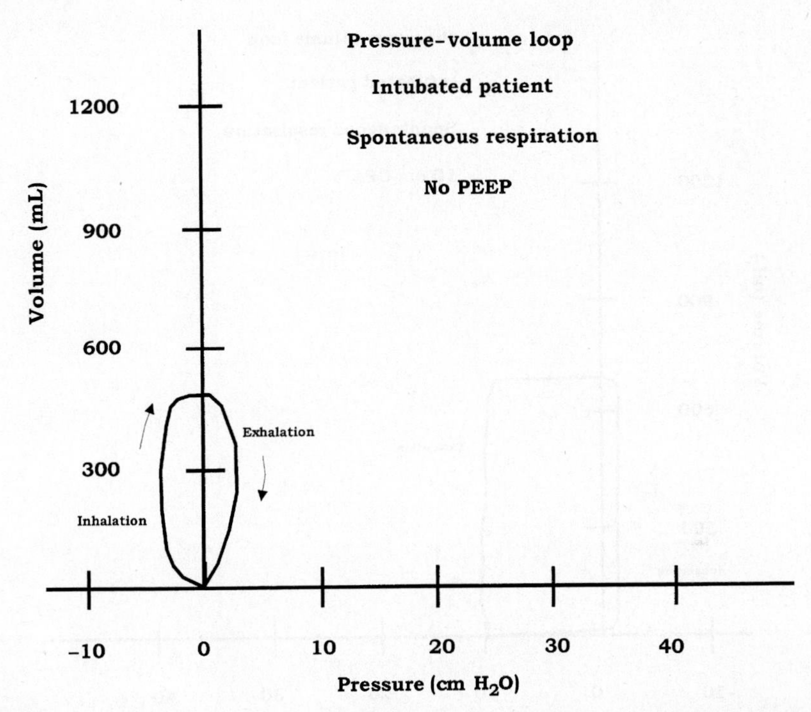

Figure 18.13 Pressure–volume loop during spontaneous respiration. During spontaneous respiration without positive end-expiratory pressure (PEEP), the pressure–volume loop begins at zero pressure and volume. During inspiration, airway pressure is negative, so the loop moves clockwise. At the end of inspiration, the negative pressure returns to zero. At this point, the loop crosses the tidal volume point on the vertical axis. During exhalation, airway pressure is positive and the loop moves to the right. At the same time, the volume drops. At the end of exhalation, the pressure and the volume return to zero. Compliance cannot be calculated from this loop because the inspiratory pressure is negative.

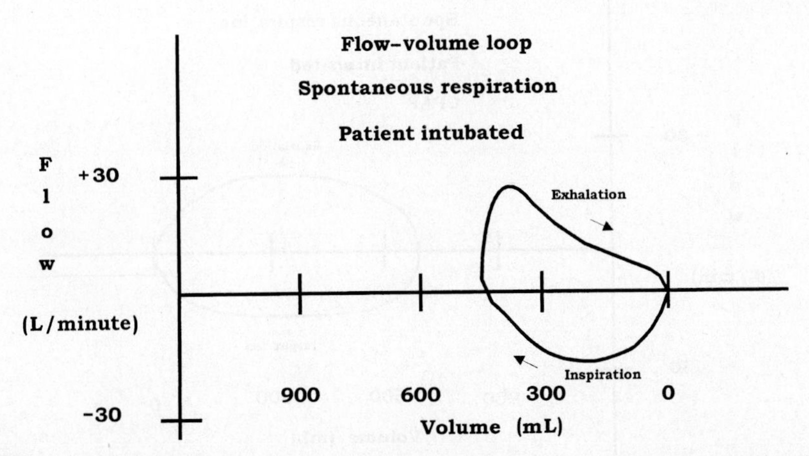

Figure 18.14 Flow-volume loop during spontaneous ventilation. During spontaneous inspiration, the peak flow occurs near the middle of inspiration. Flow during exhalation is similar to that found in volume-controlled ventilation.

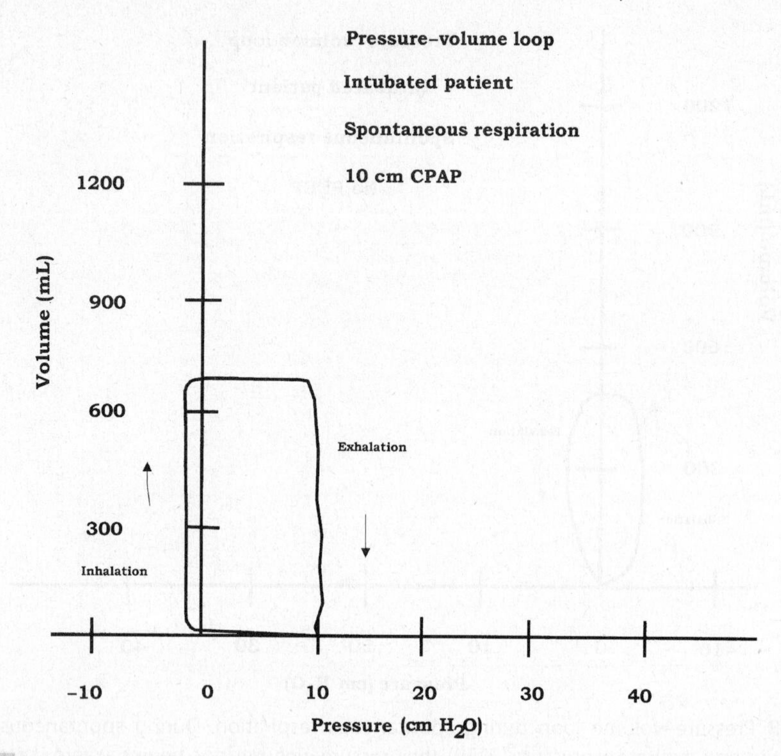

Figure 18.15 Pressure–volume loop with spontaneous respiration and 10 cm continuous positive airway pressure (CPAP). The loop starts at the CPAP value and moves to the left. Inspiration cannot begin until the pressure has become negative. At this point, the tidal volume increases rapidly. At the end of inspiration, the volume rises quickly. During exhalation, the loop moves toward the right and downward to the point of origin. This loop has a rectangular shape. The large internal area of the loop indicates increased work of breathing.

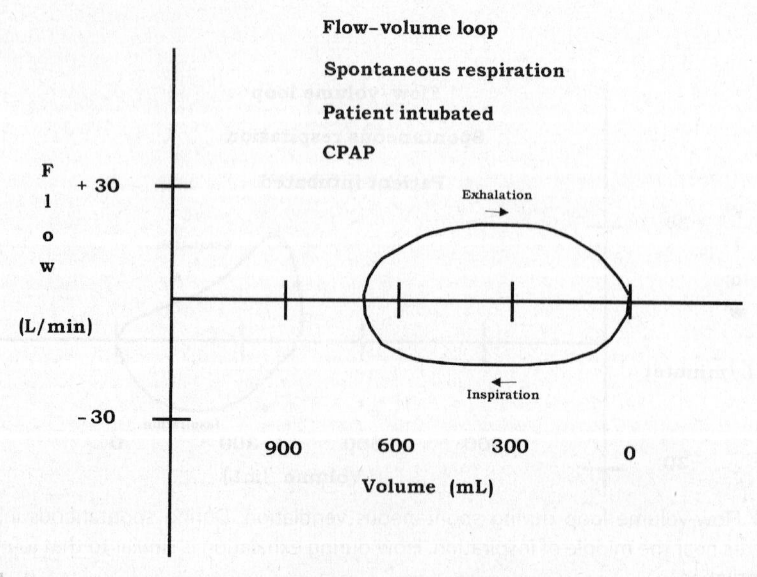

Figure 18.16 Flow-volume loop with spontaneous respiration and continuous positive airway pressure (CPAP). Both the inspiratory and exhalation portions of the loop are flattened. The exhalation portion is more rounded than that in the absence of CPAP.

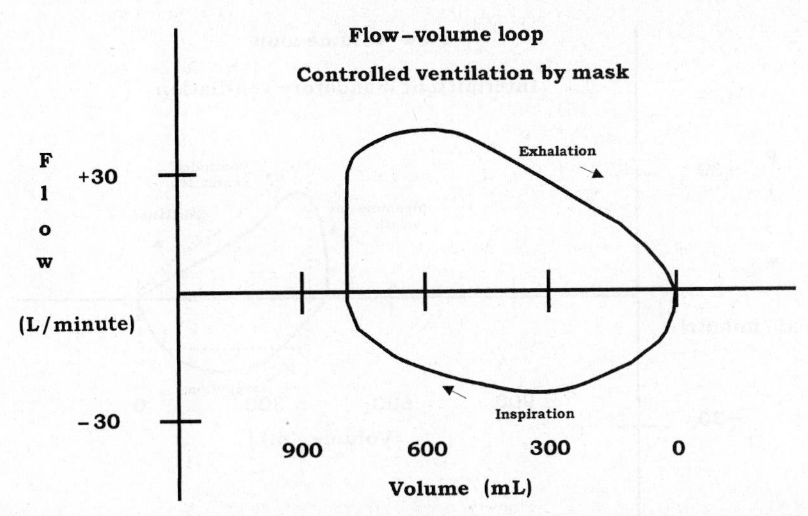

Figure 18.17 Flow-volume loop during mask ventilation. The inspiratory flow is more variable when ventilation is manually controlled than with a ventilator. The flow-volume loop is more rounded during both inspiration and exhalation. This can vary with the way the anesthesia provider squeezes the bag. During exhalation, the lower resistance that is present when there is no tracheal tube results in higher flows.

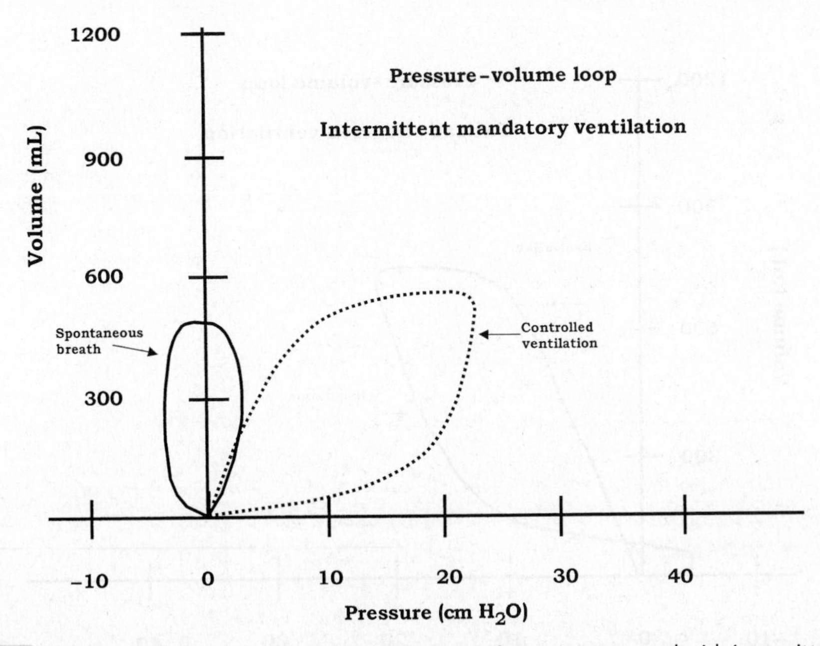

Figure 18.18 Pressure–volume loop with spontaneous ventilation interspersed with intermittent mandatory ventilation. Intermittent mandatory ventilation produces loops representing both spontaneous and controlled breaths. The loop shows both a spontaneous breath (*solid line*) and a controlled breath (*dashed line*). Monitors will usually display these loops consecutively.

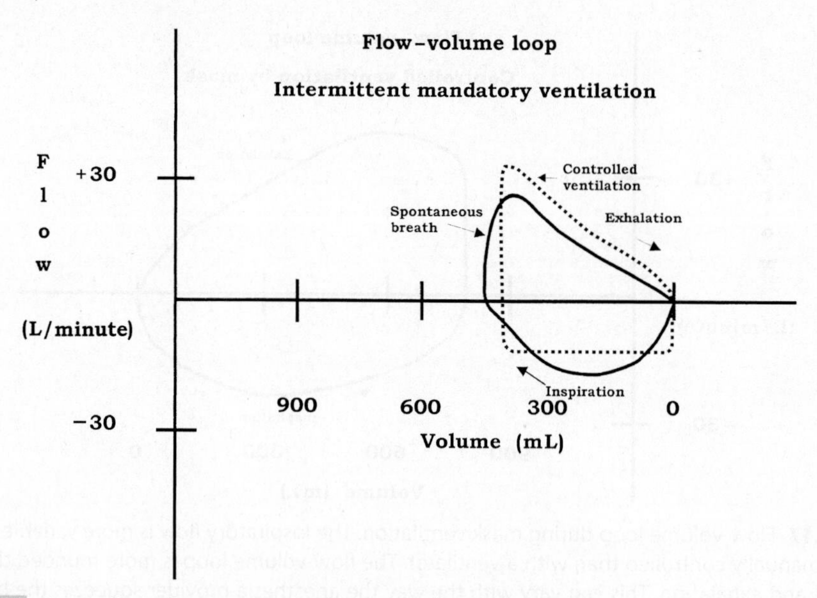

Figure 18.19 Flow-volume loop with intermittent mandatory ventilation. There is both a spontaneous breath (solid line) and a controlled breath (dashed line). Each has the characteristics of the normal loop for controlled or spontaneous respiration.

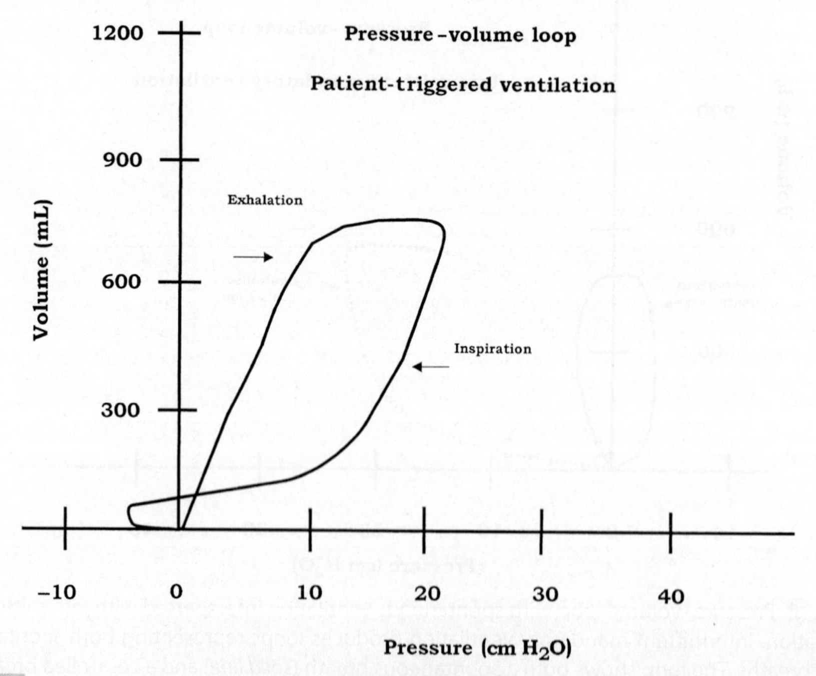

Figure 18.20 Pressure–volume loop with patient-triggered ventilation. A spontaneous breath initiates a positive-pressure breath. The loop starts out displaying negative pressure, but as the ventilator is engaged, the pressure becomes positive for the duration of inspiration. Exhalation proceeds as normal.

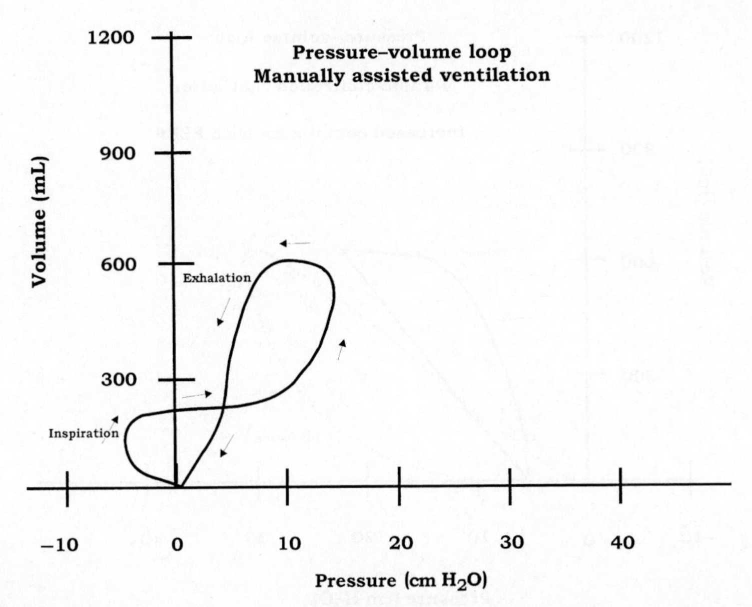

Figure 18.21 Pressure–volume loop with manually assisted ventilation. If the spontaneously breathing patient is not producing a satisfactory tidal volume, respiration can be assisted manually. As the patient begins to inspire, a negative pressure is seen. Then, the bag is squeezed and the pressure becomes positive. The shape of the inspiratory portion will depend on how and when the bag is squeezed. Exhalation may also vary, depending on manual pressure on the bag during exhalation.

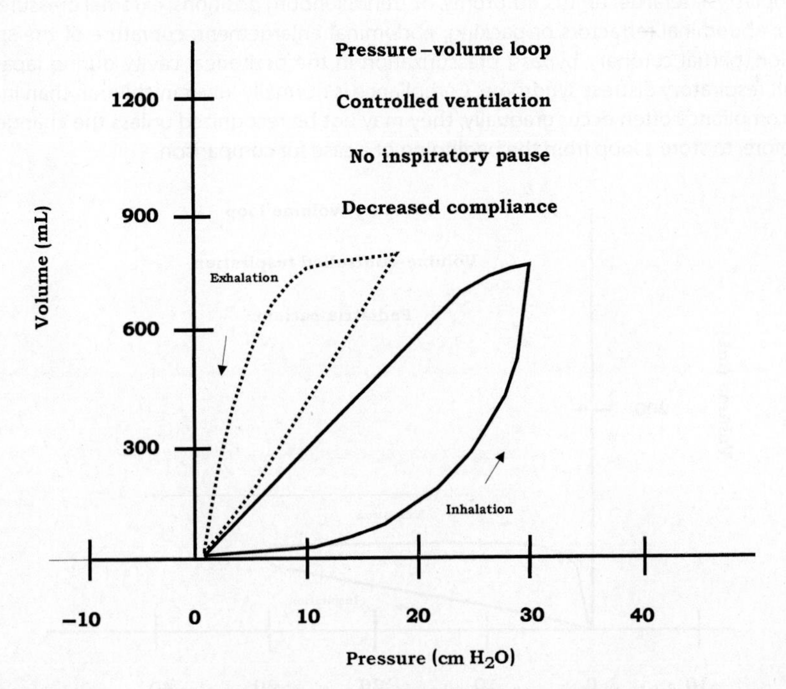

Figure 18.22 Pressure–volume loop with decreased compliance. The solid line represents decreased compliance. The dashed line shows the loop with normal compliance. A major advantage of pressure–volume loops is their ability to detect changes in compliance. If the lungs or chest wall becomes stiffer, increased pressure will be needed to deliver the same tidal volume. This causes the pressure–volume loop to be displaced clockwise.

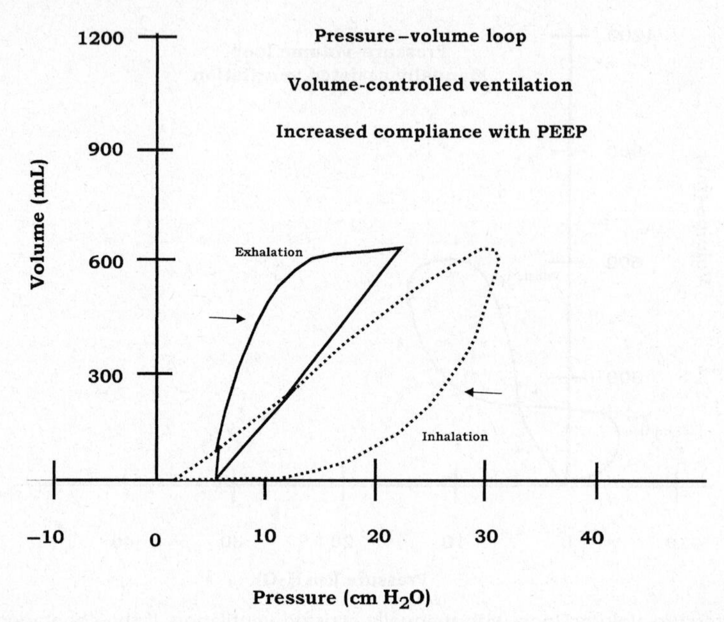

Figure 18.23 Pressure–volume loop with decreased compliance is improved by using positive end-expiratory pressure (PEEP). The *dotted line* represents decreased compliance. The addition of PEEP (*solid line*) moves the beginning point to the PEEP value and improves compliance. Decreases in compliance can result from inadequate muscle relaxation; air embolism; diseases and tumors that invade large areas of the lung or alter its distensibility; narcotics; bronchial intubation; bronchoconstriction; pneumothorax; reduction pneumoplasty; lateral decubitus, lithotomy, or Trendelenburg positions; external pressure on the chest or abdomen; abdominal retractors or packing; abdominal enlargement; curvature of the spine; obesity; prone position; partial coronary bypass; pressurization in the peritoneal cavity during laparoscopic surgery; or adult respiratory distress syndrome. Compliance is normally lower in children than in adults. Since changes in compliance often occur gradually, they may not be recognized unless the change is large. It is useful, therefore, to store a loop from the beginning of a case for comparison.

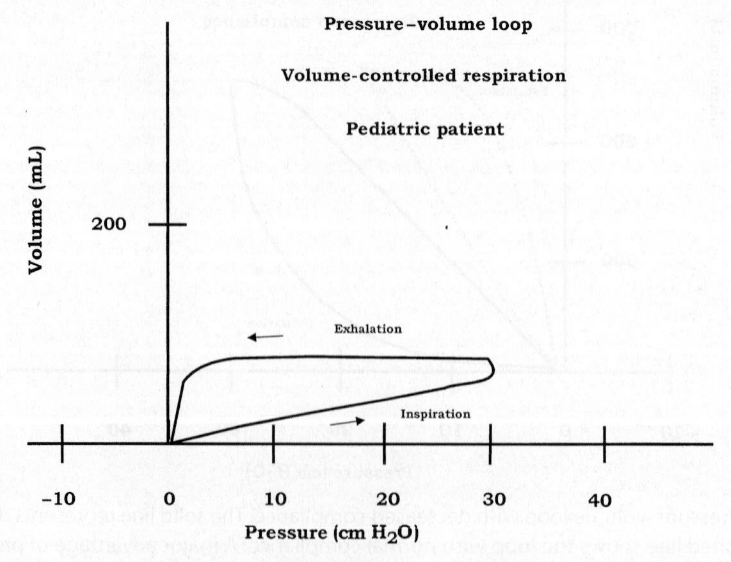

Figure 18.24 Pressure–volume loop in a pediatric patient. Compliance is lower in children than in adults because of the small tidal volumes. Higher pressures are needed to overcome the resistance of smaller tracheal tubes.

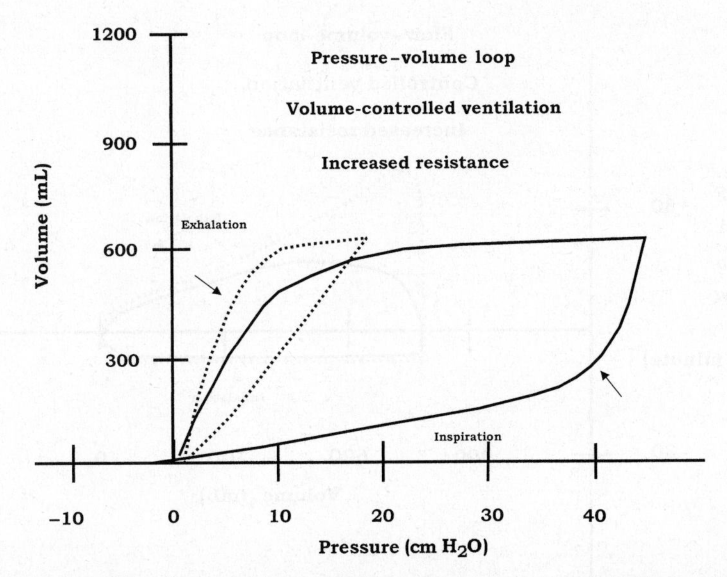

Figure 18.25 Pressure–volume loop with an increase in resistance. During controlled ventilation, increased resistance means that higher inspiratory pressures will be required to deliver a given flow. Tidal volume may be reduced. As shown in this figure (*solid line*), the pressure–volume loop is shifted to the right and downward with a large internal area. The pressure falls rapidly after inspiration is complete. The loop may be open if there is air trapping.

An increase in resistance may be caused by tracheal tube obstruction (kinking, dislodgment, or secretions), bronchoconstriction, and airway collapse from the loss of elastic recoil or by obstruction in a large airway caused by secretions, blood, foreign body, neoplasm, inflammation, or using a tracheal tube that is too small. While mild bronchospasm causes only slight changes in the loop, there will be greater changes in both the inspiratory and exhalation portions as it increases. With severe expiratory resistance, expiratory flow may stop abruptly before the next mechanical inflation. The effects of treatment of bronchospasm can be assessed by observing the loop.

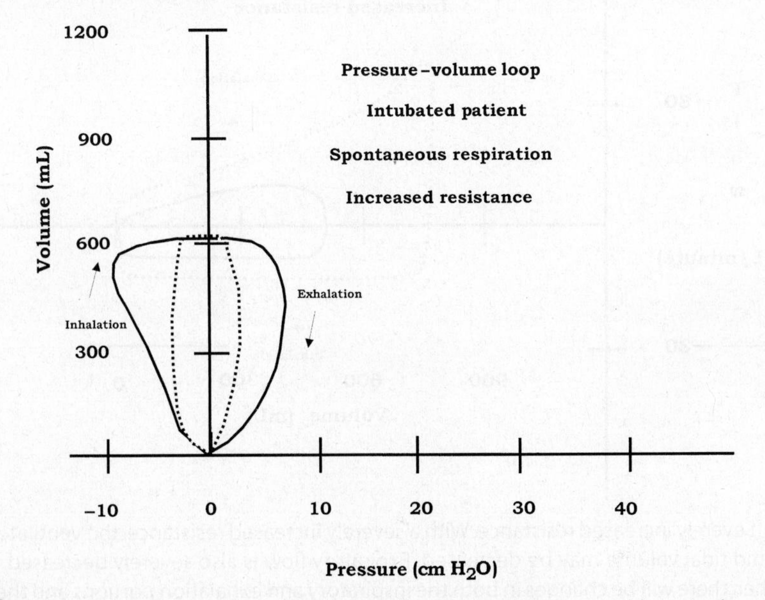

Figure 18.26 Spontaneous respiration with increased resistance. The normal loop is shown with dotted lines. With increased resistance greater pressure (more negative during inspiration, positive during exhalation) will be needed to move the same volume of gas.

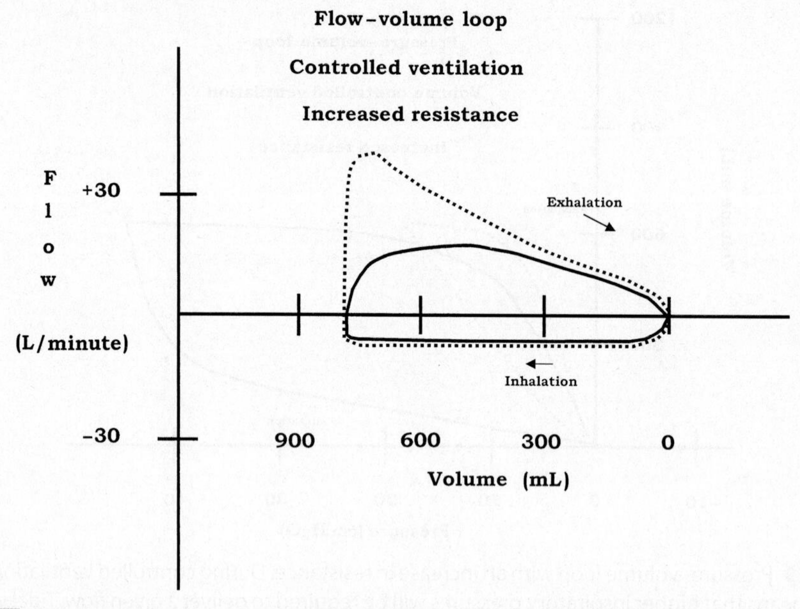

Figure 18.27 Flow-volume loop with volume-controlled ventilation and increased resistance. The dotted line represents normal resistance. When resistance is increased, the flow-volume loop will show decreased flow throughout exhalation.

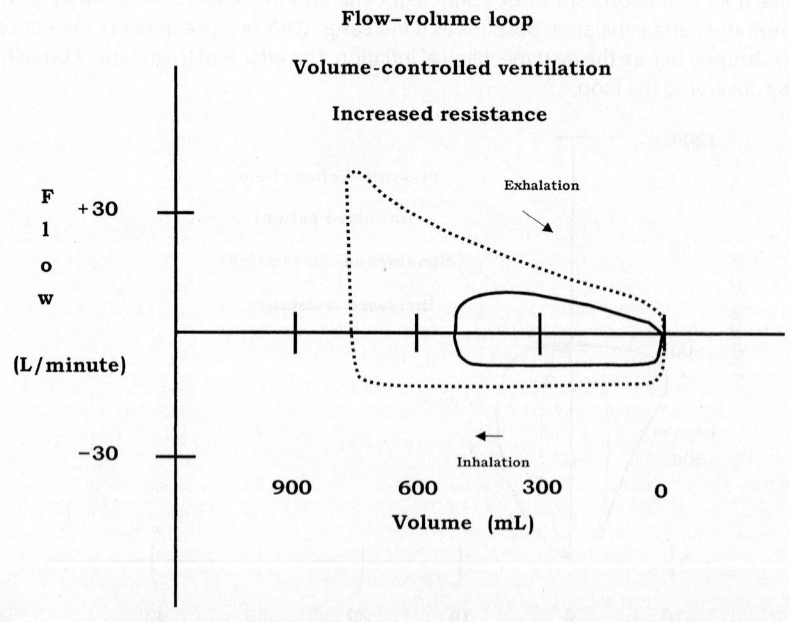

Figure 18.28 Severely increased resistance. With a severely increased resistance, the ventilator cannot fully compensate and tidal volume may be decreased. Expiratory flow is also severely decreased. As resistance increases further, there will be changes in both the inspiratory and exhalation portions and the tidal volume may be decreased. With severe expiratory resistance, expiratory flow may stop abruptly before the next mechanical inflation.

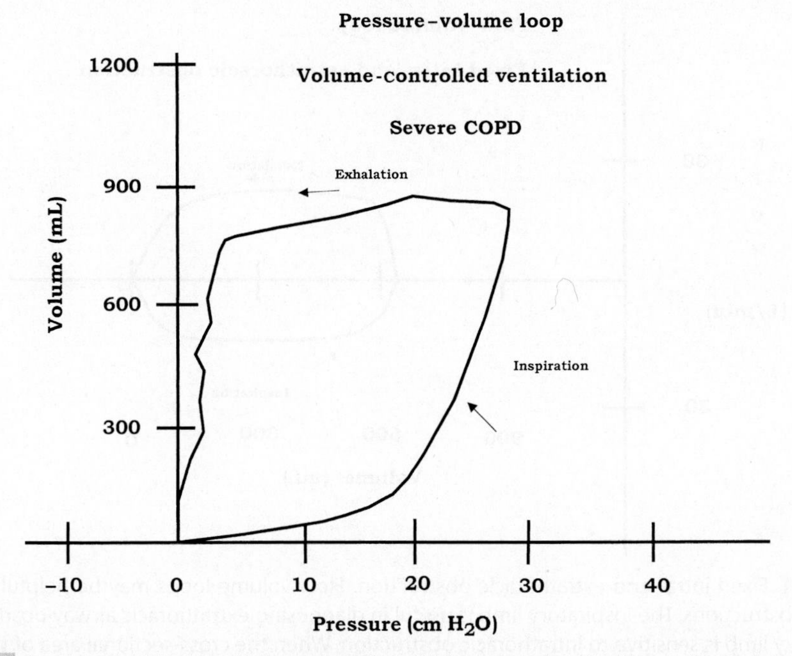

Figure 18.29 Increased resistance during exhalation. With severe chronic obstructive pulmonary disease (COPD), resistance during exhalation is greatly increased. Emphysema is characterized by a progressive loss of elastic tissue in the lung. Patients with COPD have no problem with inflating the lungs but must work to exhale. During mechanical ventilation, patients with airflow obstruction may develop inadvertent positive end-expiratory pressure (PEEP) (auto-PEEP, occult or intrinsic PEEP, dynamic hyperinflation, air trapping) if there is not enough time for complete exhalation. If the patient cannot exhale completely before the next inspiration, there will be an open loop, as shown.

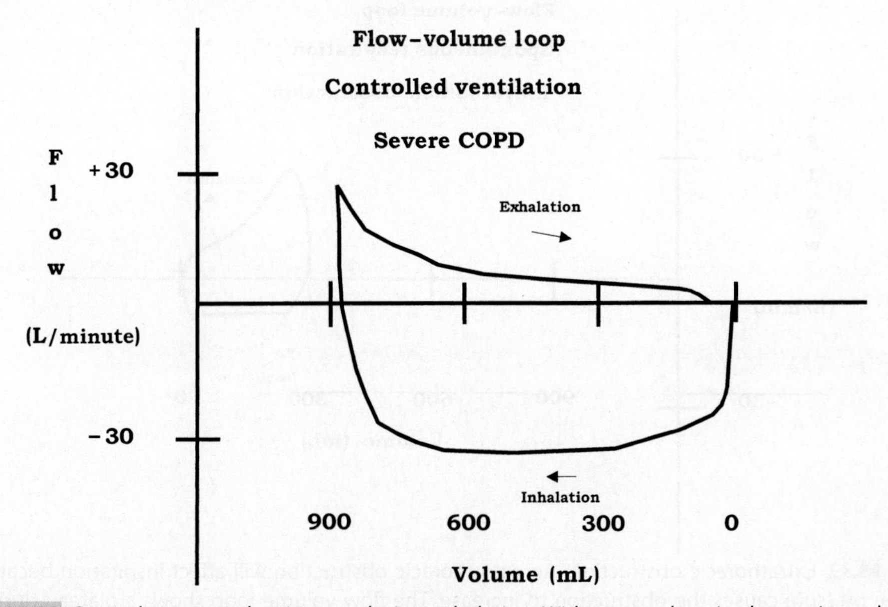

Figure 18.30 Severely increased resistance during exhalation. With severe chronic obstructive pulmonary disease (COPD), expiratory flow is greatly reduced. The loop may be open if the patient does not have sufficient time to exhale completely. Interrupted expiratory flow may suggest the presence of intrinsic positive end-expiratory pressure (PEEP) (auto-PEEP).

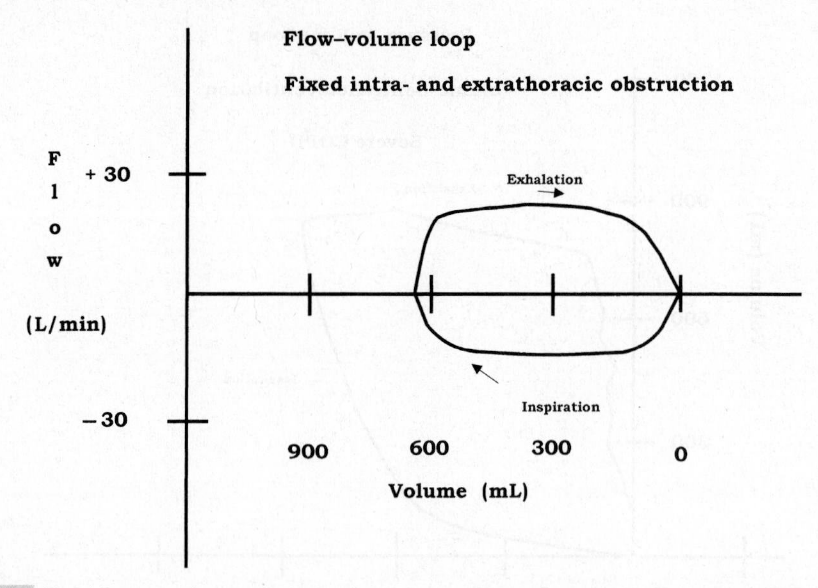

Figure 18.31 Fixed intra- and extrathoracic obstruction. Flow-volume loops may be helpful in identifying airway obstructions. The inspiratory limb is useful in diagnosing extrathoracic airway obstruction, and the expiratory limb is sensitive to intrathoracic obstruction. When the cross-sectional area of the airway is decreased to a critical level, characteristic patterns of flow occur with spontaneous ventilation. Typically, the flow rate will plateau. The flow rate at this plateau will depend on the cross-sectional area of the flow-limiting segment in the airway.

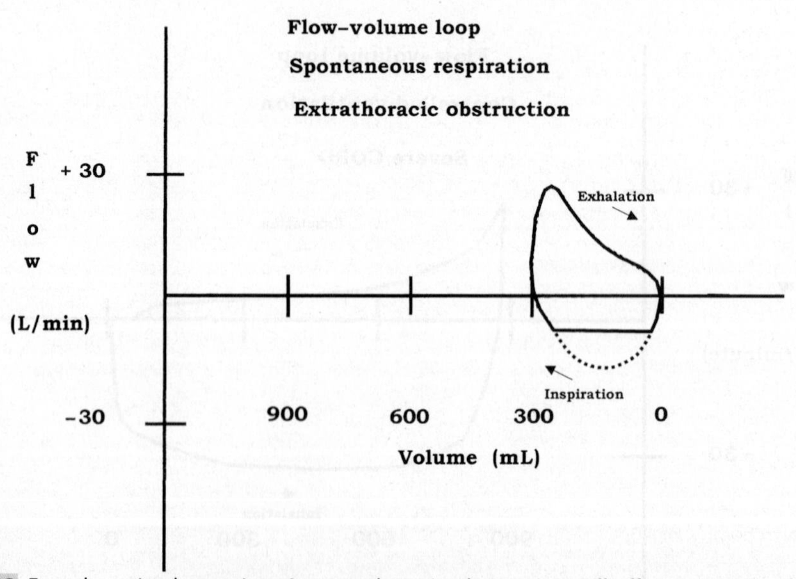

Figure 18.32 Extrathoracic obstruction. An extrathoracic obstruction will affect inspiration because the negative pressure causes the obstruction to increase. The flow-volume loop shows a plateau during the inspiratory phase. During exhalation, positive pressure in the airway will keep the airway open at the site of the lesion, leaving the expiratory curve unaffected.

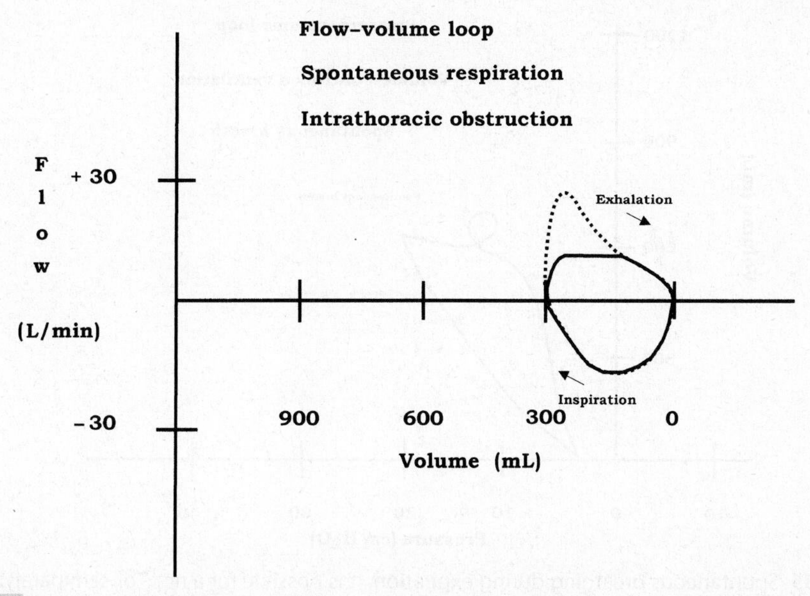

Figure 18.33 Intrathoracic obstruction. With an intrathoracic obstruction (such as a tumor in the trachea or a mediastinal mass), inspiratory flow may be relatively normal. During expiration, intrathoracic pressure becomes positive and decreases the airway diameter so that the expiratory flow is reduced. This causes a plateau in the expiratory portion of the loop.

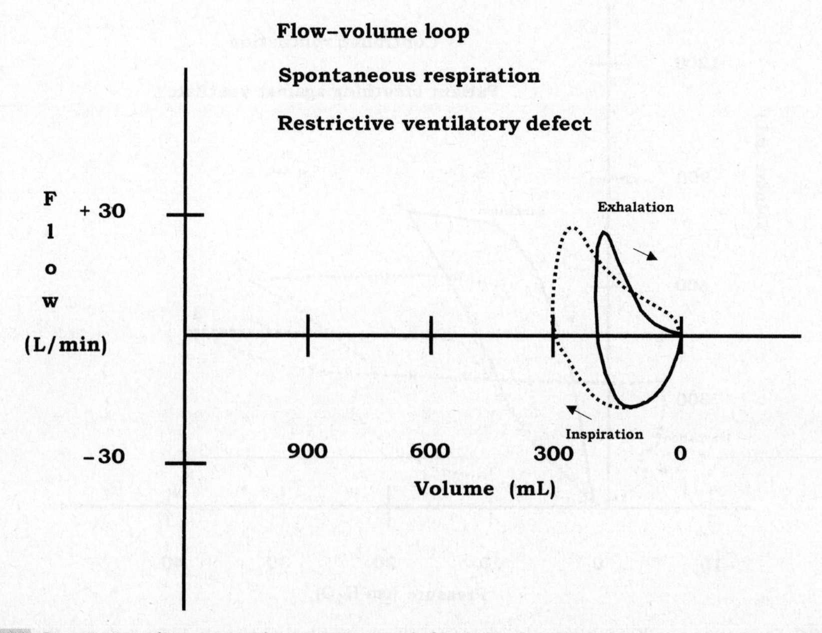

Figure 18.34 Restrictive disease. With a restrictive defect, the increase in elastic recoil is associated with higher expiratory flow. As the process becomes more severe and lung volumes are decreased, the flow-volume curve becomes tall and narrow. The dotted line shows a normal loop.

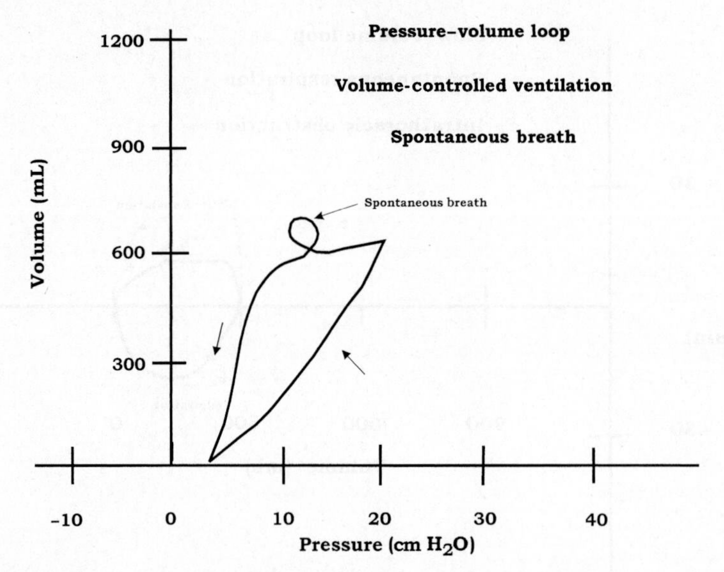

Figure 18.35 Spontaneous breathing during expiration. It is possible for a non- or semiparalyzed patient to breathe spontaneously during controlled ventilation. This can occur at any time during the respiratory cycle. This figure shows a pressure–volume loop with a spontaneous breath during exhalation. As the spontaneous breath starts, the pressure drops below the expected level whereas the volume rises above the usual curve. As the spontaneous breath is exhaled, the pressure increases briefly and the volume drops rapidly. The remainder of the loop follows the expected shape.

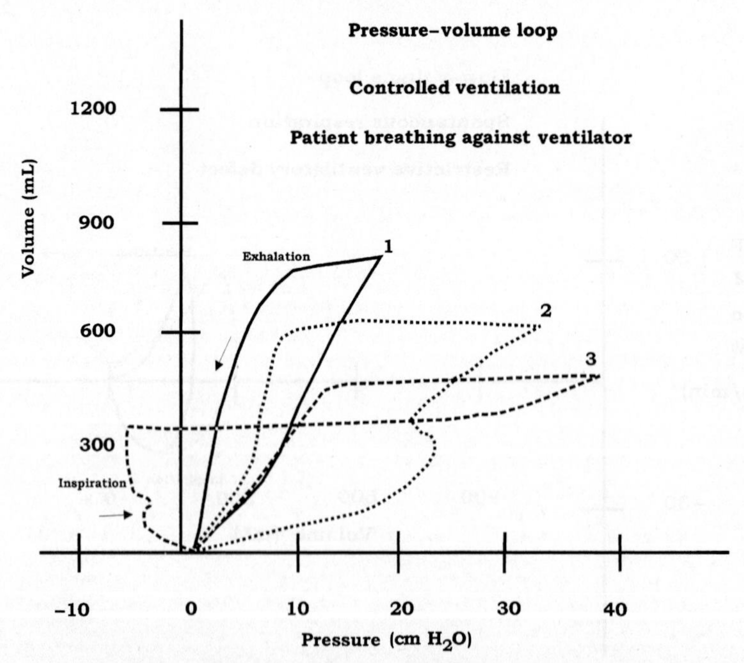

Figure 18.36 Spontaneous breathing during controlled ventilation. Loop 1 represents the normal loop during volume-controlled mechanical ventilation. Loop 2 shows a spontaneous breath during inspiration. The pressure drops and the volume increases briefly. There is a decrease in compliance that may be caused by an increase in tension in the chest wall muscles. In loop 3, the patient inhales at the beginning of the respiratory cycle, so the loop moves to the left of the vertical axis. As the ventilator cycles, the breathing system pressure rapidly becomes positive as the patient attempts to exhale against the ventilator's inspiration. There is a further decrease in compliance.

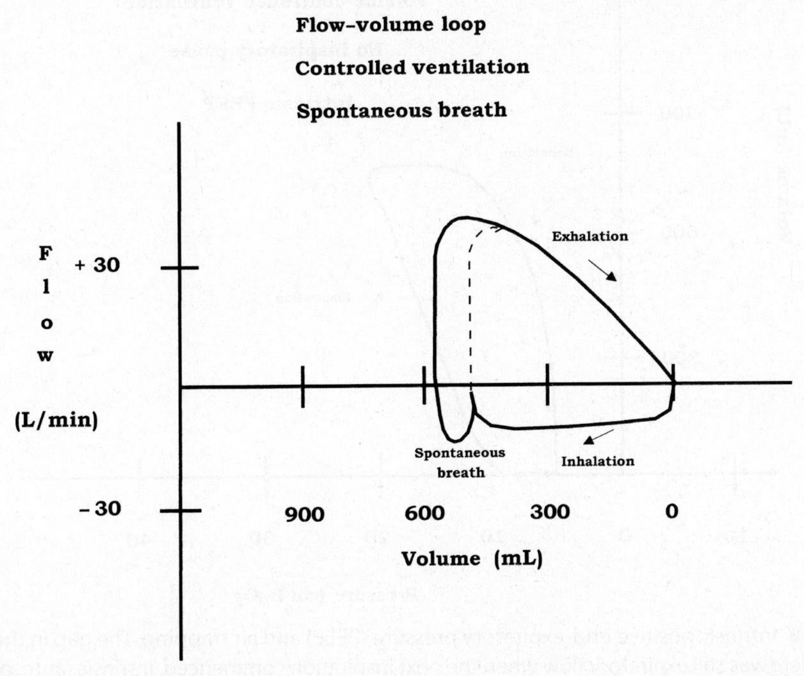

Figure 18.37 Spontaneous breathing during inspiration. This figure shows a flow-volume loop with the patient taking a spontaneous breath when the ventilator cycle is near the end of inspiration. Instead of returning to zero at the end of inspiration, the flow increases. There is a small increase in volume as well. The *dotted line* represents the normal loop.

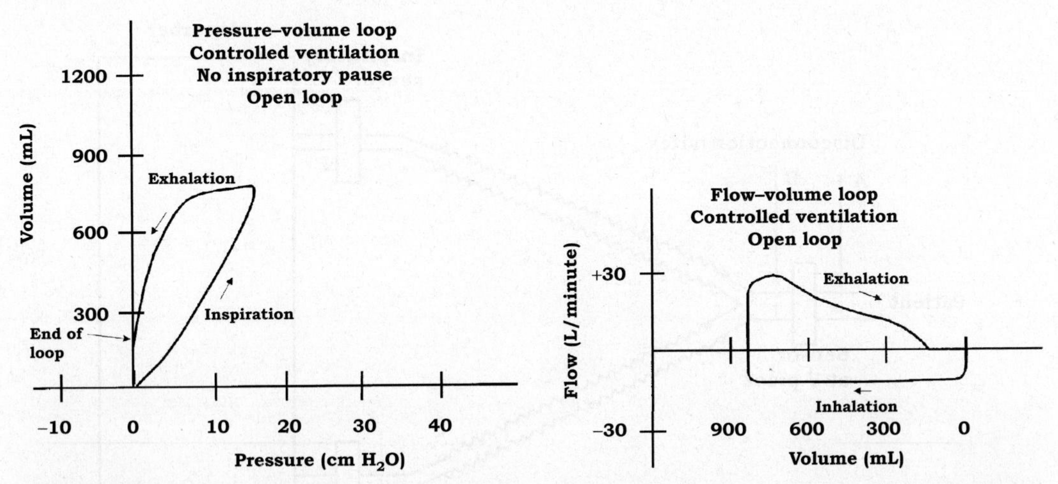

Figure 18.38 Open loop. Both a pressure–volume and flow-volume loop are illustrated. A loop should return to its starting point at the end of the respiratory cycle. An open loop has a gap between the end and starting points, indicating that the exhaled volume is less than the inspired volume. While the pressure–volume loop appears to close, it actually returns to zero pressure along the vertical axis rather than at the starting point. The point where the exhalation part of the loop reaches zero pressure indicates the difference in the inspired and exhaled volumes. Most often, an open loop occurs because there is a leak. Leaks often occur after lung reduction or other thoracic surgery. An open loop is often seen with mask anesthesia, an uncuffed tracheal tube, or a supraglottic airway device. Incorrect calibration should also be considered. An open loop may result from incomplete exhalation caused by chronic obstructive pulmonary disease, increased resistance caused by apparatus (including a double-lumen tube), a tension pneumothorax, lung retraction, or a flap-valve obstruction in a large airway.

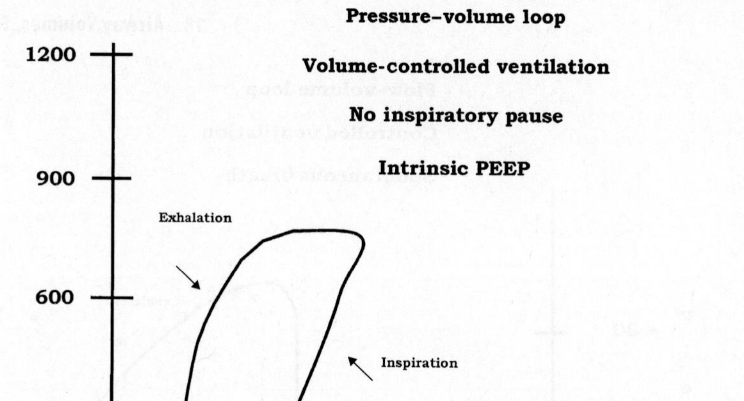

Figure 18.39 Intrinsic positive end-expiratory pressure (PEEP) and air trapping. The gap in the loop indicates that there was still expiratory flow when the next inspiration commenced. Intrinsic (auto, occult) PEEP results from a difference between the actual expiratory time and the time required for complete exhalation of the tidal volume so that some air is trapped in the lungs. It may be generated by a very short expiratory time and/or slow expiration due to high resistance or abnormally high compliance. Air trapping is likely to occur in patients with airflow limitation, inverse ratio ventilation, or when using a high respiratory rate.

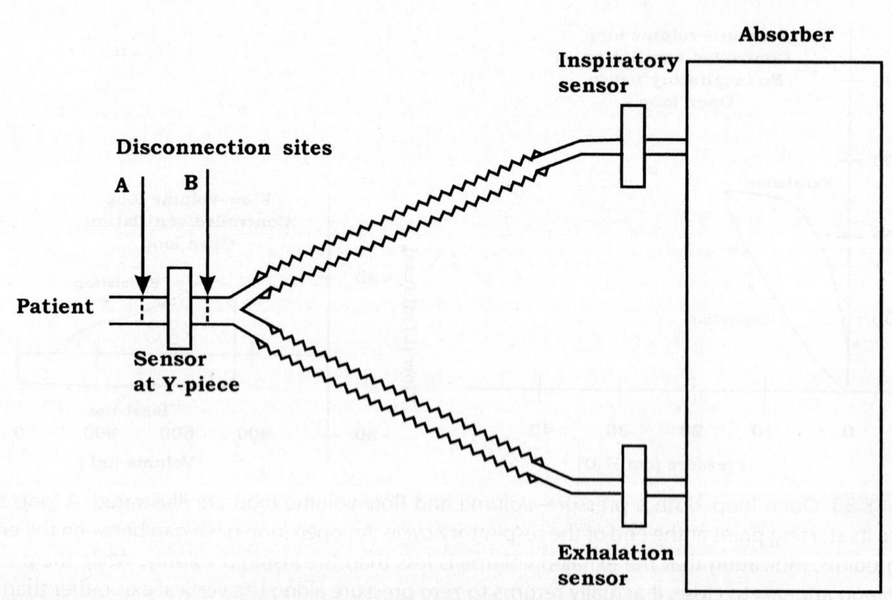

Figure 18.40 Disconnections between the Y-piece and the patient. If the disconnection is at **A** and the patient is spontaneously breathing, no loop will be generated. If respiration is controlled and the patient is not spontaneously breathing, half of a loop (the inspiratory portion) would be generated. (See **Fig. 18.41**.) If the disconnection is at **B** and the patient is spontaneously breathing, a loop normal for spontaneous breathing would be generated. If the respiration was controlled, no loop would be generated. If the sensors are at the absorber and there is no sensor at the Y-piece, a disconnection at **A** or **B** would show a half loop during controlled or spontaneous respiration.

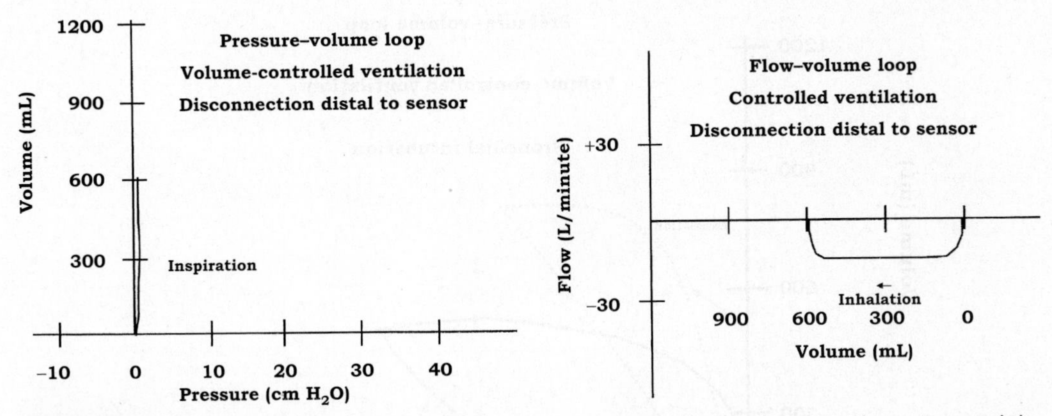

Figure 18.41 This figure shows the loops generated from a disconnection between the patient and the sensor with controlled ventilation. There will be flow during inspiration, but not exhalation, so only half of a loop will be generated.

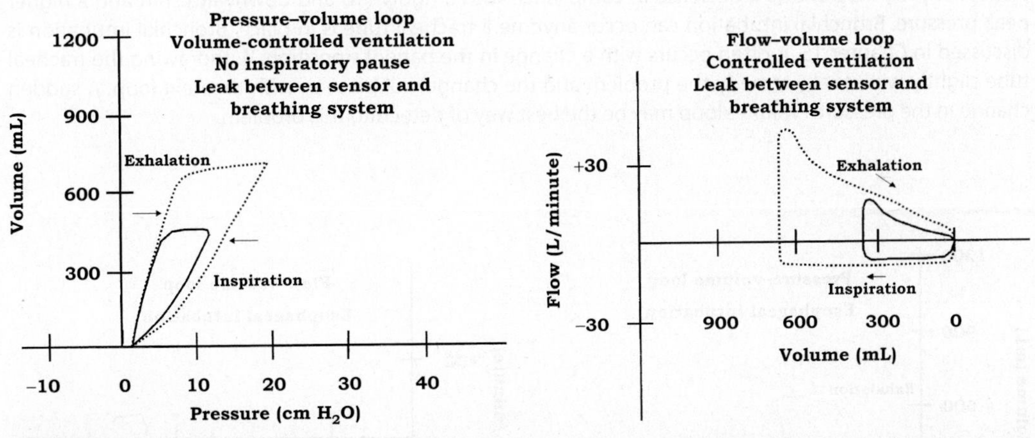

Figure 18.42 Leak between the sensor and the breathing system. These loops show a leak but not a complete disconnection. The dotted line represents the normal loop and the solid line after a leak where gas is lost during inspiration. Both loops are normal in shape but show a decrease in tidal volume and peak airway pressure and flow.

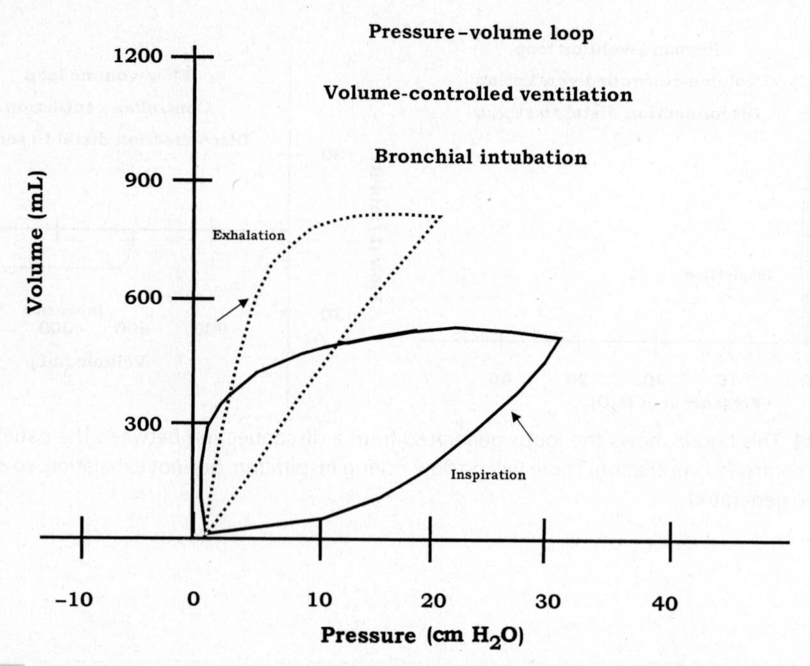

Figure 18.43 Bronchial intubation. The dotted line shows a normal loop. The solid line represents bronchial intubation. The loop shows a decrease in compliance with a rightward and downward shift and a higher peak pressure. Bronchial intubation can occur anytime a tracheal tube is in place. Bronchial intubation is discussed in Chapter 15. It often occurs with a change in the patient's position. Withdrawing the tracheal tube slightly will usually remedy the problem and the change will be seen with the next loop. A sudden change in the pressure–volume loop may be the best way of detecting this problem.

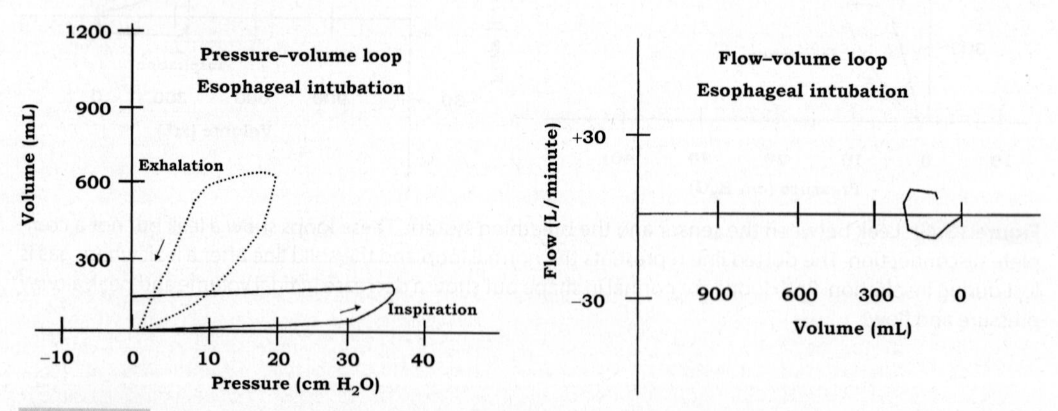

Figure 18.44 Esophageal intubation. With esophageal intubation, the pressure–volume loop will usually show a decrease in compliance (*solid line*), although compliance may be normal or increased. Gas that enters the stomach and is not returned will create an open loop. The flow-volume loop will be distorted and show small inspiratory and expiratory volumes.

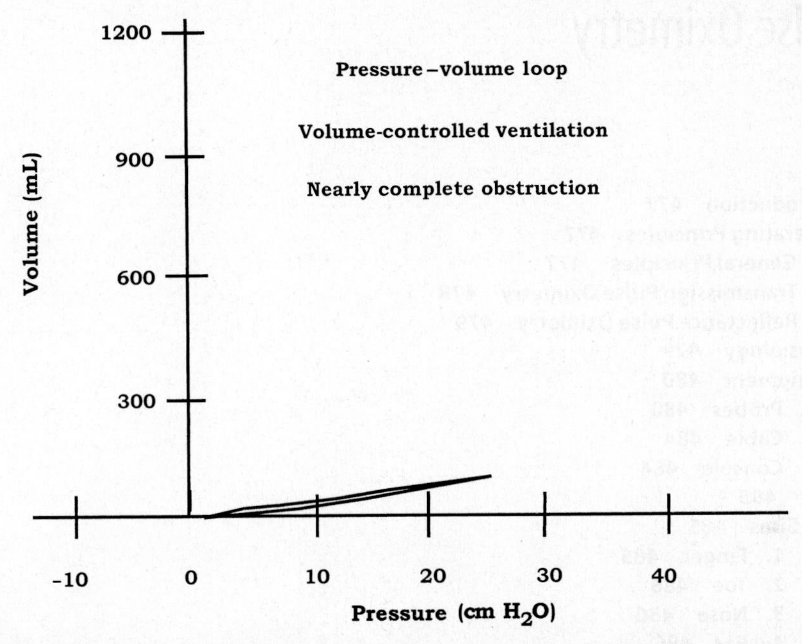

Figure 18.45 Obstructed tracheal tube. A nearly completely obstructed tracheal tube or incorrectly placed supraglottic airway device will result in a pressure–volume loop that shows a high pressure level with little or no tidal volume. This is usually a signal that the device should be removed and reinserted.

SUGGESTED READINGS

Dorsch J, Dorsch S. Airway volumes, flows, and pressures. In: Understanding Anesthesia Equipment. Fifth edition. Philadelphia: Wolters Kluwer/Lippincott Williams & Wilkins, 2008:728–774.

Raphael DT. The low-pressure alarm condition: safety considerations and the anesthesiologist's response. APSF Newslett 1998–1999;13(4):33–40.

Robinson RJS. The use of side-stream spirometry to assess air leak during and after lung volume reduction surgery. Anesthesiology 1999;91:571–573.

19 Pulse Oximetry

I. Introduction

A. Pulse oximetry, sometimes called the fifth vital sign, is a noninvasive method of measuring hemoglobin saturation (Spo_2) by using a light signal transmitted through tissue. A low Spo_2 can provide warning that hypoxemia is present before other signs such as cyanosis or a change in heart rate are observed. In addition to measuring oxygen saturation, pulse oximeters with additional wavelengths are now able to measure carboxyhemoglobin (HbCO, COHb), methemoglobin (metHb), and hemoglobin concentrations.

B. A study of closed claims of anesthetic-related malpractice cases determined that a combination of pulse oximetry and capnography could have prevented 93% of avoidable mishaps. The American Society of Anesthesiologists (ASA) and American Association of Nurse Anesthetists have made the assessment of oxygenation a standard for intraoperative and postoperative monitoring. In 2005, requirements for a variable pitch pulse tone and that the low Spo_2 alarm be audible were added to the ASA monitoring standards. In some states, using pulse oximetry is mandatory.

II. Operating Principles

A. General Principles

1. A pulse oximeter estimates Spo_2 from the differential absorption of red and infrared light in blood. Reduced hemoglobin absorbs more light than oxyhemoglobin in the red band, whereas oxyhemoglobin absorbs more light in the infrared band (**Fig. 19.1**). The pulse oximeter computes the ratio between these two signals and relates this ratio to the arterial oxygen saturation by an empirical algorithm.
2. A pulse oximeter discriminates between arterial blood and other components by determining the change in transmitted light caused by arterial blood flow. It pulses red and infrared LEDs ON and OFF several hundred times per second. The rapid sampling rate allows the peak and trough of each pulse wave to be

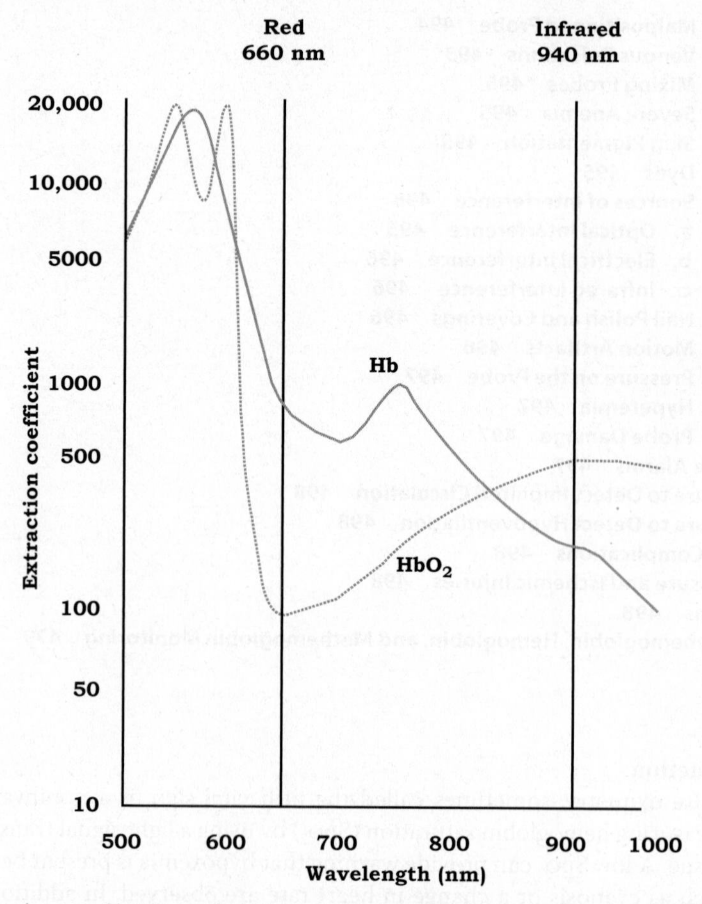

Figure 19.1 Absorbance of light as a function of wavelength. The extinction coefficient is a measure of the tendency of a substance to absorb light. At the red wavelengths (650 to 750 nm), reduced hemoglobin absorbs more light than does oxyhemoglobin. In the infrared region (900 to 1000 nm), the reverse is true.

recognized. At the trough, the light is transmitted through a vascular bed that contains mainly capillary and venous blood. At the peak, it shines through all this plus arterial blood. A photodiode collects the transmitted light and converts it into electrical signals. The emitted signals are amplified and then processed.

3. Fractional oxygen saturation (% HbO_2) is the ratio of oxyhemoglobin to the sum of all hemoglobin species present, whether available for reversible binding to oxygen or not. Functional oxygen saturation (SaO_2) is the ratio of oxyhemoglobin to all functional hemoglobins. These must be determined using an in vitro oximeter. For patients with low dyshemoglobin levels, the difference between fractional saturation and functional saturation is very small. When dyshemoglobin levels are elevated, the two values can vary greatly and pulse oximeter readings may not agree with either the true fractional or functional saturation values.
4. If any other substances that absorb light are also present in the blood, pulse oximeter calibration may become invalid.

B. Transmission Pulse Oximetry

The most common type of pulse oximeter is the transmission oximeter. With this technology, light is transmitted through a vascular bed and detected on the opposite side of that bed.

C. Reflectance Pulse Oximetry

1. Reflectance oximetry relies on light that is reflected (backscattered) to determine oxygen saturation. The probe has both an LED and a photodetector on the same side (see **Fig. 19.12**).

CLINICAL MOMENT Transmission pulse oximetry probes are not accurate when used in the manner of reflectance oximetry and vice versa.

2. With reflectance pulse oximetry, the signals are weaker than those in transmission oximetry, so the photodiode area needs to be as large as possible. The tissue must be well perfused to obtain a strong signal. Heating the measurement site and applying pressure may be helpful. Vasoconstriction can cause overestimation of the oxygen saturation. If the probe is located over an artery or a vein, the reading may be artifactually low.

III. **Physiology**

A. Efficient oxygen transport relies on the ability of hemoglobin to reversibly load and unload oxygen. The relationship between oxygen tension and oxygen saturation is seen in the oxyhemoglobin dissociation curve (**Fig. 19.2**).

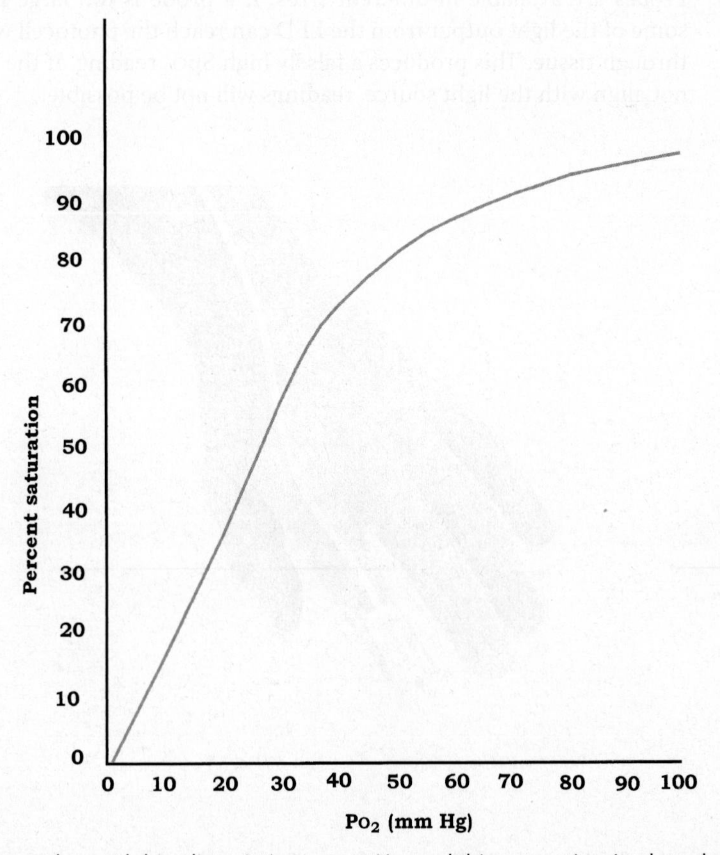

Figure 19.2 The oxyhemoglobin dissociation curve. Hemoglobin saturation is plotted as a function of oxygen tension.

B. Between 90% and 100% saturation, the partial pressure of oxygen in arterial blood (Pao_2) will be 60 torr or more. Below 90% saturation, the curve becomes steeper and small drops in saturation correspond to large drops in oxygen partial pressure. If a problem develops, there may not be much time before the oxygen level becomes dangerously low.

IV. Equipment

A. Probes

1. The probe (sensor, transducer) is the part that comes in contact with the patient. It contains one or more LEDs (photodiodes) that emit light at specific wavelengths and a photodetector (photocell, transducer). The LEDs provide monochromatic light. This means that they emit a constant wavelength throughout their life, so they never need recalibration. LEDs cause relatively little heating and are so inexpensive that they may be used in a disposable probe.
2. **Figures 19.3** to **19.8** show several types of probes. Probes may be reusable or disposable. A disposable probe is usually attached using adhesive. Reusable probes either clip on or are attached using adhesive or Velcro. Disposable probes may be easier to use, but reusable probes are more economical as long as personnel are careful not to damage them. Self-adhesive (band, wrap) probes are less susceptible to motion artifact and less likely to come off if the patient moves than those that clip on. Clip-on probes sometimes do not provide adequate shielding from ambient light.
3. Probes are available in different sizes. If a probe is too large for the patient, some of the light output from the LED can reach the photocell without passing through tissue. This produces a falsely high Spo_2 reading. If the photocell does not align with the light source, readings will not be possible.

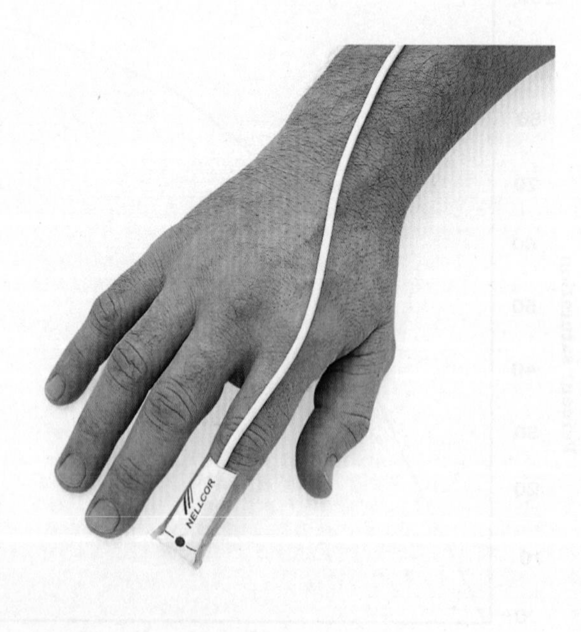

Figure 19.3 Disposable flexible probe in place on a finger. (Reprinted with permission from Nellcor Puritan Bennett, Inc., Pleasanton, CA.)

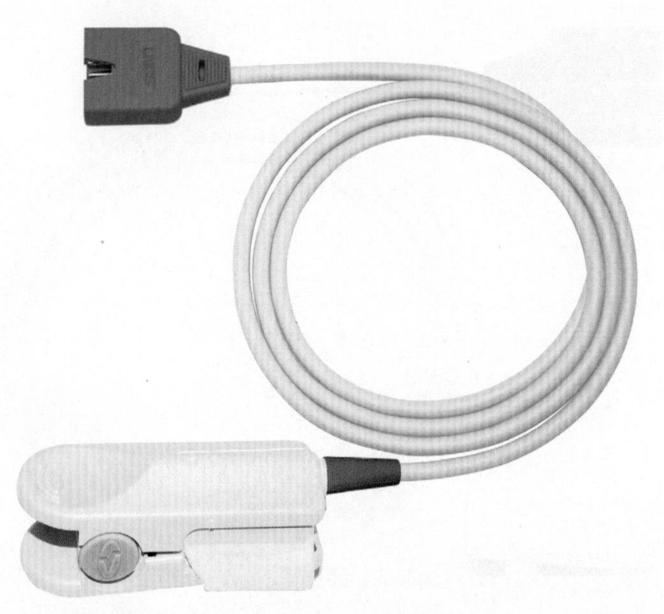

Figure 19.4 Reusable probe. This is most commonly used on a finger or toe. In infants, this type of probe can be placed on part of the hand or foot. These probes offer good shielding from ambient light. (Photograph courtesy of Masimo Corporation, Irvine, CA.)

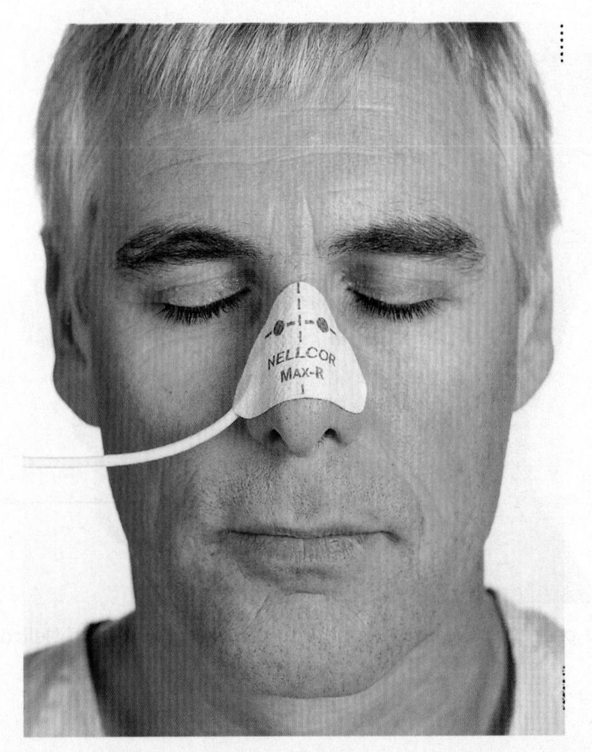

Figure 19.5 Disposable nasal probe in place. The clip from a disposable oxygen mask may be used to improve contact and to hold the probe in place. (Reprinted with permission from Nellcor Puritan Bennett, Inc., Pleasanton, CA.)

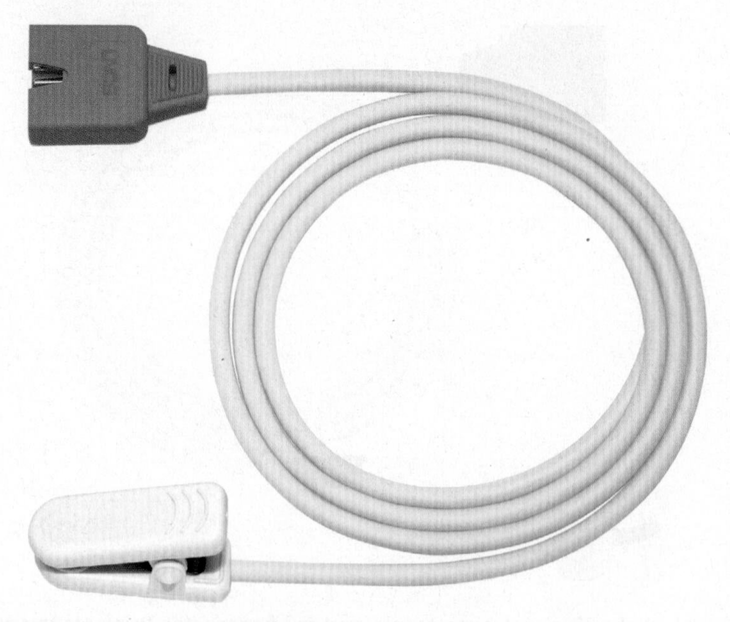

Figure 19.6 Reusable probe designed for use on the ear. This may be used on other locations, including the cheek. (Photograph courtesy of Masimo Corporation, Irvine, CA.)

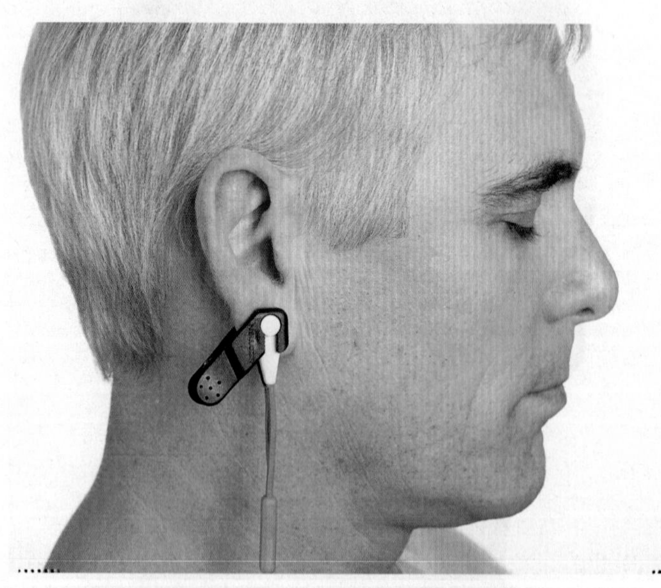

Figure 19.7 Reusable probe on the ear. (Reprinted with permission from Nellcor Puritan Bennett, Inc., Pleasanton, CA.)

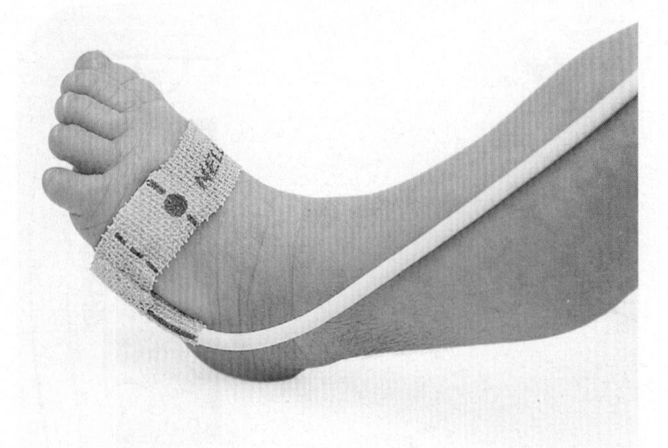

Figure 19.8 Disposable wraparound probe on the foot. (Reprinted with permission from Nellcor Puritan Bennett, Inc., Pleasanton, CA.)

CLINICAL MOMENT Attaching the reusable probe to the oximeter case when not in use will reduce damage and make it easier to find.

4. To reduce contamination, a glove, glove finger, or other covering may be used either over the application site or over the probe. Extraneous light can be eliminated by covering the probe with an opaque material such as a surgical towel, gauze, finger cot, blanket, alcohol wipe packet, or other foil shield. These coverings may also help to stabilize the probe. Mitts that keep out ambient light are available (**Fig. 19.9**).

CLINICAL MOMENT If there is difficulty in obtaining a satisfactory reading, reducing the extraneous light on the probe may improve the situation.

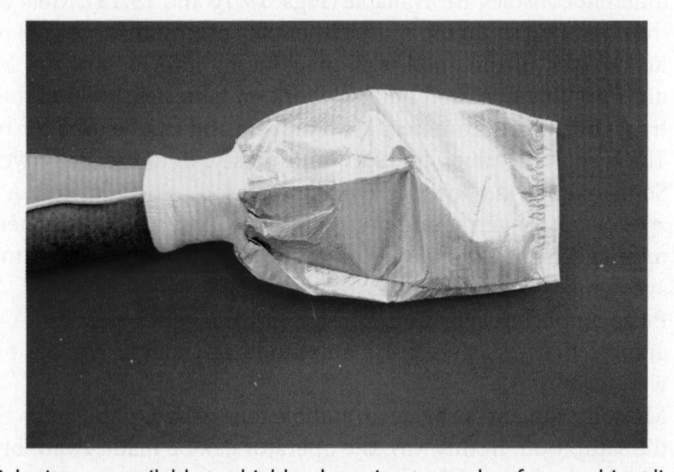

Figure 19.9 Special mitts are available to shield pulse oximeter probes from ambient light.

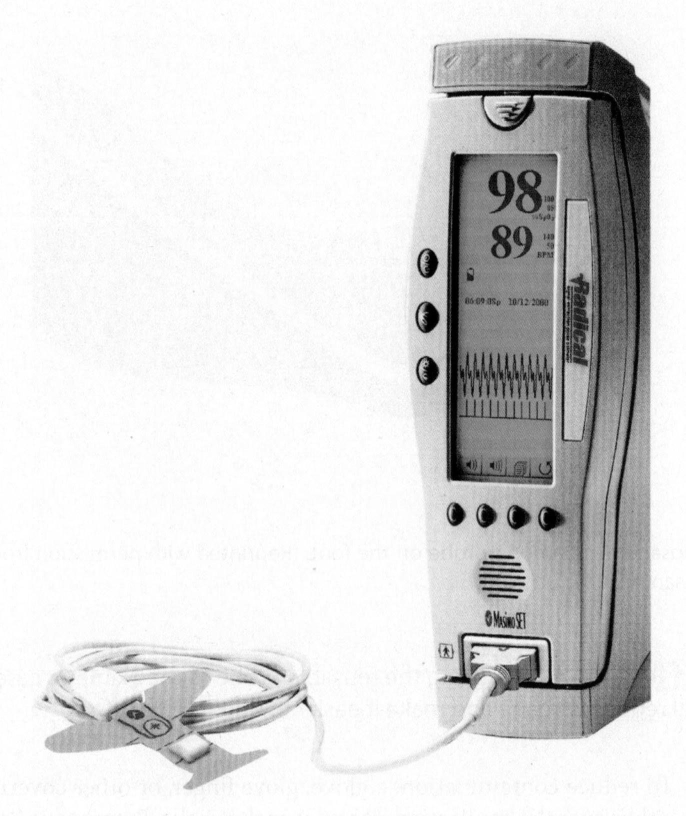

Figure 19.10 Small handheld, battery-operated pulse oximeters are often used, especially during patient transport. This unit is plugged in its recharger. (Photograph courtesy of Masimo Corporation, Irvine, CA.)

B. Cable

The probe is connected to the oximeter by an electrical cable. Cables from different manufacturers are *not* interchangeable, although the plug may fit into another manufacturer's monitor.

C. Console

1. The console is where the signal is processed and the values are reported. Many different consoles are available (**Figs. 19.10** and **19.11**). Most oximeters used in the operating room today are either part of a multifunctional physiologic monitor or part of the anesthesia machine monitoring system. Most stand-alone units are line operated but will work on batteries, making them useful during transport. Some oximeters are handheld and can be used for transport.
2. The displayed values for Spo_2 and pulse rate are usually weighted averages. Some oximeters allow the averaging period to be adjusted. A mode that averages over a longer period of time may be more accurate if there is much probe motion. Changes in pulse rate or saturation will be reflected more rapidly if the averaging is done over a shorter period of time.
3. Pulse amplitude may be represented by a signal indicator. Other units use a graphic that indicates pulse amplitude and may provide a plethysmographic waveform.
4. Most instruments provide an audible tone with variable pitch that changes with the saturation. In this way, the operator can be made aware of changes in Spo_2 without looking at the oximeter. There is usually a means to control audible signal volume.

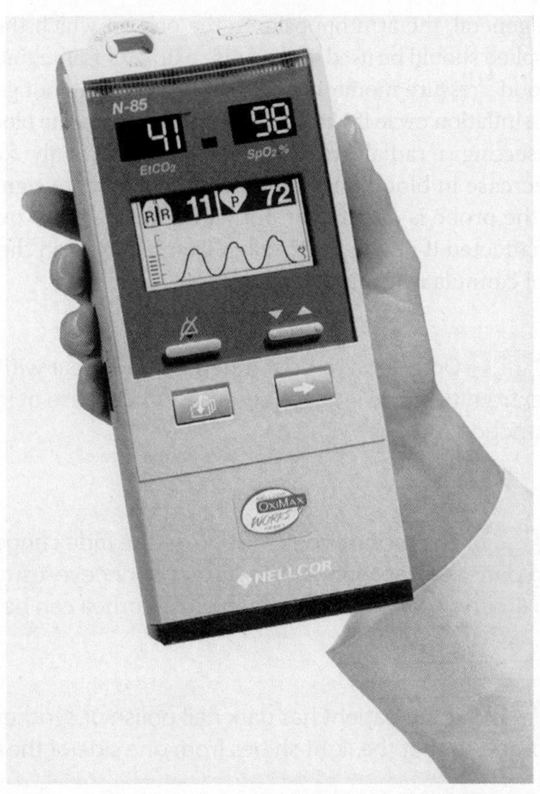

Figure 19.11 Combined pulse oximeter and carbon dioxide monitor. (Reprinted with permission from Nellcor Puritan Bennett, Inc., Pleasanton, CA.)

CLINICAL MOMENT The ASA Standards for Basic Monitoring require that the variable pitch tone be audible when the pulse oximeter is in use.

5. Alarms are commonly provided for low- and high-pulse rates and low and high saturation. Many units generate an alarm when the probe is not properly applied to the patient or if for some other reason the signal is inadequate.
6. Most pulse oximeters offer trend data. Interfaces for hardcopy recording and data management systems are usually available.

V. **Use**

A. Sites

1. **Finger**

a. The pulse oximeter probe is most commonly placed over one of the fingers (**Fig. 19.3**). This location offers a low failure rate and good accuracy. If there is poor circulation, a finger block, digital pulp space infiltration, or a vasodilator may improve performance. Vigorously rubbing the fingertip may temporarily improve circulation in the area.

b. Arm position may affect the reading. In most patients, the Spo_2 falls after the monitored arm is raised. It may also fall when the arm is lowered.

c. Motion artifacts are less frequent when the probe is placed on one of the larger fingers. The little finger may be useful if the patient has a particularly large hand. The probe may be placed over a finger that has a burn.

d. In general, the arm opposite to the one on which the blood pressure cuff is applied should be used. If the pulse oximeter is integrated with the noninvasive blood pressure monitor, the pulse oximeter will not generate an alarm during the inflation cycle if placed on the same arm as the blood pressure cuff.

e. Inserting a radial artery catheter is commonly followed by a transient decrease in blood flow and loss of an adequate signal for a pulse oximeter if the probe is on a finger of that hand, but pulse oximeter performance is unaffected if readings are taken from a finger on the arm in which an arterial cannula is present.

CLINICAL MOMENT Occasionally, poor function may occur with probe attachment on the same extremity as the intravenous infusion because of local hypothermia and vasoconstriction.

CLINICAL MOMENT The probe should not be on the index finger during recovery. An awakening patient often will want to rub his or her eye, usually with the index finger. If the oximeter probe is on that finger, the cornea can be scratched.

CLINICAL MOMENT If the patient has dark nail polish or synthetic fingernails, position the probe so that the light shines from one side of the finger to the other side.

2. **Toe**

   The toe is an alternative site when the finger is not available or the signal from the finger is unsatisfactory. Detecting desaturation will not be as rapid with the sensor on the toe, as with more centrally placed probes. The toe may provide a more reliable signal in patients who have had a lower extremity block.

3. **Nose**

   a. The nose is usually a convenient location. Nasal probes respond more rapidly to changes in saturation than probes placed on extremities. The bridge (**Fig. 19.5**), wings of the nostrils, and the nasal septum have all been used.

   b. Accuracy at the nose is controversial. It has been recommended under conditions such as hypothermia, hypotension, and vasoconstrictor drug infusion. In hypothermic patients, the nasal septum was found to be a more reliable site than the finger. Some studies have found that nasal probes often give grossly erroneous results and have a higher failure rate than other sites during poor perfusion. If the patient is placed in the Trendelenburg position, venous congestion may occur at the nose, causing the pulse oximeter to display artificially low saturations.

4. **Ear**

   a. An ear probe (**Fig. 19.6**) may be held in place by a plastic semicircular device hung around the ear. Stabilizing devices such as headbands may be useful. The earlobe should be massaged for 30 to 45 seconds with alcohol or a vasodilator. EMLA cream can be applied for 30 minutes prior to probe application to increase perfusion.

b. An ear probe can be particularly useful when there is finger motion. Response time is faster with an ear probe than with a finger probe, and an ear probe may perform better than a finger probe when perfusion is poor. The ear is relatively immune to sympathetic system vasoconstrictive effects. Ear probes may give more erroneous readings than finger probes in patients with tricuspid incompetence or a steep head-down position.

5. **Tongue**

a. A tongue probe can be made by placing a malleable aluminum strip behind a flexible probe and bending it around the tongue. A disposable probe wrapped around the tip of the tongue in the sagittal plane may also be used. Reflectance pulse oximetry has been used on the superior surface of the tongue. The mouth should be closed.

b. The tongue may be especially useful in patients who have burns over a large percentage of their body surface. Desaturation and resaturation are detected at the tongue quicker than at the finger or toe.

c. A lingual probe is more resistant to signal interference from electrosurgery than probes placed on peripheral sites but may be difficult to maintain in place during emergence from anesthesia. Tongue quivering may mimic tachycardia. Other problems are venous congestion from a head-down position and excessive oral secretions.

6. **Cheek**

a. A probe with a metal strip backing or a clip-on ear probe can be used on the cheek or lips. Probes specially designed for this site are available.

b. Probes at this location detect increases and decreases in saturation more quickly than finger or toe probes. Buccal oximetry has been found to be effective during hypothermia, decreased cardiac output, increased systemic vascular resistance, and other low pulse pressure states. This site may be useful in patients who have burns. Disadvantages include difficult placement, poor acceptance by patients emerging from anesthesia, and artifacts during airway maneuvers.

7. **Esophagus**

The esophageal probe uses reflectance oximetry technology. The esophagus, a core organ, is better perfused than the extremities during poor peripheral perfusion states and may provide a more reliable site for pulse oximetry in a patient with hemodynamic instability. It reflects changes in arterial saturation more quickly than peripheral sites such as the finger. This site may be useful for patients who have extensive burns in whom conventional probes would be difficult to place. It has been used successfully in neonates and children.

8. **Forehead**

a. A flat reflectance pulse oximeter sensor can be used on the forehead (**Fig. 19.13**). It should be placed just above the eyebrow so that it is centered slightly lateral of the iris. The sensor site should be cleaned with alcohol before applying the sensor. Pressure on the probe from a headband or a pressure dressing may improve the signal.

b. The forehead is usually easily accessible and associated with few motion artifacts. It is less affected by vasoconstriction from cold or poor perfusion than the ear or finger. Saturation changes can be detected more rapidly at the forehead than at the finger. Venous blood pooling because of compromised return to the heart may cause low-saturation readings. It should not be used if the patient is in the Trendelenburg position.

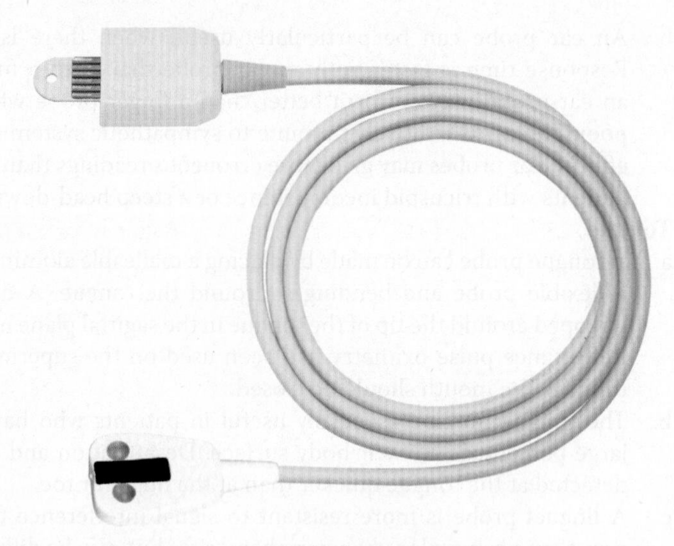

Figure 19.12 Reflectance pulse oximeter probe. The light source and the sensor are situated next to each other. (Photograph courtesy of Masimo Corporation, Irvine, CA.)

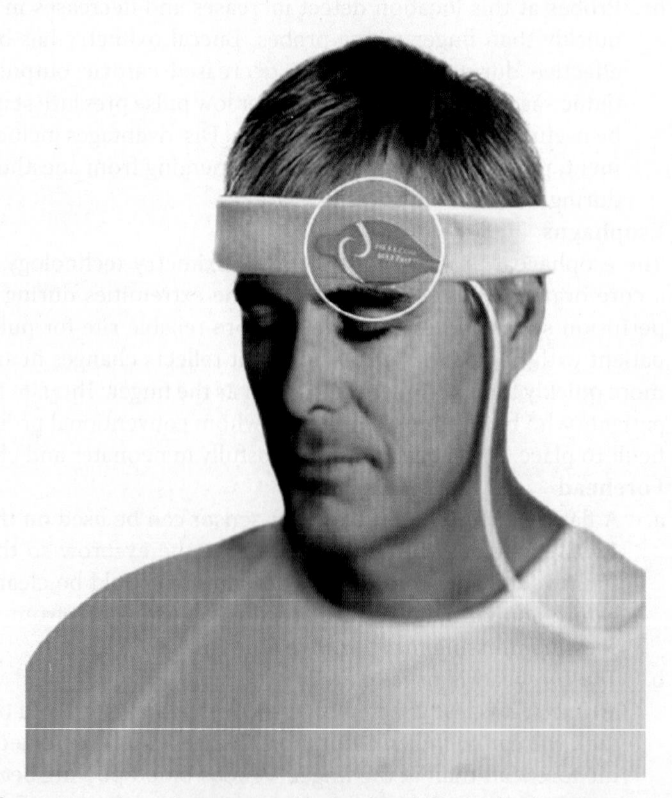

Figure 19.13 Reflectance pulse oximeter on the forehead. Note the headband securing it in place. (Photograph courtesy of Masimo Corporation, Irvine, CA.)

B. Fixation

1. Proper probe placement is crucial for good performance. A malpositioned probe can result in false-positive or false-negative alarms. Probes can be totally or partially dislodged without this being noticed.
2. Adhesive probes may stay on better than clip-on probes. It may be beneficial to tape a probe in place when it will be inaccessible during surgery, but it is important to avoid arterial or venous compression. Wrapping the monitoring site loosely with gauze may help to fix the probe in position. Another method is to slip the cut finger from a glove over the probe. The probe should be protected from bright light (**Fig. 19.9**).

C. Stabilizing the Signal

The search that the pulse oximeter goes through when a probe is initially applied (or dislodged) includes sequential trials of varying light intensity in an effort to find a signal strong enough to transmit through the tissue but not so strong that the detection system is saturated. Once a pulse is found, there is usually a few more seconds delay while Spo_2 values for several pulses are averaged.

CLINICAL MOMENT Appearance of a satisfactory waveform is an indication that the readings are reliable. Comparing the pulse rate shown by the oximeter with that by an electrocardiograph monitor is also an indication that saturation readings are reliable. A discrepancy between the pulse rates frequently indicates probe malposition or malfunction. A discrepancy can also occur during certain dysrhythmias.

D. Reusing Disposable Probes

Because disposable probes are costly, many institutions reuse them. Although concerns about this have been expressed, several studies show that the failure rate of reprocessed probes is equal to or less than that of new probes and the accuracy is not affected.

VI. Applications

A. Monitoring Oxygenation

1. **Anesthetizing Areas**
   a. Oxygen desaturation can occur anytime during anesthesia, regardless of the anesthesia provider's skills and experience. Pediatric patients are especially at risk. Most severe desaturations occur during induction or emergence from anesthesia. Studies have shown that the incidence of hypoxemic events and myocardial ischemia is reduced when pulse oximetry is used.
   b. Oximetry is useful in managing one-lung anesthesia to help to determine whether the measures taken to increase the oxygen saturation are necessary or effective.
   c. Oximetry is useful for patients undergoing regional and monitored care anesthesia. Often, the signs of hypoxia are confused with restlessness from an inadequate block. Instead of supplying oxygen and assisting respiration, additional sedation is often provided, which compounds the problem. Using oximetry, the patient's oxygenation status can be assessed and measures taken to improve Spo_2 when indicated.
   d. Pulse oximetry may be useful to confirm correct tracheal tube placement when a functional carbon dioxide monitor is not available. If oxygen saturation rises after intubation and ventilation, correct tube placement is likely.

CLINICAL MOMENT Preoxygenation may delay the onset of desaturation with an esophageal intubation. By the time this desaturation occurs, the clinician may not be thinking about incorrect tracheal tube placement.

e. Other problems that can cause oxygen saturation to drop include fat embolism, amniotic fluid embolism, pulmonary edema, breathing system disconnections and leaks, aspiration, tracheal tube obstruction, hypoxic gas mixture, oxygen delivery failure, hypoventilation, anaphylaxis, bronchospasm, pneumothorax, malignant hyperthermia, and pulmonary embolism. Causes of hypoxia related to equipment are discussed in Chapter 10.

CLINICAL MOMENT Pulse oximetry may help to detect inadvertent bronchial intubation but is not reliable, particularly if an elevated inspired oxygen concentration is being used. The absence of desaturation does not rule out bronchial intubation. Methods to detect bronchial intubation are discussed in Chapter 15.

2. **Postanesthesia Care Unit**
   The postanesthesia care unit (PACU) is another location where desaturation is common. Routine oxygen administration to postoperative patients may not be necessary when they are monitored with pulse oximetry. Before leaving the recovery room, a trial using room air while monitoring oxygen saturation may provide an indication that oxygen therapy needs to be continued beyond the PACU or that the patent needs to be retained in the unit for a longer time.
3. **Transport**
   Unrecognized oxygen desaturation may occur while the patient is being transported between the operating room and the PACU and between other areas. Pulse oximetry is included on most transport monitors, and portable pulse oximeters are available.
4. **Patients Receiving Postoperative Opioids**
   The Anesthesia Patient Safety Foundation has advocated use of continuous monitoring of oxygenation (generally pulse oximetry in nonventilated patients receiving patient-controlled analgesia, neuraxial opioids, or serial doses of parenteral opioids) (1).

B. Monitoring Peripheral Circulation

1. Pulse oximetry can detect arm positions that compromise circulation. A pulse oximeter attached to a toe can help to warn of decreased perfusion in the foot in patients in the lithotomy position. Monitoring oxygen saturation during shoulder arthroscopy has been recommended as a test for brachial artery compression. However, an adequate pulse signal may be present with brachial plexus compression.
2. Patients with limb fractures may have compromised circulation distal to the fracture. Pulse oximetry may serve as a useful guide to blood flow to that area. Pulse oximetry may not be helpful in warning that a compartment syndrome is developing, because arterial pulse diminution is a late sign.
3. Patients who undergo mediastinoscopy are at risk for brachiocephalic artery and aortic arch compression between the mediastinoscope and the sternum.

Arterial compression may be detected by measuring pulse wave amplitude on a pulse oximeter.

4. Pulse oximetry may be used to evaluate the effect of a sympathetic block as indicated by increased peripheral blood flow.

C. Determining Systolic Blood Pressure

A pulse oximeter can be used to determine the systolic blood pressure. The blood pressure cuff is applied to the same arm as the pulse oximeter. The cuff is inflated slowly, and the pressure at the point at which the waveform is lost is noted. It also can be determined by inflating the cuff well past the systolic pressure and looking for the onset of a signal as the cuff is deflated. One study found that the best agreement with Korotkoff sounds and noninvasive blood pressure equipment occurred when the average of blood pressures estimated at the disappearance and reappearance of the waveform was taken as the systolic pressure.

D. Avoiding Hyperoxemia

In premature neonates, oxygen administration may be associated with the development of retinopathy and other pathological conditions. Pulse oximetry can aid in titrating inspired oxygen by detecting hyperoxemia. The high Spo_2 alarm should be set at 95% or lower for this purpose.

VII. **Advantages**

A. Pulse oximetry is accurate, and accuracy does not change with time. Numerous studies have shown that the difference between saturation determined by pulse oximetry and arterial blood gas analysis is clinically insignificant above an Spo_2 saturation value of 70%. Most manufacturers claim that errors are less than ±3% at saturations above 70%. This accuracy should be sufficient for most clinical purposes, except possibly neonatal hyperoxia. Pulse oximetry readings are not affected by anesthetic gases or vapors.

B. Pulse oximetry is accurate in patients with dysrhythmias, provided the Spo_2 is stable and the plethysmogram is noise free and has reasonable amplitude. The Spo_2 may be correct even if the pulse rate is not.

C. Pulse oximetry has a fast response time, especially compared with transcutaneous measurements. Readout typically begins within a few heartbeats after the probe is applied. This is a distinct advantage over transcutaneous monitoring, which requires a prolonged warm-up time.

D. Pulse oximetry is noninvasive, which allows it to be used as a routine monitor. It is readily accepted by awake patients, so it can be applied before anesthesia begins.

E. Continuously monitoring the quality of the peripheral pulse may be helpful in determining whether a hypotensive patient has good cardiac output. If blood pressure is low and pulse signal strength is high, the patient is probably vasodilated but perfusing adequately. If, however, both blood pressure and pulse strength are low, perfusion may be inadequate.

F. Perfusion is indicated by the pulse signal strength, and oxygenation is indicated by saturation. Most oximeters will signal if the blood flow is not adequate to provide a saturation value. This is helpful in determining a truly low saturation value, as opposed to one caused by low blood flow.

G. Applying the probe is easy and fast. A variety of different probes are available for different site applications.

H. Changes in pulse tone with varying saturation allow the user to be continuously updated on Spo_2 without taking his or her eyes off the patient. Tone modulation allows hypoxic episodes to be recognized more quickly than if a fixed tone were used. Most anesthesia providers can detect the direction (but not the magnitude) of a change in saturation by listening to the change in the pulse tone pitch.

I. The wide variety of probe configurations confers broad clinical applicability to all types of patients, including preterm infants. The ability to use various vascular beds ensures access during surgery.

VIII. Limitations and Disadvantages

A. Failure to Determine the Oxygen Saturation

There is a small but definite incidence of failure with pulse oximetry. Factors that are reported to increase failure rates include ASA physical status 3, 4, or 5 patients; young and elderly patients; orthopedic, vascular, and cardiac surgery; electrosurgery use; hypothermia; hypotension; hypertension; duration of intraoperative procedure; chronic renal failure; low hematocrit; and motion at the sensor site. The actual failure rate varies with the monitor. A pulse oximeter may zero out, meaning that it displays "00" for the Spo_2 and pulse rate values when it fails to produce a measurement or it might display "–" for the values. Some pulse oximeters blank the display or give a message such as "Low Quality Signal" or "Inadequate Signal." Others freeze the display.

B. Poor Function with Poor Perfusion

1. Pulse oximeters require adequate pulsations to distinguish light absorbed from arterial blood from venous blood and tissue light. Readings may be unreliable or unavailable if there is a loss or diminution of the peripheral pulse (proximal blood pressure cuff inflation, external pressure, improper positioning, hypotension, hypothermia, Raynaud's phenomenon, cardiopulmonary bypass, low cardiac output, hypovolemia, peripheral vascular disease, a Valsalva maneuver such as seen in laboring patients, or infusion of vasoactive drugs).
2. Methods to improve the signal include applying vasodilating cream, performing sympathetic and digital nerve blocks, administering intra-arterial vasodilators, and warming cool extremities. Using a better perfused site such as the cheek, tongue, nasal septum, or esophagus may be helpful. Improved signal technology by newer pulse oximeters can improve performance during low perfusion.

C. Difficulty Detecting High Oxygen Partial Pressures

At Pao_2 values above 90 mm Hg, small changes in saturation are associated with relatively large changes in Pao_2 (**Fig. 19.2**). Thus, it has limited ability to distinguish high but safe levels of arterial oxygen from excessively elevated levels.

D. Delayed Hypoxic Event Detection

1. While the pulse oximeter response time is generally fast, there may be a significant delay (lag) between a change in alveolar oxygen tension and a change in the oximeter reading. It is possible for arterial oxygen to reach dangerous levels before the pulse oximeter alarm is activated. Setting the low Spo_2 alarm threshold just below the oxygen saturation will decrease the delay.
2. Delayed response can be related to probe location. Desaturation is detected earlier when the probe is placed more centrally. Lag time will be increased with poor perfusion. Venous obstruction, peripheral vasoconstriction, cold, and motion artifacts can result in increased time to detect hypoxemia.
3. The algorithms used to prevent false alarms may increase the delay in detecting hypoxic events. A pulse oximeter may respond to a noisy or weak signal by simply holding on to an old value. Increasing the time over which the pulse signals are averaged also increases the delay time.

E. Erratic Performance with Dysrhythmias

Irregular heart rhythms can cause the pulse oximeter to perform erratically. During aortic balloon pulsation, diastolic pressure augmentation exceeds that of systolic pressure. This leads to a double- or triple-peaked arterial pressure waveform that confuses the pulse oximeter, so it may not provide a reading.

F. Inaccuracy

1. **Different Hemoglobins**

Most pulse oximeters are designed to detect only two species of hemoglobin: reduced and oxygenated. Whole blood often contains other moieties. This disturbs the wavelength absorbance ratio used to determine oxygen saturation.

a. Methemoglobin

1) Normally less than 1% of the total hemoglobin, metHb is an oxidation product of hemoglobin that forms a reversible complex with oxygen and impairs the unloading of oxygen to tissues. Methemoglobinemia can be congenital or acquired. Drugs causing methemoglobinemia include nitrobenzene, benzocaine, cetacaine, and dapsone. Methemoglobin absorbs light equally at the red and infrared wavelengths that are used by most pulse oximeters. When compared with functional saturation, most pulse oximeters give falsely low readings for saturations above 85% and falsely high values for saturations below 85%. The discrepancy between Spo_2 and functional saturation increases as the level of metHb increases and functional hemoglobin saturation decreases.

2) If there are conflicting results between the pulse oximeter and arterial blood gas analysis, methemoglobinemia should be suspected and the diagnosis should be confirmed by multiple wavelength co-oximetry. The standard blood gas analysis is not capable of detecting and measuring metHb. A relatively new pulse oximeter capable of accurately measuring metHb as well as HbCO is now available.

b. Carboxyhemoglobin

1) Carboxyhemoglobin, formed when hemoglobin is exposed to carbon monoxide (CO), has an absorption spectrum similar to that of oxyhemoglobin, so most pulse oximeters will overread Spo_2 by the percentage of HbCO present.

2) An increase in HbCO may occur during laser surgery in the airway, but the levels are not high enough to keep pulse oximetry from reliably estimating saturation. Carbon monoxide production in association with dry carbon dioxide absorbent is discussed in Chapter 5.

3) Pulse oximeters that can measure HbCO accurately are now available (**Fig. 19.14**).

c. Fetal Hemoglobin

Most studies show that fetal hemoglobin (Hb F) does not affect the accuracy of pulse oximetry to a clinically important degree, although very high levels may cause it to read slightly low.

d. Hemoglobin S

Using pulse oximetry in patients with sickle cell disease is controversial. Several investigators have concluded that pulse oximetry is very inaccurate in these patients, which makes it unreliable for detecting serious hypoxemia. Other studies have found pulse oximetry to be sufficiently accurate to be useful.

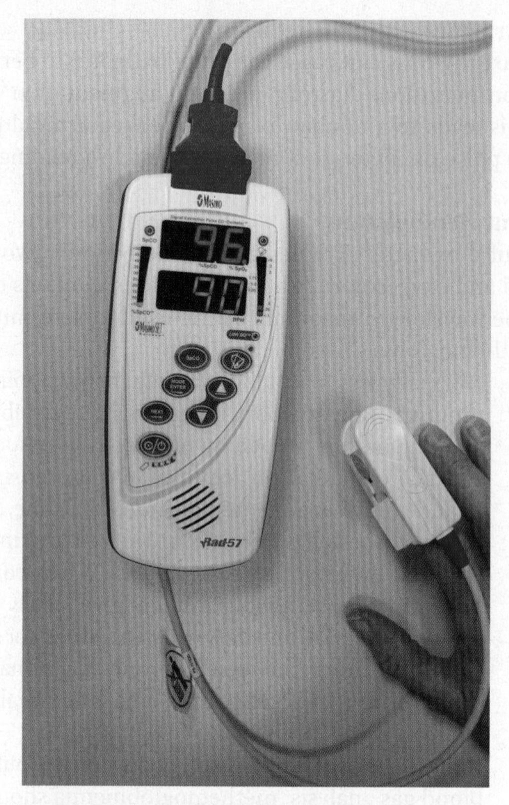

Figure 19.14 Combined pulse oximeter and carbon monoxide monitor.

e. Sulfhemoglobin

Sulfhemoglobinemia may be caused by drugs such as metoclopramide, phenacetin, dapsone, and sulfonamides. It causes the pulse oximeter to display artifactually low oxygen saturation.

2. **Bilirubinemia**

Severe hyperbilirubinemia can cause an artifactual elevation of metHb and HbCO when using in vitro oximetry but does not affect pulse oximetry readings.

3. **Low Saturations**

Pulse oximetry becomes less accurate at low oxygen saturations. This inaccuracy is greater in patients with dark skin. It should be used with caution in patients with cyanotic heart disease. Measuring Pao_2 or Sao_2 at low saturations is recommended for important clinical decisions.

4. **Malpositioned Probe**

If the probe is not properly positioned, it may allow the light from the emitter to the detector to only graze the tissue instead of passing through it. This penumbra effect reduces the signal-to-noise ratio and may result in spurious Spo_2 values in the low 90s in normal patients. If the patient is hypoxic, the oximeter may overestimate the true value. Using a probe that is too large or too small may result in inaccurate readings. Long fingernails can cause inaccurate positioning. To avoid this problem, the probe position should be checked frequently and inaccessible locations avoided.

5. **Venous Pulsations**
   a. Pulse oximeter technology assumes that the pulsatile components of light absorbance are due to arterial blood. Prominent venous pulsations may lead to underestimating the Spo_2. Pulse rate determination may be correct. The error may be worse when probes are used on the head but less when the probe is placed on the finger. In patients with low systemic vascular resistance, the pulse oximeter may underread the saturation, possibly because the oximeter is sensing pulsatile venous flow.
   b. High airway pressures during artificial ventilation may cause phasic venous congestion, which may be interpreted by the oximeter as a pulse wave. In some cases, it may be necessary to turn the ventilator OFF to obtain a correct reading.
6. **Mixing Probes**
   Spo_2 measurements may not be accurate if one manufacturer's probe is used with a different manufacturer's instrument.

CLINICAL MOMENT Although probes from one manufacturer may fit the connector of another manufacturer's oximeter, this does not mean that they will function properly. Do not use probes that are not recommended by the oximeter manufacturer.

7. **Severe Anemia**
   The pulse oximeter may overestimate Spo_2 in patients with severe anemia, especially at low saturations.
8. **Skin Pigmentation**
   Although some earlier studies showed that pulse oximeter readings were slightly high in patients with dark skin, newer studies have shown that pigmentation does not make a significant difference in pulse oximeter accuracy.
9. **Dyes**
   a. Certain dyes including methylene blue, indocyanine green, lymphazurin (isosulfan blue), indigo carmine, nitrobenzene, and patent blue when injected intravenously, intra-arterially, into lymphatics, intradermally, or into the uterine cavity can result in decreases in Spo_2 without actual decreased saturation. In vitro oximetry may also be affected by dyes. Usually, the interference lasts only a few minutes but may persist much longer, even hours, when lymphatics are injected. The pulse oximeter reaction to exogenous dyes has been used as a means of confirming intravascular catheter placement. Dye is injected into the catheter, and the pulse oximeter is observed.
   b. Fingerprinting ink will cause a low saturation reading. Henna, a stain used by some women on the fingers and toes, can cause a low saturation reading. Blue finger paints may cause low Spo_2 readings.
10. **Sources of Interference**
    a. Optical Interference
       1) Light flickering at frequencies similar to the frequencies of the LEDs, including sunlight, fluorescent lights, operating room lights, infrared heating lamps, infrared radiant warmers, light sources for various scopes, xenon lamps, bilirubin lights, phototherapy, or surgical imaging instruments, can enter the photodetector and result in

inaccurate or erratic readings. Sensitivity to light may be increased with reduced pulse amplitude. Although excessive ambient light usually prevents the oximeter from tracking the pulse, it can result in apparently normal but inaccurate measurements in some instances. One clue that optical interference is occurring is inconsistency between the pulse rate from the pulse oximeter and the electrocardiographic monitor.

2) The effects of optical interference can be minimized by selecting the correct probe, applying the probe so that the detector is across from the LEDs, making certain the probe remains properly positioned, and shielding the probe from light and other nearby probes (**Fig. 19.9**).

b. Electrical Interference

Electrical interference from an electrosurgical unit can cause the oximeter to give an incorrect pulse count (usually by counting extra beats) or falsely register a decrease in oxygen saturation, especially in patients with weak pulse signals. Manufacturers have made significant progress in reducing their instruments' sensitivity to electrical interference. Some monitors display a notice when significant interference is present. Some freeze the Spo_2 display during such interference, which may give a false sense of security. Steps to minimize electrical interference include locating the electrosurgery grounding plate as close to and the oximeter probe and console as far from the surgical field as possible; routing the cable from the probe to the oximeter away from the electrosurgery apparatus; and operating the unit in a rapid response mode. The electrosurgical apparatus and pulse oximeter should not be plugged into the same power circuit.

c. Infrared Interference

Neuronavigational equipment may affect the performance of a pulse oximeter (2). Shielding the probe with an aluminum foil will eliminate this problem.

11. **Nail Polish and Coverings**

Some shades of brown, black, blue, and green nail polish or onychomycosis (a yellowish gray color caused by fungus) may cause significantly lower saturation readings. Synthetic nails or dirt under the nail may interfere with pulse oximetry readings.

CLINICAL MOMENT If fingernail polish or covering prevents proper function, position the probe side to side across the finger.

12. **Motion Artifacts**

a. Motion of the probe can cause an artifact that the pulse oximeter is unable to differentiate from normal arterial pulsations. Motion artifacts create both false-positive (false alarm) and false-negative (missed hypoxemia) errors. Changing alarm thresholds to reduce one of these errors will often increase the incidence of the other type of error. Motion artifacts are less common with newer generation pulse oximeters.

b. Motion is usually not a problem during general anesthesia, but if the patient is shivering, has a condition such as Parkinson's disease, or is moving about or being transported, artifacts can be significant. Evoked potential monitors and nerve stimulators can produce motion artifacts if the pulse oximeter probe is on the same extremity. Motion artifacts have been caused by patients tapping their fingers while under regional anesthesia.

13. **Pressure on the Probe**
    Pressure on the probe may result in inaccurate Spo_2 readings without affecting pulse rate determination.

CLINICAL MOMENT If the probe needs to be taped or secured in place, the tape should not be go completely around the finger or toe.

14. **Hyperemia**
    If a limb becomes hyperemic after blood flow is interrupted, the oxygen saturation shown by the pulse oximetry may be artificially low. A pulse oximeter placed near a blood transfusion site may show transient decreases in oxygen saturation with rapid blood infusion.
15. **Probe Damage**
    A damaged pulse oximeter probe can cause the oxygen saturation to be higher than the actual value. The use of a cleaning agent not recommended by the manufacturer on a reusable probe can result in damage to the probe.

CLINICAL MOMENT When removing a probe from the patient at the conclusion of a case, the probe should be placed on something that will prevent it from falling onto the floor and being damaged. Do not throw the probe on the floor.

G. False Alarms
1. A high percentage of pulse oximetry alarms are spurious or trivial. Most false alarms are caused by motion artifact, poor signal quality, probe displacement, external pressure, or interference. False alarms are a more significant problem outside the operating room because patients are commonly moving and sometimes have poor perfusion. There are many sources of electronic and optical interference outside the operating room.
2. False alarms may encourage the care provider to take inappropriate actions such as disabling the alarm, setting the limits to inappropriate values, or lowering the alarm volume. Alarm misinterpretation can either result in failure to treat hypoxemia or lead to unnecessary treatment.
3. Newer pulse oximeters designed to reduce motion-related artifacts can significantly reduce the incidence of false alarms.
4. Delaying the time between detecting low Spo_2 and alarm activation, using a longer averaging time, and setting the Spo_2 alarm limit lower can reduce the number of false alarms but may increase the time before detecting hypoxemia. With some pulse oximeters, turning OFF the low-pulse rate alarm prevents false alarms when the blood pressure cuff is inflated.

CLINICAL MOMENT Some false alarms can be avoided by simple measures such as putting the probe on a different extremity than the blood pressure cuff and in a location where it is unlikely to be affected by external pressure.

H. Failure to Detect Impaired Circulation

The presence of a pulse oximeter signal and a normal reading does not necessarily imply that tissue perfusion is adequate. Some pulse oximeters show pulses despite inadequate tissue perfusion or even when no pulse is present. Ambient light may produce a false signal.

CLINICAL MOMENT Pulse oximetry is not reliable in diagnosing impaired perfusion with increased intracompartmental pressures.

I. Failure to Detect Hypoventilation

Hypoventilation and hypercarbia may occur without a decrease in hemoglobin oxygen saturation, especially if the patient is receiving supplemental oxygen (1).

CLINICAL MOMENT The pulse oximeter provides late detection of hypoventilation for a sedated patient receiving supplemental oxygen. Other methods to detect hypoventilation should be used in these patients.

CLINICAL MOMENT Pulse oximetry cannot be relied on to detect leaks, disconnections, or esophageal intubation.

IX. Patient Complications

A. Pressure and Ischemic Injuries

Injuries ranging from persistent numbness to ischemic injury at the site on which a probe was placed have been reported. These risks are increased by prolonged probe application, compromised extremity perfusion, and tight probe application. Frequent site examination and moving the probe to different sites reduce the likelihood of injury. A patient with large fingers should not have a circumferential probe placed on the finger.

CLINICAL MOMENT If the pulse oximeter signal appears to be weak, the site should be checked for increased pressure.

B. Burns

1. Injuries ranging from reddened areas to third-degree burns under pulse oximeter probes have been reported. Considering the millions of long-term applications, the incidence of these burns is quite low.
2. A burn can result from incompatibility between the probe from one manufacturer and the pulse oximeter of another. A number of pulse oximeter probes have connectors that fit different pulse oximeters, but the two may not be compatible. Using a damaged probe can result in a burn. A pulse oximeter probe may provide an alternate pathway for electrosurgical currents.
3. To avoid burn injuries, frequent probe site inspection and site rotation are recommended. When a probe is placed on a finger or toe, the light source should be placed on the nail rather than on the pulp. If the pulse oximeter display

freezes, the cause should be investigated. Only probes recommended by the oximeter manufacturer should be used.

4. Burns that are associated with pulse oximetry during magnetic resonance imaging (MRI) resulting from induced skin current beneath looped cables acting as antennae have been reported. During MRI, the danger of burns can be reduced by the following measures:
   a. All potential conductors should be checked before use to ensure that there is no frayed insulation, exposed wires, or other hazards.
   b. All unnecessary conductive materials such as unused surface coils should be removed from the MRI system bore before patient monitoring is initiated.
   c. The probe should be placed as far from the imaging site as possible.
   d. Cables, leads, or wires from monitoring devices should be positioned so that no loops are formed.
   e. If possible, no potential conductors should touch the patient at more than one location.
   f. A thick layer of thermal insulation should be placed between any wires or cables and the patient's skin.
   g. Monitoring devices that do not appear to be operating properly should be removed from the patient.

X. **Carboxyhemoglobin, Hemoglobin, and Methemoglobin Monitoring**

A. Carbon monoxide can accumulate in the breathing system from various sources, including the reaction between anesthetic agents and desiccated absorbent (see Chapter 5). It is difficult to determine whether CO is present in the inspired gases when the patient is anesthetized.

B. Methemoglobinemia is more common than might be suspected.

C. A pulse oximeter also capable of measuring both HbCO and metHb with a single sensor is available. The instrument utilizes an eight-wavelength sensor to distinguish between the various entities.

D. Pulse oximeters with the ability to measure the patient's hemoglobin are now available.

REFERENCES

1. Weinger MB. Dangers of postoperative opioids. APSF workshop and white paper address prevention of postoperative respiratory complications. APSF Newslett 2006–2007;21(4):61, 63–67.
2. Mathes AM, Kreuer S, Schneider SO, et al. The performance of six pulse oximeters in the environment of neuronavigation. Anesth Analg 2008;107:541–544.

SUGGESTED READINGS

Barker SJ, Curry J, Redford D, Morgan S. Measurement of carboxyhemoglobin and methemoglobin by pulse oximetry. Anesthesiology 2006;105:892–897.

Dorsch J, Dorsch S. Pulse oximetry. In: Understanding Anesthesia Equipment. Fifth edition. Philadelphia: Wolters Kluwer/Lippincott Williams & Wilkins, 2008:775–804.

Moyle J. Pulse Oximetry. Second edition. Indianapolis, IN: Wiley-Blackwell, 2002.

20 Neuromuscular Transmission Monitoring

MUSCLE RELAXANTS ARE EMPLOYED IN anesthesia to provide muscle relaxation and/or abolish patient movement. Numerous studies have documented enormous variations in patients' responses to muscle relaxants. Disease states and perioperative medications can modify the responses to these drugs. Neuromuscular block (NMB) depth should be monitored whenever muscle relaxants are used to avoid overdosage or underdosage during surgery and residual NMB during recovery.

I. Equipment

Monitoring NMB is accomplished by delivering an electrical stimulus near a motor nerve and evaluating the evoked muscular response.

A. Stimulator

Several stimulators are shown in **Figure 20.1**. Most are battery operated with a means to check the battery status. A stimulator may be in a module in a multiparameter monitor. The ability to deliver information to an automated record should be considered when choosing a stimulator. This is available on the newer stimulators.

1. **Current**
   a. Current, not voltage, is the determining factor in nerve stimulation. Because skin resistance may change, only a stimulator that automatically adjusts its output to maintain a constant current can ensure constant stimulation with changes in skin resistance.
   b. If a motor nerve is stimulated with sufficient current, all of the muscle fibers supplied by that nerve will contract. The current required for this is called the *maximal current.* In the clinical setting, stimuli of greater than maximal (supramaximal) intensity are used to ensure that maximal stimulation is delivered if resistance increases. A 30-mA current will produce a supramaximal response in most patients when the ulnar nerve is stimulated. Higher currents are needed with the posterior tibial nerve. Patient discomfort increases with increasing stimulating current, so a submaximal current may be better for awake patients or those recovering from anesthesia.

CLINICAL MOMENT Higher than usual currents may be needed in patients with edema or diabetes.

   c. A current display is useful to alert the user that there is a disconnection, broken lead, weak battery, or poorly conducting electrodes. These problems will cause the current to be reduced. Some stimulators have an alarm to warn when the selected current is not being delivered.
2. **Frequency**
   Stimulus frequency is usually expressed in hertz (Hz), which is cycles/second. One Hz is 1 cycle/second, and 0.1 Hz is equal to 1 stimulus every 10 seconds.
3. **Waveform**
   The stimulus waveform should be rectangular and monophasic. Biphasic waves may produce repetitive stimulation, which can underestimate NMB depth.
4. **Duration**
   The duration should be 300 milliseconds or less. If the pulse duration is more than 0.5 milliseconds, a second action potential may be triggered.
5. **Stimulation Patterns**
   a. Single Twitch
      1) Single-twitch (T_1) stimuli are usually delivered at a frequency of 0.1 or 1 Hz.

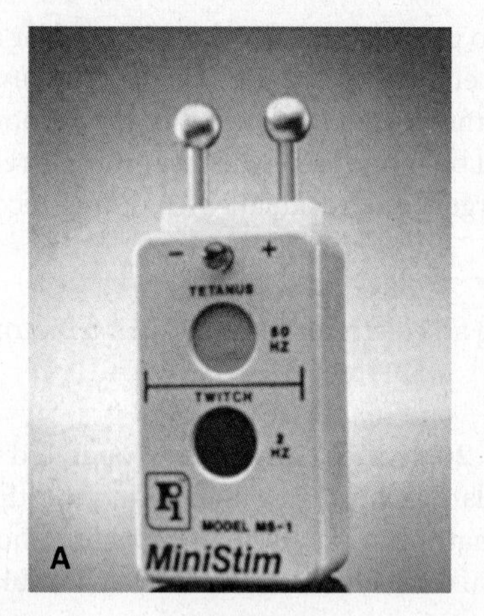

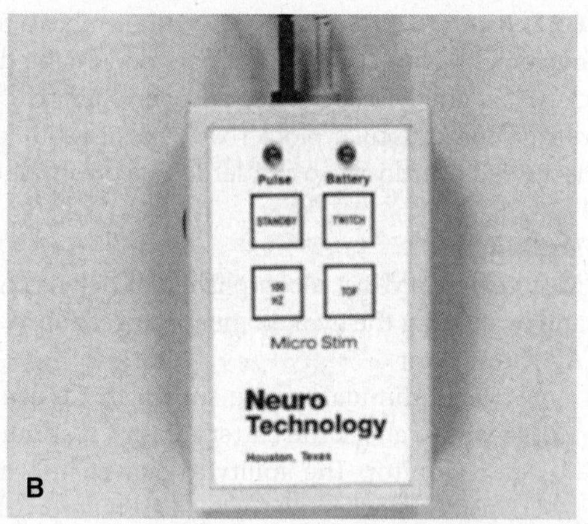

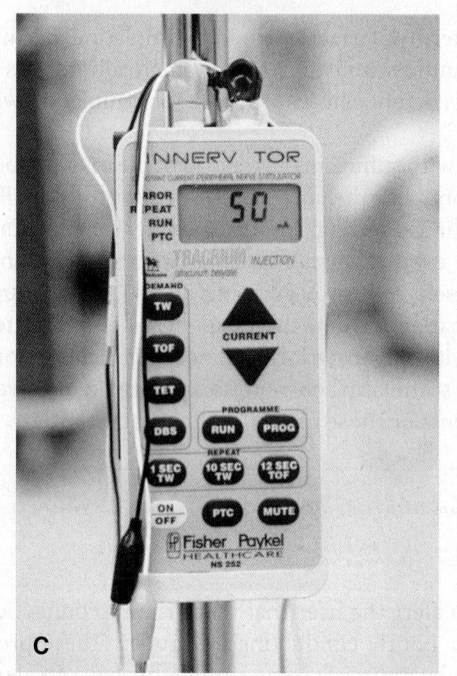

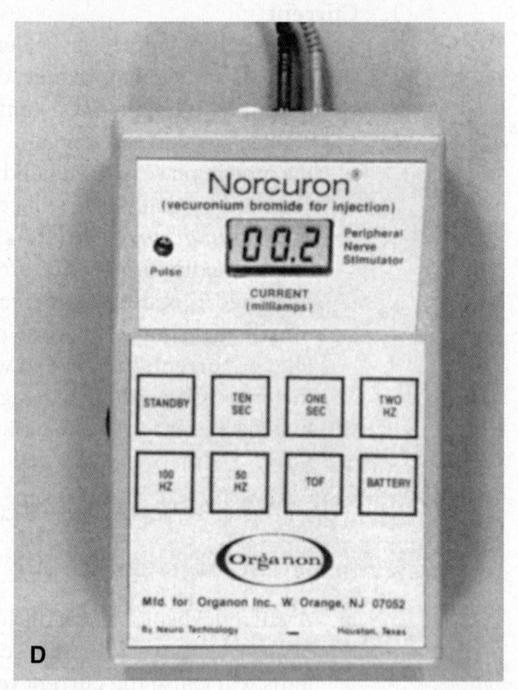

Figure 20.1 Neuromuscular stimulators. **A:** This simple device has only two patterns of stimulation: tetanus and single twitch. The delivered current cannot be varied and is not displayed. Note the metal ball electrodes. (Courtesy of Professional Instruments, a subsidiary of Life Tech, Inc.) **B:** This unit has three modes of stimulation: single stimulus (twitch), tetanus, and TOF. The current is varied by using a rheostat at the side, but there is no display of the current being delivered. **C:** This unit has four patterns of stimulation: single twitch (available at 0.1 and 1 Hz), TOF (which can be repeated automatically every 12 seconds), 50-Hz tetanus, and DBS. It also is capable of delivering the stimulus pattern for obtaining a PTC. The selected current is displayed in the window. Failure to deliver this current will cause a mark to be displayed to the right of the word *ERROR*. Note that the connections for the lead wires are of different colors. **D:** This unit has three modes of stimulation: single stimulus (which can be delivered at 0.1, 1, or 2 Hz), tetanus (which is available at a frequency of 50 to 100 Hz), and TOF. Stimulus current is varied by using a rheostat at the side. The delivered current is displayed in a window, to the left of which is an indicator that lights when a stimulus is being delivered. A battery status check button is present.

CLINICAL MOMENT Using a single twitch more frequently than once every 10 seconds is associated with a progressively diminished response and could result in overestimating the NMB.

2) The control response strength is noted (**Fig. 20.2A**). The strengths of subsequent twitches are then compared with the control and expressed as a percentage of the control (single-pulse or single-twitch depression, $T_1\%$, $T_1\%$, $T_1{:}T_c$). With both a nondepolarizing block and a depolarizing block, there will be a progressively depressed response as the block develops.

CLINICAL MOMENT A lower body temperature will cause a reduced response.

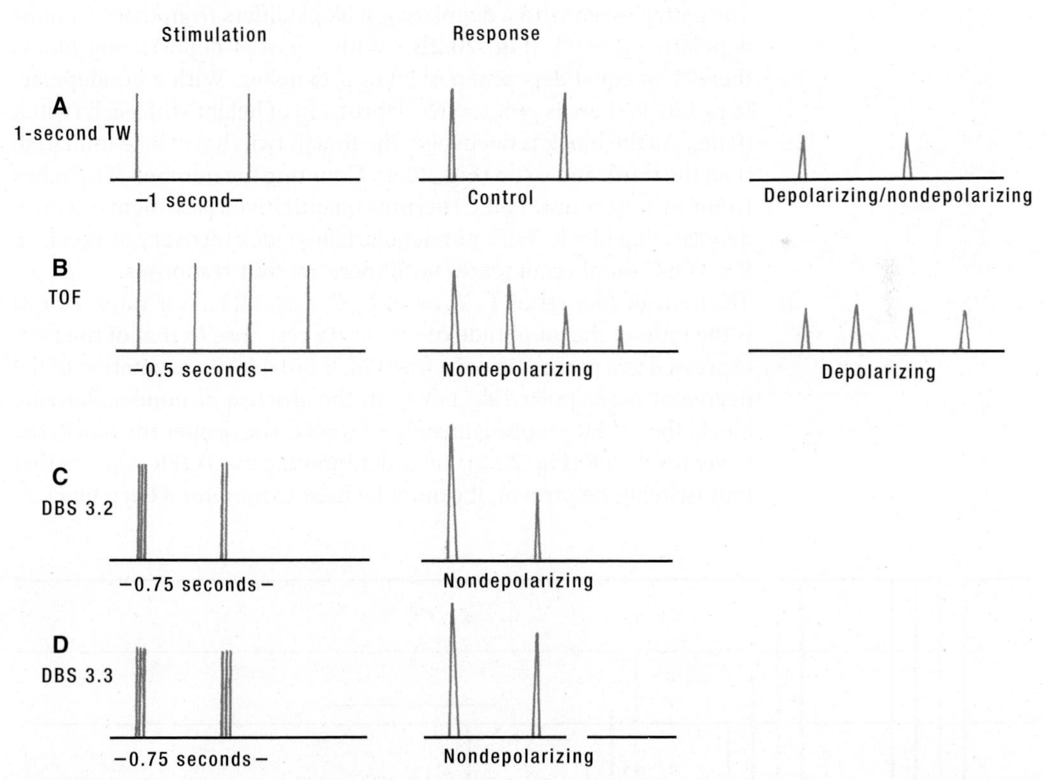

Figure 20.2 Patterns of stimulation and response. **A:** Single-stimulus stimulation at 1 Hz (1 stimulus/second). The height of the control twitches are noted. With either a depolarizing or a nondepolarizing block, twitch height is decreased. **B:** Train-of-four stimulation. Four successive single stimuli are delivered with 0.5-second intervals. With a nondepolarizing block, there will be progressive depression of the response with each stimulus (fade). With a depolarizing block, the responses will be depressed equally. **C,D:** Double-burst stimulation. Three stimuli are delivered at 50 Hz, followed 0.75 seconds later by two or three similar stimuli. There will be depression of the response to the second burst with a nondepolarizing block. Note the increased height of the response to the first burst compared with that seen with TOF stimulation. TW, time weight; TOF, train of four; DBS, double-burst stimulation.

3) The single stimulus is useful to establish a supramaximal stimulus and to identify whether conditions satisfactory for intubation have been achieved. It can be used (in conjunction with a tetanic stimulus) to monitor deep levels of NMB [the posttetanic count (PTC), discussed below].
4) There are several disadvantages associated with single-twitch simulation. There needs to be a control. It cannot distinguish between a depolarizing block and a nondepolarizing block. Most important, the return of response to the control level does not guarantee full recovery from NMB.

b. Train of Four
   1) Train of four (TOF, $T_{4,}$ T_4/T_1) consists of four single pulses of equal intensity delivered at intervals of 0.5 seconds (**Fig. 20.2B**). TOF should not be repeated more frequently than every 10 to 12 seconds. Many modern stimulators do not allow the TOF to be repeated more often.
   2) Before any relaxant has been given, all four responses are the same. The pattern seen with a depolarizing block differs from that of a nondepolarizing block (**Fig. 20.2B**). With a partial depolarizing block, there is an equal depression of all four twitches. With a nondepolarizing block, there is progressive depression of height with each twitch (fade). As the block is deepened, the fourth twitch will be eliminated, then the third, and so on (**Fig. 20.3**). Counting the number of twitches (train-of-four count, TOFC) permits quantitative assessment of a nondepolarizing block. With nondepolarizing block recovery or reversal, the TOFC number increases until there are four responses.
   3) The train-of-four ratio (T_r, T_4 ratio, T_4:T_1, T_r%, TR%, TOF ratio, TOFR) is the ratio of the amplitude of the fourth response to that of the first, expressed as a percentage or a fraction. It provides an estimation of the degree of nondepolarizing NMB. In the absence of nondepolarizing block, the TOFR is approximately 1 (100%). The deeper the block, the lower the TOFR (**Fig. 20.3**). Since determining the TOFR requires that four twitches be present, it cannot be used to monitor a deep block.

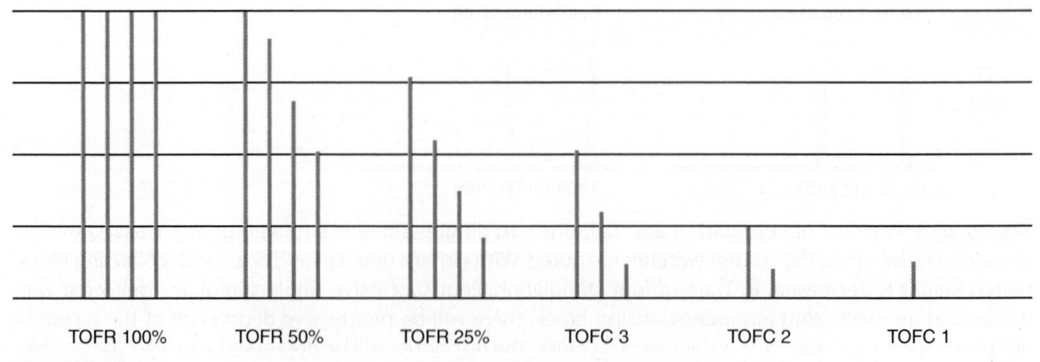

Figure 20.3 Onset and progressive deepening of nondepolarizing block using train-of-four stimulation. When there is no neuromuscular block present, all four responses are equal. With onset of the block, there is progressive depression of twitch height with each twitch (fade). As the block progresses, the last twitch is lost and the TOFC is less than 4. TOFR, train-of-four ratio; TOFC, train-of-four count.

4) TOF has several advantages. It is a more sensitive indicator of residual NMB than a single twitch. A control is not necessary. It can distinguish between a depolarizing block and a nondepolarizing block and is valuable in detecting and following the development of a phase II block following succinylcholine administration.
5) The main disadvantage of TOF is its poor performance at both extremes of NMB, deep relaxation, or near complete recovery.

CLINICAL MOMENT Tactile or visual evaluation of the TOFR is of little value above a ratio of 0.4 to 0.5.

CLINICAL MOMENT A TOFR of 0.9 or more should be achieved before the patient awakens.

c. Tetanus
1) Tetanus is a rapidly repeated (50, 100, or even 200 Hz) stimulus. In the absence of NMB, tetanus causes sustained stimulated muscle contraction. With a depolarizing block, the response will be depressed in amplitude but sustained. With a nondepolarizing block, the response is depressed in amplitude and the contraction is not sustained (fade or decrement). With profound NMB, there is no response. Fade after 50-Hz tetanic stimulation is a more sensitive index of NMB than a single twitch but not sufficiently sensitive to be used for assessing adequate recovery.
2) The most commonly used frequency is 50 Hz, because it stresses the neuromuscular junction to the same extent as a maximal voluntary effort. Using a frequency of 100 Hz allows more sensitivity in evaluating residual paralysis and is more useful in monitoring profound NMB.
3) The tetanic stimulus duration is important because it affects fade. The standard duration is 5 seconds. Tetanic stimulation should not be repeated more often than every 2 minutes. Some newer stimulators limit how frequently it can be used.
4) Posttetanic facilitation (potentiation, PTF) is a temporary increase in response to stimulation following a tetanic stimulus. It is seen with a nondepolarizing but not a depolarizing block. It is maximal at around 3 seconds and lasts up to 2 minutes.
5) When the NMB is so profound that there is no response to a single twitch or TOF stimulation, it may be possible to estimate NMB by using the PTC. This is performed by administering a tetanic stimulus of 50 Hz for 5 seconds. After a 3-second pause, single-twitch stimuli are applied at 1 Hz and the number of (posttetanic) responses is counted. The number of twitches elicited increases as the NMB depth decreases.
6) A significant disadvantage of tetanic stimulation is that it is very painful and should be avoided in the conscious patient.

d. Double-Burst Stimulation
1) Double-burst stimulation (DBS, minitetanus) consists of two short bursts of 50-Hz tetanic stimuli separated by 750 milliseconds. DBS

should not be repeated at intervals of less than 12 seconds. Caution should be exercised when switching between double-burst and TOF stimulation. Up to 92 seconds may be required before these responses stabilize.

2) DBS has been used mainly to detect residual NMB. Studies show that fade (response to the second burst weaker than that to the first) is more readily detected with DBS than with TOF using visual or tactile monitoring. It has also been used for intraoperative assessment of NMB. Another use of DBS is to assess deep block, since the first twitch in double burst can be detected at deeper block levels than the first twitch in TOF.

3) DBS causes more discomfort than TOF stimulation but less than tetanic stimulation. It can be used at submaximal currents. This causes less discomfort and, in most cases, is more reliable than testing with supramaximal stimuli.

B. Electrodes

Stimulation is achieved by placing two electrodes along a nerve and passing a current through them. Stimulation can be carried out either transcutaneously with surface electrodes or percutaneously with needle electrodes.

1. **Surface Electrodes**

Surface (gel, patch, pad) electrodes have adhesive surrounding a gelled foam pad in contact with a metal disc, with an attachment for the electrical lead. They are readily available, easily applied, disposable, self-adhering, and comfortable. The electrodes can be used to monitor the electrocardiographic (ECG) tracing. The electrode–skin resistance decreases with a large conducting area, as do skin burns and pain. A large conducting area may make it difficult to obtain supramaximal stimulation and may stimulate multiple nerves. If this problem occurs, it may be better to use pediatric electrodes.

2. **Needle Electrodes**

Metal-hub needles can also be used. These electrodes run the risk that the needle may penetrate the nerve. They are not well accepted by awake patients.

3. **Polarity**

Stimulators produce a direct current by using a negative electrode and a positive electrode. The polarity of the outlet sockets should be indicated on the stimulator. Usually, the positive electrode is red and the negative is black. Maximal effect is achieved when the negative electrode is placed directly over the most superficial part of the nerve being stimulated. The positive electrode should be placed along the course of the nerve, usually proximally to avoid direct muscle stimulation.

CLINICAL MOMENT If electrode polarity is unknown, the connections can be reversed to determine which arrangement evokes the greater response.

II. **Methods to Evaluate Evoked Responses**

A. Visual

Visual assessment can be made to count the number of responses present with a TOF stimulus, to determine the PTC, and to detect fade with TOF or DBS. PTF can also be assessed. Studies have shown that it is difficult to visually determine the TOFR or to compare single-twitch height to its control accurately.

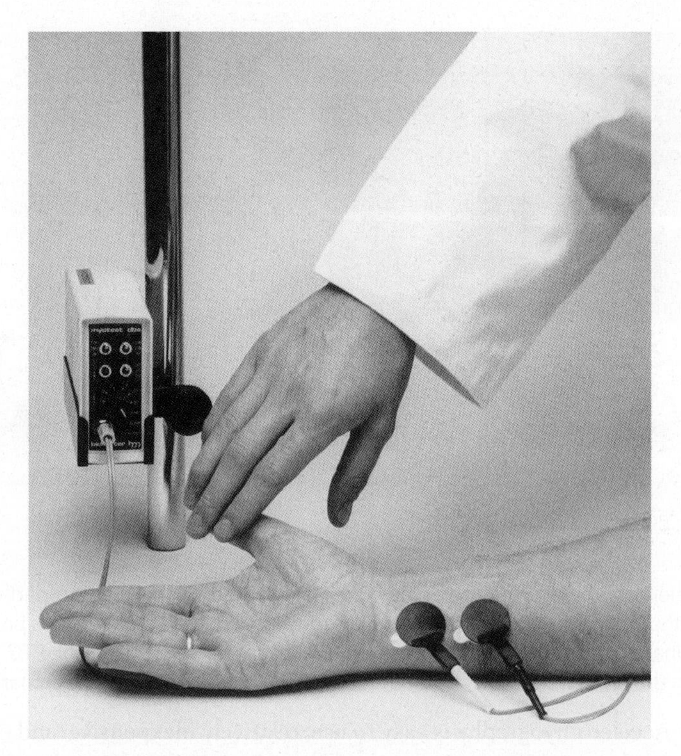

Figure 20.4 For tactile evaluation of thumb adduction, the hand is supine and a slight preload is applied. (Photograph courtesy of Biometer, Odense, Denmark.)

B. Tactile

Tactile evaluation is accomplished by placing the evaluator's fingertips over the stimulated muscle and feeling the contraction strength (**Fig. 20.4**). It is more sensitive than visual monitoring for assessing NMB by using TOF. It can be used to evaluate the presence or absence of responses and/or fade with TOF, double-burst, and tetanic stimulation. The PTC can also be determined. If there is a response to all four stimuli with TOF stimulation, the TOFR can be estimated. Unfortunately, it is difficult for even trained observers to detect TOF fade tactilely unless the TOFR is below 40%. Detecting fade tactilely is somewhat better with DBS but cannot be depended on to detect residual paralysis.

CLINICAL MOMENT NMB is easier to evaluate when the evaluator uses the patient's dominant hand.

C. Acceleromyography

1. Acceleromyography (ACG, AMG), utilizes a thin piezoelectric transducer in a suitable housing fixed to a digit or muscle part (**Fig. 20.5**). When the digit or muscle moves, a voltage proportional to the acceleration is generated. This is converted into an electrical signal.
2. This method requires that the muscle being stimulated has unrestricted movement. An elastic preload can be applied to return the moving part to its original position. ACG can be used to assess NMB in the hand, with the patient's arm tucked at the side as long as the finger can move freely.

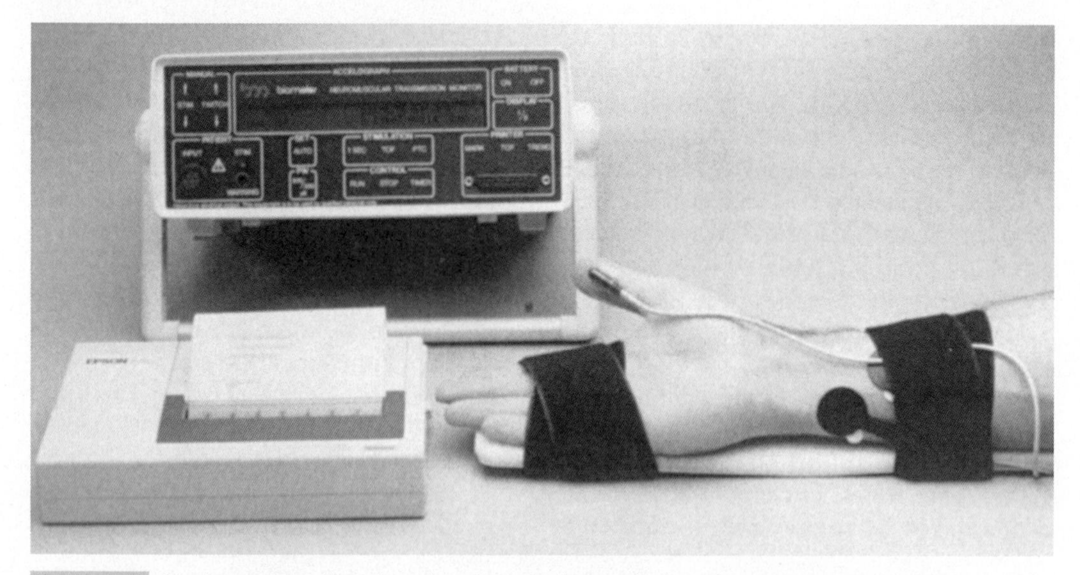

Figure 20.5 Accelerography. The piezoelectric wafer is attached to the moving part—in this case, the thumb. When the thumb moves, an electrical signal proportional to the acceleration is produced. The monitor allows determination of single-twitch depression, TOF count or ratio and/or the PTC. Responses can be displayed by using the printer. (Courtesy of Biometer International A/S, Odense, Denmark.)

3. Acceleromyography is easy to use, relatively inexpensive, and can be interfaced to transmit information to an electronic record. It does not require a preload. It gives more accurate results than visual or tactile evaluation and can be applied to a variety of muscles.
4. Using ACG results in better detection of residual NMB than visual or tactile methods or clinical tests.

D. Kinemyography

1. Kinemyography (KMG) utilizes a bending sensor that is placed between the thumb and the forefinger (**Fig. 20.6**). The core of the single-use sensor is a piezoelectric material. When the material changes shape, the electrical charge in the material is redistributed and this leads to an electron flow to balance the charges. This flow is proportional to the amount of distortion. The hand need not be immobilized as long as the thumb and the forefinger can move freely.

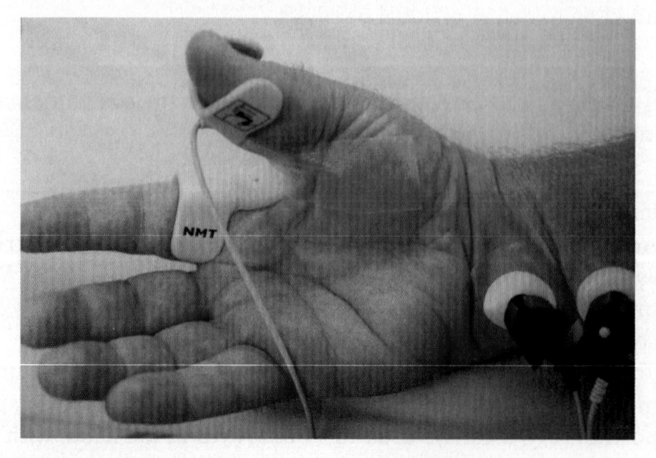

Figure 20.6 Sensor for kinemyography. The sensor is secured with tape.

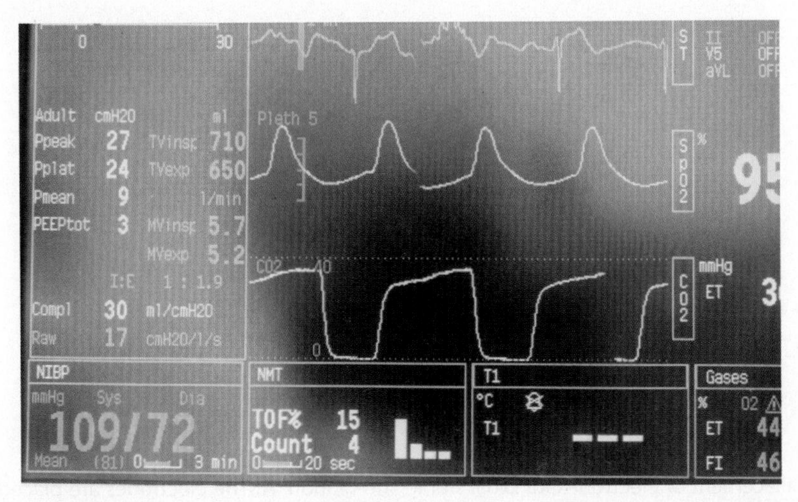

Figure 20.7 The train-of-four (TOF) count and ratio are shown on the monitor. The scale at the bottom shows the frequency of stimulation (every 20 seconds) and how much time has elapsed since the last stimulus. This information comes from a kinemyograph.

2. This technology can be used to measure TOF, double burst, and single twitch. The results are displayed on the monitor screen (**Fig. 20.7**).
3. KMG has been shown to provide satisfactory results for clinical purposes.
4. KMG can be used only to measure NMB at the adductor pollicis muscle and there is only one probe size. Also, a problem with this technology has been reported (1, 2). The numerical TOF% may show inadequate recovery, whereas the responses displayed on a bar graph appear to be identical.

III. **Choice of Monitoring Site**

The stimulated nerve should be away from the surgical field. If visual or tactile monitoring is to be used, the location must be accessible to the anesthesia provider. If a muscle in an arm or a leg is used, blood pressure should be measured on a different extremity. An arteriovenous shunt does not contraindicate that arm being used to monitor NMB. If the patient has an upper-motor-neuron lesion, a nerve in an affected (paretic) extremity should not be used, because it may falsely show resistance to nondepolarizing drugs. If possible, the nerve stimulator electrodes should be placed on an extremity different from the pulse oximeter probe to avoid motion artifacts on the oximeter.

A. Ulnar Nerve

1. The ulnar nerve is most commonly used, and the adductor pollicis (thumb) muscle is most commonly monitored. Because this muscle is on the side of the arm opposite the site of stimulation, there is little direct muscle stimulation.
2. The ulnar nerve can be stimulated at the elbow, wrist, or hand (**Fig. 20.8**). Stimulation at the wrist will produce thumb adduction and finger flexion. Stimulation at the elbow also produces hand adduction. At the wrist, the two electrodes should be placed along the medial aspect of the distal forearm, approximately 2 cm proximal to the proximal wrist skin crease with the negative electrode distal (**Fig. 20.8A**). There the ulnar nerve is superficial. Alternately, the positive electrode may be placed on the dorsal side of the wrist. At the elbow, the electrodes should be placed over the sulcus of the epicondyle of the humerus (**Fig. 20.8B**). Caution must be exercised to ensure that the electrodes do not cause ulnar nerve compression. The electrodes may also be placed on the hand, with the negative electrode on the palm between the thumb base and

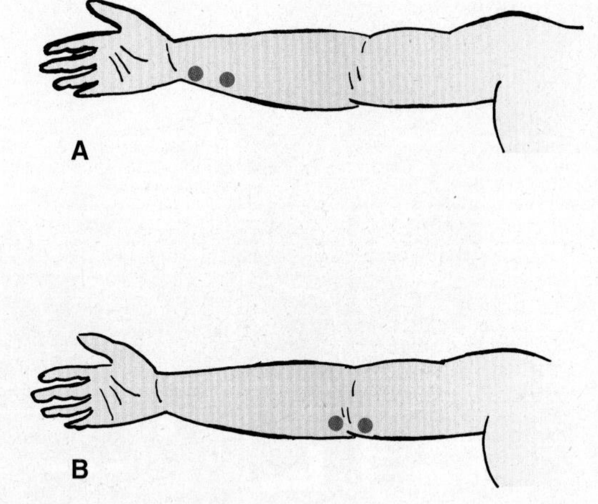

Figure 20.8 Placement of electrodes for ulnar nerve stimulation. **A:** The electrodes are placed along the ulnar aspect of the distal forearm. **B:** The electrodes are placed over the sulcus of the medial epicondyle of the humerus.

the second finger and the positive electrode in the same position on the dorsal side of the hand.

3. For tactile assessment, the thumb should be held in slight abduction and the observer's fingertips placed over the distal phalanx in the direction of movement (**Fig. 20.4**). Preloading the thumb with a rubber band may improve visual assessment.
4. When monitoring the adductor pollicis muscle, it is important to realize that the onset and duration of NMB at the larynx and the diaphragm are shorter than those at peripheral muscles. These muscles are relatively sensitive to NMB.

B. Median Nerve

The median nerve is larger than the ulnar but less superficial. It can be stimulated at the wrist by placing the electrodes medial to where the electrodes would be placed for ulnar nerve stimulation or at the elbow adjacent to the brachial artery. This results in thumb adduction.

C. Tibial Nerve

To stimulate the tibial nerve at the popliteal fossa, two stimulating electrodes are placed along the lateral side of the popliteal fossa. The gastrocnemius muscle is stimulated. Using this muscle may cause significant leg movement, which may distract the surgeon.

D. Posterior Tibial Nerve

1. To stimulate the posterior tibial nerve, electrodes are placed behind the medial maleolus and anterior to the Achilles tendon at the ankle (**Fig. 20.9**). Stimulation causes plantar flexion at the foot and the big toe. ACG can be used at this site.
2. The posterior tibial nerve offers many advantages. It is especially useful in children (in whom it may be difficult to find room on the arm because of other monitors or invasive lines) and when the hand is inaccessible or for other reasons such as amputation, burns, infection, or head and neck procedures.
3. Compared with the ulnar nerve, the posterior tibial nerve displays a slower onset of relaxation. Most studies show little difference in the time to recovery from neuromuscular relaxation.

E. Peroneal Nerve

To stimulate the peroneal (lateral popliteal) nerve, electrodes are placed on the lateral aspect of the knee (**Fig. 20.10**). It may be necessary to try different positions

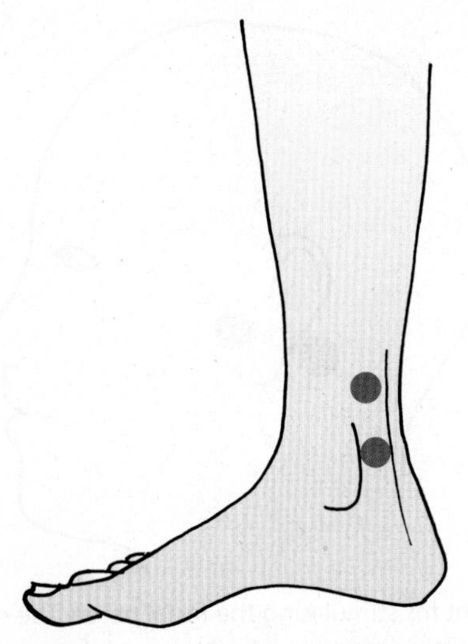

Figure 20.9 Placement of electrodes for stimulating the posterior tibial nerve. The negative electrode is placed behind the medial malleolus, anterior to the Achilles tendon. The positive electrode is placed just proximal to the negative electrode. Stimulation causes plantar flexion of the great toe.

to achieve the best response. Stimulation causes the foot to dorsiflex. Compared with the ulnar nerve, the peroneal nerve shows a slower onset of relaxation and the muscles show greater resistance to NMB.

F. Facial Nerve

The facial nerve enervates the muscles around the eye. It is most useful for detecting the onset of relaxation in the muscles of the jaw, larynx, and diaphragm. ACG can be used with the facial nerve.

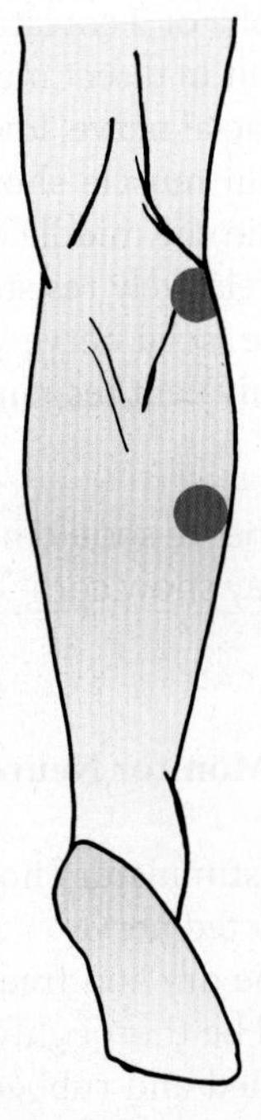

Figure 20.10 Electrode placement for stimulating the peroneal (lateral popliteal) nerve. The electrodes are placed lateral to the neck of the fibula. Stimulation causes dorsiflexion of the foot.

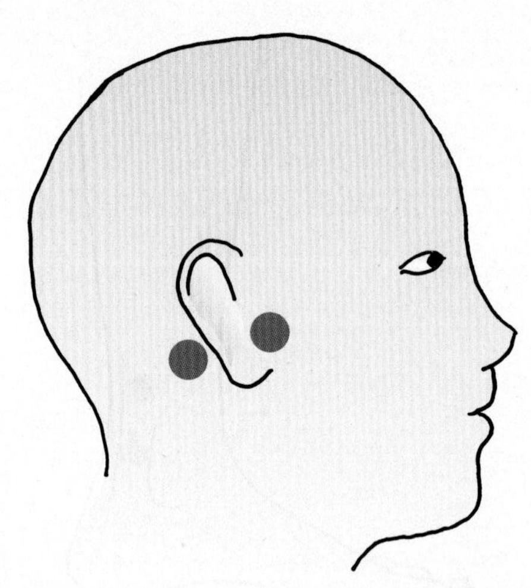

Figure 20.11 Electrode placement for stimulating the facial nerve. The negative electrode is placed anterior to the earlobe. The positive electrode is placed posterior or inferior to the earlobe.

1. Several electrode configurations have been used for stimulating the facial nerve.
   a. The negative electrode is placed just anterior to the inferior part of the ear lobe, and the other electrode is placed just posterior or inferior to the lobe (**Fig. 20.11**). Stimulation at these sites will make it more likely that muscle contractions are the result of nerve stimulation rather than direct muscle stimulation.
   b. Another way the facial nerve can be stimulated is to place one electrode lateral to and below the lateral canthus of the eye and the other electrode anterior to the earlobe or 2 cm lateral to and above the lateral canthus. This placement may result in direct muscle stimulation.
2. When stimulating the facial nerve, low currents (20 to 30 mA) should be used. The corrugator supercilii muscle should be observed. With ACG, the transducer should be placed in the middle of the superciliary arch.
3. The facial muscles are relatively resistant to NMB drugs. Therefore, managing NMB by stimulating the facial nerve will result in greater relaxation than that from a limb nerve if equivalent responses are used.

CLINICAL MOMENT The facial nerve should not be used to assess recovery from NMB because the responses may show complete recovery while significant NMB is still present.

IV. Using the Nerve Stimulator to Monitor Neuromuscular Block

A. Before Induction

1. Prior to induction, the stimulator should be connected to electrodes that are positioned over the selected nerve.
2. Electrode sites should be dry and free of excessive hair or scar tissue or other lesions. The skin should be thoroughly cleansed with a solvent such as alcohol and then completely dried and rubbed briskly with a gauze pad until a slight redness is visible.

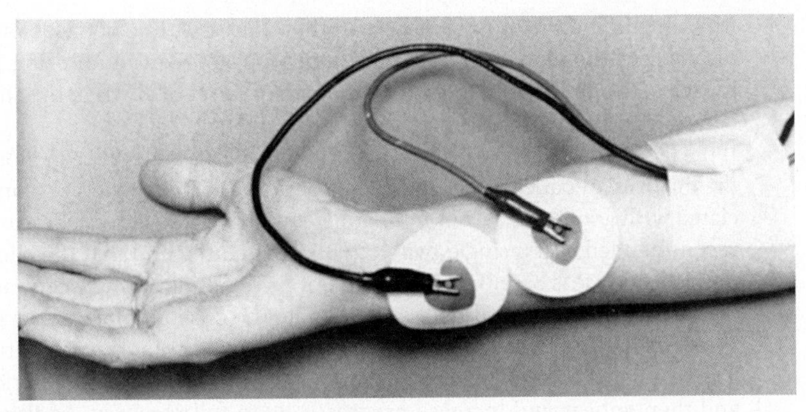

Figure 20.12 Electrodes in place. Creating loops and securing the wires with tape will decrease the likelihood that the wires will be pulled off the electrodes.

CLINICAL MOMENT Wiping the skin with alcohol and rubbing with an abrasive before the electrode is applied will remove insulating skin oils and lower resistance.

3. The electrodes should be checked to verify that the gel is moist. It is important to avoid spreading the gel or overlapping adhesive while placing the electrodes. After the leads are attached to the electrodes, tape should be placed over the leads to prevent movement. It is a good practice to create a loop to prevent electrode displacement (**Fig. 20.12**).

B. Induction

Nerve stimulation should be delayed until the patient is asleep. After induction but before administering any muscle relaxants, the stimulator should be turned ON and set to deliver single-twitch stimuli at 0.1 Hz. Applying stimulation more frequently will make it appear that the NMB onset time is shorter. The stimulator output should be increased until the response does not increase with increasing current and then increased 10% to 20%. If maximal stimulation is not achieved with a current of 50 to 70 mA, the electrodes should be checked for proper placement.

C. Intubation

1. Complete relaxation of the jaw, laryngeal and pharyngeal muscles, and diaphragm is needed for optimal intubating conditions and to reduce the risk of trauma. It should be kept in mind that the response to intubation is a function of both muscular block and the level of anesthesia. It is possible to intubate a patient with less than complete paralysis if sufficient anesthetic depth is present.
2. The onset of NMB is faster in centrally located muscles such as the diaphragm, facial, laryngeal, and jaw muscles than peripheral muscles such as the adductor pollicis.
3. The diaphragm, eye muscles, and most laryngeal muscles are more resistant to nondepolarizing relaxants than peripheral muscles. The diaphragm is resistant to succinylcholine, though the laryngeal muscles are sensitive to it. The masseter muscle is relatively sensitive to both nondepolarizing and depolarizing relaxants. It often reacts with increased tone instead of relaxation to succinylcholine, particularly in children.

4. Monitoring the eye muscle response will reflect the time of onset and the level of NMB at the airway musculature more closely than monitoring peripheral muscles, which will underestimate the rate of onset of NMB in the airway musculature and may overestimate the degree of block.
5. If the facial nerve cannot be used, a peripheral nerve will suffice in most cases. In the majority of patients, disappearance of the adductor pollicis response is associated with good to excellent intubating conditions. Whatever nerve is used, it is recommended that a single twitch at 0.1 Hz be used and that the clinician wait until a response is barely perceptible before attempting laryngoscopy and intubation. More rapid stimulation may accelerate the onset of block at the stimulated site. DBS has been used to indicate optimal conditions for tracheal intubation.
6. The response to stimulation will usually disappear for a variable period of time and then appear and increase progressively to full recovery. Additional relaxants should not be given until there is evidence of some recovery to make certain that the patient does not have an abnormal response. It is not necessary to wait for complete recovery before giving additional relaxants.

D. Maintenance

1. During maintenance, the stimulator can be used to titrate the relaxant dosage to the needs of the operative procedure, so both under- and overdosage are avoided. Too deep an NMB may make it difficult to reverse the relaxant at the termination of the anesthetic. Underdosage may result in inadequate relaxation or undesirable patient movement. In a study of closed claims against anesthesiologists, eye injuries constituted 3% of claims. Patient movement was the mechanism of injury in 30% of these cases, and a nerve stimulator was not used in any of these patients.
2. The degree of NMB required during a surgical procedure depends on many factors, including the type of surgery, the anesthetic technique, and anesthetic depth. It is important to correlate the reaction to nerve stimulation with the patient's clinical condition because there may be a discrepancy between the relaxation depth of the monitored muscles and those at the surgical site. If the surgeon believes that relaxation is inadequate, the anesthesia provider should confirm that the stimulator is working properly. If it does not display the delivered current, electrodes may be placed on the user's arm and a low current used to confirm proper functioning.
3. TOF is commonly regarded as the most useful pattern for monitoring NMB during maintenance. The goal for most cases in which abdominal muscle relaxation is required should be to maintain at least one response to TOF stimulation in a peripheral nerve. If no response is present, further administration of relaxants is not indicated. If two responses are present, abdominal relaxation may be adequate using balanced anesthesia. Presence of three twitches is usually associated with adequate relaxation if a volatile anesthetic agent is used. Deeper levels of NMB may be required for upper abdominal or chest surgery or if diaphragmatic paralysis is needed. If the facial muscles are used, at least one twitch should be added to the mentioned recommendations.
4. Muscle relaxants are sometimes administered in cases such as eye or intracranial surgery or laser surgery on the vocal cords to guarantee that movement does not occur. To ensure total diaphragmatic paralysis, the NMB should be so intense that there is no response to posttetanic stimulation in a peripheral muscle (i.e., the PTC is zero). One approach is to give a bolus of a short-acting muscle relaxant when the PTC is 1. Alternatively, the twitch response at a

muscle more resistant to NMB may be monitored and a dose of relaxant given as soon as there is any response.

E. Recovery and Reversal

CLINICAL MOMENT Assessment of neuromuscular blockade should be performed before the patient emerges from anesthesia. Accurate assessment in the unanesthetized patient is more difficult.

1. At the end of a procedure, a stimulator allows the anesthesia provider to determine whether or not the block is reversible and adjust the reversal agent dose, if required, to the patient's requirement. Numerous studies have shown that significant residual NMB persisting into the postoperative period is a common occurrence. Using a nerve stimulator may detect residual NMB, which could lead to life-threatening complications.
2. When relaxation is no longer required, administration of NMB drugs should be discontinued. As recovery progresses, the responses to TOF will progressively appear and then fade will disappear. The ease of reversing a nondepolarizing block is inversely related to the degree of block at the time of reversal. The time depends on the relaxant that was used.
3. Recovery is governed by sensitivity of the muscle and the rate at which the drug disappears from the plasma.

CLINICAL MOMENT It is best to use a peripheral muscle to monitor recovery, because its complete recovery would indicate that residual muscular weakness contributing to problems with airway patency or respiration is unlikely. The probability of detecting fade with the index finger is greater than if the thumb or great toe is used.

4. In the past, many investigators thought that a TOFR of 0.7 was adequate. However, a normal response to hypoxemia, protection from pulmonary complications, and the absence of eyelid heaviness, visual disturbances, difficulty swallowing, or patient anxiety may require a higher ratio. It is now recommended that the TOFR at the adductor pollicis be at least 90%.

CLINICAL MOMENT Residual NMB cannot be reliably detected by TOF stimulation if visual and/or tactile monitoring is used. Detection may be somewhat better when using DBS but is most reliably accomplished by ACG.

5. Clinical criteria in an unanesthetized patient have been used to ascertain whether the return of muscle strength is adequate. These include the ability to (a) open the eyes for 5 seconds and not experience diplopia, (b) sustain tongue protrusion, (c) sustain head lift for at least 5 seconds, (d) sustain hand grip, (e) sustain leg lifting in children, (f) cough effectively, and (g) swallow. A more sensitive test may be the ability to resist removing a tongue blade from clenched teeth. Clinical criteria in an anesthetized patient include an adequate tidal volume and an inspiratory force of at least 25 cm H_2O negative pressure. These clinical criteria do not exclude clinically significant residual paralysis.

F. Postoperative Period

Even if a nerve stimulator has not been used during an operation, it can be of use in the postoperative period to detect residual paralysis. If the patient is not fully anesthetized, it is preferable to use less than supramaximal stimulation. This decreases the discomfort associated with stimulation and may improve the visual assessment accuracy.

V. **Hazards**

A. Burns

Burns have been reported when using a stimulator with metal ball electrodes. Needle electrodes may be associated with local tissue burns from electrosurgical units because they provide good contact with minimal resistance for exit of high-frequency current over a small area of skin. Severe burns resulting in permanent loss of hand function caused by a nerve stimulator have been reported.

B. Nerve Damage

The pressure of an electrode on a nerve can result in palsy.

C. Pain

Patient discomfort will be reduced by using lower currents and avoiding tetanic stimulation or DBS when the patient is not fully anesthetized.

D. Electrical Interference

Using a nerve stimulator may cause changes in the ECG tracing or interfere with an implanted pacemaker.

E. Incorrect Information

With some stimulators, when the batteries are low, only three pulses are generated during TOF stimulation. This could lead to incorrect interpretation of the degree of NMB.

REFERENCES

1. Kopman AF. The Datex-Ohmeda M-NMT module: a potentially confusing user interface. Anesthesiology 2006;104: 1109–1110.
2. Paloheimo M. The Datex-Ohmeda M-NMT module: a potentially confusing user interface. In reply. Anesthesiology 2006;104:1110–1111.

SUGGESTED READINGS

Ali HH. Criteria of adequate clinical recovery from neuromuscular block. Anesthesiology 2003;98:1278–1280.

Claudius C, Viby-Mogensen J. Acceleromyography for use in scientific and clinical practice. A systematic review of the evidence. Anesthesiology 2008;10:1117–1140.

Dorsch J, Dorsch S. Neuromuscular transmission monitoring. In: Understanding Anesthesia Equipment. Fifth edition. Philadelphia: Wolters Kluwer/Lippincott Williams & Wilkins, 2008:805–825.

Hemmerling TM. Brief review: Neuromuscular monitoring: an update for the clinician. Can J Anesth 2007;54:58–72.

Naguib M, Kopman AF, Ensor JE. Neuromuscular monitoring and postoperative residual curarization: a meta-analysis. Br J Anaesth 2007;98:302–316.

Torda RA. Reviews. Monitoring neuromuscular transmission. Anaesth Intensive Care 2002;30:123–133.

21 Alarm Devices

I. Introduction

A. The purposes of an alarm are to transfer information, enhance vigilance, and warn of a potential or actual abnormal or unusual condition. It is essential that there be a means to alert personnel to a change or potential change in monitored variables that reflect the condition of the patient or equipment, because there will always be occasions when operator vigilance will be lowered or attention reduced while performing other tasks.

B. The number of alarms in anesthetizing areas has greatly increased. To add to further confusion, alarm sounds may come from sources other than anesthesia apparatus, such as electrosurgical equipment, lasers, hearing aids, phones, and beepers.

II. Terminology

A. *Alarm Condition Delay*: Time from the occurrence of a triggering event to the time the alarm system determines that an alarming condition exists.

B. *Alarm Signal Generation Delay*: Time from the onset of an alarming condition to the generation of its alarm signals.

C. *Alarm Limit*: Threshold used by an alarm system to determine an alarm condition.

D. *Alarm Off*: State of indefinite duration in which an alarm system or part of an alarm system does not generate alarm signals.

E. *Alarm Paused*: State of limited duration in which the alarm system or part of the alarm system does not generate alarm signals.

F. *Alarm Preset*: Set of stored configuration parameters, including selection of algorithms and initial values for use.

G. *Alarm Reset*: Operator action that causes the cessation of an alarm signal for which no associated alarm condition currently exists.

H. *Alarm Settings*: Alarm system configuration, including but not limited to alarm limits, the characteristics of any alarm signal inactivation states, and the values of variables or parameters that determine the alarm system function.

I. *Alarm Signal*: Signal generated by the alarm system to indicate the presence of an alarm condition.

J. *Alarm System*: Parts of medical electrical equipment that detect alarm conditions and, as appropriate, generate alarm signals.

K. *Audio Off*: State of indefinite duration in which the alarm system or part of the alarm system does not generate an auditory alarm signal.

L. *Audio Paused*: State of limited duration in which the alarm system or part of the alarm system does not generate an auditory alarm signal.
M. *Default Alarm Preset*: Alarm preset that can be activated by the alarm system without operator action.
N. *False-Negative Alarm Condition*: Absence of an alarm condition when a valid triggering event has occurred.
O. *False-Positive Alarm Condition*: Presence of an alarm condition when no valid triggering event has occurred.
P. *High Priority*: Indicates that an immediate operator response is required.
Q. *Information Signal*: Any signal that is not an alarm signal or a reminder signal. Examples include the pulse oximeter tone or electrocardiograph, the waveform of the electrocardiograph, and the heart rate numeric.
R. *Intelligent Alarm System*: Alarm system that makes logical decisions on the basis of monitored information without operator intervention. Intelligent alarm system methodologies include analysis of trends, limit comparisons, data redundancy, data fusion, rules, fuzzy logic controllers, and neural networks.
S. *Latching Alarm Signal*: Alarm signal that continues to be generated after its triggering event no longer exists until stopped by deliberate operator action.
T. *Low Priority*: Indicates that operator awareness is required.
U. *Medium Priority*: Indicates that prompt operator response is required.
V. *Reminder Signal*: Periodic signal that reminds the operator that the alarm system is in an alarm signal inactivation state.
W. *Inhibit, mute, silence,* and *suspend* have been used in past terminology for alarms. Unfortunately, different meanings were attributed to these terms. For this reason, these terms will not be used.

III. Alarm Prioritization

A. All alarms are not equally important. The information that an alarm conveys may represent an emergency, the potential for an emergency, or just an unusual condition requiring awareness. Prioritized alarms help to differentiate life-threatening situations from those that are less urgent. Alarm condition priorities are shown in **Table 21.1**. It may be possible to increase the priority of an alarm, but the priority cannot be decreased.
B. A high-priority alarm indicates a condition that requires immediate action. Examples include asystole, ventricular fibrillation, cardiac support device (intra-aortic balloon pump, cardiopulmonary bypass machine) failure, high airway pressure, extreme hypoxemia, and sustained high-energy radiation.
C. Medium priority implies a potentially dangerous situation that requires a prompt response. Examples include many cardiac arrhythmias, high or low blood pressure, apnea (unless prolonged or associated with hypoxemia), mild hypoxemia, and high or low carbon dioxide levels.
D. A low-priority alarm indicates that only operator awareness is required. Examples include failure of an infusion pump for maintenance intravenous fluids and failure of an enteral feeding pump.
E. The object of prioritization is to minimize distraction from less important alarms during an emergency. It has been suggested that only the alarm sound corresponding to the most urgent of the prevailing alarm conditions should be annunciated; all other sounds should be temporarily audiopaused. Once the most urgent alarm condition is resolved, the sound corresponding to the next highest priority condition would then be initiated. This priority interlock should be limited to audible annunciations; lower priority visual signals need not be suppressed because they are relatively unobtrusive.

Table 21.1 Alarm Condition Priorities

Potential Result of Failure to Respond to the Cause of Alarm Condition	Onset of Potential Harm[a]		
	Immediate[b]	Prompt[c]	Delayed[d]
Death or irreversible injury	High priority	High priority	Medium priority
Reversible injury	High priority	Medium priority	Low priority
Minor injury or discomfort	Medium priority	Low priority	Low priority or no alarm signal

An information signal may be used to indicate the potential for delayed minor injury or discomfort.
[a]Onset of potential harm refers to when an injury occurs and not to when it is manifested.
[b]Having the potential for the event to develop within a period of time not usually sufficient for manual corrective action.
[c]Having the potential for the event to develop within a period of time that is usually sufficient for manual corrective action.
[d]Having the potential for the event to develop within an unspecified time that is greater than that given under "prompt."
From International Standards Organization. Medical Electrical Equipment—Parts 1-8: General Requirements for Safety. Collateral Standard: General Requirements, Tests and Guidelines for Alarm Systems in Medical Electrical Equipment and in Medical Electrical Systems (ISO-IEC 60601-1-8). Geneva, Switzerland: International Standards Organization, 2003.

IV. Audible Signals

A. The primary purpose of auditory alarm signals is to get the operator's attention. In addition, they should help the operator identify the onset of an alarm condition, the urgency of the required response, and the device that generated the alarm signal.

B. An audible signal will attract attention faster and more reliably than a visual one. Ideally, this should be indicated in a timely, nonstartling, and nonirritating fashion. Unfortunately, the qualities that cause sounds to attract attention also tend to make them intrusive or startling. Some are so unpleasant that the response may be to pause or deactivate the audible signal.

CLINICAL MOMENT Loud noise in the operating room can make audible alarms difficult or impossible to hear and recognize. Try to keep the noise level in the operating room to a minimum.

C. Once an audible signal has been perceived, the next step is to identify its origin. This is important because many monitors are not in the clinician's immediate field of view, and the operator cannot always turn around to view them. Many anesthesia providers have trouble identifying the source of audible alarms. Inability to identify an alarm source may delay or prevent the appropriate remedial action. Speech audible alarms are easily identified with respect to the source and are easier to remember than abstract sounds.

D. After an audible signal has succeeded in capturing attention, audio pausing will provide time to correct the situation. The continuous presence of an audible signal can degrade task performance and impair detection of new alarm conditions and the ability to distinguish between existing and new alarm conditions. The visual signal should stay activated until the condition that triggered the alarm is corrected. If another alarm condition occurs while an alarm is audio paused, both audible and visual signals associated with that alarm should be activated.

Table 21.2 Characteristics of Alarm Indicator Lights

Alarm Category	Indicator Color	Flashing Frequency
High priority	Red	1.4–2.8 Hz
Medium priority	Yellow	0.4–0.8 Hz
Low priority	Cyan or yellow	Constant

CLINICAL MOMENT If the audio alarm signal is turned OFF or to a volume too low to be heard, an alarm condition may not be recognized and a dangerous situation may be allowed to persist.

V. Visual Signals

A. Visual signals help the operator to locate the alarm source and to identify the specific alarm condition. Their principal drawback is that they can go unrecognized for a much longer time than audible signals. Symbols for visual alarm signals in compliance with the international standard are shown in **Figure 21.1**.

B. **Table 21.2** shows the color and flashing requirements for alarm indicator lights or graphical simulation of indicator lights in compliance with the international standard. **Figure 21.2** shows some visual signals.

VI. Alarm Organization

Alarm messages sometimes arrive in an unorganized pattern. A single, integrated display may aid alarm identification because the anesthesia provider needs to look in only one place to identify problems.

VII. Alarm Limits

A. An alarm limit (set point, threshold value, threshold, setting) may be nonadjustable, operator-adjustable, or determined by an algorithm. The alarm standard requires that if an operator-adjustable alarm limit is provided, the limit shall be indicated continuously or by operator action so that it can be determined if the set values are appropriate for the patient and the procedure (**Figs. 21.3** and **21.4**).

B. Default alarm limits can be set by the manufacturer, the healthcare facility, or the operator. They may be default values or may be bracketed around the value of a monitored variable at a point in time, recent values of a monitored variable, or a control setting.

C. Ensuring that an alarm is activated before a dangerous condition has occurred without creating frequent spurious alarms requires intelligence on the part of both the alarm system and the operator. Wide limits result in fewer false alarms but increase the risk of missing a true alarm (good specificity but poor sensitivity).

CLINICAL MOMENT With pressure and volume alarms during artificial ventilation, a low alarm limit setting may result in a partial disconnection or a small leak being missed.

CLINICAL MOMENT Constrictions in the breathing system that increase resistance can cause the airway pressure to remain above a low-alarm set point, although a total disconnection would probably not be missed.

Graphic	Description
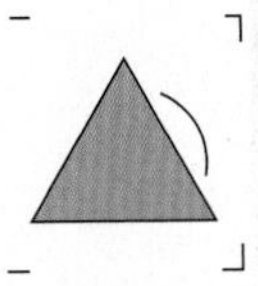	ALARM CONDITION *Note 1:* The alarm condition may be indicated inside, beside, or below the triangle. *Note 2:* If there is a need to classify alarm conditions according to priority, this may be indicated by adding one, two, or three optional elements (e.g., ! for low priority, !! for medium priority, and !!! for high priority).
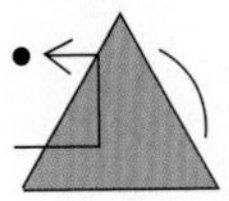	ALARM RESET *Note:* The alarm condition may be indicated inside, beside, or below the triangle.
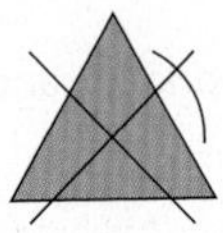	ALARM OFF This is to identify the control for alarm OFF or to indicate that the alarm system is in the alarm OFF state. *Note 1:* The alarm condition may be indicated inside, beside, or below the triangle. *Note 2:* The symbol may also be used to identify equipment that has no alarm system.
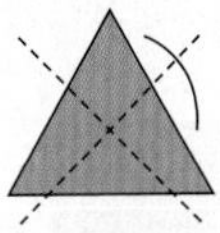	ALARM PAUSED This is to identify the control for alarm paused or to indicate that the alarm is in the alarm OFF state. *Note 1:* The alarm condition may be indicated inside, beside, or below the triangle. *Note 2:* A numerical time remaining counter may be placed above, below, or inside the triangle.
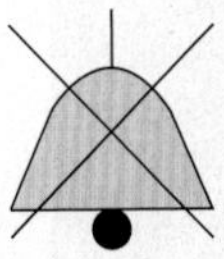	AUDIO OFF This is to identify the control for audio OFF or to indicate that the alarm system is in the audio OFF state. *Note:* The alarm condition may be indicated inside, beside, or below the bell.
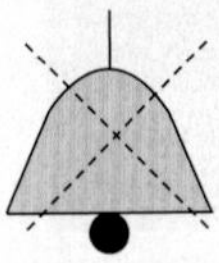	AUDIO PAUSED This is to identify the control for audio paused or to indicate that the alarm system is in the audio-paused state. *Note 1:* The alarm condition may be indicated inside, beside, or below the bell. *Note 2:* A numerical time remaining counter may be placed above, beside, or below the bell.

Figure 21.1 Graphic symbols for alarm systems. (From International Standards Organization. Medical Electrical Equipment—Parts 1-8: General Requirements for Safety. Collateral Standard: General Requirements, Tests and Guidelines for Alarm Systems in Medical Electrical Equipment and in Medical Electrical Systems (ISO IEC 60601-1-8). Geneva, Switzerland: International Standards Organization, 2003.)

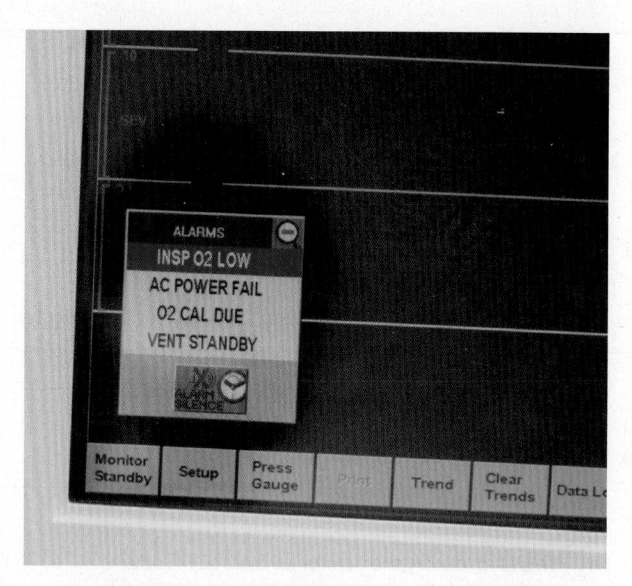

Figure 21.2 Visual alarm signals. Red indicates high priority, yellow medium priority, and yellow or white a low-priority alarm condition.

CLINICAL MOMENT To prevent unnecessary alarms from sounding, some clinicians set the alarm limits in a wide range around the normal values. This can prevent both an alarm from sounding and a potentially hazardous situation being recognized quickly. Alarm limits need to be set close to the normal values.

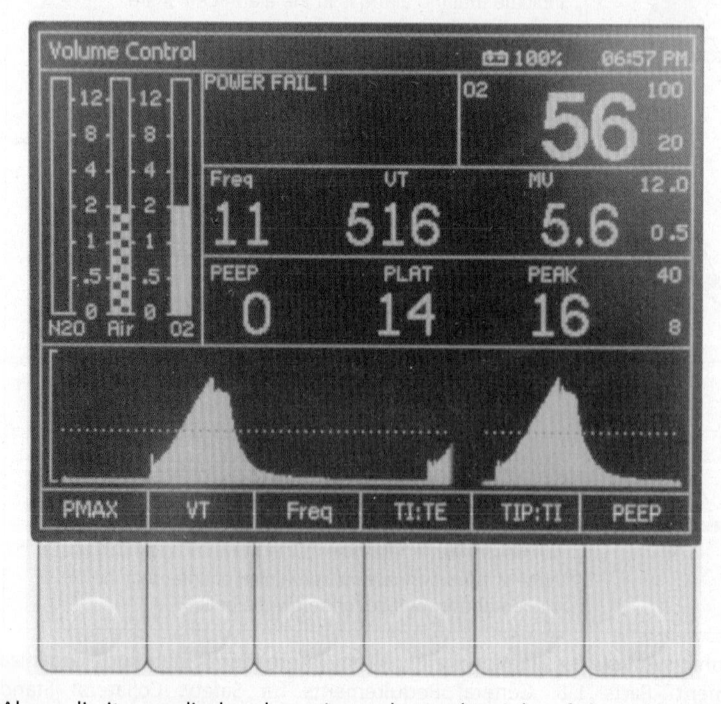

Figure 21.3 Alarms limits are displayed continuously on the right of the values for the parameters. (Photograph courtesy of Draeger Medical, Inc., Lubeck, Germany.)

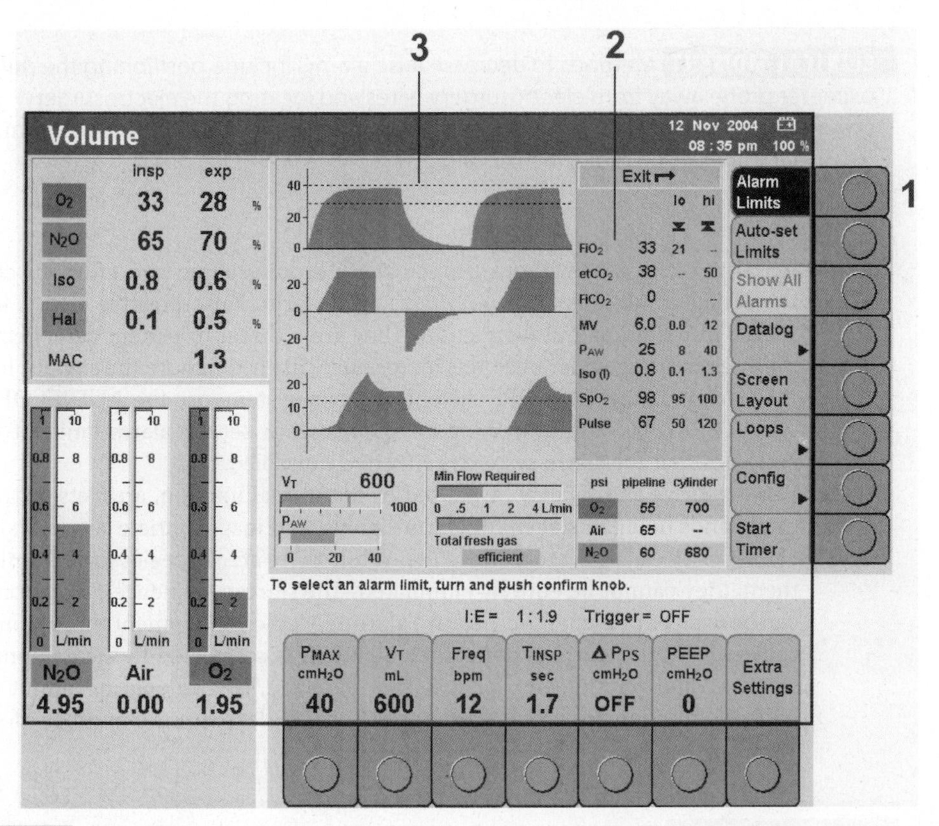

Figure 21.4 The complete set of alarm values is displayed. To display the menu of alarm limits, the alarm limits soft key (*1*) is pressed. The menu (*2*) lists the parameters, their current measured values (larger numbers), and the current low- and high-alarm limits. The alarm limits also appear on the curves as *dashed lines* (*3*). (Photograph courtesy of Draeger Medical, Inc.)

D. Some clinicians simply use the limits set by the last person who used the device. Others keep the thresholds close to the manufacturer preset limits.

CLINICAL MOMENT Recording the alarm limits on the anesthesia log may help to remind the clinician to verify whether the limits are reasonable and also offers some evidence that the alarm was activated.

CLINICAL MOMENT The only time that an alarm should be deliberately disabled is during cardiopulmonary bypass. It is important to restore the alarm after the conclusion of the bypass.

VIII. False Alarms

Actual alarm malfunctions are rare. The anesthesia provider can reduce the number of false-positive and false-negative alarms by carefully preparing the patient interface, securely attaching probes, selecting monitors with artifact-rejection capabilities, using reasonably (but not excessively) wide limits, and tailoring the alarms to the patient and operation needs.

CLINICAL MOMENT Methods to decrease false alarms include positioning the pulse oximeter probe away from electrosurgery wires and locating the electrosurgery grounding pad as far away from the pulse oximeter probe and electrocardiogram (ECG) electrodes as possible.

A. False-Positive Alarms

1. An alarm activated without proper cause requires time and effort to check the actual conditions and audio pause the alarm. False-positive alarms are a source of irritation and distraction. They are a threat to patient care, because the anesthesia provider becomes increasingly likely to ignore the signals, lower the alarm volume, turn OFF the entire alarm system, use the AUDIO OFF or AUDIO PAUSE without looking for the cause, or set the alarm limits at such extremes that the alarm system is effectively disabled.
2. False-positive alarms may be caused by alarm malfunction, artifacts, extraneous sounds being mistaken for alarm signals, and inappropriate set points.
3. False-positive alarms are a fact of life. While there are strategies for minimizing them, they cannot be entirely eliminated. The startup sequence on equipment can be used to prevent false-positive alarms. Medical equipment that automatically enables the alarm system when a patient is connected to the equipment, when a valid physiologic signal is first detected, or through an "admit new patient" function activated by the operator will decrease the number of such alarms.

CLINICAL MOMENT False-positive alarms may be reduced by changing alarm limits at certain times. For example, the heart rate alarm limit might be set higher during intubation than during maintenance.

CLINICAL MOMENT The ALARM PAUSED state can be used to avoid nuisance alarm signals while performing an action that is likely to cause an alarm condition. Examples of such actions are intentional breathing system disconnection to perform airway suctioning, opening a transducer to air for zero calibration, intubation, and trying to restore spontaneous breathing at the end of a case.

4. Monitors with artifact rejection, such as pulse oximeters with motion-resistant algorithms, can decrease the number of false-positive alarms. Filtration in the algorithm that is monitoring for an alarm condition often causes delay in the alarm condition. For instance, a heart rate monitor can average the R-R interval for several heartbeats. An abrupt change in R-R intervals will not immediately cause an alarm condition, because it will take several consecutive heartbeats for the calculated heart rate to exceed the alarm limit. Some ECG monitors have automatic lead switching so that monitoring can continue even if one or two electrodes come OFF. This can decrease false-positive alarms.
5. False alarms can be reduced by integrating monitors. An example is synchronizing the pulse oximeter and noninvasive blood pressure monitor so that if the oximeter probe is on the same arm as the blood pressure cuff, there will be no alarm if no pulse is detected on cuff inflation. Another example is the pulse

oximeter and ECG. Spo_2 values are rejected unless the pulse rate measured on the oximeter matches that on the ECG.

B. False-Negative Alarms

1. If an alarm system fails to generate a signal when it should (false negative), the patient's safety may be threatened. An alarm condition may be rejected or missed because of spurious information produced by the patient, the patient–equipment interface, other equipment, or the equipment itself. Another cause is the alarm being turned OFF. Subsequent users may not be aware that it has been turned OFF. Automatic enabling is present on many newer monitors. Once a monitored parameter is sensed, the alarm becomes active. This eliminates the problem of forgetting to turn an alarm ON or not being aware that an alarm has been turned OFF by a previous user. Reminder signals should reduce the chance that an alarm system is unintentionally left in the ALARM OFF state.

CLINICAL MOMENT False-negative alarms may be caused by speaker failure, setting the audible volume too low, or setting the alarm limits too widely.

2. False-negative alarms may be reduced by not setting the limits too widely, using the AUDIO PAUSE or ALARM PAUSE state rather than the AUDIO OFF state, and checking alarm systems at regular intervals to detect problems such as a faulty loudspeaker or low-audible volume that can result in an audible signal not being heard.

CLINICAL MOMENT Many monitors allow the alarm threshold(s) to be set by the operator. The further the threshold is set from the measured value, the more likely it is that a false-negative alarm will occur.

SUGGESTED READINGS

Dorsch J, Dorsch S. Alarm devices. In: Understanding Anesthesia Equipment. Fifth edition. Philadelphia: Wolters Kluwer/Lippincott Williams & Wilkins, 2008:828–835.

Edworthy J, Hellier E. Alarms and human behavior: implications for medical alarms. Br J Anaesth 2006;97:12–17.

22 Noninvasive Blood Pressure Monitors

I. Introduction

Blood pressure is a significant indicator of cardiovascular function. Frequent blood pressure determinations during anesthesia aid drug titration and fluid management and warn of conditions such as hypotension that could affect patient safety. There are a number of devices that automatically measure blood pressure noninvasively (indirectly).

II. Intermittent Blood Pressure Monitors

Intermittent, noninvasive blood pressure (NIBP) measurement requires a distensible cuff or bladder enclosed in an unyielding cover. The cuff is placed around a limb and inflated, and blood flow through the underlying artery is obstructed. The cuff is then deflated in a controlled manner so that the pressure applied to the artery decreases. Pulsations are detected, and the results are displayed or recorded as blood pressure. Most devices also display pulse rate.

A. Operating Principles

1. The majority of automated noninvasive monitors employ oscillometry. The cuff is inflated above the point where pressure oscillations occur. As the cuff is deflated, pressure pulsations (oscillations) caused by arterial wall movement are transmitted to the cuff. The magnitude of these oscillations increases to a maximum and then decreases (**Fig. 22.1**). A sensor in the monitor measures these oscillations. After the determination is complete, the remaining air in the cuff is rapidly exhausted.

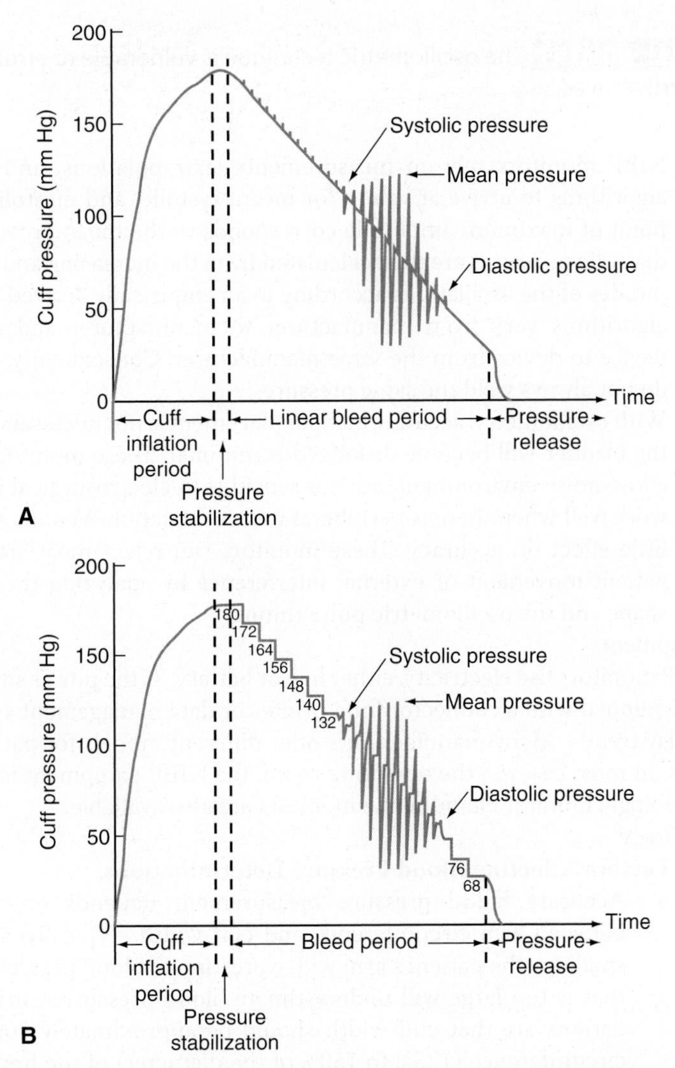

Figure 22.1 **A,B:** Sequence of oscillometric blood pressure determination. Cuff deflation may be linear (*A*) or in steps (*B*). Pressure oscillations increase in magnitude, then decrease. The oscillations are analyzed to determine systolic, mean, and diastolic pressures. (Reprinted with permission from Nellcor Puritan Bennett, Pleasanton, CA.)

2. During the first cycle, the cuff is inflated to a predetermined pressure that is held constant while the monitor attempts to detect oscillations. If significant pulsations are still present, the cuff is inflated further. When first turned ON, most automatic blood pressure monitors stop inflation at 160 torr or less. On pediatric units, a lower pressure is used. If the initial cuff pressure is greater than necessary to determine systolic pressure, the monitor may decrease this pressure during the following cycles. If the initial pressure is too low, the monitor will increase it during the next cycle. When no oscillations are detected, the pressure in the cuff is decreased in a stepwise or linear manner (**Fig. 22.1**).

CLINICAL MOMENT The oscillometric technique is vulnerable to error in patients with arrhythmias.

3. NIBP monitors rely on measurements, extrapolations, and clinically tested algorithms to arrive at values for mean, systolic, and diastolic pressures. The point of maximum amplitude corresponds to the mean pressure. Systolic and diastolic pressures are then calculated from the increasing and decreasing magnitudes of the oscillations according to an empirically derived algorithm. These algorithms vary from manufacturer to manufacturer and sometimes from device to device from the same manufacturer. Consequently, different devices do not always yield the same pressures.
4. With oscillometry, accurate bladder placement is not necessary and the risk that the bladder will become dislodged is minimal. These monitors do not require a low-noise environment, are not sensitive to electrosurgical interference, and work well when there is peripheral vasoconstriction. Venous engorgement has little effect on accuracy. These monitors can reject most artifacts caused by patient movement or external interference by analyzing the pulse waveform shape and the oscillometric pulse timing.

B. Equipment

NIBP monitors use electricity, either line or battery, as the power source. Many units are equipped with a connector for a printer or data management system. Some can display trends. Many manufacturers offer different models for patients of different sizes. In most cases in the operating room, the NIBP equipment is a module in the physiologic monitor. Stand-alone monitors are also available.

C. Accuracy

1. **Factors Affecting Blood Pressure Determinations**
   a. Accurate blood pressure measurement depends on the relationship between arm circumference and cuff width. Typically, a cuff that is too small for the patient's arm will overestimate blood pressure whereas a cuff that is too large will underestimate blood pressure. Current recommendations are that cuff width should be approximately 40% to 50% of the circumference (125% to 150% of the diameter) of the limb midpoint. It is important that different cuff sizes be readily available. If a sufficiently large cuff is not available, it may be possible to place a cuff more distally on the limb. The forearm or wrist may be used when the upper arm is inaccessible and/or a standard blood pressure cuff does not fit. The lower leg may also be used.
   b. The site where the cuff is placed affects the measured pressure. The systolic pressure tends to increase and diastolic pressure tends to decrease with more peripheral sites. Increased vascular tone may result in an increased pulse pressure. Vascular disease and peripheral vasoconstriction may cause reduced pressures at distal locations.

CLINICAL MOMENT If the cuff and the patient's heart are not at the same level, a correction must be made. For each 10 cm of vertical height, 7.7 mm Hg (for every inch, 1.80 mm Hg) above or below the heart level should be added to or subtracted from the measured pressure.

CLINICAL MOMENT The beach chair position, used for orthopedic shoulder arthroscopic procedures, is associated with decreased cerebral pressure under anesthesia and has been associated with catastrophic intraoperative strokes (1). The measured blood pressure must be corrected to account for the height of the brain above the measurement site. Blood pressure values less than 80% of the preoperative resting values should be treated aggressively to enhance the margin of safety and deliberate hypotension must be avoided.

2. **Correlation with Other Blood Pressure Determination Methods**
   a. Indirect pressure readings never exactly match invasive pressures. Many feel that the standard for comparison should be the pressure measured directly in an artery, most commonly the radial. Unfortunately, simultaneous measurements often cannot be made. Another reason for pressure differences is that direct and indirect monitors measure different physical properties. The direct method measures both the systolic and diastolic pressures and estimates the mean. Oscillometry measures the mean and estimates the systolic and diastolic pressures.
   b. Many studies have compared pressures obtained with NIBP monitors with those obtained directly. In general, the correlation is best in normal, healthy patients and least accurate at the extreme levels of blood pressure. Although errors can occur in either direction, oscillometric devices tend to overestimate low pressures and underestimate high pressures.
   c. Most studies have concluded that an NIBP monitor is not sufficiently accurate if vasoactive drugs are being administered, although in critically ill patients, it may be useful for trending purposes. With moderate to severe hypotension, the automated machine often cycles repeatedly before indicating a failure to measure.

D. Use
   1. If possible, the cuff should not be applied to the limb in which an intravenous infusion tube is placed because infused fluids and drugs will be slowed down or blocked and the increased pressure may cause blood to flow retrograde into the infusion tubing or cause blood or fluid extravasation. In some cases, it may be possible to place the cuff distal to the infusion site. If used on the arm, the cuff should be placed as high as possible and the inflation tubes should exit proximally. If the upper arm is very large or conically shaped, it is better to measure blood pressure at another location such as the forearm, thigh, or lower leg.

CLINICAL MOMENT Many blood pressure cuffs are placed too near the elbow. Locating the cuff close to the axilla will lessen the risk of neuropathies.

CLINICAL MOMENT The cuff should not be applied over a superficial nerve, bony prominence, or joint.

CLINICAL MOMENT When using an automated blood pressure monitor, the arm under the cuff should be covered with a soft wrap. If the arm is not wrapped, there can be petechiae, skin breakdown, or nerve damage under the cuff. Often, the patient complains more about this discomfort than that from surgery.

2. Before applying the cuff, all residual air should be expelled. The cuff should be applied snugly enough to allow only one finger to be slipped under it. Too tight a cuff may cause discomfort and venous distention. Too loose a cuff may cause falsely elevated readings and may prevent the monitor from determining the blood pressure. The cuff should be placed and several inflations made while the patient is awake to elicit complaints.
3. Blood pressure measurements should be made no more frequently than clinically necessary. When rapid changes in blood pressure are anticipated, a 1- or 2-minute cycle time offers no advantage over a 5-minute cycle time but the shorter time may increase the complication rate.

CLINICAL MOMENT The cuff site and extremity should be inspected periodically during prolonged applications. It is a good practice is to occasionally switch the cuff to another site, if possible, especially during long surgical procedures.

E. Complications

1. **Damage to Underlying Tissues**

   Petechiae, erythema, edema, thrombophlebitis, and skin avulsion at the cuff site have been reported. Patients taking anti-inflammatory drugs, steroids, or anticoagulants and patients with thin or redundant skin are especially susceptible to the development of petechial hemorrhages.
2. **Neuropathies**

   Neuropathies of the median, ulnar, and radial nerves have been reported. All resolve spontaneously. Excessive movement makes it difficult for the device to determine pressures, so it will cycle more often, possibly to higher pressures. This can contribute to nerve injuries.
3. **Compartment Syndrome**

   Cases of compartment syndrome associated with prolonged use have been reported. In one case, the patient had hyperactivity and tremor. In another, the blood pressure was labile, causing the monitor to cycle longer and with higher pressures than usual. In a third case, the cuff was applied across the antecubital fossa.
4. **Mechanical Problems**

   Failure of an NIBP monitor is common. A leaking cuff, hose, or connector is a fairly common reason.
5. **Artifacts**

   Oscillometric devices are sensitive to both intrinsic and extrinsic motions. Intrinsic motion artifacts are caused by deliberate patient motion, shivering, tremors, convulsions, restlessness, or vigorous skin preparation. Extrinsic motion artifacts are caused by actions that compress the cuff, such as bumping by personnel or equipment or massaging the arm where the blood pressure cuff is located. Monitors that synchronize with the electrocardiogram can reduce artifacts.

CLINICAL MOMENT External pressure on the blood pressure cuff will make it difficult to produce a good pressure reading.

F. Advantages

1. **Automaticity**
   a. A major advantage of NIBP devices is that they can determine pressures regularly and frequently on an automatic basis. During busy times, this is very helpful, saving time and allowing clinicians to perform other tasks.
   b. Automatic devices eliminate most of the factors that cause errors when blood pressures are determined manually, such as variable concentration, reaction times, hearing acuity, ambient noise, confusing auditory and visual cues, variable deflation rates, background noise, variable sound interpretation, preference for certain digits, and bias from knowledge of previous readings. They may eliminate some of the mistrust that some individuals have when others measure the blood pressure manually.
2. **Simplicity**
   Automatic NIBP monitors are simple to use. They do not require extensive training to set up or maintain.
3. **Noninvasiveness**
   In comparison with direct measurements, NIBP monitors are less expensive, simpler, and avoid most of the risks (ischemic damage, emboli) associated with direct techniques.
4. **Reliability**
   NIBP monitors are reliable devices that generally do not require a lot of maintenance or experience a lot of downtime.

G. Disadvantages

1. **Unsuitable Situations**
   While noncontinuous blood pressure monitoring is helpful in establishing trends, it is unsuitable for detecting rapid changes in blood pressure. If rapid changes are anticipated, a continuous method should be used.
2. **Patient Discomfort**
   Patient discomfort is often associated with a prolonged cycle time. Cycle time will be prolonged with a large cuff, hypertensive patients, poor peripheral circulation, a leak in the cuff or monitor, low blood pressure, dysrhythmias, or motion artifacts.
3. **Clinical Limitations**
   Automated blood pressure devices do not work well in extreme heart rate and pressure conditions. In extreme conditions, even mean pressure may not be measurable. These monitors are often not as reliable as needed for use in ambulances and helicopters.

REFERENCE

1. Cullen D. Beach chair position may decrease cerebral perfusion. Catastrophic outcomes have occurred. APSF Newslett 2007;22:25, 27.

SUGGESTED READINGS

Dorsch J, Dorsch S. Noninvasive blood pressure monitors. In: Understanding Anesthesia Equipment. Fifth edition. Philadelphia: Wolters Kluwer/Lippincott Williams & Wilkins, 2008:837–844.

Stebor AD. Basic principles of noninvasive blood pressure measurement in infants. Adv Neonatal Care 2005;5:252–261.

23 Ultrasonic Equipment

I. Introduction

A. The use of ultrasound in anesthesia for regional blocks, blood vessel cannulation, and other procedures has increased dramatically. The ability to actually see complex and varied anatomical features (nerves, blood vessels, and surrounding structures) is a major improvement over using surface anatomy (which can vary widely) and guessing where structures are located (especially in patients with difficult external anatomy) or using "clicks" or "pops" as an indication of correct needle placement.

B. This chapter's purpose is to acquaint the clinician with the basics of ultrasound equipment, its uses, and possible problems. To use this technology well, an in-depth understanding of the relevant anatomy is indispensable. Discussing techniques for blocking specific nerves and cannulating specific vessels is beyond the scope of an equipment textbook. The reader is referred to textbooks and articles that describe these techniques.

II. Ultrasound Basics

As an ultrasound wave travels through a medium, some of it reflects back to the source as an echo. The timing and energy of the echo will be related to the depth and the physical nature of the structure encountered by the wave (Fig. 23.1). Structures differ in their ability to reflect sound waves. Hypoechoic structures do not reflect sound waves well and appear gray to black. Anechoic (echo-free) structures appear black. Hyperechoic structures reflect sound waves well and appear light to white. These differences allow ultrasound equipment to image various anatomical features and fluids.

III. Ultrasound Equipment

A. Overview

1. There is great variability in ultrasound equipment. The latest systems are compact, portable, and easy to set up and use. Advances in technology now allow smaller and deeper structures to be imaged. Another advance is increasing automaticity so that the user no longer has to make adjustments in frequency and gain.

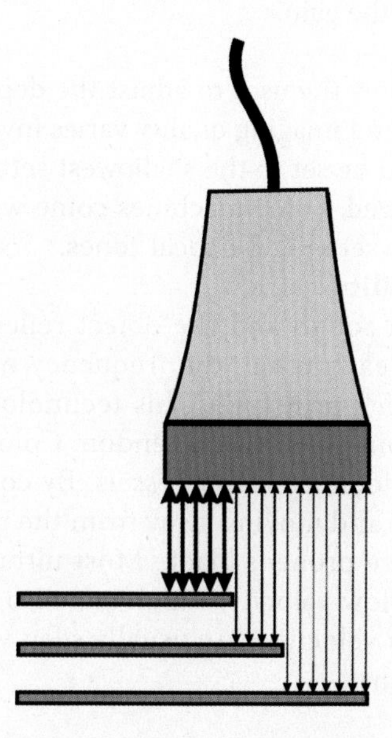

Figure 23.1 As the sound wave is reflected off deeper structures, a weaker echo is generated, as illustrated by the relative thickness of the lines.

2. The choice of an ultrasound system should depend on the available resources and user's needs. A battery pack to power the system without being plugged into main power may be available. The system should offer a choice of probes. Color- and pulse-wave Doppler imaging capability is very useful to accurately identify blood vessels.
3. Irrespective of size or function, six common components are used in all ultrasound machines: master synchronizer, pulser, transducer, processor, display device, and storage device.

B. Master Synchronizer

The master synchronizer organizes and times the flow of electrical signals within the system.

1. **Frequency**

   Increasing wave frequency allows higher resolution (i.e., the amount of details on the image) but limits the tissue penetration. High frequencies are most useful for viewing superficial structures. Lower frequencies allow visualization at greater depth but provide less resolution. Newer ultrasound systems automatically change the frequency as depth (which is set by the operator) changes.
2. **Contrast**

   Modern machines allow the user to adjust the contrast (dynamic range compression). Increasing the contrast makes white images whiter and black images darker. This may produce a better view of the edges of anatomical structures. Decreased contrast makes everything look gray.
3. **Gain**

   Ultrasound systems allow the user to adjust the brightness (gain) of the entire image. Increasing the gain makes the entire image whiter. Increasing the gain too much creates a snowy background in which structures become indistinguishable. In general, the gain should be set so that most of the background is black and only the structures of interest are easily seen. Many machines automatically adjust the gain.
4. **Depth**

   All machines allow the user to adjust the depth to which the ultrasound penetrates. Ultrasound imaging quality varies inversely with penetration depth, so the depth should be set to the shallowest setting at which all the structures of interest are imaged. Some machines come with preset focal zones, and some allow the user to set multiple focal zones.
5. **Doppler Capability**

   If the source of sound and the object reflecting that sound are moving in relationship to each other, the frequency of the reflected sound wave will change (Doppler's principle). This technology can be used to distinguish a blood vessel from a nerve or a tendon. Color-flow doppler ultrasonography can be used to identify blood vessels. By convention, blood flowing toward the probe is red and moving away from the probe is blue. Blood flowing perpendicular to the probe is black. Most ultrasound systems have a means to determine the flow velocity, which can also be used to differentiate arteries and veins. High velocities are usually seen with arteries; low velocities usually indicate veins.

C. Pulser

The pulser (beam former, pulse generator) controls the firing pattern in the transducer.

D. Transducer

1. The transducer (transmitter, probe) converts the electrical signals received from the pulser into a sequence of ultrasound pulses and converts returning acoustic pulses into electrical impulses that are sent to the processor.
2. An ultrasound beam is generated by creating an electrical field across piezoelectric crystals positioned along the transducer surface. Connected to the crystals are wires that transmit electrical impulses from the pulser during the pulse-generation phase and back to the processor when electrical impulses are generated in the crystals by the returning echos. The wire, backing material, and the crystal are housed in a case to protect them from the elements and protect the patient and operator from electrical shock.
3. The active elements can be in a straight line (linear array) or an arc (convex or curved array) (Fig. 23.2). A probe with a smaller footprint (hockey stick) may be needed for areas such as the supraclavicular region where space is limited.
4. The linear array transducer produces a rectangular image. The image is uniform in both near and far fields. There is a 1:1 relationship between the contact portion of the transducer and the image size. A curved transducer is useful when a wide field needs to be imaged. It produces a wedge-shaped ultrasound beam that fans out as it moves to greater depths. It is useful to locate landmarks such as widely separated bones.

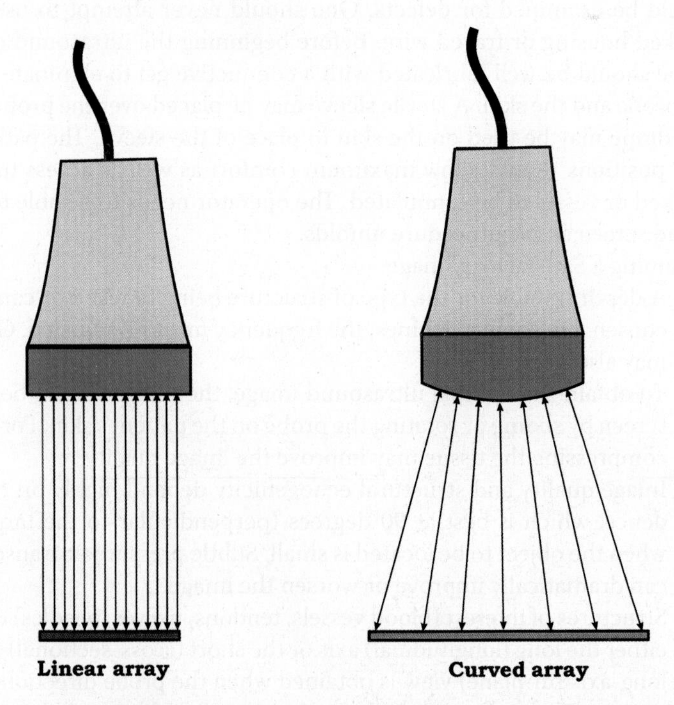

Figure 23.2 With a linear array, a rectangular image that is uniform in both near and far fields is produced. There is a 1:1 relationship between the contact portion of the transducer and the image size. The curved transducer produces an image wider than the transducer.

5. Some ultrasound systems provide an optional needle-guide device for their transducers. This secures the needle to the transducer and directs the needle in a predetermined direction.

E. Processor

The processor contains the necessary elements for conversion of the returning electrical impulses into an image and transmits it to the display.

F. Display

Once an image is formed, it is displayed on a screen in a digital format. There are a number of ways that the information can be displayed. The B-mode displays brightness and produces a body slice. This is the most commonly used mode. The A-mode displays an amplitude signal. The M-mode displays motion against time.

G. Storage Device

The storage device (archive) keeps the information for further review and to meet legal requirements. The equipment should include a high-capacity hard disk to store images and short-film sequences. A CD burner to store files and data transfer capability is desirable.

IV. Performing an Ultrasound Examination

Equipment used to perform vascular cannulation or regional anesthesia such as a marking pen and a ruler; sterile drapes; needles, syringes and local anesthetic for skin infiltration; and specific block needles/catheters should be present. As always, equipment for treating emergencies such as an intravascular injection of local anesthetic should be immediately available.

A. Probe Preparation

The probe suitable for the particular application should be selected. The probe should be examined for defects. One should never attempt to use a probe with a cracked housing or frayed wire. Before beginning the ultrasound examination, the probe should be well lubricated with a conductive gel to eliminate any air between the probe and the skin. A sterile sleeve may be placed over the probe. A sterile adhesive drape may be used on the skin in place of the sleeve. The patient's and operator's positions should allow maximum comfort as well as access to the nerve to be blocked or vessel to be cannulated. The operator needs to be able to view the ultrasound screen as the procedure unfolds.

B. Obtaining a Satisfactory Image

1. A depth suitable for the type of structure being blocked or cannulated must be chosen. On some machines, the frequency must be adjusted. Gain and contrast may also need to be set.
2. To obtain the optimal ultrasound image, the image should be centered on the screen by sliding or rotating the probe on the patient's skin. For deep structures, compressing the tissue may improve the image quality.
3. Image quality and structural echogenicity depend highly on the angle of incidence, which is best at 90 degrees (perpendicular to the target), particularly when the object to be located is small. Subtle pressure or transducer angulation can dramatically improve or worsen the image.
4. Structures of interest (blood vessels, tendons, nerves, needles) can be imaged on either the long (longitudinal) axis or the short (cross-sectional) axis (Fig. 23.3). A long-axis (in-plane) view is obtained when the probe direction is parallel to the structure being viewed. A short (cross-sectional, out-of-plane) axis is obtained when the probe is perpendicular to the structure of interest. A vessel, nerve, or needle appears as a circular structure or a dot. These structures cross the axis only once so the area of interest may be missed or the probe may need to

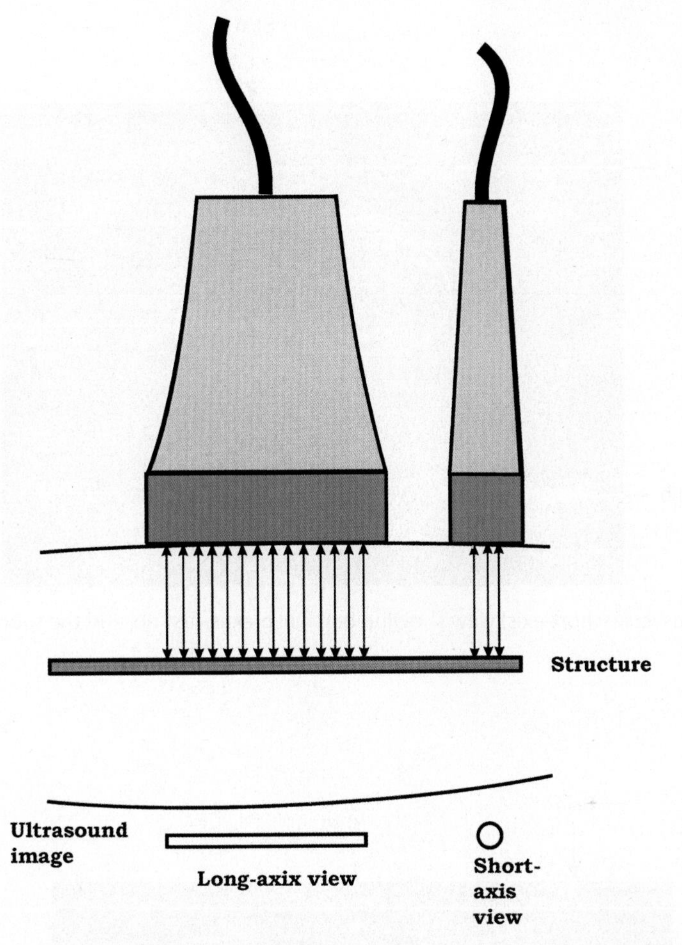

Figure 23.3 Structures may be viewed along the long axis (parallel to the structure) or the short axis (perpendicular to the structure). Along the long axis, the length of the part of the structure being viewed is equal to the width of the transducer. In the short axis, the structure is viewed in cross section and the image corresponds to the cross-sectional shape and size of the structure.

be moved along the structure. If the needle tip is not seen, it may be necessary to inject a small amount of saline, dextrose, or local anesthesia to determine whether the tip is in the field of view.

C. Tissue Identification

The next step is to visualize all the anatomical structures in the target area. All adjustable ultrasound variables (penetration depth, frequency, and gain) should be optimized. Figures 23.4 to 23.7 shows examples of ultrasonic views of various structures.

1. **Nerves and Tendons**
   a. Nerves can be imaged either using a short (cross-section) axis or a long (longitudinal) axis. Peripheral nerves may appear dark (hypoechoic) or bright (hyperechoic), depending on the nerve size, the sonographic frequency, and the ultrasound beam angle. Nerve identity can be confirmed by scanning along the known course of the nerve.
   b. On transverse scans, a nerve can be round, oval, or triangular. A single nerve can have all three shapes along its path. Unlike blood vessels, nerves are not compressible. Most peripheral nerves appear as multiple, round, or

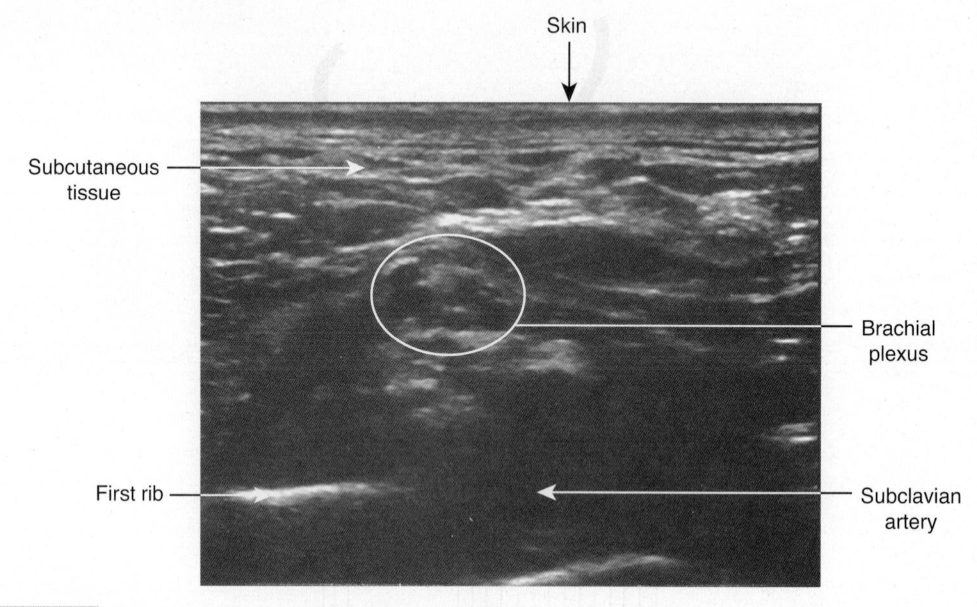

Figure 23.4 Transverse (short-axis) view showing brachial plexus, first rib, and the subclavian artery.

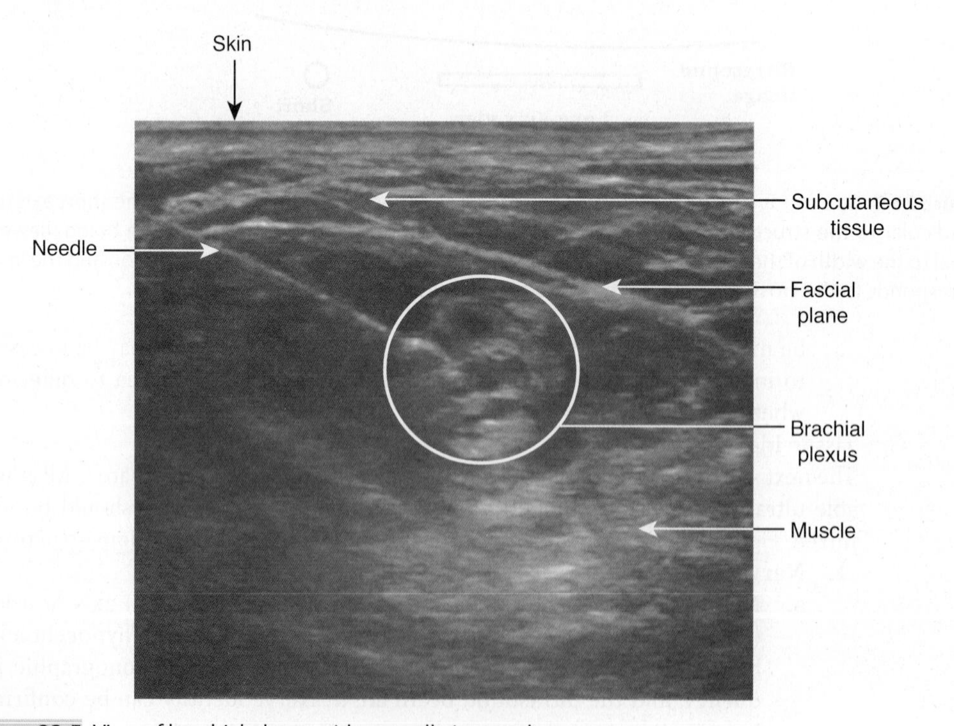

Figure 23.5 View of brachial plexus with a needle inserted.

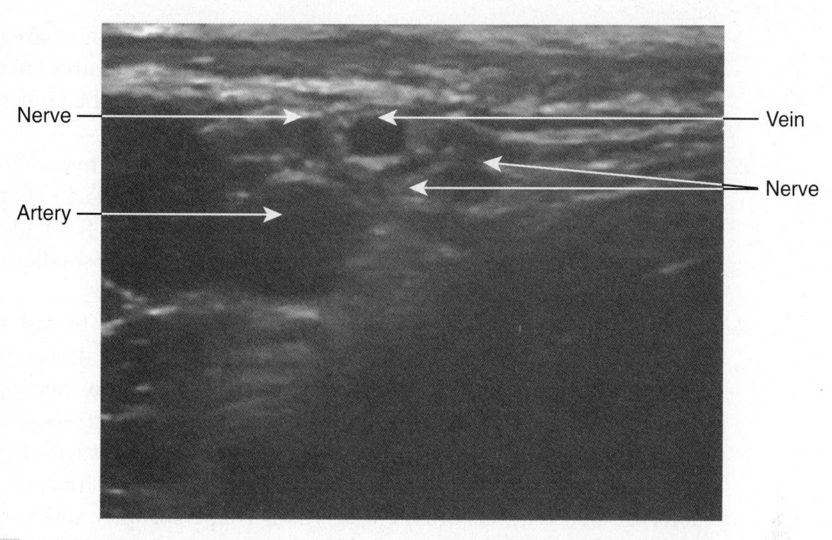

Figure 23.6 Ultrasound view showing an artery, three nerves, and a vein.

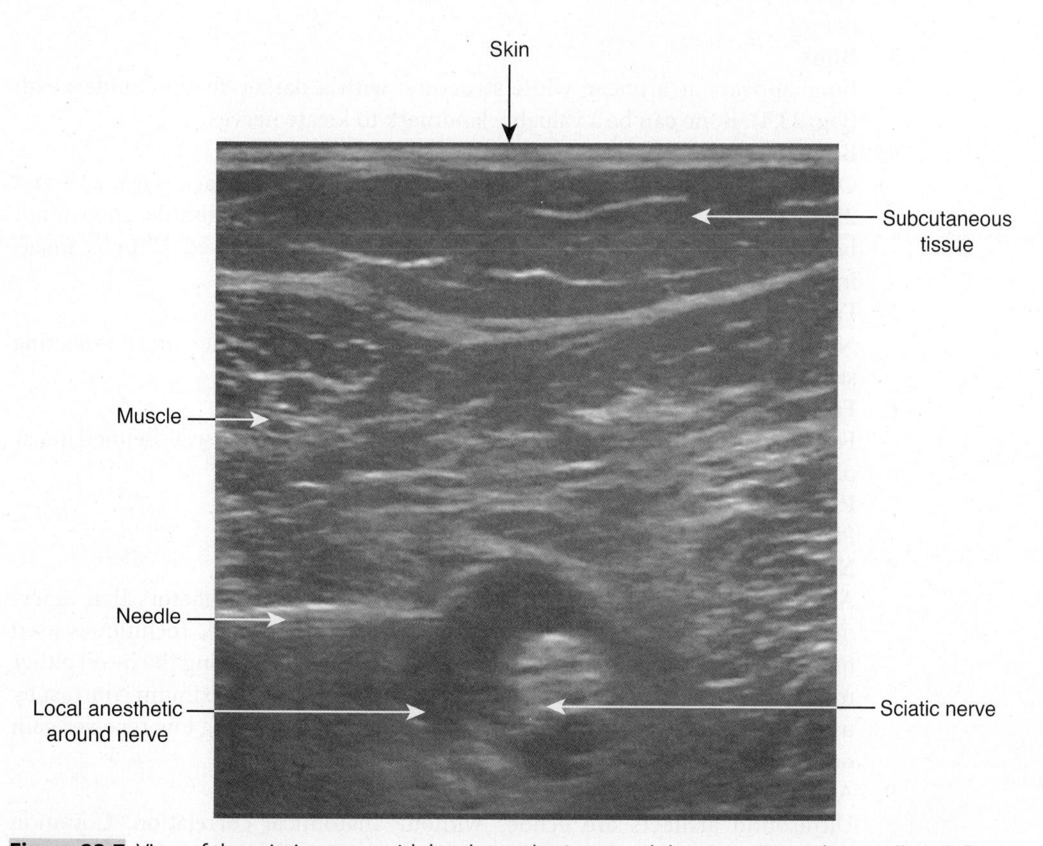

Figure 23.7 View of the sciatic nerve, with local anesthetic around the nerve. Note the needle at left.

oval hypoechoic areas encircled by a relatively hyperechoic area (honeycomb pattern) (Figs. 23.4 to 23.6). The hyperechoic structures are the nerve fascicles, whereas the hypoechoic background reflects the connective tissue between the neuronal structures.

c. In a longitudinal view, each nerve appears as a relatively hyperechoic band characterized by multiple discontinuous hypoechoic (dark) stripes separated by hyperechoic (bright) lines (fasicular pattern). A fascicular pattern is typical of large peripheral nerves and is not seen with smaller nerves or cervical nerve roots, which appear monofascicular.

d. Nerves and tendons have a similar appearance and may be indistinguishable. Tendons have fine parallel lines separated by fine darker lines on a long-axis view. The linearity is more pronounced than for nerves, and the lines are much finer. When tendons are viewed transversely, they have a fibrillar pattern, with fine linear echoes resembling fibrils with hypoechoic areas that are not as prominent. Other ways to distinguish nerves and tendons are that tendons often change their shape abruptly and only form at the end of muscles.

2. **Muscles**
   Muscles have a pinnate or featherlike appearance in the long axis (Figs. 23.5 and 23.7). There is a uniform darker pattern on the short-axis scan. There are darker spaces within the muscles and lighter colors around the muscle than on nerves.
3. **Bone**
   Bone appears as a linear, white structure, with a darker shadow underneath (Fig. 23.4). Bone can be a valuable landmark to locate nerves.
4. **Blood Vessels**
   On the short axis, a blood vessel lumen appears dark to black (Figs. 23.4 and 23.5). Arteries have a more defined circular structure, are pulsatile, and cannot be compressed. Veins are nonpulsatile and can be compressed. Doppler imaging is especially useful for identifying blood vessels.
5. **Fat**
   Normal fatty tissue is dark unless there is a tumor or other more reflecting structure.
6. **Fascia**
   Fascia reflects ultrasound well and appears lighter. There is a well-defined linear pattern that marks tissue boundaries (Fig. 23.5).
7. **Pleura**
   Pleura appears light with darker cavities.
8. **Needles**
   A needle appears light (Figs. 23.5 and 23.7). The primary factors that determine needle visibility are the insertion angle and the gauge. Techniques used to improve needle visibility include using a large needle, facing the bevel either toward or away from the ultrasonic beam, and providing maximum contrast by using a dark background. This can be accomplished by using low receiver gain or injecting a small test dose of local anesthetic.
9. **Artifacts**
   Ultrasound artifacts are echoes without anatomical correlation. Common problems include similar appearance of muscles and nerves, making them difficult to differentiate. There may be anatomical differences that make it hard to determine the source of the ultrasound image. A highly echoic target can

appear hypoechoic or become invisible on the basis of the angle of the ultrasound probe toward the target (angle of insonation). This is called anisotropy. Anisotropy is a problem because differentiation between nerves, muscles, and tendons may be difficult. Anisotropy results from a lack of ultrasonic beam reflection occurring with a loss of a 90-degree incidence angle between the probe and the structure being imaged.

V. **Clinical Uses**

A. Nerve Blocks with Only Ultrasound Guidance

1. The objective of a nerve block is to atraumatically deposit local anesthetic in the correct perineural location. The safety and efficacy of the block rests on the ability to unequivocally identify the nerve(s), needle, and spread of local anesthesia.
2. To be successful at ultrasound-guided neural blockade, one must be familiar with the relevant cross-sectional anatomy and coordinate the imaging probe with the block needle. A pilot scan should be performed to adjust the ultrasound settings and provide an overview of the anatomy.
3. A variety of needles have been developed to help make ultrasound identification easier. Large-bore needles are easier to visualize and are often used for deeper blocks. Generally 22-G needles that have blunt tips (B bevel) are used for ultrasound-guided blocks. These can be seen easily when blocking superficial nerves. For deeper applications, 17-G needles are used.
4. Subcutaneous infiltration is used to render the procedure painless.
5. The probe is held in the operator's nondominant hand and the needle in the dominant hand. The needle should be inserted with the bevel directly facing the active face of the transducer to improve needle-tip visibility.
6. There are two ways to visualize needle movement, both currently in clinical use. The inserted needle may be seen along its full length (long-axis or in-plane) or transversely (short-axis or out-of-plane) (Fig. 23.8). For single-injection nerve

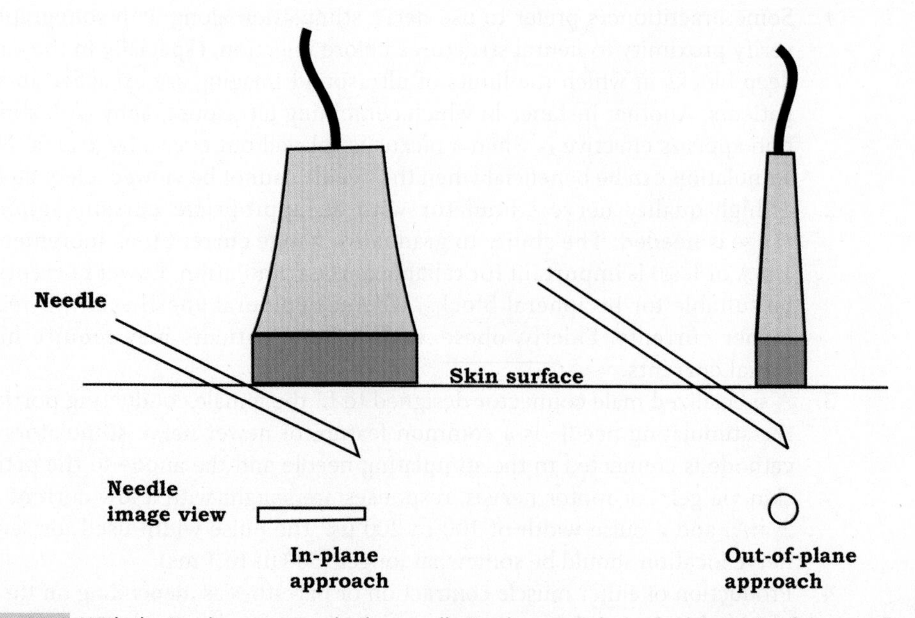

Figure 23.8 With the in-plane approach, the needle is advanced along the long axis of the needle, allowing the part of the needle under the transducer to be viewed. With the out-of-plane approach, a cross-sectional view will be seen.

blocks, the in-plane technique is most often used. For vascular cannulation and inserting a continuous nerve catheter, the out-of-plane technique is usually preferred.

7. With the in-plane approach the needle is advanced in the long axis of the transducer (Fig. 23.8). Needle tip visibility is reduced at steep angles. The transducer is manipulated as necessary to bring the needle into the imaging plane. It may be difficult to keep the needle perfectly parallel to the transducer, making frequent fine adjustments necessary. The entire part of the needle under the transducer, including the tip, should be visualized.
8. If the needle cuts across the transducer's short axis (Fig. 23.4), a cross-sectional view of the needle will be seen. This is known as the out-of-plane technique. The target is typically centered within the field of view and the depth is noted. The needle will be imaged as a small dot, which can be difficult to see. In addition, the needle will cross the ultrasound beam only once. When the needle is visualized, it may be well above or below the target nerve, depending on the insertion angle. Accurate needle tip localization is often inferred by observing local tissue movement or tissue expansion during fluid injection (Fig. 23.7).
9. It is not necessary to contact a nerve with the block needle to surround it with local anesthetic if the correct fascial planes are identified. Test injections to visualize local anesthetic distribution should be small (1 to 2 mL). When local anesthesia is injected around a nerve, a light diffusion area is often seen and the surrounding tissue will often be seen to separate and expand. Nerves will often be easier to identify after the injection of undisturbed local anesthetic and sometimes can be seen to float freely within the injected solution (Fig. 23.7). If the local anesthesia seems to collect on one side of the nerve, the block needle should be repositioned and the test injections continued. If the nerve swells, this may be evidence of an intraneural injection, so the needle should be repositioned.

B. Use in Conjunction with a Nerve Stimulator

1. Some practitioners prefer to use nerve stimulation along with sonography to verify proximity to neural structures before injection, especially in the case of deep blocks in which the limits of ultrasound imaging are exceeded in some patients. Another instance in which combining ultrasonography with stimulation appears effective is when a plexus is splayed out over a large area. Nerve stimulation can be beneficial when the needle cannot be viewed adequately.
2. A high-quality nerve stimulator with an appropriate current amplitude range is needed. The ability to gradually change current (i.e., increments of 1 mA or less) is important for reliable nerve stimulation. Lower currents will be suitable for peripheral blocks, whereas epidural anesthesia will require higher currents. Elderly, obese, and diabetic patients may require higher initial currents.
3. A specialized male connector designed to fit the female conducting portion of the stimulating needle is a common feature of newer nerve stimulators. The cathode is connected to the stimulating needle and the anode to the patient's skin via gel. For motor nerves, responses are sought with a low current (1 to 2 mA) and a pulse width of 100 to 200 μs. The pulse width used for sensory nerve location should be somewhat longer (300 μs to 1 ms).
4. Production of either muscle contraction or paresthesias, depending on the type of stimulated nerve (motor or sensory), indicates needle-tip placement near the nerve. The current intensity is decreased as the needle approaches the nerve. Once the acceptable threshold current is reached, aspiration for potential intravascular

placement is performed. With a negative aspiration, a test injection (1 to 2 mL) of local anesthetic or normal saline is performed. The muscle twitch should diminish following the test injection (the Raj test). If a nonconductive solution (e.g., dextrose in water) is injected, the current density at the needle tip will increase, with resulting maintenance or augmentation of the motor response.

C. Vessel Location and Cannulation

For peripheral venous or arterial cannulation, one operator holds the probe proximal to the insertion site in a transverse plane to the vessel to be cannulated. The vessel is then searched for its suspected anatomic position. Once found, the vessel is lined up in the middle of the probe. A second operator then ascertains the location and depth of the vessel by viewing the ultrasonographic screen. After the usual sterile preparation, the operator advances the needle into the vessel.

VI. **Advantages**

A. Improved Block Quality

Ultrasound guidance can significantly improve nerve block quality and duration for almost all types of regional anesthesia in both adult and pediatric patients. It allows successful block of nerves infrequently blocked in the past. Many nerves can be blocked at alternative, nontraditional locations or using different approaches. Onset time may be faster. In addition to providing real-time guidance of the needle toward a nerve or plexus, ultrasonography allows the anesthesia provider to witness the local anesthetic spread and, if necessary, change the needle-tip position after the initiation of an injection. Finally, continuous peripheral nerve catheters can be placed with ultrasound imaging.

B. Low Complication Rate

1. Ultrasound allows neural and nonneural structures to be directly visualized in order to ensure accurate needle placement and may decrease the incidence of complications such as pneumothorax, hematoma, organ puncture, and accidental intravascular injection. It may allow nerve blocks in patients receiving anticoagulants. Another possible benefit is a reduction in the incidence of systemic local anesthetic toxicity.
2. For patients with difficult intravenous access (obesity, history of intravenous drug abuse, chronic medical problems), using ultrasonography to guide peripheral intravenous cannulation results in a higher rate of successful cannulation, requires less time, decreases the number of percutaneous punctures, and improves patient satisfaction (1). For establishing an indwelling catheter in the radial artery, ultrasound guidance results in more frequent success rates and reduces the time required (2). Using ultrasound guidance for central venous placement also results in a significant reduction in complications (3). The National Institute for Health and Clinical Excellence has recommended using ultrasound guidance for elective central venous cannulation in both adults and children and suggested considering its use in emergency cannulation.

C. Reduced Pain

Ultrasonography can reduce patient discomfort by reducing the number of percutaneous punctures, improving the effectiveness of regional anesthesia, and avoiding paresthesias and muscle contractions during nerve stimulation.

D. Versatility

A wide variety of new techniques of regional blocks have become possible by ultrasound guidance. An advantage of ultrasound guidance is that the block may be repeated at the same site when it begins to dissipate. This is often not feasible with the nerve stimulation technique. A successful block can be achieved using ultrasonography in patients with amputated extremities or other anatomical conditions in which nerve stimulation is not practical.

E. Portability

Because the equipment is portable, it can be easily made available in various locations. Blocks can be performed without moving the patient and while maintaining the usual monitoring and therapies.

F. Cost-effectiveness (4)

Less local anesthetic may be necessary to produce an adequate nerve block. Some studies have demonstrated a shortened procedure time.

G. No Radiation Exposure

Many procedures previously requiring fluoroscopic or computed tomographic guidance can now be performed using ultrasound guidance, obviating the need for radiation exposure.

VII. Complications

A. Nerve Injury

It is difficult to evaluate nerve injury associated with ultrasound-guided nerve blocks, given the low incidence of this problem. Visualization of needle-to-nerve contact and their interaction may help reduce this problem.

B. Intravascular Local Anesthetic Injection

In spite of using correct ultrasonic technique, accidental intravascular local anesthetic injection is still possible. Causes of this problem include technical errors such as failure to evaluate structures using color-flow Doppler ultrasonography, failure to visualize the needle reaching the target, failure to use the correct ultrasound probe for the area being examined, and incorrectly identifying structures. Poor needle insertion site selection and the angle of penetration may prevent needle visualization. The needle tip could have moved into a compressed echo-invisible vein. Local anesthetic injection prior to an intravascular injection could have displaced the vein. It is important that local anesthetic spread be monitored.

VIII. Summary

Ultrasound has an established place in anesthesia. Its usefulness for nerve blocks and vascular cannulation is becoming well recognized. Many clinicians feel that ultrasound-guided nerve blocks and central venous cannulation are or soon will be the standard of care. It offers advantages in other areas as well. Ultrasonography has been used to assess the subglottic diameter, which may help in assessing the appropriate size of tracheal tube; locating the trachea in percutaneous dilatational tracheostomy in patients with difficult anatomy; and providing information for a variety of other situations, including cardiac tamponade, lymphadenopathy, pneumothorax, severe hypovolemia, presence or absence of cardiac activity during a cardiac arrest, evaluation of bladder volume, plural effusion, and vascular anatomical variations including aneurysms.

REFERENCES

1. Constantino TG, Parikh AK, Satz WA, Fojtik JP. Ultrasonography-guided peripheral intravenous access versus traditional approaches in patients with difficult intravenous access. Ann Emerg Med 2005;46:456–461.
2. Wigmore TJ, Smythe JF, Hackig MB, et al. Effect of the implementation of NICE guidelines for ultrasound guidance on the complication rates associated with central venous catheter placement in patients presenting for routine surgery in a tertiary referral centre. Br J Anaesth 2007;99:663–665.
3. Shiver S, Blalvas M, Lyon M. A prospective comparison of ultrasound-guided and blindly placed radial arterial catheters. Acad Emerg Med 2006;13:1275–1279.
4. DeConciliis G. Justifying the cost of ultrasound for blocks. How is it worth the capital investment if your facility can't bill for it. Outpatient Surg Mag 2010;9:88–89.

SUGGESTED READINGS

Bigeleisen PE. Ultrasound-Guided Regional Anesthesia and Pain Medicine. Philadelphia: Wolters Kluwer/Lippincott Williams & Wilkins, 2010.

Gray AT. Ultrasound-guided regional anesthesia. Current state of the art. Anesthesiology 2006;104:368–373.

Gray AT. Atlas of Ultrasound-Guided Regional Anesthesia. Philadelphia: Elsevier/Saunders, 2009.

Levitov A, Mayo PH, Slonim AD. Critical Care Ultrasonography. New York: McGraw Hill, 2009.

Marhofer P, Grener M, Kapral S. Ultrasound guidance in regional anaesthesia. Br J Anaesth 2005;94:7–17.

Randolph AD, Cook DJ, Gonzales CA, Pribble CG. Ultrasound guidance for placement of central venous catheters: a meta-analysis of the literature. Crit Care Med 1996;24:2053–2058.

Sites BD. Ultrasound-Guided Regional Anesthesia: Let Vision Guide You. Orlando, FL: American Society of Anesthesiologists, 2008. ASA Refresher Course No. 101.

Tsui BCH. Atlas of Ultrasound and Nerve Stimulation-Guided Regional Anesthesia. New York: Springer, 2007.

V

Equipment Related to Environmental Situations

24 Temperature Monitoring and Control

I. Indications for Temperature Monitoring

A. The monitoring guidelines of the American Society of Anesthesiologists state that every patient receiving anesthesia shall have his or her temperature monitored when clinically significant changes in body temperature are intended, anticipated, or suspected. The Standards for Nurse Anesthesia Practice state that one must monitor body temperature continuously on all pediatric patients receiving general anesthesia and, when indicated, on all other patients.

B. Temperature monitoring should be performed whenever large volumes of cold blood and/or intravenous fluids are administered; when the patient is deliberately cooled and/or warmed; during surgery of substantial duration; in hypothermic or pyrexial patients or those with a suspected or known temperature regulatory problem such as malignant hyperthermia; and patients in whom hyperthermia may be expected, including those with a fever, infection, blood transfusion, or an allergic reaction. Major surgical procedures, especially those involving body cavities, should be considered a strong indication for temperature monitoring.

II. Monitoring Technologies

A. A variety of technologies are available to measure temperature. None is suitable for all situations. Many devices simply display the temperature. These are less than optimal, because a high or low temperature may go unnoticed for some time. Most modern devices have alarms that can be set if the temperature exceeds a high or low limit. Temperature monitoring is available on most physiologic monitors used in the operating room (OR) and perioperative areas, often with the ability to measure the temperature at two different sites (**Fig. 24.1**). These usually have the ability to trend the temperature and transfer temperature information to an electronic record.

B. Technologies available today for temperature monitoring include the thermistor, in which the current measures the change in resistance of a metal oxide sensor sintered onto a wire or bead. Thermistors are small and inexpensive.

C. A thermocouple consists of an electrical circuit that has two dissimilar metals welded together at their ends. One of the two metal junctions remains at a constant

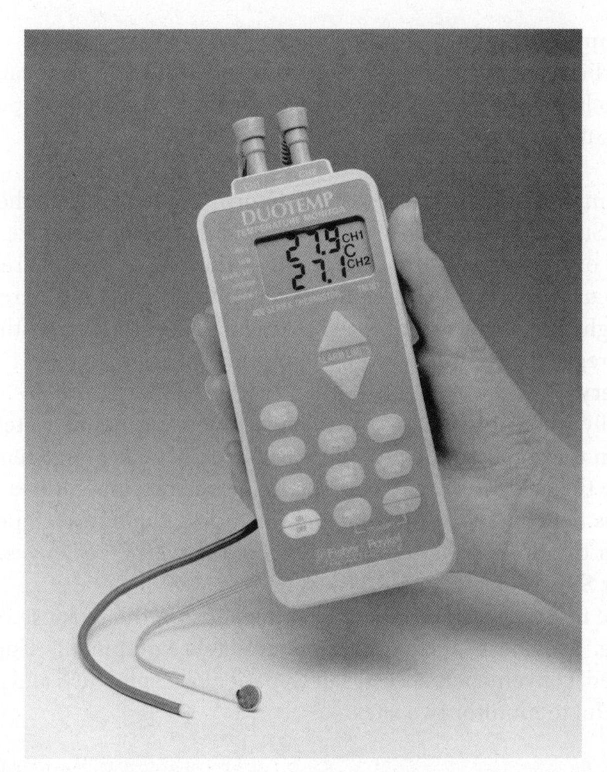

Figure 24.1 Monitor with capability for monitoring temperature at two sites and alarms. (Courtesy of Fisher Paykel Healthcare, Auckland, New Zealand.)

temperature, whereas the other is exposed to the area being measured, producing a voltage difference that is measured and converted to a temperature reading.

D. The electrical resistance of platinum wire varies almost linearly with temperature. By employing an extremely small diameter wire, rapid thermal equilibration is possible. Resistance is measured in a manner similar to a thermistor.

E. The liquid crystal thermometer has an adhesive backing with plastic-encased liquid crystals on a black background. The crystals are arranged so that letters and numbers are formed. The covering over the adhesive is removed, and the disc or strip is placed on the skin. The liquid crystal thermometer is available in two forms: one displays the skin temperature directly, and the other has a built-in correction factor (offset) so that the temperature displayed estimates core temperature. These devices are less accurate than other devices. Extreme ambient temperature, humidity, and air movement can cause inaccuracy. Other disadvantages include the need for subjective observer interpretation, the inability to interface with a recording system, difficulties with adhesion due to skin secretions, and allergic reactions to the adhesive backing. They are capable of measuring temperature only on the skin.

F. An infrared thermometer measures a portion of the infrared radiation from surfaces within its field of view. The displayed value may be the actual temperature (unadjusted, calibration mode) or with an offset to estimate temperature at another site based on selected study samples (site-equivalent mode). There are a number of problems with infrared thermometry. Measurements are intermittent. Poor penetration, improper aiming, and obstructions such as curvatures in the ear canal can result in significantly lower temperatures being reported.

III. Thermal Compartments

Although arbitrary, it is useful to divide the body into two thermal compartments: the core that includes the deep, vital internal organs and a shell of peripheral tissue that serves as insulation for the core.

A. Core

Core temperature is normally more uniform and higher than the peripheral temperatures. Sites differ as to how well they reflect core temperature. The difference may depend on the temperature change rate at that site. A site that reflects core temperature accurately when temperature change is slow may fail to reflect rapid changes. Although core temperature is tightly regulated in the unanesthetized patient, general or regional anesthesia reduces thermoregulation.

B. Periphery

Normally, thermoregulatory vasoconstriction maintains a temperature gradient between the core and the periphery of 2°C to 4°C. Regional temperature variations exist in the periphery. The correlation between temperatures measured at different sites depends on several factors, including the body temperature stability and whether or not there have been recent cold or warm challenges.

IV. Monitoring Sites

The best site for temperature monitoring depends on the purpose of the measurement, surgical site, anesthesia technique, and available equipment. Considerations should include speed, convenience, access, safety, patient acceptability, and cost-effectiveness. It may be helpful to monitor two sites.

CLINICAL MOMENT The difference in temperature between the core and a peripheral site can provide indirect information on blood flow (slow change = poor blood flow) and is helpful in guarding against an overshoot during warming or cooling.

A. Pulmonary Artery

Pulmonary artery temperature can be measured in patients who have a Swan-Ganz catheter in place. It is thought by many to be the best way to measure core body temperature. Pulmonary artery temperature generally correlates well with intrathecal and jugular bulb temperatures, even during rapid cooling and rewarming. Poor correlation with brain temperature occurs during profound hypothermia. Pulmonary artery readings are not reliable during thoracotomy or cardiopulmonary bypass.

B. Esophagus

1. Esophageal temperature can be measured by using a simple probe, an esophageal stethoscope with a thermistor (**Fig. 24.2**), or a gastric tube with a temperature sensor (**Fig. 24.3**).

CLINICAL MOMENT The temperature in the esophagus may vary up to 4°C. The esophageal temperature should be measured with the sensor located in the lower third or fourth of the esophagus. In adults, this is approximately 38 to 42 cm below the central incisors or at least 24 cm below the larynx. Placing the sensor in this position will minimize (but not completely eliminate) the effect of respired gases. When the sensor is part of an esophageal stethoscope, the ideal placement depth is 12 to 16 cm distal to the point of maximum heart sounds. If the probe is placed higher in the esophagus, the reading will be lower. If the probe is placed in the stomach, it may record temperatures higher than core, reflecting liver metabolism. The response to temperature change is slow when the probe is in the stomach.

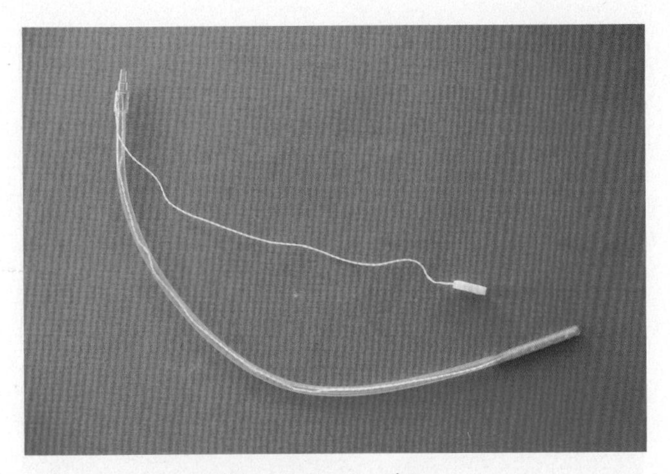

Figure 24.2 Esophageal stethoscope and temperature probe.

2. Esophageal temperature is considered core temperature by many investigators. Temperature measured in this location has shown good agreement with pulmonary artery temperature. During rapid warming or cooling, esophageal temperature shows less lag time than that measured at most other sites, although some studies found that bladder temperature showed a closer approximation to pulmonary artery temperature than the esophageal temperature. Brain temperature may be adequately reflected by esophageal temperature during mild, but not profound, hypothermia.
3. Continuous gastric suctioning will decrease esophageal temperature.
4. If an esophageal probe is used for the patient in the sitting or prone position, oral secretions can track down to the connection between the probe and monitor cable. This can lead to incorrect readings.

C. Nasopharynx

The temperature in the nasopharynx is measured with a sensor in contact with the nasopharyngeal wall. This location places the probe close to the hypothalamus. Although some studies show a good correlation between nasopharyngeal

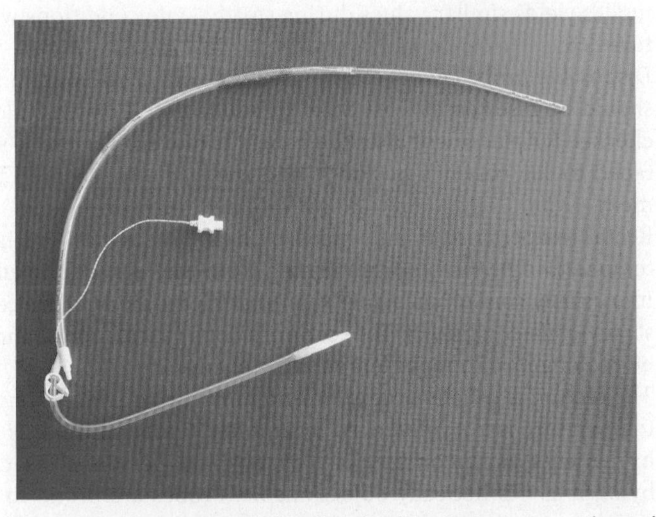

Figure 24.3 Gastric tube with temperature probe. This also functions as an esophageal stethoscope.

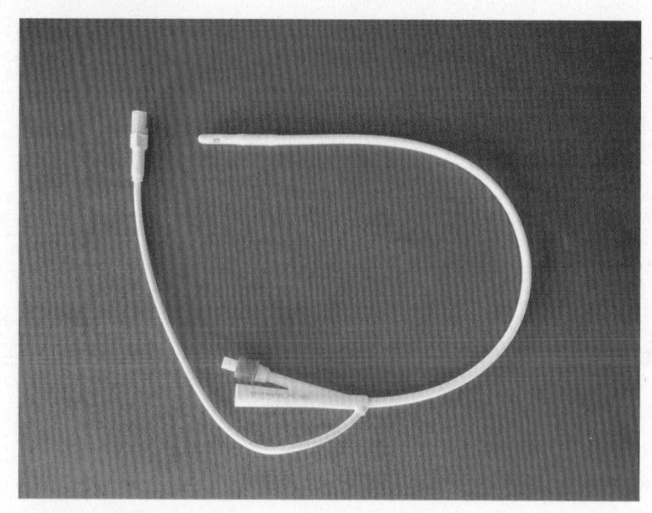

Figure 24.4 Urinary catheter with temperature sensor near the patient end.

temperature and core temperature, other studies have found the correlation less satisfactory.

D. Urinary Bladder

Urinary bladder temperature monitoring involves inserting an indwelling urinary catheter with a thermistor or thermocouple near the patient end (**Fig. 24.4**). Urinary bladder temperature usually correlates well with temperature measured at the nasopharynx, pulmonary artery, and esophagus but may lag behind during rapid warming or cooling. Correlation with these sites will be increased with a high urine flow.

E. Rectum

1. Electronic rectal thermometers may have two measurement modes: dwell or predictive. In the dwell mode, the temperature is displayed continuously. A minimum of 2 to 3 minutes is needed to reach a stable temperature. The predictive mode estimates the temperature on the basis of a temperature rise curve. It requires only 30 seconds. A comparison of measurements between the two modes yields similar values during steady-state conditions with mild temperature flux.
2. Disposable probe covers can be used to avoid cross contamination. The probe should be inserted at least 8 cm in adults and 3 cm in children. It should be checked for placement after the patient is moved. The probe should be securely taped to the patient's buttocks, and the lead wire secured to avoid displacement.
3. Rectal temperature is influenced by heat-producing flora in the rectum, the temperature of the blood returning from the legs, and insulation from feces. It is usually somewhat higher than that measured at more central sites during steady-state conditions. The rectum is not a vascular area, and the lag time may be prolonged with rapid temperature changes.
4. The rectum is usually accessible and monitoring relatively noninvasive. Rectal temperature is not influenced by ambient temperature. It is generally disliked by patients as uncomfortable, by hospital personnel as cumbersome, and by both as aesthetically objectionable. Probes are prone to come out during

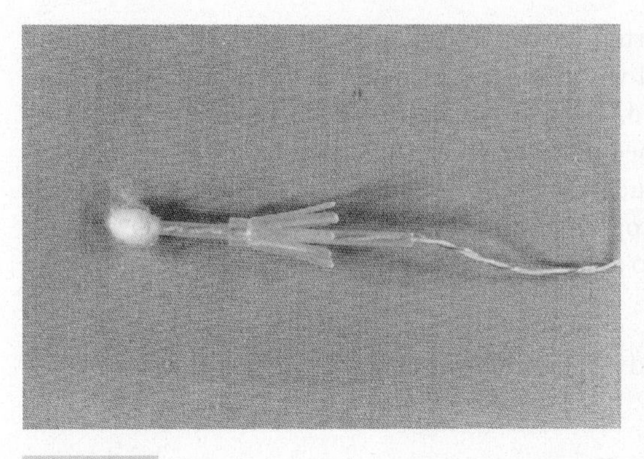

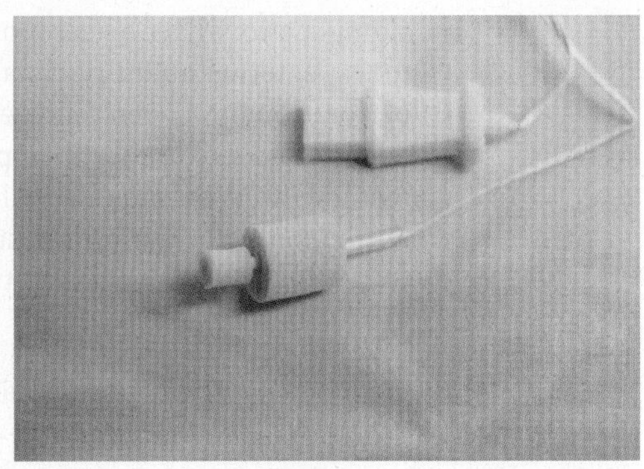

Figure 24.5 Tympanic membrane temperature probes.

recovery from anesthesia. Other disadvantages are the relative inaccessibility during surgery and the risk of bacterial contamination. Contraindications include gynecologic and urologic procedures. Bowel perforation is a risk. A pararectal abscess and pneumoperitoneum have been reported after using a rectal probe.

F. Tympanic Membrane

1. The tympanic membrane is deep within the skull and separated from the internal carotid artery by only the narrow, air-filled cleft in the middle ear and a thin bone shell. The tympanic membrane and the hypothalamus share a common blood supply, so measuring temperature at this site may reflect thermal information at the primary thermoregulation site.
2. Temperature can be measured by inserting a thermistor or thermocouple probe into the external auditory canal until it contacts the tympanic membrane (**Fig. 24.5**). Because tympanic membrane perforation is a danger, clinicians tend not to place the probe far enough into the canal. If it does not touch the membrane, the readings will not be accurate. For awake patients, appropriate placement is confirmed when the patient easily detects a gentle rubbing by the attached wire. After the probe is inserted, the aural canal should be occluded with cotton wool and covered externally to prevent ambient air movement from cooling the probe.
3. Numerous studies have shown a good correlation between tympanic membrane temperature and the temperature measured in the esophagus, pulmonary artery, or urinary bladder. Temperature may be less accurate during rapid changes. This location is considered a measurement site for core temperature.

CLINICAL MOMENT Head position can cause asymmetric changes in the tympanic temperatures. Upon assuming a lateral position, the temperature on the lower side increases whereas that on the upper side decreases.

4. Advantages of tympanic membrane temperature monitoring include cleanliness and convenience. It is tolerated by conscious patients, making it useful for postoperative monitoring. The site is readily accessible during most surgical procedures.

5. Complications have been reported. Discharge or fluid oozing from the ear, trauma to the external auditory canal with subsequent external otitis, and membrane perforation have been reported. These complications occurred before the introduction of flexible cotton-tipped probes that are less traumatic. Recommended methods to avoid trauma include otoscopic ear canal and tympanic membrane inspection before insertion, stopping insertion as soon as resistance is felt, and placement in awake patients to assess discomfort.

CLINICAL MOMENT The probe should not be inserted into the ear canal while the head is being moved.

6. Contraindications include any ear abnormality that would prevent correct placement, a skull fracture that passes through the osseous meatus, and a perforated tympanic membrane.

G. Ear Canal

1. Infrared ear thermometry (infrared emission detection thermometry, infrared tympanic membrane thermometry, infrared tympanic thermometry) is performed by inserting an otoscope-like probe into the external ear canal (**Fig. 24.6**). The tip is usually covered by a disposable cover. The device detects the amount of infrared heat emitted. The widely angled probe will measure ear canal and tympanic membrane temperature.
2. Since these thermometers are known to give temperatures lower than core temperatures, some manufacturers provide offsets to estimate the temperature at other sites. The offsets vary for different brands.
3. A tug on the ear to straighten the canal while taking a reading was found by some investigators to improve correlation with core temperatures. Other studies did not find that an ear tug was helpful. The device should be inserted with a gentle back and forth motion. A firm but gentle pressure should be applied to seal the canal from ambient air.
4. Many studies have compared temperatures obtained by infrared ear thermometers to temperatures obtained from other sites. The correlations vary from excellent to poor. There is considerable variation among different instruments

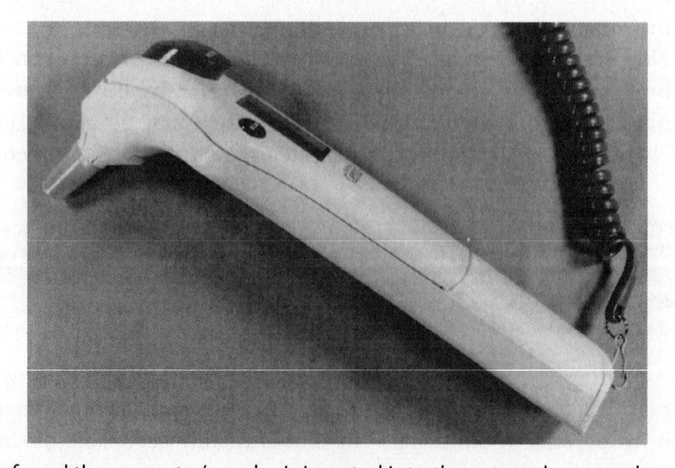

Figure 24.6 The infrared thermometer's probe is inserted into the external ear canal.

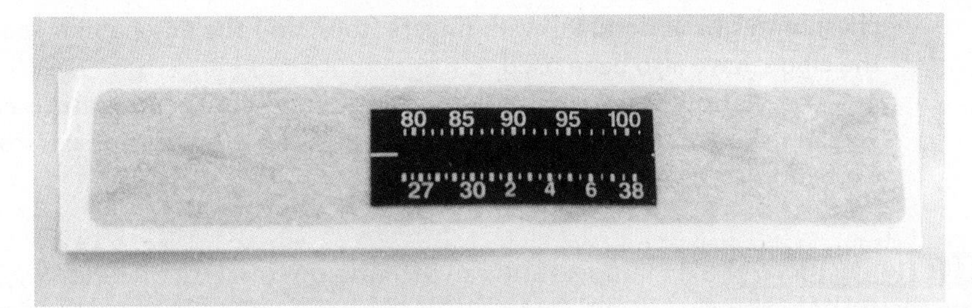

Figure 24.7 The flexible adhesive-backed strip of this liquid crystal temperature monitor has a black background. To use, the covering over the adhesive is removed, and the monitor is placed on the skin.

and with different individuals using the same instrument. A difference of 1.6°C between the two ears has been reported. Readings are affected by the ambient temperature. If the face is cooled, there will be a decreased reading. Acute otitis media will not influence the reading unless there is suppuration, in which case the reading will be increased.

CLINICAL MOMENT Ear canal temperature is a spot-check method. It is not useful for continuous monitoring.

H. Skin

1. Skin temperature can be measured by using a liquid crystal device (**Fig. 24.7**), a thermocouple, or a thermistor (**Fig. 24.8**). Some skin probes have a special backing to attach to the body and material to insulate the sensor from ambient conditions. An opaque dressing and/or tape over the sensor may decrease environmental effects.
2. Skin temperature is most commonly measured at the forehead because this site has a fairly good blood flow and there is not much underlying fat. The back,

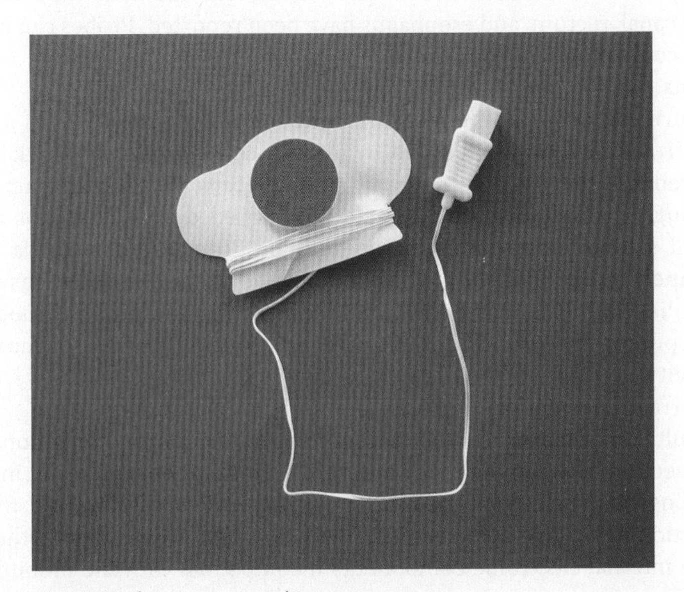

Figure 24.8 Disposable probe for measuring skin temperature.

chest, anterior abdominal wall, fingers, toes, and the antecubital space inside the elbow have also been used.

3. The correlation between skin temperature and core temperature is controversial. Skin temperature varies markedly as a function of environmental exposure.

CLINICAL MOMENT Skin temperature can increase up to 4°C to 6°C after a successful nerve block.

I. Axilla

To measure axillary temperature, a thermocouple or thermistor is positioned over the axillary artery and the arm is adducted. Equilibration may take as long as 10 to 15 minutes. Although a few studies found satisfactory correlation with more central sites, most studies show poor correlation.

J. Mouth

1. Sublingual temperature is measured by placing a probe in one of the pockets on either side of the tongue's frenulum. The patient's mouth should be closed and enough time allowed for the reading to stabilize. This area contains small muscular arteries that respond to mastication or hot or cold liquids by expanding or contracting.
2. Correlation with temperatures measured at more central sites varies somewhat but in general is fairly satisfactory. Sublingual thermometers are well tolerated by patients. Readings are not affected by the presence or absence of teeth, intubation, oxygen administration, a nasogastric tube on continuous suction, or the inspired gas temperature. Sublingual temperature may be inaccurate if the patient is a mouth breather or has tachypnea. Warm and cold ambient temperatures have a small effect on oral temperatures.

V. Hazards of Thermometry

A. Injury at the Monitoring Site

Tympanic membrane and rectal perforation and trauma to the nose, external auditory canal, rectum, and esophagus have been reported. Probes can have sharp edges that could present a hazard.

B. Burns

A burn can occur at the measurement site if the probe acts as a ground for the electrosurgical apparatus. No insulation can completely block radiofrequency currents. If there is no other satisfactory return path for the current, it can burn through insulation. Using a battery-operated device does not guarantee electrical safety, because the chassis may be grounded through a metal support. Temperature probes should be examined before use to detect insulation damage. Esophageal burns may be avoided by inserting the probe through a small tube and pulling the probe back into the tube during periods of maximal electrical activity.

C. Incorrect Information

A faulty probe can cause an incorrect temperature display. Secretions or fluids in the connection between the probe and reading instrument can result in falsely elevated readings. If the electricity in a battery-powered device is depleted, the unit may stop functioning or give incorrect information. Using probes that fit the receptacle but have internal electronic components incompatible with the monitor can give false readings.

D. Probe Contamination

Reusable temperature probes may be a source of bacterial or viral pathogens even if protective covers are used.

E. Faulty Probes

A probe should be inspected after it is removed from its packaging. A part of the sheath on an esophageal probe could break off and be aspirated.

VI. Temperature Control

A. Physiology

1. Numerous studies have shown that significant temperature changes routinely occur in anesthetized patients. Inadvertent hypothermia is by far the most common disturbance. Without specific interventions, up to 90% of patients entering the postanesthesia care unit (PACU) may be hypothermic. An exception may be patients undergoing magnetic resonance imaging (MRI), in whom the absorption of radiofrequency radiation may partially offset heat loss.
2. Core body temperature is normally maintained within a narrow range of 37 ± 0.2°C. When core body temperature goes out of this range, physiologic mechanisms to reestablish the norm are initiated. Responses to altered temperatures are less effective under anesthesia.
3. Hypothermia under anesthesia usually follows a characteristic pattern. Core body temperature decreases 0.5°C to 1.5°C during the first hour, as vasodilatation causes redistribution of body heat from the core to the periphery. Warming peripheral tissues before inducing anesthesia (prewarming) decreases the central-to-peripheral temperature gradient, thereby minimizing heat redistribution from the core to the periphery and reducing the initial decrease in core temperature. This redistribution cannot be prevented by intraoperative skin surface warming.
4. After the first hour, core temperature typically decreases at a slower rate as the body's heat loss exceeds the metabolic heat production. This is followed by a thermal plateau during which core temperature no longer significantly decreases. At this time, heat loss is in equilibrium with heat production and vasoconstriction constrains metabolic heat to the core compartment while allowing peripheral tissues to continue to cool. Patients with neuropathies have more severe hypothermia than other patients, possibly because the onset of vasoconstriction is delayed. A plateau may never be reached when regional anesthesia blocks vasoconstriction. This puts these patients at greater risk for hypothermia.
5. In postanesthetic patients, vasoconstriction inhibits rewarming. For this reason, patients should be warmed during surgery rather than allowed to cool and then "rescued" postoperatively. Warming may be accelerated by using certain drugs or with a sympathetic block.

B. Heat Loss Mechanismss

Most heat is lost via the skin surface. This loss is roughly proportional to the skin-to-environment temperature gradient and the body surface area in contact with a lower temperature environment. Pediatric patients have a high body surface area to mass ratio and thus tend to cool more quickly than adults but also rewarm more quickly.

1. **Radiation**

   Radiation is the loss of electromagnetic energy through infrared rays from the warm body to colder objects in the room that do not contact the body. It typically accounts for 65% to 70% of the body's heat loss. Radiant heat loss is a function of the difference in temperature between the patient and objects in the OR and their heat emissivity.

2. **Convection**
   The second major heat loss mechanism is convection. This is the transfer of heat to an air current. The magnitude of convective heat exchange is determined by the temperature gradient between the body and the air as well as the air velocity. Most of the heat lost by this mechanism occurs when body surfaces are exposed prior to surgical draping. Surgical drapes prevent most convective heat loss during surgery.
3. **Conduction**
   The third heat loss mechanism is conduction. Heat is lost through direct contact between the patient and colder objects such as the operating table, linens, surgical instruments, skin preparation materials, irrigation, and intravenous (IV) fluids. The heat flow is proportional to the temperature difference between the body and the colder object. Relatively little heat is lost to objects such as the OR table pad, but heat lost when cold preparatory and irrigation solutions and IV fluids are used can significantly reduce body temperature.
4. **Evaporation**
   The fourth heat loss mechanism is evaporation. Evaporation losses occur from the skin, respiratory tract, open surgical wounds, pneumoperitoneum, or wet towels and drapes that are in direct contact with the patient's body.
5. **Other Factors**
   A number of factors determine the severity of hypothermia. The surgical site is an important consideration since large cavities are subject to considerable heat loss from evaporation, whether open or laparoscopic techniques are used. Administering large quantities of cool IV or irrigation fluids will further chill the patient. Long surgical procedures, extremes of age, cachexia, female sex, and low body mass are associated with hypothermia.

C. Problems Associated with Hypothermia

Hypothermia is a potential cause of adverse patient outcomes and may be associated with life-threatening complications. Small patients and those in weakened conditions will be more susceptible to the negative effects. Maintaining patient's temperature decreases postoperative mortality and improves outcome.

1. **Metabolic Changes**
   Adverse metabolic changes include the oxyhemoglobin dissociation curve shifting to the left, metabolic product accumulation, and increased lactic acidosis.
2. **Shivering and Thermal Discomfort**
   Hypothermia is associated with postoperative shivering, which is often intense and uncontrollable. It causes patient discomfort; increased metabolic demand and cardiorespiratory work; increased intraocular and intracranial pressures; and interferes with monitoring, especially electrocardiography (ECG) and pulse oximetry. Skin temperature is equal in importance to core temperature in determining thermal comfort.
3. **Increased Recovery Time and Length of Stay**
   Most studies have shown that intraoperative hypothermia causes slower awakening and longer times in the PACU, even when temperature is not a discharge criterion. Hypothermia may cause postoperative confusion. Maintaining normothermia may shorten hospitalization.
4. **Impaired Drug Tolerance**
   Hypothermia alters drug distribution and decreases drug metabolism. This often results in higher blood concentrations and prolonged duration of action.

5. **Hypovolemia**
   Hypothermia can lead to fluid shifts from the vascular to the extracellular space and relative hypovolemia. Cold-induced diuresis can occur, adding to the problem. Patients with hypothermia have significantly greater fluid and transfusion requirements. Peripheral vasoconstriction can make it more difficult to insert peripheral venous catheters. Active local warming facilitates IV catheter insertion.
6. **Cardiovascular System Effects**
   Hypothermia enhances sympathetic activity. Peripheral vasoconstriction, which reflects the body's effort to conserve heat, can result in increased blood pressure and cardiac workload as well as ECG changes. Risks include cardiac dysrhythmias, decreased contractility, myocardial ischemia and infarction, and cardiac arrest. Hypothermia can result in increased adverse hemodynamic events and increased requirements for vasoactive drugs. Normothermia is associated with a reduction in the incidence of postoperative morbid cardiac events in patients with known risk factors for coronary artery disease. Cardiovascular system effects are modest in young, generally healthy patients.

CLINICAL MOMENT Rapidly rewarming patients with profound hypothermia can result in shock due to blood redistribution to the periphery.

7. **Effects on Coagulation**
   Hypothermia inhibits platelet function and activation of the coagulation cascade. It may be associated with increased blood loss and higher transfusion requirements.
8. **Reduced Resistance to Infection**
   Even mild hypothermia may delay healing and predispose patients to wound and other infections. An increased rate of surgical site infections can occur with mild hypothermia (1). Warming may prevent postoperative wound infection and pressure ulcers (2, 3). Maintaining normothermia in patients undergoing colorectal surgery is a performance measure of the Surgical Care Improvement Project and is recommended to decrease the risk of surgical site infections (4).
9. **Interference with Monitoring**
   Thermoregulatory vasoconstriction decreases cutaneous blood flow and may interfere with pulse oximetry and other forms of monitoring. Shivering may interfere with ECG monitoring.
10. **Increased Costs**
    Hypothermic patients have prolonged stays in the intensive care unit and healthcare facility. Normothermic heart surgery patients require decreased ventilatory support. Active warming may result in a reduction in costs (2, 3).
11. **Other**
    Cold agglutinins may be associated with infection. Vascular obstruction and even gangrene may result. Cooling may cause a decrease in urine output. The agreement of central and peripheral venous pressures deteriorates at lower temperatures. Increased pain and anxiety may be associated with hypothermia. Hypothermia may make IV cannulation more difficult.

VII. Warming Devices

A. Warming Methods

It is generally accepted that no single technique is superior in combating hypothermia. The best results are achieved by combining methods. The costs, risks, and benefits of warming should be considered for each patient, factoring in preexisting medical conditions and the surgical procedure.

1. **Forced-Air Warming Devices**
   a. Forced-air warming devices (convective warming devices, warm air blowers) entrain ambient air through a microbial filter. The filtered air is warmed using an electric heater and then blown through a hose that is connected to an inflatable patient cover. The temperature may be monitored within the warming unit or at the end of the delivery hose. Most units offer temperature selection.
   b. A variety of covers, both disposable and reusable, are available (**Figs. 24.9** to **24.12**). They have a series of holes that allow the warm, filtered air to pass through. Another design uses a fabric that allows the heated air to filter through the entire patient side of the cover.
   c. Placing a blanket or sheet over the warming blanket will result in increased heat transfer. Lower body warming is slightly more effective than upper body warming. Underbody blankets allow easy access to the patient, but they are probably useful only for very small patients.

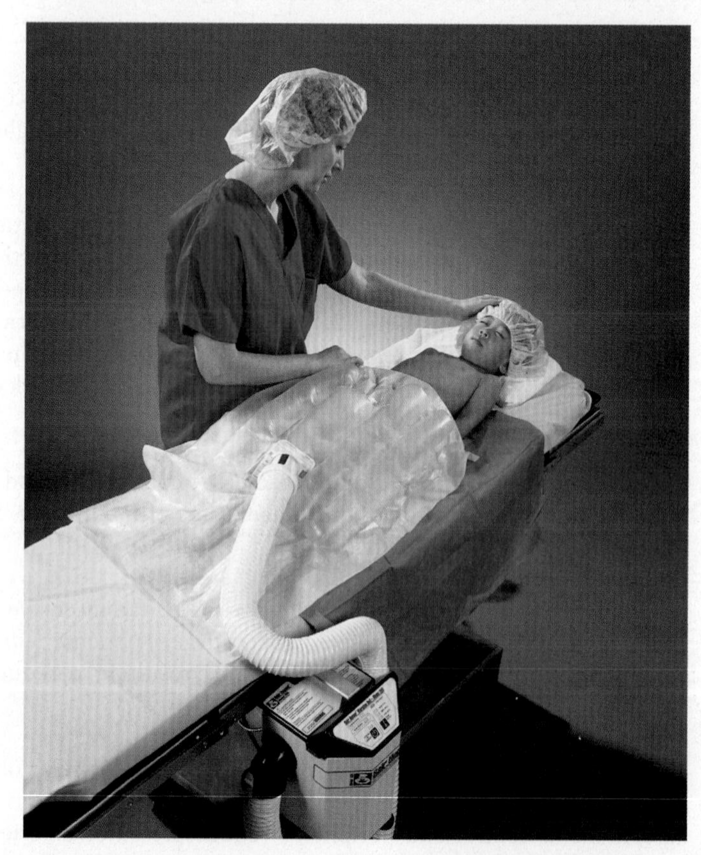

Figure 24.9 Forced air-warming device with lower body blanket. (Photograph courtesy of Arizant Healthcare, Eden Prairie, MN.)

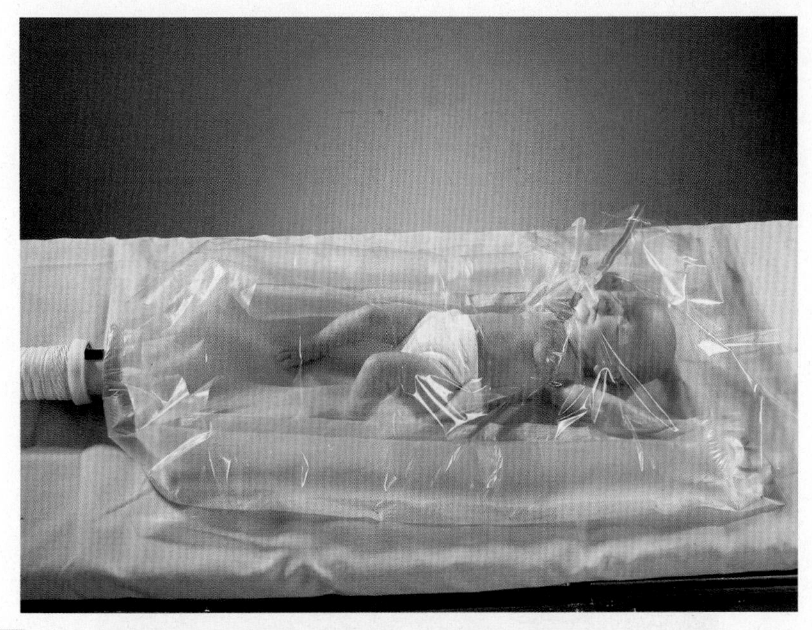

Figure 24.10 Warming blanket for a small patient. Note the plastic cover over the child. (Photograph courtesy of Arizant Healthcare, Eden Prairie, MN.)

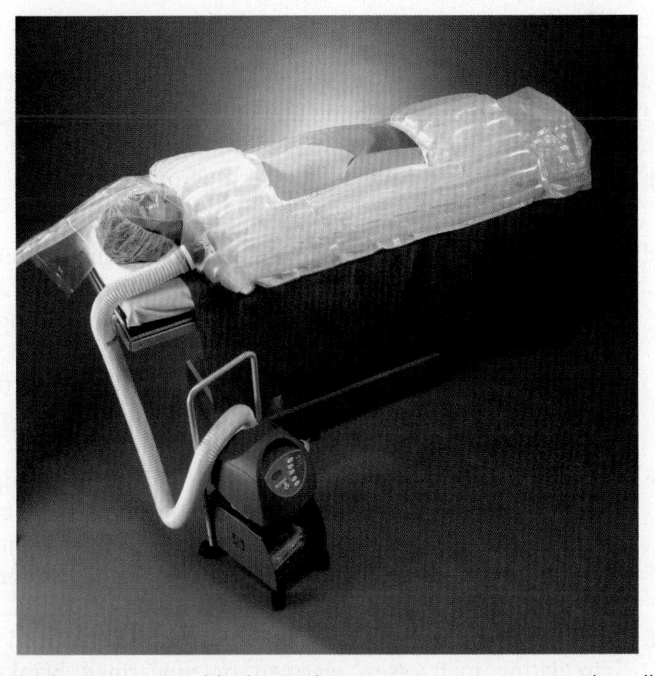

Figure 24.11 Over-the-body warming blanket with an area in center removed to allow surgical access. (Photograph courtesy of Arizant Healthcare, Eden Prairie, MN.)

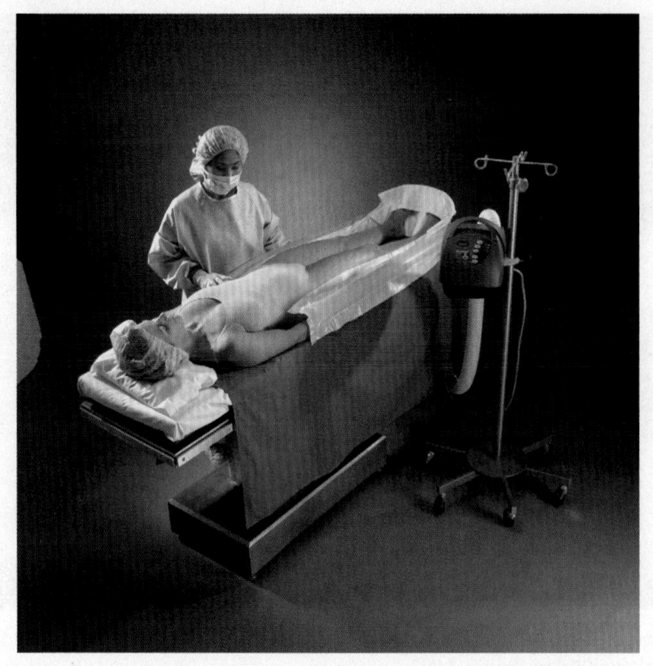

Figure 24.12 Cardiac access blanket. This provided localized warming to the legs while allowing access to both legs. (Photograph courtesy of Arizant Healthcare, Eden Prairie, MN.)

CLINICAL MOMENT While it is appealing from the viewpoint of cost control to use the hose from a forced-air warming unit without its blanket (free hosing), this should never be done. The heated air may blow onto a small area of skin, causing a burn injury. Significant burns have been reported from free hosing.

d. Numerous studies have shown that forced-air warming is effective in maintaining or increasing the patient's (including both maternal and baby) temperature, decreasing the incidence of shivering and increasing thermal comfort. It works well even when the available skin surface area to be warmed is restricted, as during orthopedic, major vascular, or abdominal operations. Forced-air warming is often used in conjunction with other warming methods.
e. Although forced-air warming is often effective in raising peripheral temperature, core temperature may not rise. This may be because of limited heat transfer between thermal compartments in vasoconstricted patients. In the patient with a neuraxial block, the vasodilatation may aid in heat transfer from the peripheral to core tissues.
f. Most studies have found forced-air warming superior to older style liquid-circulating mattresses, warmed or unwarmed blankets, radiant heat lamps, inhalation rewarming, passive insulation, electric blankets, negative-pressure warming devices, or warming IV fluids. Newer liquid-circulating devices and resistive heating devices may be as efficient as or more efficient than forced-air warming devices. Some studies have found that

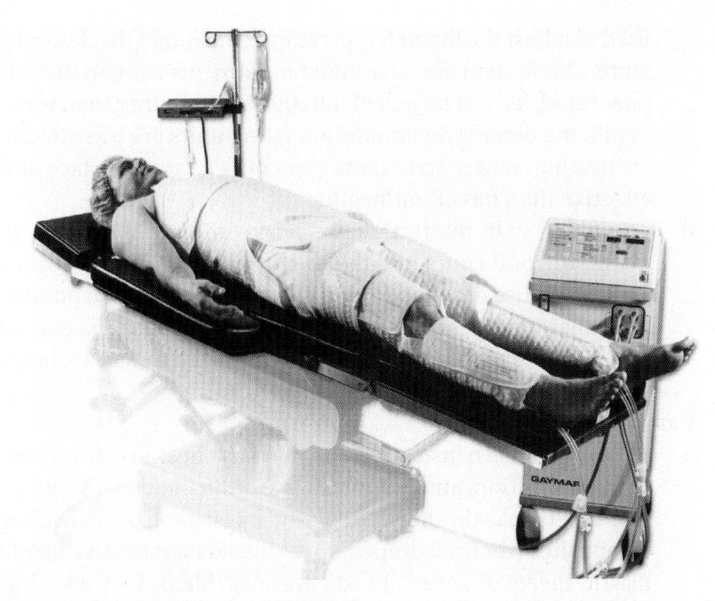

Figure 24.13 Liquid-circulating device. The patient contact part can be wrapped around various parts of the body. (Photograph courtesy of Gaymar Industries, Inc., Orchard Park, NY.)

warming IV fluids is as effective as forced-air warming in maintaining normothermia.

2. **Liquid-Circulating Devices**
   a. A liquid-circulating device consists of a heating/cooling unit and a patient contact device (mattress, pad, blanket, or wrap) connected by hose(s) (**Figs. 24.13** and **24.14**). Heated/cooled liquid circulates through the patient contact device and then back to the heating/cooling element. Some machines can supply more than one patient contact device.
   b. Some newer liquid-circulating systems use a thin disposable pad that adheres directly to the skin and is made of a material that facilitates heat conduction toward the patient. Different shapes and sizes are available, allowing attachment to various body surfaces. Most incorporate a microprocessor that controls both fluid flow and temperature. A patient temperature sensor can be

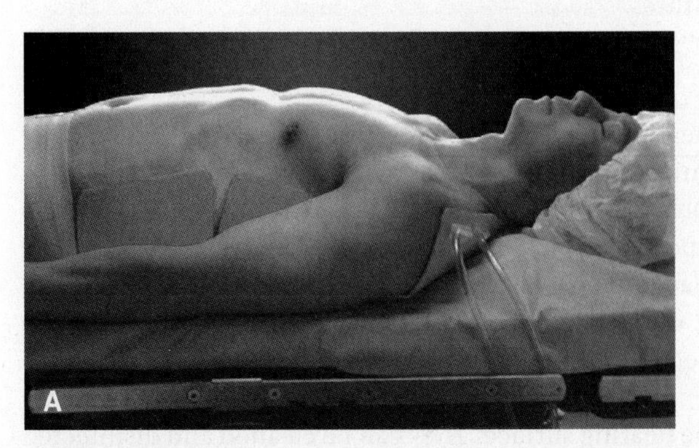

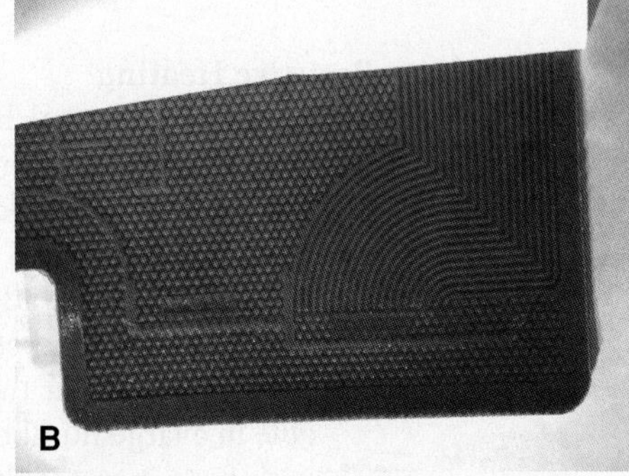

Figure 24.14 **A.** Liquid-circulating device. The patient contact part adheres to the body surface. (Picture courtesy of Kimberly-Clark). **B.** Close-up of liquid circulating device. The backing is removed, revealing the sticky side of the pad that is attached to the patient.

used to adjust the liquid temperature to maintain the desired patient temperature. One system operates under negative pressure so that if the pad is cut or punctured, air will be pulled into the system rather than water spilling out.

c. While the older style liquid-circulating units are less effective than forced-air heating, newer style units can cover a larger surface and may be more effective than forced-air heating.

d. The older style mattresses are heavy and cumbersome. It is difficult to maintain good contact with the stiff mattress and to cover a large surface area. Their use can lead to burns, especially pressure points of the patient's body that contact the blanket. Placing them above the patient may decrease the likelihood of burns. Care should be taken that the tubing does not come into contact with the patient.

3. **Passive Coverings**

a. Applying passive insulation can decrease heat loss from convection, radiation, conduction, and evaporation. Cotton blankets, surgical drapes, towels and sheets, plastic sheeting, plastic bags, and specially designed reflective composites (thermal drapes, space blankets, reflective blankets, metallized plastic sheets or sheets, head coverings, blankets, socks, leggings, etc.) are among the materials that have been used.

b. There are minimal clinical differences among the various coverings. Warming the covers or adding additional insulation layers further reduces heat loss only slightly and has not been found to be of benefit in preventing shivering. Covering as much surface area as possible is more important than the type of covering or specific area covered. Cost and convenience should be major factors when choosing covers. The costs of laundering and replacing cotton blankets must be taken into account. There are no published reports of patient injury caused by warmed hospital blankets.

c. Passive insulation reduces cutaneous heat loss but does not maintain normothermia. Applying warmed cotton blankets to the patient has been a traditional ritual in the PACU, but is ineffective in preventing hypothermia.

CLINICAL MOMENT Placing a cotton blanket over the patient as soon as possible after the patient has entered the OR will reduce initial heat loss and result in a higher body temperature than when the patient enters the PACU. Most patients consider this a humanitarian gesture.

4. **Resistive Heating**

a. Resistive electrical heating devices generate heat by passing low-voltage current through semiconductive wires or carbon fiber fabric that are attached to the patient's skin (**Fig. 24.15**) or a mattress (**Fig. 24.16**). No danger results from penetration of the fabric because the current simply flows through the adjacent fabric.

b. The reusable blanket or mattress is computer controlled to maintain the contact surface at the set temperature. Blankets and mattresses are available in a large number of configurations that can be used in various combinations to increase the heating surface. They can be cleaned and disinfected after use and reused.

c. Resistive heating has been found to be equally or more effective than most other technologies, including forced-air warming. A reported advantage

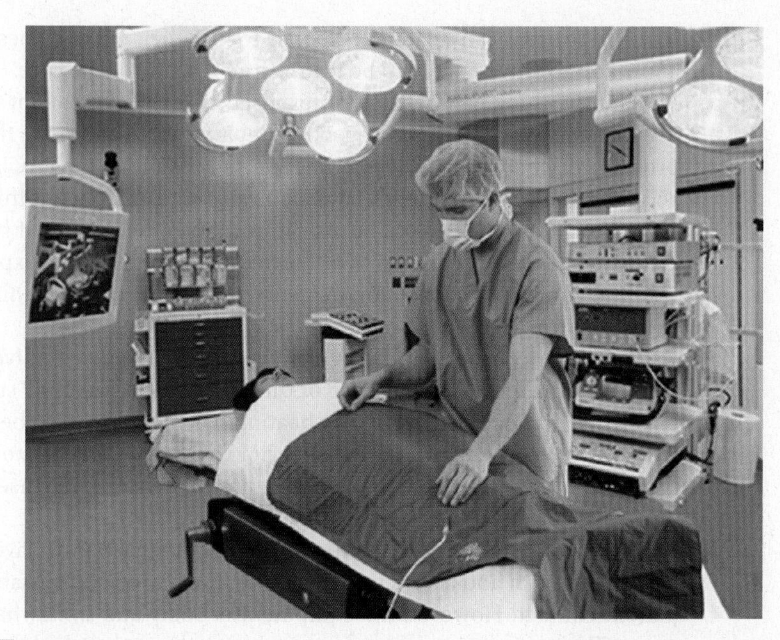

Figure 24.15 Conductive fabric patient warming device. (Photograph courtesy of Gaymar Industries, Inc., Orchard Park, NY.)

is cost saving compared with forced-air warming. It is also quieter than forced-air warming.

d. Severe thermal injuries have been reported with an electrical warming mattress. A fire may result if an electric blanket is folded and wires are broken.

5. **Radiant Heaters**

a. Radiant heaters are most effective when they heat areas that are high in arteriovenous anastomoses such as the forehead, nose, ears, hands, and

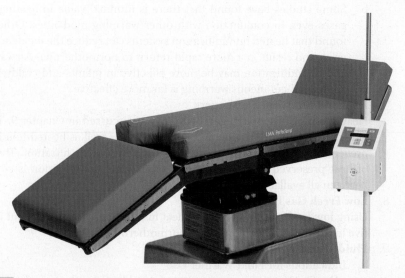

Figure 24.16 This heated mattress also has special features to prevent decubitus ulcers. (Photograph courtesy of LMA PerfecTemp., San Diego, CA.)

feet. These areas can dilate in response to local heating and anesthesia and allow applied heat energy to be transferred directly to the core.

b. Radiant warming can be used on exposed areas of the patient's skin during catheter placement, during skin preparation, and during the surgical procedure, when feasible. It may be especially useful in the PACU. The heat should shine on the patient's bare skin or at most through a thin sheet. If placed too close to the skin, burns can result, so the skin must be assessed frequently to detect early signs of thermal injury. Since skin exposure may result in cooling by convection currents, it is important to eliminate drafts in the environment.

c. Radiant heat can provide faster rewarming and reduced shivering. It is more effective in infants because of their relatively large body surface area in relation to body mass. Radiant heating has been found to be less effective than forced-air warming but superior to electric, warmed, or reflective blankets. It decreases heat loss before skin washing but increases it during washing.

d. Radiant heat lamps enable the medical and nursing staff to have an unobstructed view of and access to the patient. There are no disposables and no patient contact. However, the equipment is bulky and somewhat cumbersome. The exposure may be unacceptable to the patient and family members. It may cause burns or hyperthermia if used for long periods of time, if the radiant heat source is close to the patient's skin, or if there is a problem with the skin temperature measurement sensor. It is necessary to adjust the heater–skin distance if the operating table is raised or lowered. Patients with poor peripheral circulation may be more difficult to heat. Radiant warmers may interfere with imaging if used in an MRI unit.

6. **Heating and Humidifying Inspired Gases**

   a. Evaporative heat loss from the airway can be prevented by using warm, humidified gases (inhalation rewarming). Devices for heating and humidifying inspired gases are discussed in Chapter 9. Minimal heat transfer occurs with this method, which carries the risk of thermal injuries.

   b. Some studies have found that there is minimal value in heating inspired gases even in conjunction with other warming modalities. Other studies found that heated humidification systems can reduce the incidence of shivering and result in a more rapid return to normothermia. Airway heating and humidification may be more effective in infants and children than in adults, but cutaneous warming is far more effective.

7. **Heat and Moisture Exchangers**

   Heat and moisture exchangers (HMEs) are discussed in Chapter 9. They provide efficient humidification and work almost as well as heated humidifiers to prevent respiratory heat loss but cost less and provide filtration. The amount of heat preserved by this method is small. Heat conservation is comparable between all available HMEs.

8. **Low Fresh Gas Flows**

   Using low fresh gas flows reduces heat loss through the airways but is ineffective in maintaining intraoperative normothermia.

9. **Fluid Warming**

   a. Indications for Fluid Warmer Use

      1) Fluid warmers are used to warm blood products and IV solutions. Since the temperature of blood and IV solutions are usually well below body temperature, they can be a significant source of heat loss

when large volumes are used. Most fluid warmers have a temperature display and an alarm to alert the operator if the heater temperature or temperature of the fluid is too high. Some devices alarm if the heater temperature falls below a threshold.

2) Fluid warming can prevent the heat loss caused by infusing cold fluids but generally cannot transfer enough heat to prevent hypothermia or restore normothermia expeditiously unless extracorporeal rewarming is used. Warming a liquid improves the flow through the administration set by lowering fluid viscosity.

3) No clear guidelines about when these devices should be used exist. It is generally agreed that warming should be performed during massive and/or rapid transfusion, in patients with cold agglutinins, and for exchange transfusions in the neonate. Using fluid warmers during routine procedures is controversial. Variables that should be considered include the infusion rate, the total volume to be used, the temperature of the fluid to be infused, and other patient-warming techniques that are in use.

b. Factors Determining the Fluid Temperature at the Patient

A number of factors determine the fluid temperature when it reaches the patient. One factor is the fluid temperature before it is warmed. If very cold, the temperature may not reach the set point as it passes from the controller, particularly at rapid flow rates. If the flow rate to the patient is slow, the fluid may reach the set point but may cool in the tubing before it reaches the patient. If the flow rate is fast, it may not reach the setpoint before it is on the way to the patient. If the length of tubing between the controller and the patient is short, there is less opportunity for the fluid to cool before it reaches the patient. Some warming devices can be placed close to the site where fluid enters the patient. This prevents heat loss from ambient temperature before the fluid is administered.

c. Fluid Warming Methods

1) Fluids that do not contain dextrose may be prewarmed up to a temperature of 43°C. The warming cabinet cannot be used to heat blood.

CLINICAL MOMENT Warmed IV fluid bags must not be applied to the patient's skin for warming or positioning. They may cause burns and are an ineffective warming method.

2) In-line warming devices heat fluid as it passes from the source (a solution bag or infusion device) to the patient. The fluid may be warmed in the tubing, or it may pass through a special cassette that is placed in a dry heat warmer. There may be a water bath or miniature microwave warmer around the infusion line.

B. Cost-effectiveness

1. The influence of warming on perioperative costs depends on the patient's condition, surgical procedure, and institutional factors related to cost accounting.
2. Avoiding the negative outcomes associated with the hypothermic patient may reduce expenses. Blood loss and transfusion requirements, time to extubation, the need for drugs, the number of blankets used, and the length of stay in the PACU may be reduced. The normothermic patient is more hemodynamically stable, requiring less intensive nursing care.

3. Comparing the different methods for providing warmth to patients, it was determined that the old-style water mattress and insulating covers have the lowest return on a cost basis; IV fluid warmers were more effective but not as economical as forced-air warmers. Electric blankets may be more cost-effective than forced-air devices. If the blankets are reusable, the reprocessing costs must be considered.

C. Hazards Related to Patient Warming

1. **Softened Tracheal Tube**

Heat supplied by a convective warming device has been shown to soften a polyvinyl chloride tracheal tube. This would make the tube more likely to kink and possibly obstruct.

2. **Infection**

a. The possibility of bacterial dissemination by forced-air devices has caused some to be uncomfortable with their use. Studies indicate that there is no increased risk associated with forced-air warming devices. Recommendations to avoid this problem include using a filter in the hose, changing the filter regularly, using only manufacturer-recommended blankets, disinfecting or sterilizing the detachable hose, and not reusing coverlets.

b. A water bath can act as a source of infection. IV injection ports and tubing connections should be kept out of the water. The water should be discarded after use and the reservoir cleaned and disinfected.

c. If a leak develops in a fluid warming system, unsterile water may enter the line and be infused into the patient.

3. **Burns**

a. A report from the American Association of Anesthesiologists closed-claims database showed 54 patient burns out of 3000 total claims. Eighteen burns were caused by bags or bottles that had been heated and placed next or close to the patient's skin. Of the eight burns from electrically powered warming equipment, five resulted from circulating-water mattresses. Other reported burns were from a warming light and a heated humidifier tubing. In only one case was the heating device found to be defective. Unfortunately, burns are not usually recognized until after surgery has been completed.

b. A common patient factor in many burns is poor cutaneous blood flow. Injuries are usually most severe in areas overlying bony prominences. The risk of tissue injury is further increased when heat or pressure is combined with chemical irritation from skin-cleaning solutions, especially those containing iodine. Age is another factor. Elderly patients often have thin, delicate skin that is especially susceptible to injury. The skin of newborn patients has a reduced thickness compared with adults. This diminishes protection against external noxious events. Patients with ischemic tissue or those who undergo procedures involving cardiopulmonary bypass are likely to be at increased risk of thermal injury.

CLINICAL MOMENT Heating devices should not be used distal to a tourniquet or arterial clamp or during cardiopulmonary bypass.

c. When a warming device is used for a patient with compromised circulation, the patient's skin condition should be monitored frequently and the unit's maximum heat setting not used. Constant vigilance must be exercised to ensure that portions of heating devices not meant for direct patient contact, such as the tubing for a water blanket or a forced-air hose, do not come in contact with the patient. Solution and blanket-warming cabinet temperature should be limited to 43°C.
d. When a burn occurs, the pattern of the lesion can help to identify the cause. If a warming device has been used and the lesion conforms to that of the device's edges but no other area of the skin is involved, then it is likely that the warming device caused the lesion.

4. **Increased Transcutaneous Medication Uptake**
An increase in transdermal drug uptake may occur when the skin is heated. For this reason, transdermal medication should be applied in a location that will not be warmed or should be discontinued during heating.

5. **Hemolysis**
Blood may hemolyze if overheated. If water from a fluid-warming system leaks into blood, hemolysis may result.

6. **Current Leakage**
Liquid bath and dry heat exchangers must be well grounded. They can leak electrical current into the fluid path.

7. **Air Embolism**
a. A hazard with fluid warmers is the possibility of infusing air into the patient, as a result of bubbles created on warming the fluid (outgassing), air entrained through an infusion system, or by delivering air contained in the fluid source. The danger is greatest with pressure infusers, when fluids are infused by a pump, and when rapid, high-volume fluid administration is necessary.
b. Solution manufacturers typically put 50 to 75 mL of air into each solution container. This should be removed from the container and the tubing checked for bubbles before starting a pressurized infusion. Partially emptied fluid bags should not be reattached to the IV system.
c. Many systems provide a warning feature to alert the operator to air in the line, and traps that collect bubbles are incorporated into many disposable sets. If the trap is installed upside down, air may be transmitted to the patient. Many of these traps cannot be easily vented; once the trap becomes full, air may be delivered to the patient. Some gas-eliminating devices use a microporous membrane that allows the gas to escape without any user intervention. Another design uses a mechanism that stops the fluid flow when air is detected. Some systems allow fluid containing air to be recirculated to the reservoir chamber. No gas-eliminating device can reliably remove large amounts of air. Automatic air detection devices may fail.

8. **Interference with Bispectral Index Monitoring**
Falsely elevated bispectral index values have been reported in patients receiving forced-air warming around the head. Temporary interruption of the warm airflow may be required to get accurate readings.

9. **Pressurized Infiltration**
The use of a fluid-warming system that pressurizes the fluid can result in fluid extravasation. A compartment syndrome could occur.

REFERENCES

1. Mauermann WJ, Nemergut EC. The anesthesiologist's role in the prevention of surgical site infections. Anesthesiology 2006:105;413–421.
2. de Lissovoy G, Fraeman K, Hutchins V, et al. Surgical site infection: incidence and impact on hospital utilization and treatment costs. Am J Infect Control 2009;37(5):387–397.
3. Kirkland KB, Briggs JP, Trivette SL, et al. The impact of surgical-site infections in the 1990s: attributable mortality, excess length of hospitalization, and extra costs. Infect Control Hosp Epidemiol 1999;20(11):725–730.
4. Bratzler DW, Hunt DR. The surgical infection prevention and surgical care improvement projects: national initiatives to improve outcomes for patients having surgery. Clin Infect Dis 2006;43(3):322–330.

SUGGESTED READINGS

Dorsch J, Dorsch S. Temperature monitoring. In: Understanding Anesthesia Equipment. Fifth edition. Philadelphia: Wolters Kluwer/Lippincott Williams & Wilkins, 2008:858–870.

Dorsch J, Dorsch S. Temperature control equipment. In: Understanding Anesthesia Equipment. Fifth Edition. Philadelphia: Wolters Kluwer/Lippincott Williams & Wilkins, 2008:884–906.

Lenhardt R. Monitoring and thermal management. Best Pract Res Clin Anesthesiol 2001;17:569–581.

Sessler D. Temperature monitoring. In: Miller R, ed. Anaesthesia. Sixth edition. New York: Churchill-Livingstone, 2005:1571–1598.

Sessler DI. Temperature monitoring and perioperative thermoregulation. Anesthesiology 2008;109:318–338.

25 Operating Room Fires and Personnel Injuries Related to Sources of Ignition

I. Introduction

Although flammable anesthetics have disappeared from operating rooms, perioperative fires continue to occur. They can have devastating consequences, precipitate legal action, and take a great psychological toll on everyone involved. They usually come as a complete surprise.

Most operating room fires are of little consequence and are not reported, making the actual incidence difficult to determine. Approximately 10% to 20% of reported fires result in serious patient injury. Fuels present in the operating room include plastics that produce dense, black smoke when ignited. The smoke may contain toxins and may hinder safe patient and staff evacuation from the room. Sudden ignition can present secondary problems. It can cause a startle reflex, causing the surgeon's hand to jerk and potentially cut into unintended tissue or set other areas of the surgical site on fire.

II. The Fire Triangle

For a fire to occur, three factors (fire triangle or triad) must be present: an ignition source, a fuel, and an oxidizer to support combustion (**Fig. 25.1**). These factors need to be present in the proper proportions and under the right conditions for a fire to occur.

A. Ignition Source

1. Lasers

The acronym *laser* (light amplification by stimulated emission of radiation) defines the process by which a form of energy is converted into light energy. The term can also refer to the device that produces the light or to the light itself. Lasers use a collimated, coherent, monochromatic, intense beam of electromagnetic radiation to cut, coagulate, or vaporize tissue. The rate at which the laser energy is delivered is called the power and is measured in watts. The wattage is equal to the amount of energy, measured in joules, divided by the exposure

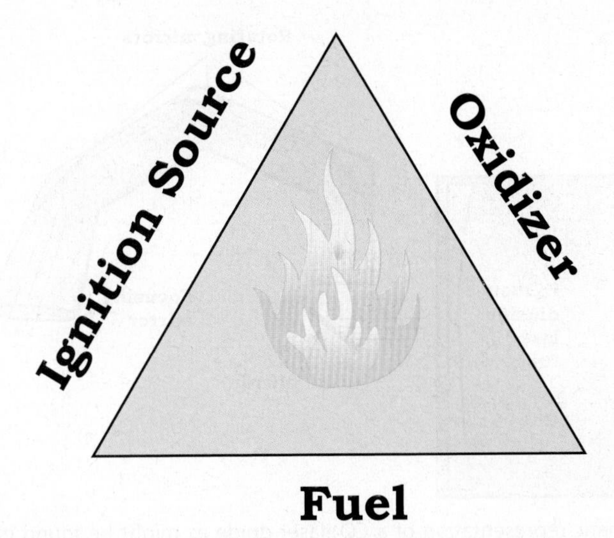

Figure 25.1 Three things are necessary for a fire to occur: an ignition source, fuel, and an oxidizer.

time measured in seconds. Laser power density is the amount of power distributed within an area in watts per square centimeter.

a. Laser System Components

1) The basic laser system components are two parallel mirrors encompassing the laser medium and a power source (**Fig. 25.2**). In addition, there may be an aiming beam.

2) The laser medium (head) holds the substance that is energized to produce light. The medium, which may be a solid, liquid, or gas, determines the emitted radiation wavelength. The laser is named after the material used as the medium.

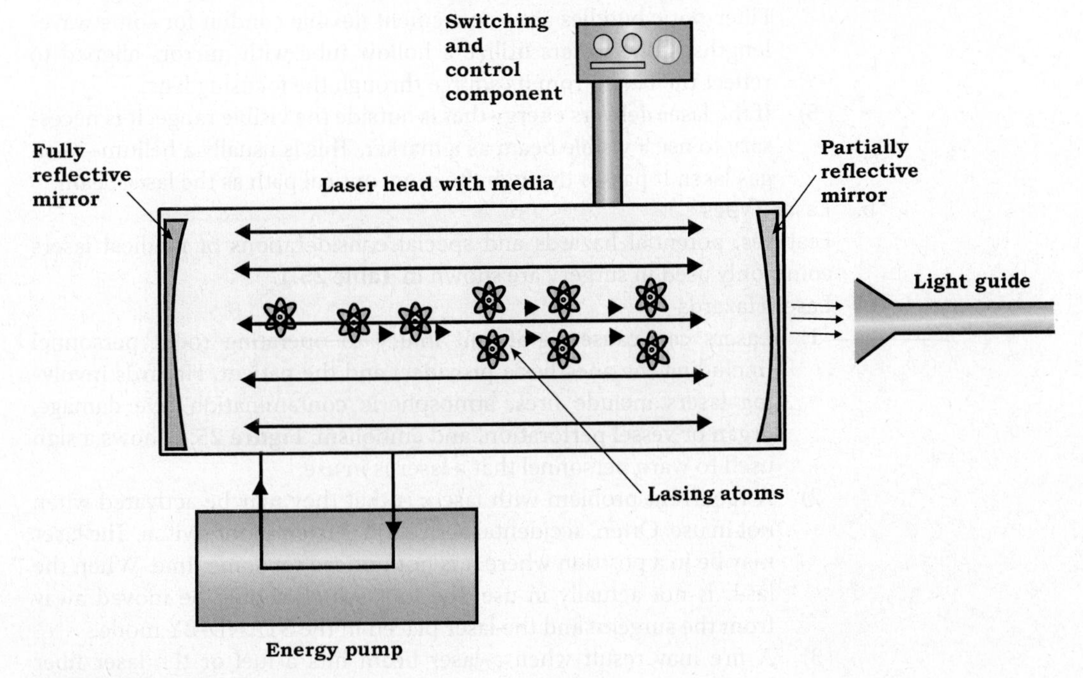

Figure 25.2 Components of a laser.

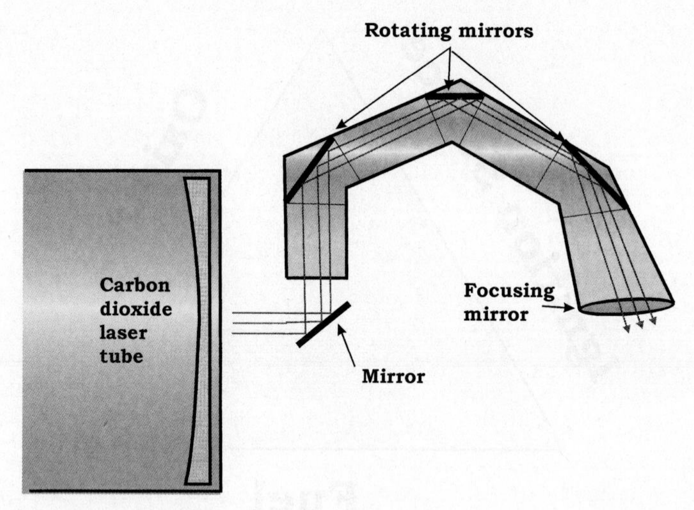

Figure 25.3 A schematic representation of a CO_2 laser guide as might be found in either an operating microscope or a handheld wand. The guide consists of hollow tubes with hinged, aligned mirrors that reflect the beam from its source through the focusing lens.

3) The power (pumping, pump, excitation) source supplies energy to the laser medium. When the power source is activated, energy is absorbed by electrons in the laser medium, which are elevated to energy levels above their ground state. They then decay to lower energy levels and emit photons that are not in phase with one another and travel in all directions. Mirrors are used to reflect and increase the emission energy. One of the mirrors is not 100% reflective and allows a small portion of the light to escape.
4) A light guide (delivery system) directs the laser beam (**Fig. 25.3**). Fiber-optic bundles are a convenient flexible conduit for some wavelengths. Other lasers utilize a hollow tube with mirrors aligned to reflect the beam from its source through the focusing lens.
5) If the laser delivers energy that is outside the visible range, it is necessary to use a visible beam as a marker. This is usually a helium–neon gas laser. It passes through the same optical path as the laser beam.

b. Laser Types

Features, potential hazards and special considerations of medical lasers commonly used in surgery are shown in **Table 25.1.**

c. Laser Hazards

1) Lasers can cause significant injury to operating room personnel (including the anesthesia provider) and the patient. Hazards involving lasers include fires, atmospheric contamination, eye damage, organ or vessel perforation, and embolism. **Figure 25.4** shows a sign used to warn personnel that a laser is in use.
2) A recurrent problem with lasers is that they may be activated when not in use. Often, accidental activation is from a foot switch. The laser may be in a position where it is not noticed for some time. When the laser is not actually in use, the foot switch should be moved away from the surgeon and the laser placed in the STAND-BY mode.
3) A fire may result when a laser beam hits a fuel or the laser fiber becomes damaged. Ignition can be almost instantaneous. While most

Table 25.1 Commonly Used Lasers and Associated Personnel Hazards

Laser Medium	Features	Potential Hazards to the Eye	Special Considerations
CO_2	Readily absorbed by all biologic materials, independent of pigmentation. Tissue destruction is proportional to its water content. Produces a very superficial tissue effect.	Injury to the eye will be confined to the cornea. There is no risk to the retina. Since the laser is absorbed by plastic and glass, ordinary eyeglasses with sideguards can be used for eye protection.	Fires involving both tracheal tubes and supraglottic devices have been reported with this laser.
Nd-YAG	Can be transmitted through fiber-optic fibers. Poorly absorbed by water but well absorbed by pigmented tissue.	Retinal damage can occur. Opaque green eyewear or eyewear with clear lenses with a special coating should be worn.	Because it is taken up by pigment, colored markings on tracheal tubes are more likely to be damaged than clear portions. Blood or mucus on or in the tracheal tube makes the tube less resistant to the laser beam. Fires have been reported from an Nd-YAG laser passed through the channel of a flexible bronchoscope. The rigid bronchoscope is recommended for use with this laser, although the flexible scope may be needed to treat hard-to-reach areas.
KTP	Passes through clear substances but is absorbed by hemoglobin and other pigments.	Retinal damage may occur. Special eyewear with red filter should be worn.	
Argon	Beam is selectively absorbed by red, orange, and yellow pigments and strongly absorbed by hemoglobin and melanin. Fiber-optic bundles can be used to transmit the laser beam.	Retinal damage may occur. Special opaque orange goggles/eyewear should be worn.	

From Klarr P. Laser complications. In: Atlee J, ed. Complications in Anesthesia. Philadelphia: WB Saunders, 1999:588–590.

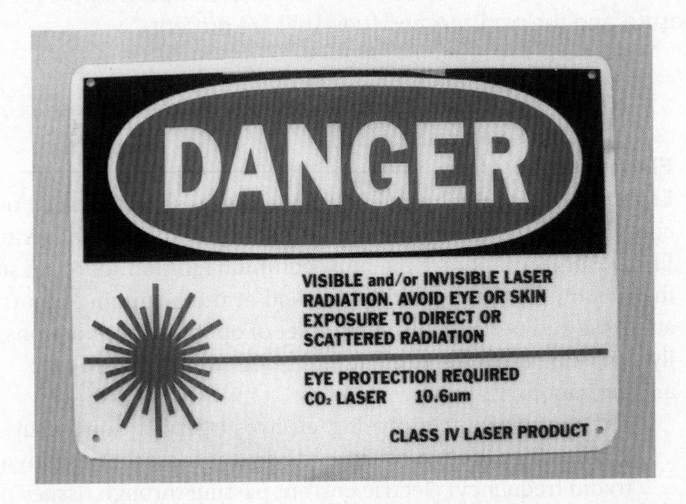
DANGER
VISIBLE and/or INVISIBLE LASER
RADIATION. AVOID EYE OR SKIN
EXPOSURE TO DIRECT OR
SCATTERED RADIATION
EYE PROTECTION REQUIRED
CO2 LASER 10.6um
CLASS IV LASER PRODUCT

Figure 25.4 Sign warning that laser is in use. Note that the laser class is mentioned on the sign.

ignition sources must be in contact with a material to cause ignition, a laser can supply heat to a fuel up to several meters away or under several layers of material.

CLINICAL MOMENT A surface drape can be penetrated by the laser but not ignite. Materials under the drape may then ignite and burn without being noticed for several minutes.

CLINICAL MOMENT The laser beam can be reflected from a metal surface, causing a burn or igniting material in a remote location.

d. Laser Risk Classification

1) A classification system reflecting laser risks to the patient and personnel has been developed. The higher the class, the more stringent the protection needed.
2) Lasers that are totally enclosed or that give extremely low energy output fall into class 1. These are safe to view.
3) Low-risk lasers are in class 2. Their risk is approximately equivalent to staring at the sun or other bright lights that can cause central retinal injury. These are not hazardous unless someone overcomes his or her natural aversion response to bright light.
4) Class 3 lasers are divided into two subcategories: 3a and 3b. These lasers are a hazard even if viewed only momentarily. Class 3a lasers pose a moderate ocular hazard. Class 3b lasers are extremely hazardous. Even momentarily viewing is potentially hazardous to the eye. They may also be a hazard to the skin.
5) Class 4 lasers pose serious skin, eye, and fire hazards. Most lasers used in surgery are class 4 lasers.

CLINICAL MOMENT Class 3b and 4 lasers represent significant ignition hazards. The ignition risk of other classes of lasers will depend on how they are focused, the time of exposure, and the oxidizers and fuels that are present.

6) A metal instrument can become overheated with prolonged laser use and could cause a burn.

2. **Electrosurgery Unit**

Electrosurgery (radio frequency) apparatus is so widely used that there is often complacency about reading the instruction manual or following safe practices. Electrosurgery units are the most common ignition source in surgical fires. The instruction manual should be studied at the beginning of a training program and reviewed periodically. A brief set of operating instructions should be readily available on the instrument.

a. Terminology

The vocabulary concerning electrosurgery is somewhat confusing. This chapter defines electrosurgery devices as those that employ a high-frequency (radio frequency) electric current passing through tissues to cut, coagulate, or provide a blend of cutting and coagulation. Electrocautery devices utilize a heated wire or blade, usually at the end of a probe, for coagulation. Most electrocautery devices are battery operated.

b. Modes
   1) There are three modes available on modern electrosurgery devices. The cutting mode uses a continuous, undampened sine wave. Heating is rapid and produces high temperatures that explode cells that come in contact with the electrode. This produces a cut in the tissue.
   2) The coagulation mode features short bursts of a dampened sine wave. Less heat is produced since the current is not continuous. Tissue desiccation occurs, and the ends of blood vessels are sealed.
   3) The blend (cut-coagulation) mode employs a waveform and voltage between the cutting and coagulation cycle. The relative amount of cutting or coagulation depends on the lengths of the voltage bursts. Several blend settings may be available on an electrosurgical unit.

c. Types
   1) Monopolar
      (i) There are three basic components in a monopolar electrosurgery unit: generator, active electrode, and dispersive electrode (**Fig. 25.5**). Electrons flow from the generator to the active electrode and through the patient to the dispersive electrode, sometimes incorrectly called the *grounding pad*, via the lowest impedance pathway that it can find.
      (ii) The electrically powered generator (power unit) creates a radio frequency current that passes through the active electrode. The effect on tissue depends on the current intensity, the current type, the duration of exposure to the current, the hand piece being used, and the dispersive electrode. Coagulation requires longer contact with the probe than cutting. As electrical energy

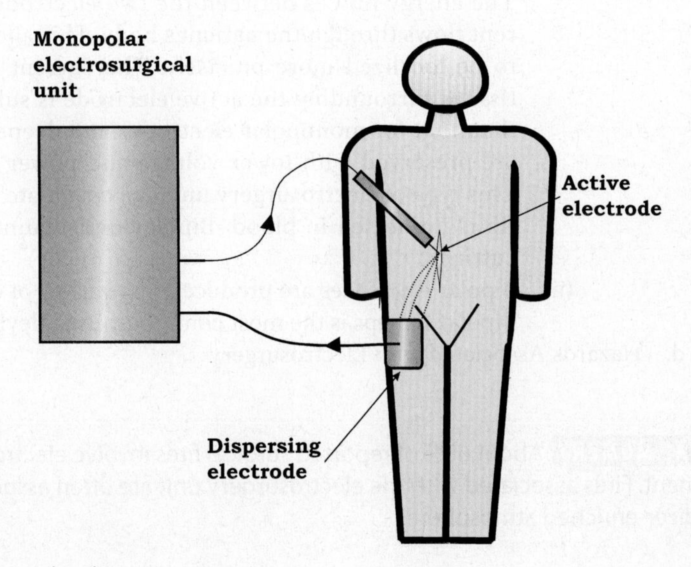

Figure 25.5 Monopolar electrosurgery unit.

is applied to the tissue, charring occurs. Since char has high impedance, more current dissipates directly to the dispersive electrode and the effect is reduced.

(iii) The active electrode has a handle and is connected to the generator by a flexible wire. The tip configuration determines its ability to desiccate tissue. A needle-tip electrode concentrates more power on tissue contact than does a paddle or ball-shaped electrode. At a given electrode voltage, the paddle-shaped tip provides a higher power at the edge than on the flat portion.

(iv) The dispersive (inactive, return) electrode collects the current from the patient and returns it to the generator to complete the circuit. The large contact pad surface provides low impedance. Most pads presently in use are pregelled with a sticky surface. With some electrosurgery units, two dispersive electrodes ("split pads") are used.

(v) Modern electrosurgical units possess a return electrode (contact quality) monitoring system. This ensures that the patient is connected to the return electrode. Current flowing to the active electrode is measured and compared with current returning from the dispersive electrode. If the currents are not balanced, the unit is deactivated. If the machine is equipped with "split pads," the unit will not function unless both pads are in contact with the patient. A more recent innovation is active electrode monitoring. This continuously monitors the electrical circuit and automatically shuts down the generator and sounds an alarm if dangerous electrical leakage occurs. Newer generators can sense dramatic changes in tissue impedance or temperature changes at the return electrode.

2) Bipolar

(i) The bipolar electrosurgery unit is composed of a generator and two electrodes located within millimeters of each other. The energy flow is between the two electrodes and no current flows through the patient's body. This allows the energy to be localized more precisely. The current density in the tissues surrounding the active electrode is substantially less than that for monopolar electrodes and deeper tissue layers are preserved with lower voltage and power requirements. This type of electrosurgery unit can coagulate even when the tip is immersed in blood. Bipolar units cannot be used for cutting.

(ii) Bipolar electrodes are produced in a variety of configurations. Bipolar forceps is the most commonly used device.

d. Hazards Associated with Electrosurgery

CLINICAL MOMENT About 68% of reported surgical fires involve electrosurgical equipment. Fires associated with the electrosurgery unit are often associated with an oxidizer-enriched atmosphere.

CLINICAL MOMENT Alcohol-based solutions can ignite under the drapes when electrosurgery is used.

1) Mishaps with the electrosurgery unit often involve faulty return electrodes, improper electrode placement, or alternative low-impedance pathways. Among the low-impedance alternative pathways are electrocardiogram (ECG) electrodes, temperature probes, urinary catheters, metallic parts on surgical tables, heating pads, and pulse oximeters.
2) When the electrosurgery unit is used, heat vaporizes tissue or expels tissue embers from the tip. In room air, tissue vapors do not ignite, and embers are quickly extinguished. In an oxidizer-enriched atmosphere, the vapors can ignite into a brief flame and burn until they are consumed. A flare of evolved gases can directly ignite any convenient fuel. The electrical wires associated with the electrosurgery electrode may develop a short circuit, which could result in a fire.

3. **Argon Beam Coagulator**
The argon beam (enhanced) coagulator (ABC) is solely a coagulating instrument. Radio frequency monopolar current is delivered through ionized argon gas flow. The flow is altered as the power is changed. The tip does not touch the tissue. If the tip is more than 1 cm from the tissue surface, only a gentle stream of argon will flow. When the tip is 1 cm or less from the tissue surface, the active mode occurs. If the nozzle tip glows red, the tip is too close to the tissue or the power setting is too high.
4. **Fiber-optic Illumination System**
A fiber-optic illumination system consists of a light source and light-transmitting cable. The cable is connected to an endoscope, headlight, or other equipment. These light sources can provide several hundred watts of visible, infrared, and ultraviolet light. The power is typically focused into a fiber-optic cable of small diameter that can deliver a high-power density.

CLINICAL MOMENT The term *cold light*, used to describe light from a fiber-optic source, is incorrectly assumed by many to mean that heat is not generated. Actually cold light refers to light in which the amount of infrared radiation has been reduced. The infrared radiation is usually reduced in the surgical instrument and not in the light source. The infrared light is transmitted to the surgical instrument by the cable.

CLINICAL MOMENT Many surgeons remove the fiber-optic cable from the endoscope and let it rest on the drape. The cable end can retain a significant amount of heat after being disconnected from the light source and, if unprotected, can start a fire.

5. **Defibrillator**
When a defibrillator is activated, a spark may be generated if insufficient force is applied to the paddles; if the paddle pad is too small; if the paddles are

applied over an irregular surface or bony prominence or near an ECG electrode; when insufficient, excess, or the wrong kind of gel is used; or if there is another conductive medium between the paddles. If disposable defibrillation pads are used to increase electrical conduction between the paddle and the patient, an arc can occur if the paddle surface is not completely on the pad, if the pad is smaller than the paddle, if there is a fold in the pad, or if the pad is dry.

CLINICAL MOMENT When ventilating a patient just prior to defibrillation or cardioversion, remove the mask and move it away from the patient. Turning the oxygen OFF during defibrillation is also recommended.

6. **Pressure Regulators**
   a. When gas is allowed to flow from a high-pressure to a low-pressure chamber, recompression can cause a rapid rise in temperature. Materials that cannot withstand both 100% oxygen and high temperatures will ignite. This hazard has been associated mostly with oxygen regulators that have aluminum parts.
   b. Another cause of heat in a pressure regulator is particle impact from contaminants. Teflon tape, chips from seal materials, or hydrocarbon contaminants may be present.
7. **Surgical Lights**
   Surgical lights can be a source of ignition. If the light does not have the proper mechanism to dissipate infrared radiation or if that mechanism fails, energy levels high enough to cause burns or fires can occur. If an oxygen or nitrous oxide hose contacts a surgical light, the hose can be ruptured.
8. **Other Ignition Sources**
   An electrical fire can occur in any environment where there is electrical equipment. A short circuit can occur in an anesthesia machine. In one reported case, a short circuit in a laryngoscope with a rechargeable handle caused flames to shoot from the charging end of the handle. Electrical arcing in surgical booms has been reported to cause fires. Other reported sources of ignition include resectoscopes, heat lamps, heated probes, pneumatic tourniquets, dental and orthopedic burrs, saws and drills, heated-wire breathing tubes, and humidifiers.

B. Fuels

A fuel is anything that can burn, including most things that come in contact with patients as well as patients themselves. Fuels abound in the operating room.

1. **Tracheal Tubes**
   a. The risk and characteristics of a tracheal tube fire will depend on the type of tube used. In most cases, ignition requires that the tube be penetrated. The fire begins on the inside rim of the penetrated area and then spreads both with and against the oxidizing gas flow.
   b. Polyvinyl chloride (PVC) tubes are combustible in an oxidizer-enriched atmosphere with a carbon dioxide (CO_2) laser. Once ignited and penetrated, a PVC tube can sustain a torch-like flame. PVC tubes without markings are relatively resistant to the Nd-YAG laser, but markings increase the risk. If there is blood, mucus, or saliva on the tube, the risk of fire is increased. The injuries associated with PVC tube fires are more severe than those with other types of tubes.

c. Red rubber tubes are combustible with the CO_2, potassium titanyl phosphate (KTP), and Nd-YAG lasers. A major problem is the inability to see through the tube. Should an intraluminal fire develop, it may go undetected longer than with other tubes. Damage to the tracheobronchial tree after an intraluminal fire may be less severe with a red rubber tube than with a PVC tube. Red rubber tubes are less likely to soften, deform, or fragment if ignited than are other tubes. Another advantage is that they can be quickly removed from the patient. A high-pressure cuff deflates more quickly than a low-pressure cuff.
d. A silicone tube is more resistant to penetration by a CO_2 laser than other tubes. If ignited, a silicone tube rapidly turns into brittle ash that crumbles easily and may be aspirated, raising the possibility of future problems with silicosis. Acute injuries are less severe than with red rubber and PVC tubes.
e. A number of ready-to-use laser-resistant tubes and tube wraps are available and are discussed in Chapter 15. It is important to remember that "laser-resistant" does not mean "laser-proof." Laser-resistant tubes can ignite, especially if the manufacturer's warnings, precautions, or directions for use are not followed.

CLINICAL MOMENT If a laser-resistant tube is used with a laser other than that for which it was designed or a flammable part such as the cuff is in contact with the laser beam, it can catch fire. Confirm that the type of tube to be used is appropriate for the laser that is being used.

CLINICAL MOMENT Laser-resistant tubes are usually not resistant to other heat sources such as an electrocautery or electrosurgery tip.

2. **Supraglottic Airway Devices**
The relative resistance of supraglottic airway devices to ignition depends on their composition. Those devices that are made of silicone rubber such as the LMA-Classic, LMA-Flexible, and LMA-ProSeal are significantly more resistant to the CO_2 laser than PVC tracheal tubes. Many disposable supraglottic devices are made of PVC and are probably as susceptible to fires as tracheal tubes with the same composition.

CLINICAL MOMENT No manufacturer currently approves its supraglottic airway device for laser surgery in the airway.

3. **Surgical Products**
a. Surgical drapes, towels, and dressings are common fuel sources for operating room fires. Often, the drape is ignited from another fire. While many drapes are resistant to ignition in room air, the oxidizer-enriched atmosphere that is often present may cause them to burn vigorously.
b. Disposable drapes may be particularly difficult to deal with during a fire because they are often water repellent. Dousing the area with water may

even spread the flame. Laser-resistant drapes are available. Some synthetic drapes will melt rather than ignite when a laser beam hits them.

c. There are numerous reports of surgical sponges, gauze pads, and swabs being ignited. Wet sponges may be used to protect a tracheal tube from a laser beam. However, if they are allowed to dry out, they become flammable.

4. **Adhesive Substances**
   Adhesive tape can be the fuel for a fire. Collodion and benzoin are flammable.
5. **Skin Preparatory Solutions**
   Flammable volatile organic solutions are often used to cleanse the skin prior to surgery. If the liquid or vapor is contacted by an ignition source, a flame can result. Alcohol-based solutions are especially flammable. They can infiltrate and pool under the drapes. When this happens, they are slow to dissipate.

CLINICAL MOMENT Alcohol-based fires have a flame that is difficult to see. Often, the result of the flame be the first indication of a fire.

6. **Intestinal Gases**
   Gases that accumulate in the bowel (especially hydrogen, hydrogen sulfide, and methane) can be the fuel for a fire or explosion if an electrosurgery unit is used to open the bowel. Proper bowel preparation may prevent this. Sufficient oxygen to support combustion is normally not present in intestinal gas. However, nitrous oxide may diffuse into the intestinal lumen, creating a flammable mixture.
7. **Oxygen Cannulae**
   Oxygen cannulae are made of plastic that can burn. They carry 100% oxygen. If touched by a hot electrosurgery probe or a laser beam, they burn readily. Even if not directly contacted, the area around them may be so oxygen-rich that a small spark can turn into a burning ember that can ignite the cannula.

CLINICAL MOMENT Most patients who receive oxygen through a face mask or catheter do not require 100% oxygen. Oxygen can be mixed with air to lower the oxygen concentration (see **Fig. 25.6**) or an air flowmeter can be used (**Fig. 25.7**). The patient's oxygen saturation can be measured using pulse oximetry to ensure adequate oxygenation.

8. **Lubricants and Ointments**
   Petroleum-based ointments that are used in an oxidizer-enriched atmosphere will ignite when enough heat to cause vaporization is present. Water-based lubricants will not burn and can be used to coat hair to make it fire-resistant.
9. **Body Hair**
   Body hair, including eyelashes, moustaches, and beards, can be involved in a fire. Surface flame propagation occurs where there are fine surface fibers of fabric or body hair. In the presence of an oxidizer, these fine fibers can be ignited. Often, the skin or underlying fabric is not burned. The surface fire races in the direction of the oxygen source, where the oxygen supply tubing may be ignited.

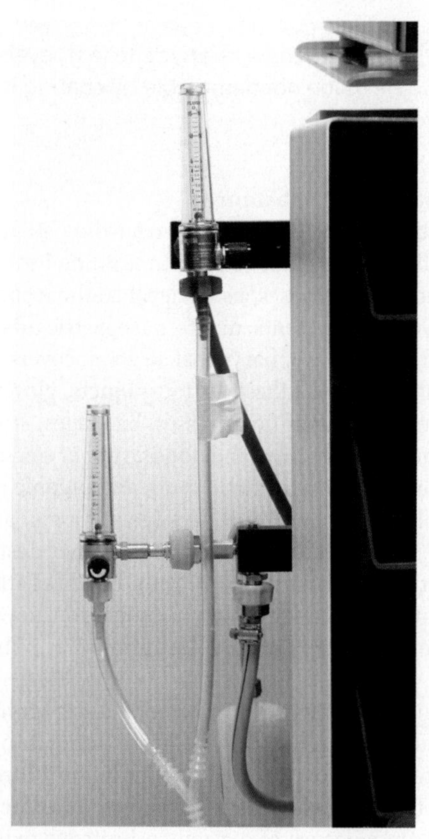

Figure 25.6 Gas from an oxygen flowmeter and an air flowmeter can be connected to produce a gas with an oxygen concentration of less than 100%.

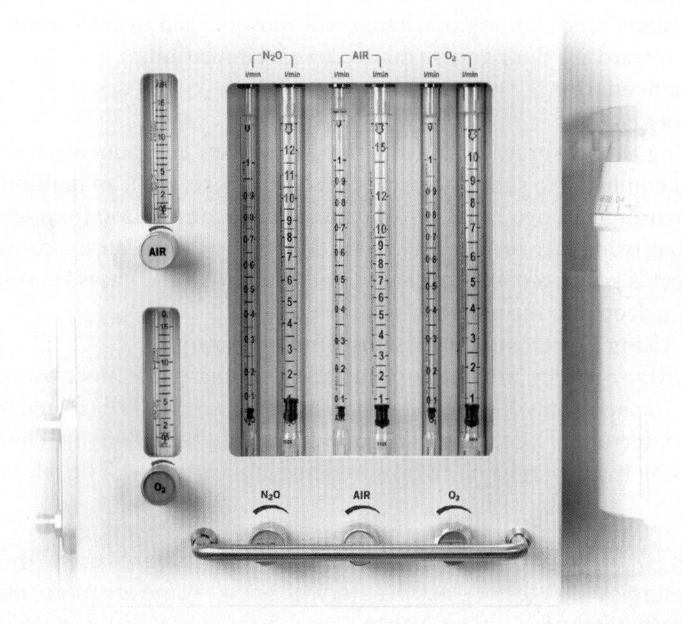

Figure 25.7 This machine has accessory (courtesy) flowmeters for both air and oxygen, allowing administration of a gas with an oxygen concentration of less than 100%. (Photograph courtesy of Datascope, Montvale, New Jersey.)

CLINICAL MOMENT Hair near the operative site (e.g., eyebrows, beards, and moustaches) should be made nonflammable by coating it thoroughly with a water-based lubricating jelly.

10. **Other Combustible Substances**
    a. A number of articles used in or near the patient can serve as the flammable material. These include (but are not limited to) oxygen tubings, endoscopes, smoke evacuator hoses, esophageal stethoscopes, breathing tubes, reservoir bags, eye patches, stents, masks, nasogastric tubes, enteric feeding tubes, rubber and plastic nasopharyngeal airways, covers, paper products, blood pressure cuffs, aerosol adhesives, tourniquets, gloves, stethoscope tubing, throat packs, egg crate foam mattresses, bandages, stockinettes, dressings, pillows, glue, gowns, straps, caps and hoods, rubber electrosurgical unit probe sheaths, shoe covers, local anesthetic spray, and organic gas from a necrotic tumor.
    b. Alcohol-based hand sanitizers (gels, foams, and liquids) are highly flammable. They should be stored in a cabinet designed for flammable materials. A study published in 2003 found no fires attributable to hand sanitizers. The National Fire Protection Association now allows alcohol-based hand sanitizer dispensers in corridors and other public areas.

C. Oxidizers
   1. With an oxidizer-enriched atmosphere, a fire ignites easily, burns more vigorously, spreads more rapidly, and is more difficult to extinguish. The oxidizers of greatest interest are oxygen and nitrous oxide. Nitrous oxide supports combustion and in the process releases the energy of its formation, providing increased heat. Thus, any mixture of oxygen and nitrous oxide will support combustion. Air will also support combustion, because it contains oxygen.
   2. Because oxygen is heavier than air, it collects in low-lying areas, including drape folds. Some materials such as drapes and towels absorb and retain oxygen for some time. Tenting the drapes will allow oxygen to drain away from the patient toward the floor and be diluted by air circulation.

III. **Common Scenarios**

A. Airway Fires

During airway surgery, all of the three necessary components are in close proximity: a combustible substance (tracheal tube, gauze, etc.), an ignition source (laser or electrosurgery apparatus), and gas to support combustion (oxygen with or without nitrous oxide). An airway fire is particularly serious because a considerable amount of heat is generated in a small area, and the smoke and gases from such a fire can be blown deep into the patient's lungs.

1. **Using Electrosurgery during Tracheostomy**

   Many airway fires have occurred while using the electrosurgery unit during tracheostomy. Often, the patient is being given 100% oxygen in anticipation of interrupted ventilation and/or because of the underlying clinical condition. If the tracheal tube or cuff is contacted, an oxidizer will be released.

CLINICAL MOMENT There is no tracheal tube that is safe for use with electrosurgical devices or electrocautery, although some are more resistant to ignition than others.

2. **Using Electrosurgery in the Mouth**
   Using electrosurgery in the oral cavity may result in a fire. The tracheal tube is often the fuel source, but other items such as a sponge or patient tissue may be involved.

CLINICAL MOMENT If there is a leak around the tracheal tube, gauze in the throat will dry out and become oxidizer-enriched more quickly.

3. **Laser-Induced Tracheal Tube Fire**
   a. The likelihood that a laser beam will contact the tracheal tube during airway procedures is high. The tube may be exposed to either the direct or reflected laser beam. Flaming tissue in close proximity to the tube may cause it to ignite.

CLINICAL MOMENT The cuff is the most vulnerable part of the tracheal tube. Laser-resistant tubes do not have laser-resistant cuffs.

   b. During lower airway surgery, the tracheal tube tip should be placed just below the vocal cords so that it is as far away from the operative site as possible.

B. Other Head and Neck Fires
Head and neck fires can occur during local anesthesia procedures when electrosurgery apparatus is used. Often, oxygen is being administered and it may diffuse into the surgical area. Any flammable item in the vicinity can catch fire. Electrocautery in the presence of supplemental oxygen during facial surgery can result in serious injury during monitored anesthesia care.

C. Fires Involving Pressure Regulators
While not a frequent occurrence, an oxygen regulator fire can be disastrous. These fires may result from adiabatic compression or particle ignition in which debris is blown from the cylinder into the regulator with sufficient energy to cause ignition. Improperly assembling a pressure regulator may also result in a fire.

D. Intraperitoneal Fires
Several explosions have been reported during laparoscopy when nitrous oxide was used as the insufflating gas. Nitrous oxide in the inspired gases will diffuse into the peritoneal cavity and may reach a high enough concentration to support combustion. Fires have also resulted from inflating the peritoneal cavity with an O_2–CO_2 mixture instead of pure CO_2.

CLINICAL MOMENT The Pin Index Safety System (Chapter 1) will not prevent a tank containing a mixture of oxygen and CO_2 rather than a tank containing 100% CO_2 from being installed on the laparoscopic apparatus. The index hole positions for 100% CO_2 and any concentration of CO_2 greater than 7% are the same.

E. Fires during Defibrillation
Oxygen is always used during resuscitation, and the source is often disconnected and placed near the head. This may allow oxygen to flow over the defibrillation electrodes. A spark caused by placement of the defibrillator paddle or electrode close

to an ECG electrode or poor contact between the patient's skin and the defibrillator paddle or electrode may ignite hair or other combustible materials in the area.

CLINICAL MOMENT During defibrillation or cardioversion, the oxygen source must be moved away from the patient.

F. Anesthesia Machine Fires

Modern anesthesia machines are computer driven and thus have multiple electronic components that could malfunction and cause a fire.

IV. **Personnel Risks**

A. Smoke Hazards

1. Potentially hazardous airborne contaminants are formed from vaporized tissue when a laser is used. These by-products have the potential to be mutagenic, carcinogenic, teratogenic, or vectors for viral infection. Electrosurgery devices and bone saws can produce vaporized fragments with the same hazards.
2. Inhaling potentially hazardous airborne contaminants can be kept to a minimum by scavenging the smoke. This helps to give the surgeon a clearer view of the surgical field and removes offensive and irritating odors. Various surgical smoke evacuators are available.

CLINICAL MOMENT To be most effective, the smoke evacuator nozzle should be positioned as close as possible to the operative field. The evacuator should be functional before, during and for at least 30 seconds after tissue is vaporized.

3. Personnel masks should be removed and discarded as soon as possible after use. Standard surgical masks filter out particles down to about 3 μm in diameter. The laser plume has particles as small as 0.31 μm. High-efficiency masks can filter particles down to 0.30 μm, but they are difficult to breathe through and lose their efficiency when wet.

B. Ocular Injuries

1. The laser beam may travel some distance so the hazard area may not be limited to the immediate surgical area and may present a risk to operating room personnel. The surgeon is not highly susceptible to injury because of the safety devices built into the instrument. However, if the instrument is accidentally activated, the surgeon will be exposed to the same hazards as other personnel.
2. The eye is especially vulnerable to injury. Because CO_2 laser beams are absorbed within the first 200 μm of tissue, they are a hazard to the cornea. Argon, KTP, and Nd-YAG lasers are more likely to cause damage to the retina. The extent of damage will depend on the part of the retina that is affected. Permanent vision loss may result.
3. All personnel in the area where a laser is used should wear appropriate protective eyewear. This may include goggles, face shields, spectacles, or prescription eyewear with special materials or reflective coatings or both, selected to reduce the potential ocular exposure. The safety eyewear should be marked according to the wavelength/laser type (**Fig. 25.8**). The patient's eyes should be closed and covered with saline-soaked gauze or a nonshiny metal shield. Awake patients should wear goggles specific for the laser being used. Windows in the room should be covered and a warning sign placed on the operating

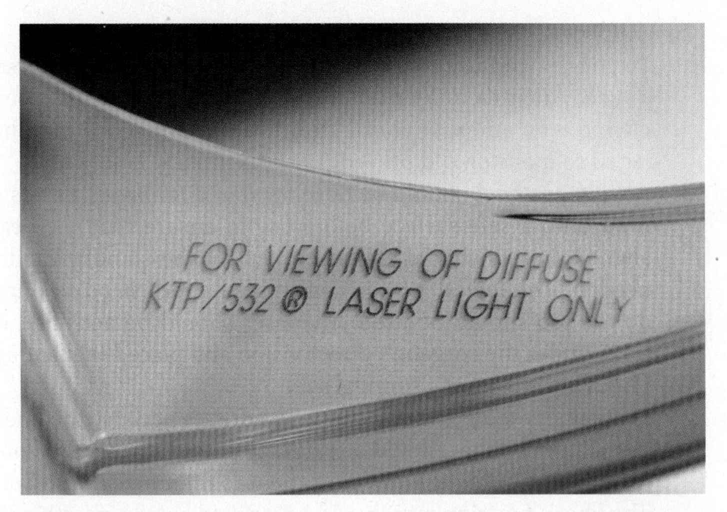

Figure 25.8 All laser-protective eyewear should be clearly and permanently labeled.

room door at the eye level (**Fig. 25.4**). Spare eyewear should be available at all entrances.

CLINICAL MOMENT Be certain that the protective eyewear being used is appropriate for the laser type in use.

CLINICAL MOMENT Orange laser goggles will block out blue light so that blue items appear gray. This may hinder color coding for identifying labels and reading colored monitor screens.

CLINICAL MOMENT Eyewear is not designed for looking directly at a laser beam.

C. Electrical Shock

1. Another concern is electrical shock from the electrosurgery device. A common practice among surgeons is to allow an assistant to touch the distal end of a forceps with the active electrode of the electrosurgery apparatus. This action makes the forceps the active electrode. A glove may not offer sufficient protection from the electrical circuit. Holes appear in as many as 15% of gloves.
2. There are ways to minimize the risk of shock while using electrosurgery. The active electrode should be firmly in contact with the forceps before it is energized. The person holding the forceps should try to contact as large an area as possible to spread the charge concentration.

V. **Fire Prevention**

The best way to deal with fires is to prevent them from starting. Fires can be avoided by not allowing the three elements of the fire triad to come together at the same time.

A. Controlling Ignition Sources

One way to reduce fires is to properly use equipment that might act as an ignition source. It is important to read instruction manuals and to alter techniques to fit these instructions.

1. **Lasers**
   a. Personnel who use lasers should take a certified laser course. They should practice their technique on inanimate objects and gain experience in association with an experienced clinician. Specific personnel should be designated to monitor and prevent laser hazards.
   b. A laser protocol should be developed and followed. Lasers should be test fired onto a safe surface before use to ensure that the beam is properly aligned. Lasers should always be kept in the standby mode except when needed. The lowest power density and shortest pulse duration that will do the job should be used. The laser should be activated only when the tip is under the surgeon's direct vision and placed in standby mode before removing it from the surgical site.
   c. Laser fibers should not be clipped to drapes because the fibers may be broken. The laser fiber should be carefully passed through an endoscope before introducing the scope into the patient to minimize the risk of fiber damage. The fiber's functionality should be verified before inserting the endoscope.
   d. After a laser contact tip is used, it will remain hot for several seconds. Blind entry into cavities with this tip should be avoided. The risk of tracheal tube ignition will be lowered if the laser is activated during the expiratory pause.
2. **Electrosurgery Unit**
   a. The electrosurgery unit should not be used during tracheostomy. Bleeding should not be treated by electrosurgery after a flammable dressing has been applied.
   b. A bipolar electrosurgery unit should be used whenever possible. This will reduce the current density in the tissues surrounding the active electrode and minimize the potential for direct coupling. Bipolar units work at lower voltages and are not associated with insulation failure.
   c. Monopolar units should have a means to monitor the return electrode or active electrode. This will minimize the risk of stray electrosurgical burns. Before each use, the electrosurgery unit and associated safety features should be inspected for damage and tested to ensure that the unit is functioning correctly. If it is not working properly or is damaged, the unit should be immediately removed from service. The unit should be protected from spills. Unintentional activation may occur if fluids enter the generator. The alarm system should be checked before applying the dispersive electrode. The active electrode should have a tip that is secure, because a loose tip may cause a spark. Pregelled dispersive electrode pads should be checked for uniform gel distribution and exposed wires before being applied to the patient. Outdated or previously opened but unused dispersive electrode pads should not be used, because the gel can undergo electrolysis and/or desiccation. If a dispersive electrode pad requiring gel is used, the pad should be checked carefully to identify any dry spots on its surface before it is placed on the patient.
   d. After the patient has been positioned, the connection between the patient and the unit should be established by placing the dispersive electrode on a site that is highly vascular with a large muscle mass. The dispersive electrode should be the appropriate size for a patient (i.e., neonate, infant, pediatric, adult) and never cut to reduce its size.
   e. The dispersive electrode should be applied to clean, dry skin over a large, well-perfused muscle mass as close to the operative site as practical, avoiding bony

prominences, scar tissue, tattoos, or skin over a metal prosthesis or distal to a tourniquet. Excessive hair should be removed before applying the dispersive electrode, because hair will insulate the pad from the patient. The pad's entire surface area should maintain uniform body contact. There should not be any tenting, gaping, or moisture under the pad because this will interfere with adhesion to the skin and decrease the contact surface. The dispersive electrode conductive status should be checked if any tension is applied to the cord or if the patient is repositioned after the pad is applied. A dispersive electrode should not be reused.

f. ECG electrodes should be placed as far as possible from the operative site or dispersive electrode to minimize the current flow through the electrodes and monitor the flow to the dispersive electrode.
g. If insulated electrosurgical electrode probes are required, only commercially available insulated probes should be used. Insulating sleeves cut from catheters or other materials should not be used to sheathe probes.
h. The lowest power settings that are effective for the surgical procedure, as determined by the surgeon in conjunction with the manufacturer's recommendation, should be used.

CLINICAL MOMENT The entire circuit should be checked for proper continuity if the operator requests higher power settings because of ineffectual results.

i. The electrosurgery unit should be activated only when the tip is under the surgeon's direct vision and only by the person using it. Cords should not be clamped or wound around any objects. The electrosurgery probe should be kept clean with wet gauze pads to minimize the risk that adherent tissue may incandesce or flame. A rough surface pad can also be used. The electrosurgical pencil should be placed in a protective holster and the electrosurgical unit placed in standby mode whenever it is not in active use. Unnecessary foot switches should be removed so that they are not accidentally activated.
j. During laparoscopic surgery, all-metal or all-plastic cannulae should be used and not a hybrid cannula system (i.e., a combination of plastic and metal cannulae). Electrosurgery electrodes should not be used inside metal suction irrigators.
k. The electrosurgical unit should be deactivated before removing it from the surgical site. Even after deactivation, the probe tip may retain enough heat for a few seconds to melt plastics or ignite some fuels, so it should be placed inside a clean, well-insulated holder or broken off. In addition to protecting the tip, this makes it more difficult to accidentally activate the switch on the probe handle. The tip should be broken, and a safety cover should be placed over the tip and activation switch before the device is discarded.

3. **Argon Beam Coagulation**

All safety measures observed for the electrosurgical unit should be observed for argon beam coagulation. The electrode should not be placed in direct contact with tissue. The hand piece should be moved away from the patient's tissue after each activation. The argon gas flow and the argon coagulator should be activated simultaneously. Air should be purged from the argon gas line before each procedure.

4. **Fiber-optic Light Sources**
All connections in a fiber-optic system should be made before the light source is activated, because the end of the cable can cause a fire. An active fiber-optic cable should not be placed on flammable material. The light source should be turned OFF before disconnecting the cable. The end of a fiber-optic cable can retain a significant amount of heat after being disconnected from the light source. Therefore, it is important to be careful where the end of a fiber-optic cord is placed.
5. **Heated Humidifiers**
Only a breathing tube and a heating circuit labeled for use with a specific humidifier should be used. Heated breathing circuits should not be covered with sheets, blankets, towels, clothing, or other material. The circuit should not rest on surfaces such as the patient, operating table, blankets, or medical equipment. Instead, a boom arm or tube tree should be used to support them. A heated-wire breathing circuit should not be turned ON before gas flow through the breathing tube has been initiated.

CLINICAL MOMENT If there is no flow (as during cardiopulmonary bypass) a heated humidifier must be turned OFF.

6. **Defibrillators**
When using a defibrillator, care should be taken to hold the paddles firmly and position them properly. Disposable conductive pads should be larger than the paddle's metal surface and be within their expiration date. This will prevent arcing when the paddles are activated. ECG electrodes should be applied as far as possible from the defibrillation pads.
7. **Electrical Faults**
All electrical cords should be inspected regularly for cuts and nicks in the insulation, frayed insulation, and loose connections at the plug or receptacle ends. All plugs should be pushed completely into the receptacles to prevent prong-to-prong arcing.

B. Managing Fuels
1. **Tracheal Tubes**
a. Nonintubation Techniques
Since the tracheal tube is often the source of a fire, anesthetic techniques that do not require a tracheal tube will eliminate one component of the fire triad. These include apnea and spontaneous breathing. With the apneic technique, the patient is ventilated using a mask or tracheal tube and these are withdrawn as the laser is used. After a short apneic period, ventilation is reinstated. This is repeated as long as necessary to perform the surgical procedure.
b. Filling the Cuff with Saline
1) The cuff is the most vulnerable part of the tracheal tube, regardless of the tube or cuff material. Fluid in a cuff acts as a heat sink and makes the cuff less easy to perforate. Filling the cuff with a lidocaine jelly plus saline mixture not only prevents the cuff from being ignited but may also plug small holes in the cuff resulting from a laser hit. If the cuff is perforated, a jet of fluid may extinguish the fire.

2) Care must be taken to remove all air from the cuff, because any remaining air will settle in the most superior part of the cuff, which is the part most likely to be hit by the laser beam. Adding methylene blue or other biocompatible and highly visible dye to the saline will help the surgeon recognize a perforated cuff.

c. Protective Wrappings
The tube can be covered with a protective wrapping. Merocel wrap (Laser-Guard™) was found to be acceptable for surgical levels of the CO_2, KTP, and Nd-YAG lasers. Merocel-wrapped tubes are not more combustible if they are coated with blood. Reflected laser beams have not been a problem with this wrap. This product is easier to apply than metallic tapes.

d. Protecting the Cuff with Wet Covers
As a further precaution, moist cottonoids, sponges, or pledgets can be placed on the cuff. Cotton gauze is a good choice because it stays wet longer than other covers and has low energy transmission. Wet gauze will also protect the shaft. These have been found to be especially helpful with the CO_2 laser. The Nd-YAG, KTP, and argon lasers may allow some energy to penetrate the pledget and rupture the cuff.

CLINICAL MOMENT It is important that wet covers is kept moist. Laser beam hits may dry them. Further hits can cause the cottonoids and/or cuff to ignite. All these must be retrieved after surgery.

e. Special Tracheal Tubes
1) No laser-resistant tracheal tube is completely safe from all types of lasers under all conditions. All can be damaged or ignited by lasers for which they are not intended or by high laser energies. Some are made more combustible by blood. Tubes sold for use with lasers should indicate the type of laser for which they are suited as well as the conditions (power, power density, spot size, oxygen concentration) under which the tube is safe to use. Strict adherence to manufacturer's warnings and directions is essential.
2) If the Nd-YAG laser is used through a fiber-optic bronchoscope passed through a tracheal tube, it is best to use an unmarked PVC tube. The tracheal tube tip should be as far from the operative site as possible.
3) Double-cuff tubes are no more resistant to leaks that will occur after cuff puncture but do allow a seal to be maintained if one cuff remains intact. The second cuff remains vulnerable to puncture.
4) There are disadvantages associated with laser-resistant tubes. They are more expensive than PVC and red rubber tubes. Some laser-resistant tubes are so stiff that it is difficult to pass a stylet or use them with a specialized laryngoscope such as the Bullard laryngoscope (Chapter 14). Therefore, a difficult intubation may become even more challenging when these tubes are needed. Since these tubes are often used for patients who have had previous laryngeal surgery, the anatomy may be distorted, making intubation especially difficult.

f. Using Smaller Tracheal Tubes
Small-diameter tracheal tubes require higher power densities for ignition than large-diameter tubes because the higher gas flow cools smaller tubes more quickly than larger tubes. Also, the smaller the tube, the less likely it is to be hit by an ignition source.

g. Making the Tracheal Tube Easy to Remove
The tube should be fixed so that it can be removed quickly, if necessary. If the tube is to be removed, this should be done immediately after ignition to minimize damage to the airway and lungs. If the tube continues to burn, it may be very difficult to remove. Some tracheal tubes break apart as they burn. If the tube is wrapped, the wrapping may break into pieces that could lodge in the airway.

CLINICAL MOMENT PVC tubes with fluid-filled cuffs are more difficult to remove than red rubber tubes. The fastest way to deflate a fluid-filled cuff is to remove the contents with a syringe rather than cutting the pilot balloon.

h. Wetting Fuels
Using wet towels, packers, or sponges around the surgical site can keep materials near the site from igniting. Gauze or sponges used with uncuffed tracheal tubes to minimize gas leakage into the pharynx and sponges, gauze, and pledges (and their strings) used to protect the tracheal tube cuff should be moistened and not allowed to dry.

i. Proper Preparation Practices
Water-based solutions should be used to decontaminate the skin prior to surgery, whenever possible. If alcohol-containing solutions must be used, a minimum amount should be used and applied like paint and not in a thick, runny coat. The solution should not be applied in a manner that allows dripping, pooling, or wicking. If solution drips away from the surgical site, it should be immediately blotted with a gauze sponge before it can soak into any absorbent material. Any soaked materials should be removed. Preparatory solution that is pooled on skin (in the umbilicus or cricoid notch) may be removed with a sterile sponge. Draping should be delayed to allow the solution to fully vaporize and become diluted in room air. This could take 10 minutes or longer. Incise (adhesive, occlusive) drapes should be used, if possible, to isolate head and neck incisions from oxygen-enriched atmospheres and from flammable vapors beneath the drapes. If the incised material does not adhere to the patient, the preparatory solution is likely wet and the patient should be redraped after the prepared area is fully dry.

j. Correct Product Choices
1) It is important to consider the fire potential when choosing equipment. The anesthesia provider should be aware of the circumstances under which a fire can occur and strive to use products that have the lowest flammability under conditions where it will be used.
2) Fire/laser-resistant drapes should be used when exposure to ignition is possible. It is important that the drape be tested with the type of ignition source that is to be used. Laser-resistant anesthesia circuit

protectors and drapes are available. These are aluminized to deflect the laser beam. There is still the possibility that the beam may be reflected onto a flammable surface and start a fire.

3) Using a metallic Y-piece and elbow will ensure that tracheal tube combustion will not spread to the anesthesia breathing system.

k. Other Measures

A number of other measures may be beneficial in preventing a fire. The tracheal tube should be withdrawn to above the surgical site during tracheotomy. Using positive end-expiratory pressure (PEEP) may decrease the risk of airway fire in some cases. Nursing personnel can reduce the combustible load in the room by removing disposable paper wrappers and covers before surgery begins. Not only does this reduce the fuel in the room but it also reduces the waste, which must be disposed as "red bag" that incurs higher disposal costs.

C. Minimizing Oxidizer Concentrations

1. The fire risk can be reduced by removing or isolating the oxidizer from the surgical area or minimizing its concentration.
2. During defibrillation, all sources of oxygen should be completely removed from the area around the patient.
3. Oxygen should be administered only when indicated and in no higher concentration than is needed (as guided by oxygen saturation monitoring).
4. Some anesthesia machines have an air flowmeter (**Fig. 25.7**). An oxygen and an air flowmeter can be connected using a Y-piece (**Fig. 25.6**) or a blender used to supply a gas with an oxygen concentration more than 21% but less than 100% to the patient.
5. If the machine has an air flowmeter, a mixture of oxygen and air can be set and delivered to the common gas outlet. If the common gas outlet can be accessed, a nasal cannula can be mated to the outlet by using a 5-mm tracheal tube connector. If the common gas outlet cannot be accessed, a circle system can be attached to the machine, the adjustable pressure-limiting valve closed, and the selector switch set to BAG. A nasal cannula can then be attached to the Y-piece. This arrangement may cause the continuous positive pressure alarm to be activated.
6. If possible, the oxygen flow should be discontinued for at least 1 minute before heat-producing surgical instruments are used. When the heat source is no longer in use and any tissue embers are extinguished, oxygen administration can be resumed.
7. During head and neck surgery, a barrier should be established between the oxygen-enriched atmosphere beneath the drapes and the surgical field, if possible. This can often be accomplished with an adhesive (incise, occlusive) drape. When gas is used to ventilate the area under the drapes and prevent CO_2 accumulation, the lowest acceptable concentration of oxygen should be used.

CLINICAL MOMENT If sticky plastic drapes are used to form a barrier, the sticky side that extends over the tracheal tube and/or breathing system should be covered with sponges or a cloth so that the tracheal tube or breathing system does not stick to the drape, which could cause inadvertent extubation when the drape is removed.

8. Forming an open tent with the drapes will prevent gases from collecting and allow the oxygen to dissipate. Since oxygen is slightly heavier than room air as long as there is some way for the oxygen to get in and out of a space, it will tend to flow toward the floor. Actively scavenging the space beneath drapes with a suction device will lower the oxygen concentration. Devices that combine oxygen delivery with suction to prevent oxygen buildup under the drape have been described.
9. A forced-air warming machine (Chapter 24) can be used to provide a high flow of air around the patient's head while a nasal cannula delivers 100% oxygen to the patient, or a fan can be used to blow the accumulated oxygen away from the patient.
10. Although using lower inspired oxygen concentrations will reduce the ignition risk, it will not totally prevent it. If there is a significant leak around the tracheal tube, the anesthesia provider may fill the reservoir bag by pushing the oxygen flush. This will result in an elevated oxygen concentration. A more appropriate response would be to increase the fresh gas flow while maintaining the same inspired oxygen concentration or to replace the tracheal tube.
11. When electrosurgery is used in the oral cavity, using a cuffed tracheal tube will minimize the oxidizer level. If an uncuffed tube must be used, an occlusive pharyngeal pack moistened with a nonflammable liquid will reduce the gas flow into the oral cavity. Insufflating the mouth with a gas such as helium, CO_2, or nitrogen will reduce the oxidizer concentration. The oropharynx can be scavenged with suction.

D. Preventing Pressure Regulator Fires

Fires in pressure regulators can be minimized by not allowing them to become contaminated with oil, grease, or other combustible materials or cleaned with a flammable agent such as alcohol. Before a regulator is fitted to a cylinder, particles should be cleared from the cylinder outlet by removing the protective cap or seal and slowly and briefly opening ("cracking") the valve with the port pointed away from the user and any other persons. A cylinder valve should always be opened slowly to allow heat to be dissipated as the gas is recompressed. Consideration should be given to replacing aluminum regulators with those made from brass. Rules for handling cylinders are discussed in Chapter 1.

VI. Fire Plan

A. Each healthcare facility should formulate a plan for dealing quickly with an operating room fire. Surgical teams should be trained and participate in practice drills for keeping minor fires from getting out of control and managing fires that do get out of control. They should know the location and proper use of alarm boxes, gas shutoff valves, and fire extinguishers (**Fig. 25.9**). Evacuation procedures should be reviewed periodically.

CLINICAL MOMENT During a Joint Commission on Accreditation of Healthcare Organizations inspection, it is common for the examiner to ask clinicians where the gas shutoff valves are and the location of fire extinguishers and fire alarms.

B. The acronym **RACEE** (**R**escue the individual involved in the fire; **A**ctivate the alarm; **C**onfine the fire; **E**xtinguish the fire; and **E**vacuate if required) can be used when there is a fire. It is important to immediately call for help, decide who is going to fight the fire, when it will be appropriate to leave the room, and how to care for the patient during the fire.

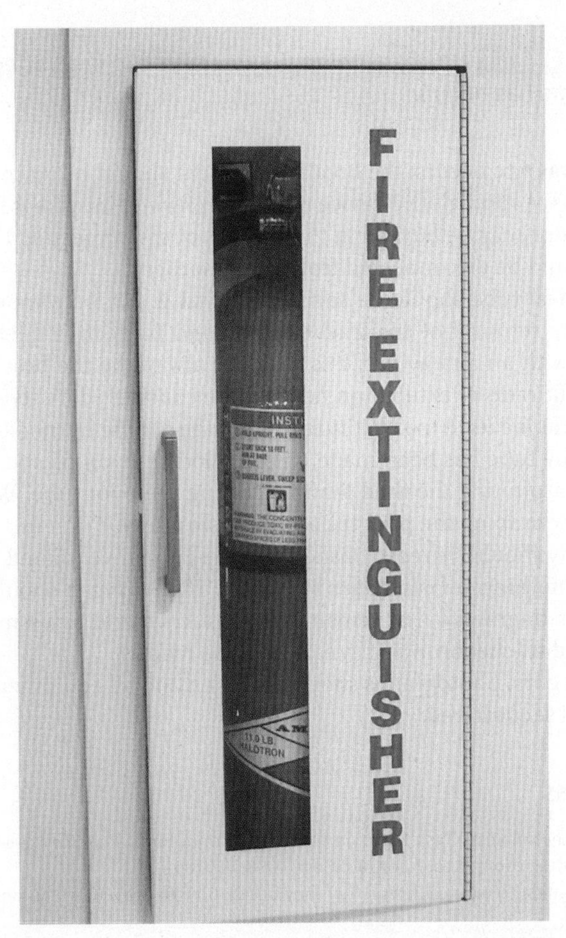

Figure 25.9 Fire extinguishers should be in conspicuous locations, well known to all operating room staff members.

C. Burning material on or in the patient often can be extinguished by hand or with a nonflammable liquid (e.g., saline from a basin on the scrub table) or a wet cloth. During laser surgery of the airway, at least two syringes filled with sodium chloride should always be available to extinguish a fire. Larger areas can be smothered with a blanket or wet towel. Fire blankets are not recommended. If the drape is water resistant, water poured on it will be ineffective. The fire will burn on the underside. The only effective technique is to pull the burning materials away from the patient.

D. Fires that involve electrical components are best handled by unplugging the device and removing it from the room.

E. The flows of oxygen, nitrous oxide, or air to any involved equipment should be turned OFF, if this can be accomplished without injury to personnel or the patient. Most patients can tolerate short periods of oxygen deprivation. The patient should be ventilated with air and intravenous agents used to maintain anesthesia until all possible sources of fire are suppressed. It may be necessary to close the oxygen and nitrous oxide shutoff valves to the affected room. Cylinder valves should be closed and all cylinders removed from the area. If supplemental oxygen is necessary to oxygenate the patient, the patient should be moved to the nearest area where oxygen can be safely used.

CLINICAL MOMENT Do not squeeze the reservoir bag in an attempt to blow the fire out after a fire has begun.

F. If an airway fire occurs, the breathing system should be disconnected from the tracheal tube or supraglottic device to stop gas flow. If this site is not easily accessible or the operator may be burned in the process of disconnecting the tube, the breathing tubes should be disconnected from the absorber.

G. The tracheal tube should be secured so that it can be removed quickly. Although immediate removal of the tracheal tube and protective devices is usually recommended with an airway fire, this may not always be the best course of action. The risk:benefit ratio of extubation needs to be considered. A stylet or airway exchange catheter can be used to substitute a new tube for the burned tube. If the decision to remove the tube has been made, saline-filled cuffs on plastic tubes can be deflated faster by aspirating the fluid than by cutting the pilot tube. With red rubber tubes, simply unclamping the pilot tube is the fastest way.

H. The airway should be reestablished and the patient ventilated with air until it is certain that nothing remains burning. Then, 100% oxygen should be administered. A search for fragments that remain in the trachea and assessment of damage to the larynx and tracheobronchial tree should be made.

I. If a fire occurs, photographs should be taken and all equipment used during the fire saved and sequestered.

SUGGESTED READINGS

American Society of Anesthesiologists Task Force on Operating Room Fires. Practice advisory for the prevention and management of operating room fires. Anesthesiology 2008;108:786–801.

Anonymous. A clinician's guide to surgical fires. How they occur, how to prevent them, how to put them out. Health Devices 2003;32:5–24.

AORN Guidance Statement: Fire Prevention in the Operating Room. 2005. http://www.ashe.org/ashe/codes/nfpa/pdfs/aorn_firesafety.pdf

Dennis V. 7 hot spots in electrosurgery. Outpatient Surg Mag 2005;6:49–53.

Dorsch J, Dorsch S. Operating room fires and personnel injuries related to sources of ignition. In: Understanding Anesthesia Equipment. Fifth edition. Philadelphia: Wolters Kluwer/Lippincott Williams & Wilkins, 2008:907–929.

Ehrenwerth J. A Fire in the Operating Room! It Could Happen to You. Orlando, FL: American Society of Anesthesiologists, 2008. ASA Refresher Course No. 115.

Gross JB. Less Jolts from Your Volts: Electrical Safety in the Operating Room. Orlando, FL: American Society of Anesthesiologists, 2008. ASA Refresher Course No. 104.

Lee J. Update on electrosurgery. Outpatient Surg Mag 2002;3:44–53.

Lees DE. Operating room fires: still a problem? ASA Newslett 2002;66:33–34.

McKee K. A guide to testing your electrosurgery instruments. Outpatient Surg Mag 2001;11:59–64.

Meltzer B. Issues in electrosurgery. Outpatient Surg Mag 2001;11:51–61.

National Fire Protection Association. NFPA 10, Standard for Portable Fire Extinguishers. 2007 edition. Cheshire, CT: National Fire Protection Association.

Pfenninger J. ABCs of electrosurgery. Outpatient Surg Mag 2004;5:45–50.

Prasad R, Quezado Z, St. Andre A, et al. Fires in the operating room and intensive care unit: awareness is the key to prevention. Anesth Analg 2006;102:172–174.

Wasek S. Preventing surgical fires. Outpatient Surg Mag 2003;4:28–35.

26 Equipment Checkout and Maintenance

I. Introduction

A. A checkout procedure is analogous to the preflight check for airline pilots and is intended to determine whether equipment is present, properly functioning, and ready for use. Failure to perform an adequate equipment checkout is a factor in many critical incidents and can lead to patient injury, death, or "near misses." Proper checking can reduce equipment-related morbidity and mortality and educate the anesthesia provider about equipment. Defects may be found even just after preventive maintenance has been performed.

B. Failure to perform a proper check before use is common. Many anesthesia providers are unable to identify intentionally created faults. With intensive training, performance improves but high rates of correct completion are not achieved.

II. Available Checklists

A. Manufacturer's Checklist

All manufacturers provide a detailed checkout in their user manual that accompanies the anesthesia machine. This checkout is typically very detailed and if strictly followed would likely find almost any problem. The user manual should be carefully studied whenever a machine that is new to the anesthesia provider is used or questions concerning the machine arise. Unfortunately, these procedures are often overly complicated, so in practice it is often abridged or skipped altogether.

B. 1993 FDA Checkout

The Food and Drug Administration (FDA), working with representatives of the anesthesia community and industry, developed a preuse checkout procedure, which was published in 1986. Unfortunately, this list was too complicated for most users. A simplified, more user-friendly version was published in 1993. It is shown in **Table 26.1.**

C. 2008 ASA Checkout

1. The American Society of Anesthesiologists (ASA) in conjunction with manufacturers, the American Association of Nurse Anesthetists, and other interested parties in 2008 published a new checklist that recognizes that newer, computer-

Table 26.1 Anesthesia Apparatus Checkout Recommendations, 1993[a]

This checkout, or a reasonable equivalent, should be conducted before administration of anesthesia. These recommendations are valid only for an anesthesia system that conforms to current and relevant standards and includes an ascending bellows ventilator and at least the following monitors: capnograph, pulse oximeter, oxygen analyzer, respiratory volume monitor (spirometer), and breathing system pressure monitor with high- and low-pressure alarms.

Emergency Ventilation Equipment

*1. *Verify that backup ventilation equipment is available and functioning*

High-Pressure System

*2. *Check the oxygen cylinder supply*
  a. Open the oxygen cylinder and verify that it is at least half full (about 1000 psig)
  b. Close the cylinder

*3. *Check the central pipeline supplies*
Check that the hoses are connected and pipeline gauges read about 50 psig

Low-Pressure System

*4. *Check the initial status of the low-pressure system*
  a. Close the flow control valves and turn vaporizers OFF
  b. Check the fill level and tighten vaporizers' filler caps

*5. *Perform a leak check of the machine's low-pressure system*
  a. Verify that the machine master switch and flow control valves are OFF
  b. Attach a "suction bulb" to the common (fresh) gas outlet
  c. Squeeze the bulb repeatedly until fully collapsed
  d. Verify that the bulb stays *fully* collapsed for at least 10 seconds
  e. Open one vaporizer at a time, and repeat the above-mentioned parts c and d
  f. Remove the suction bulb and reconnect the fresh gas hose

*6. *Turn the machine master switch ON as well as all other necessary electrical equipment*

*7. *Test the flowmeters*
  a. Adjust the flow of all gases through their full range, checking for smooth operation of floats and undamaged flow tubes
  b. Attempt to create a hypoxic oxygen–nitrous oxide mixture and verify correct changes in flow and/or alarm

Scavenging System

*8. *Adjust and check the scavenging system*
  a. Ensure proper connections between the scavenging system and both the APL (pop-off) valve and the ventilator relief spill valve
  b. Adjust the waste gas vacuum flow, if possible
  c. Fully open the APL valve and occlude the Y-piece
  d. With minimum oxygen flow, allow the scavenger reservoir bag to collapse completely and verify that the absorber pressure gauge reads about zero
  e. With the oxygen flush activated, allow the scavenger reservoir bag to distend fully and then verify that the absorber pressure gauge reads less than 10 cm H_2O

Breathing System

*9. *Calibrate the oxygen monitor*
  a. Ensure that the monitor reads 21% in room air
  b. Verify that the low oxygen alarm is enabled and functioning
  c. Reinstall the sensor in the circuit and flush the breathing system with oxygen
  d. Verify that the monitor now reads more than 90%

10. *Check the initial status of the breathing system*
  a. Set the selector switch to BAG mode
  b. Check that the breathing circuit is complete, undamaged, and unobstructed
  c. Verify that the carbon dioxide absorbent is adequate
  d. Install the breathing circuit accessory equipment (e.g., humidifier, PEEP valve) that is to be used during the case

11. *Perform a leak check of the breathing system*
  a. Set all gas flows to zero (or minimum)
  b. Close the APL (pop-off) valve, and occlude the Y-piece
  c. Pressurize the breathing system to about 30 cm H_2O by oxygen flush
  d. Ensure that the pressure remains fixed for at least 10 seconds
  e. Open the APL (pop-off) valve and ensure that the pressure decreases

Manual and Automatic Ventilation Systems

12. *Test the ventilator systems and unidirectional valves*
  a. Place a second breathing bag on the Y-piece
  b. Set the appropriate ventilator parameters for the next patient
  c. Switch to the automatic ventilation (VENTILATOR) mode
  d. Turn the ventilator ON and fill the bellows and breathing bag by oxygen flush
  e. Set the oxygen flow to minimum and other gas flows to zero
  f. Verify that during inspiration, the bellows delivers appropriate tidal volume and that during expiration, the bellows fills completely
  g. Set the fresh gas flow to about 5 L/minute
  h. Verify that the ventilator bellows and the simulated lungs fill and empty appropriately without sustained pressure at end expiration
  i. Check for proper action of the unidirectional valves
  j. Exercise the breathing circuit accessories to ensure proper function
  k. Turn the ventilator OFF and switch to manual ventilation (BAG/APL) mode
  l. Ventilate manually and ensure inflation and deflation of artificial lungs and appropriate feel of system resistance and compliance
  m. Remove the second breathing bag from the Y-piece

Monitors

13. *Check, calibrate, and/or set alarm limits of all monitors.*
  Capnometer
  Pulse oximeter
  Oxygen analyzer
  Respiratory volume monitor (spirometer)
  Pressure monitor with high- and low-airway alarms

Final position

14. *Check the final status of the machine.*
  a. Vaporizers OFF
  b. APL valve open
  c. Selector switch to BAG
  d. All flowmeters to zero
  e. Patient suction level adequate
  f. Breathing system ready to use

[a]If an anesthesia provider uses the same machine in successive cases, the steps marked with an asterisk (*) do not need to be repeated or may be abbreviated after the initial checkout.

driven anesthesia machines include an automated checkout procedure, which is primarily a breathing system and ventilator function test. Unfortunately, some clinicians believe that the automated checkout covers the entire machine and breathing system.

2. The 2008 checkout listed the following requirements for safe anesthesia delivery:
   a. Reliable oxygen delivery in any appropriate concentration up to 100%.
   b. A reliable means to deliver positive-pressure ventilation.
   c. Presence of functional backup ventilation equipment.
   d. Positive pressure in the breathing circuit that can be released in a controllable manner.
   e. The ability to administer anesthetic vapor, if desired.
   f. Suction available and adequate for use.
   g. The ability to conform to practice standards for monitoring.
3. These items must be checked at the beginning of the day and after the anesthesia machine is moved or serviced or vaporizers are changed. Following this checklist will typically require less than 5 minutes at the beginning of the day and less than 2 minutes between successive cases.
4. The essential steps in the checklist are presented in **Table 26.2.** This list recognizes the ability of a qualified anesthesia technician instead of, or in addition to, the anesthesia provider to test certain functions.
5. This checkout depends on the individual institution to fill in the details of how each machine and item will be checked. The details will depend on the particular anesthesia machine being used. The manufacturer's checkout should be consulted and incorporated into the checkout as much as possible. Because of the variety of machines that are in use or will be introduced, only generalities can be provided in this text. The user must determine which parts are checked automatically and add those that are not covered.

D. Checkout Concepts

1. Both the 1993 and 2008 checkouts require the anesthesia provider to check various areas but do not indicate how the check is to be performed. To complicate things even further, the new anesthesia machines with automated checkout procedures cover only part of the requirements. Often they prompt the anesthesia provider to check other items but do not give details on how to do so.
2. To explain how various items care can be checked, the 1993 checkout will be used as a model. When an alternate test method is given, the advantages and deficiencies of that method will be pointed out.
3. This checkout is designed for a workstation with a circle system, ventilator, capnograph, oxygen analyzer, respiratory volume meter, and airway pressure monitor. Clinicians who use equipment that does not conform to this configuration (e.g., a Mapleson system) will need to modify the procedure. Such modifications should have appropriate peer review. The manufacturer's user manual should be consulted for special procedures.
4. A copy of the checkout procedure should be kept in, on, or near the anesthesia machine. A record that the checklist was used should be made and kept. It should include a place for the anesthesia provider and the anesthesia technician to sign after the checkout has been successfully completed. A printed checklist may result in a more organized and systematic approach than a mental checklist.

Table 26.2 ASA Guidelines for Preanesthesia Checkout[a]

Item No.	Item	Responsible Party
1.	Verify that the auxiliary oxygen cylinder and the manual ventilation device (bag-valve-mask unit) are available and functioning	Anesthesia provider and anesthesia technician
2.	*Verify that patient suction is adequate to clear the airway	Anesthesia provider and anesthesia technician
3.	Turn the anesthesia delivery system ON and confirm that AC power is available	Anesthesia provider or anesthesia technician
4.	*Verify the availability and functionality of required monitors, including alarms	Anesthesia provider or anesthesia technician
5.	Verify that pressure in the oxygen cylinder on the anesthesia machine is adequate for the intended use or location	Anesthesia provider and anesthesia technician
6.	Verify that piped gas pressures are equal to or greater than 50 psig.	Anesthesia provider and anesthesia technician
7.	*Verify that vaporizers are adequately filled and that the filler ports are tightly closed.	Anesthesia provider or anesthesia technician
8.	Verify that there are no leaks in the gas supply pipelines between the flowmeters and common gas outlet (low pressure system)	Anesthesia provider or anesthesia technician
9.	*Test scavenging system function	Anesthesia provider or anesthesia technician
10.	Calibrate, or verify calibration of, the oxygen monitor and check the low oxygen alarm	Anesthesia provider or anesthesia technician
11.	*Verify that the carbon dioxide absorbent is fresh and not exhausted	Anesthesia provider or anesthesia technician
12.	*Perform breathing pressure and leak testing	Anesthesia provider and anesthesia technician
13.	*Verify that gas flows properly through the breathing circuit during inspiration and exhalation	Anesthesia provider and anesthesia technician
14.	*Document completion of the checkout procedure	Anesthesia provider and anesthesia technician
15.	Confirm adequate ventilator settings and evaluate readiness to deliver anesthesia care (ANESTHESIA TIME OUT)	Anesthesia provider

[a]The steps marked with an asterisk (*) must be carried out before each subsequent case. Other steps may be omitted or abbreviated when this machine is again used that day.

III. General Considerations in Electronic Checking

A. Many anesthesia machines provide an electronic checking procedure (**Fig. 26.1**). When the machine is turned ON, it reminds the user to start the checkout. Before an electronic checkout is performed, all components that are to be used for the anesthetic should be in place. If the breathing tubing is to be extended, it should be extended to the desired length. During the checking procedure, the machine may prompt the anesthesia provider to make certain adjustments such as opening or closing the adjustable pressure-limiting (APL) valve, occluding the Y-piece, or adjusting the gas flows.

B. These electronic checking procedures test the electronic as well as some mechanical components of the anesthesia machine. In addition they may gather information (resistance, compliance, and leaks) on the breathing system [**Fig. 26.1B**]). They may also remind the user to check functions that are not included in the automatic checkout.

C. Most machines have a mechanism to limit or skip the electronic checkout in emergency situations. Many clinicians routinely use this to bypass the checkout. This is

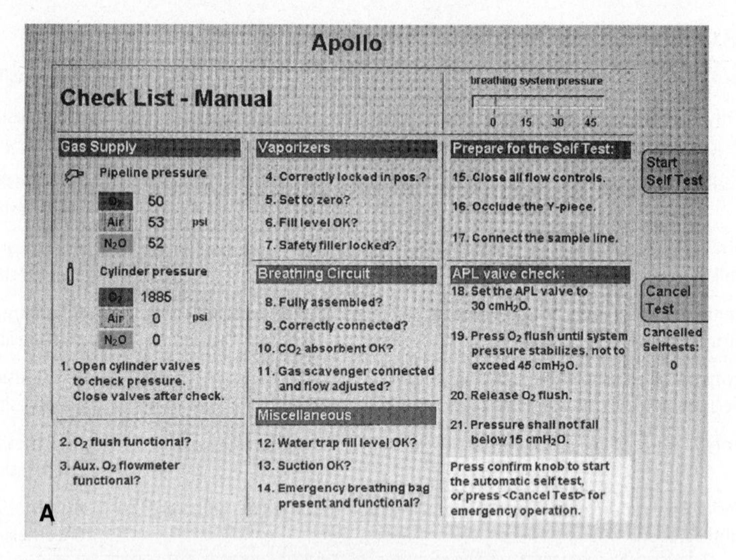

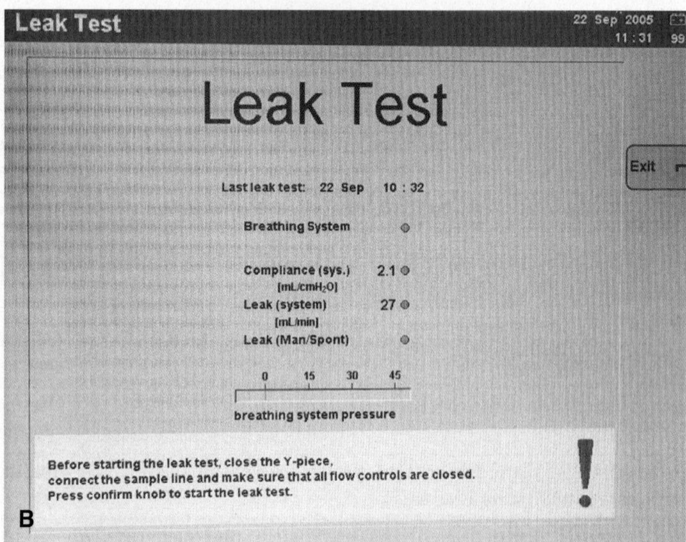

Figure 26.1 Electronic checkout procedure on a newer model anesthesia machine. **A.** The procedure lists several steps that the user must do before the Self Test is begun as well as other things (suction, emergency ventilation bag, water trap level) the user should check. **B.** The test procedure may provide information (compliance, leak rate) about the breathing system after the self test is complete. (Picture courtesy of Drager Medical, Lubeck, Germany).

not a good practice. The electronic check provides a more comprehensive check than most anesthesia providers perform and may detect some problems that would not otherwise have been found.

CLINICAL MOMENT If the electronic checkout is bypassed, this will be recorded in the memory of the computer. In the event of an adverse outcome, this information may be queried during legal proceedings. Some machines will not allow more than 10 consecutive bypasses without a full checkout being performed.

CLINICAL MOMENT If an anesthesia machine has been held in a ready-to-use (standby) state for emergencies, it should be turned OFF at least once every 24 hours and restarted with a new checkout procedure.

IV. Daily Checks before Beginning Anesthesia

A. Emergency Ventilation Equipment

1. **Resuscitation Bag**

   a. Although rare, certain malfunctions can render the anesthesia machine inoperative. Sometimes, the problem cannot be quickly diagnosed or corrected. In this situation, a manual resuscitator (Chapter 7) will allow the user to provide positive-pressure ventilation while the problem is corrected or the machine replaced.

   b. The resuscitator should be inspected for signs of wear such as cracks or tears. Even a new disposable resuscitation bag may have been improperly assembled or defective. A reservoir bag should be placed over the patient port (**Fig. 26.2**). Squeezing the resuscitation bag should cause the reservoir bag to inflate. After the reservoir bag is fully inflated and the resuscitation bag has been released, the reservoir bag should easily deflate.

   c. The patient port should be occluded and the bag squeezed (**Fig. 26.3**). Pressure should build up rapidly. If there is a pressure-limiting device, it can be checked by connecting a pressure manometer between the patient port and the bag, using a T-fitting. If there is an override mechanism on the pressure-limiting device, this should be checked.

   d. To check that the bag refill valve opens, the bag should be squeezed, the patient port occluded, and then the bag released. The bag should reexpand rapidly. Attaching an oxygen source is not necessary.

   e. If the resuscitator has a closed reservoir (Chapter 7), its function can be checked by performing several compression-release cycles with no oxygen

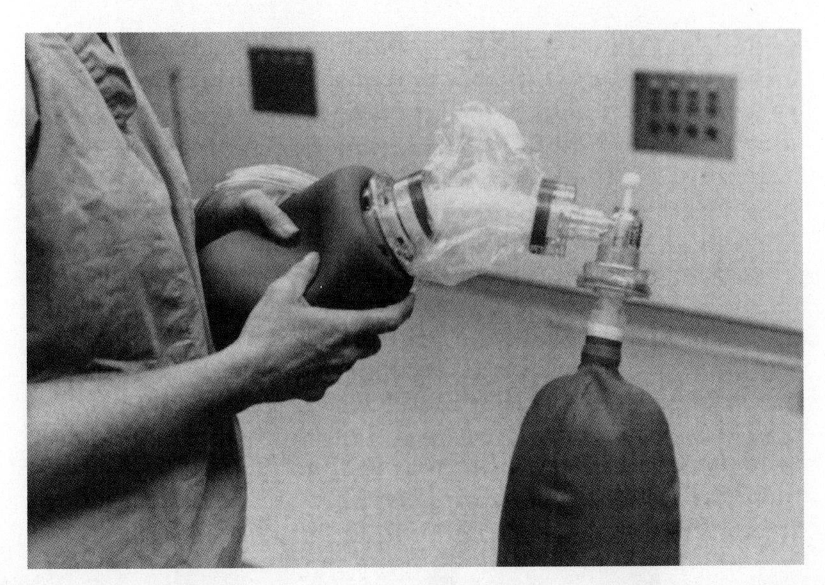

Figure 26.2 The resuscitation bag is further checked by placing a reservoir bag over the patient port. Squeezing the resuscitation bag should cause the reservoir bag to inflate. The reservoir bag should then deflate easily when it is squeezed.

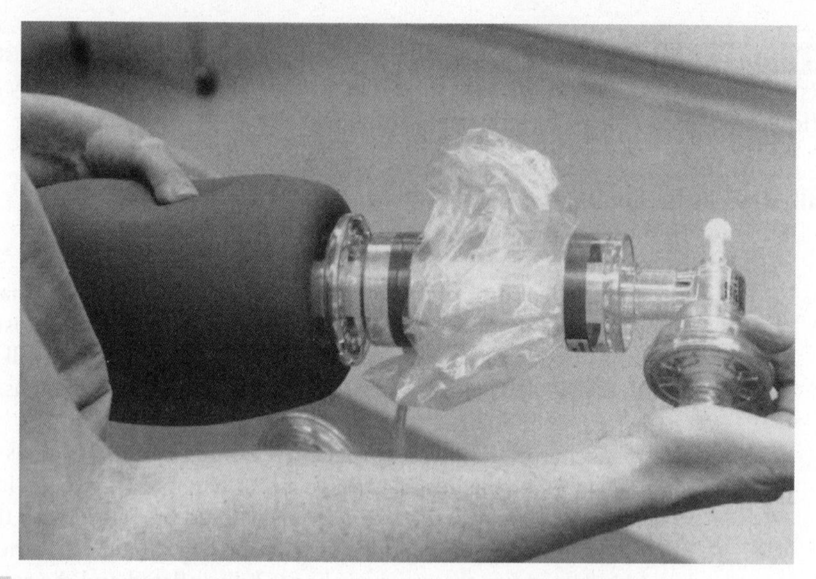

Figure 26.3 Squeezing the resuscitation bag with the patient port occluded.

flow into the reservoir. The reservoir should deflate, but the resuscitation bag should continue to expand. This procedure verifies that the air inlet valve functions with an empty reservoir.

2. **Oxygen Source**

   A source of oxygen to connect to the resuscitation bag should be available. An oxygen flowmeter attached to the pipeline outlet (**Fig. 26.4**), a cylinder with regulator, or the courtesy flowmeter on the anesthesia machine

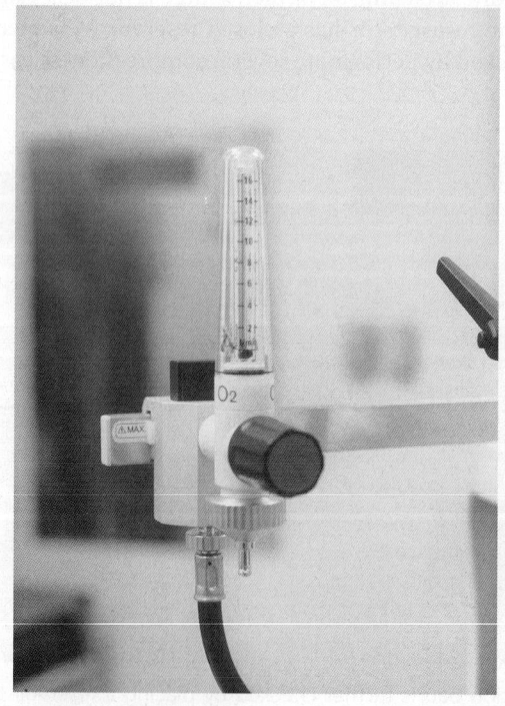

Figure 26.4 A flowmeter that is separate from the anesthesia machine can provide a source of oxygen in an emergency.

(Chapter 3) can be used. These should be checked to confirm that gas is delivered.

CLINICAL MOMENT The courtesy flowmeter on the anesthesia machine may or may not be connected to the cylinder on the machine as well as the pipeline supply. If oxygen from the courtesy flowmeter cannot be drawn from the cylinder on the machine in the event of pipeline failure, a separate cylinder with a pressure regulator and flow-metering device needs to be immediately available.

3. **Difficult Airway Equipment**
   If there is any indication that maintaining the patient's airway or performing tracheal intubation will be difficult, a difficult airway cart should be in the room. Whatever device is expected to be used needs to be present, assembled, and in working order.

B. Suction
   Adequate suction can be determined by placing the end of the suction tubing on the underside of the thumb with the hand at shoulder height (**Fig. 26.5**). The tubing should stay attached without support. A rigid suction catheter (Yankauer) should be immediately available.

C. Gas Supplies
   1. **Cylinder Pressure (High-Pressure System)**
      a. Cylinders should be checked for correct mounting. If there is an expiry label on a cylinder, it should be checked for currency. Yokes should be scanned to make certain that any yoke not containing a cylinder is fitted with a yoke (blanking) plug (Chapter 3). All tags should indicate *full* or *in use*.
      b. Before proceeding further, all flow control valves should be closed by turning them completely clockwise. Excessive torque should be avoided. Opening a cylinder or connecting a pipeline hose when a flow control valve is

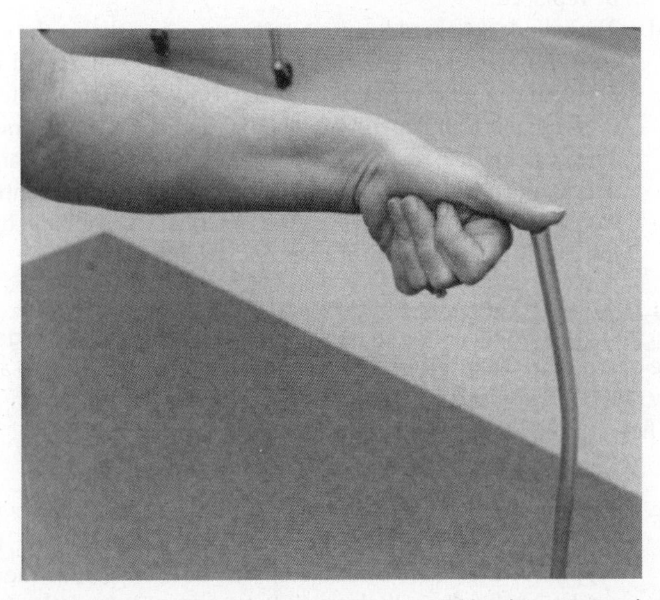

Figure 26.5 Test of suction. The strength of the vacuum is tested by determining that the weight of the suction tubing can be supported at shoulder height by the seal between the tubing and the underside of a finger. If the vacuum is unsatisfactory, the tubing will not remain in contact with the finger.

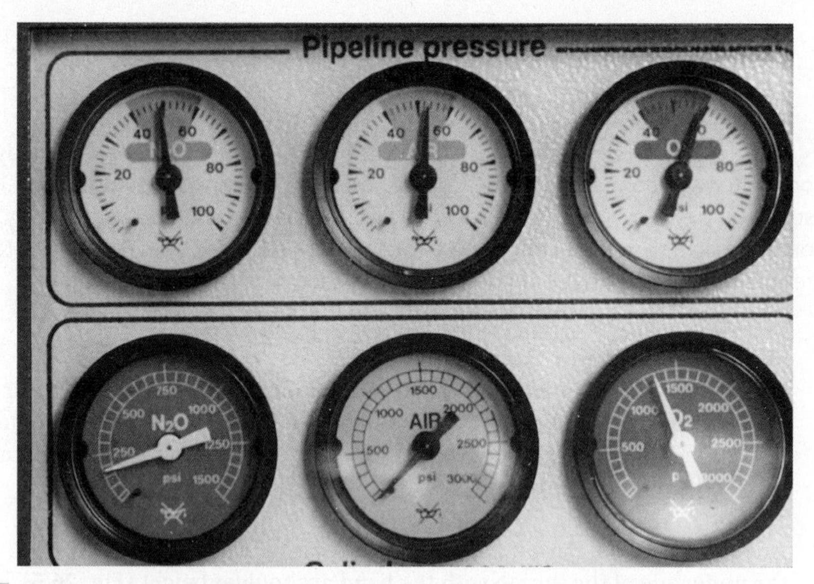

Figure 26.6 **Top row:** Pipeline pressure gauges. **Bottom row:** Cylinder pressure gauges.

open may cause the indicator to shoot up to the top of the tube and be damaged, stuck at the top, or not noticed.

c. Cylinder pressure is checked by turning the valve slowly counterclockwise while observing the related pressure gauge (**Fig. 26.6**). If a hissing sound occurs, there is a leak at its connection to the yoke. If tightening the cylinder in the yoke fails to stop the sound, the cylinder valve should be closed. Check that the cylinder is correctly placed in the yoke and that the washer is present and undamaged. If the hissing sound persists, the cylinder should be replaced.

d. The cylinder(s) should contain sufficient gas so that in the event of a problem with the pipeline supply, life support can be maintained until the pipeline problem can be corrected or more cylinders obtained. How low a pressure is acceptable will depend on whether additional cylinders are readily available, how low a fresh gas flow can be used, whether mechanical ventilation is necessary and what type of ventilator is present. Some ventilators use oxygen to drive the bellows. Others use air or a mixture of air and oxygen as the driving gas. A piston ventilator does not require driving gas.

CLINICAL MOMENT A full E cylinder will contain about 625 L of oxygen with a pressure of around 2000 psig. One full cylinder will last between 3.0 and 3.5 hours at a flow rate of 3 L/minute if a gas-driven ventilator is not in use. If a 1 L/minute oxygen flow is used, oxygen will be supplied for 625 minutes.

e. The authors believe that 500 psig in an oxygen cylinder is adequate, provided cylinders will not be the primary oxygen supply (i.e., there is a pipeline supply). A mechanical ventilator that uses oxygen as the drive gas should not be used if the cylinder supply is in use. The anesthesia provider should be aware of the steps needed to conserve oxygen.

CLINICAL MOMENT When the cylinder is to be the primary oxygen supply, the cylinder should be full and an additional cylinder should be immediately available.

CLINICAL MOMENT If the oxygen cylinder valve remains open after the pressure has been checked, oxygen will automatically be used if the pipeline fails or if the pressure drops below the regulated cylinder pressure. This may not be noticed by the anesthesia provider until the cylinder is empty and there is no oxygen available. If the cylinder is turned OFF and the pipeline pressure fails, there will be an alarm on newer machines and the nitrous oxide flow (if in use) will be interrupted. The operator can then open the cylinder valve, institute measures to conserve oxygen, and send for additional oxygen cylinder(s).

f. It has been suggested that merely checking a cylinder for adequate pressure is not enough. The check valve that prevents cylinder gas from being used when the pipeline is connected may stick, preventing flow from the cylinder if the pipeline is not in use. To check this valve, the pipeline hoses should be disconnected and flow at the flowmeters demonstrated after the cylinder is opened. This will also test the nonreturn valves in the pipeline hose inlet (see Chapter 3). If this valve fails, gas from the cylinder could flow retrograde into the gas pipeline system. If no gas flow occurs from the end of the pipeline hose when the pipeline hose is disconnected and the cylinder is turned ON, the check valve is functioning properly.

g. If it is planned to use a gas other than oxygen, it is reassuring to know that a cylinder supply is available on the machine. Some institutions do not purchase anesthesia machines with yokes for air and nitrous oxide, reasoning that since these gases are not essential to patient safety, backup cylinders are not necessary. As discussed in Chapter 1, the contents of a nitrous oxide cylinder are not reflected by the pressure unless all of the liquid has evaporated and the cylinder is nearly empty. The pressure gauge will continue to read 745 psig until all the liquid has vaporized. If the pressure is less than 600 psig, the nitrous oxide cylinder is nearly empty and should probably be replaced.

h. Empty or near-empty cylinders should be labeled as empty and replaced with full cylinders (see Chapter 1).

2. **Pipeline Pressure (Intermediate Pressure System)**
It is a good idea to disconnect the pipeline hoses from the machine at night to allow the anesthesia machine to be moved for cleaning and reduce gas loss from leaks. If this is the case, the hoses need to be reconnected to the pipeline system at this point. Fittings should hold firmly, no leaks should be audible, and the hoses should be arranged to prevent occlusion. The pipeline pressure indicators (**Fig. 26.6**) should read 345 to 380 kPa (50 to 55 psig) after the hoses are attached.

D. Low-Pressure System Check
The low-pressure system includes the flowmeters, vaporizers, and anything else between the flow controls and the machine outlet.

1. **Vaporizers**
The liquid level in each vaporizer should be checked, adding more agent if needed. Filler caps and drain valves should be tight. All the vaporizers should

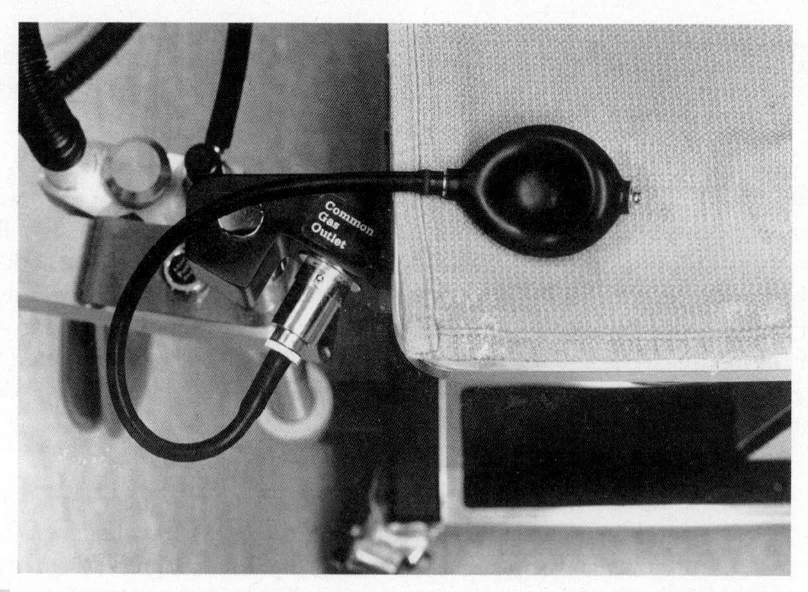

Figure 26.7 The suction bulb is attached to the common gas outlet and squeezed until it is collapsed. It should remain collapsed for at least 10 seconds. Following this, each vaporizer in turn should be turned ON and the maneuver repeated.

be tested to make certain that they cannot be lifted from their mountings and are not tilted.

2. **Leaks**
   a. General Considerations
      1) Selecting an appropriate leak check can be difficult, because some anesthesia machines have a check valve either at the common gas outlet or just downstream of the vaporizers. This prevents gas in the breathing system from flowing back into the machine.
      2) The minimum mandatory oxygen flow present on some older machines will make it difficult to detect small leaks. The leak test must be performed without the basal flow. To accomplish this, the machine needs to be turned OFF.
      3) Irrespective of which test is used, the leak test should be performed with the vaporizers turned OFF and then be repeated with each vaporizer separately turned ON to its minimum setting. If this is not done, the machine may pass the test for leaks, but a leak associated with a vaporizer or its mounting will be missed.
   b. Negative Pressure Test
      1) The negative pressure test uses a suction bulb to create a negative pressure in the machine. The bulb is attached to a 15-mm adaptor, which fits the anesthesia machine common gas outlet (**Fig. 26.7**). This device is available commercially or can be constructed by taking a sphygmomanometer bulb, reversing the air inlet valve in the bulb, and connecting one end of a short tubing to the bulb and the other to a 15-mm tracheal tube adaptor. Alternately, the device can be constructed from the bulb pump from a disposable intravenous blood administration set.
      2) To perform the test, all flowmeters are turned OFF. If there is a minimum mandatory oxygen flow, the entire machine must be turned

OFF. Squeezing the bulb until it is remains collapsed creates a negative pressure in the machine. If the bulb remains collapsed for 10 seconds or longer, there is no significant leak present. If there is a leak, the bulb will quickly inflate.

3) This test should be repeated with each vaporizer turned ON. The suction bulb is then removed and the fresh gas hose is reconnected.
4) This negative pressure leak test will work for all makes and models of machines, whether there is a check valve or not. For this reason, it is sometimes called the *universal leak test*. It differentiates between breathing system leaks and leaks in the machine. Unfortunately, it is not possible to use this test on some new anesthesia machines because the common gas outlet is not accessible. The electronic checkout may determine that a leak is present in the low-pressure system.

c. Combined Breathing System and Machine Leak Test
1) The following test can be used to check for leaks in the breathing system and the parts of the machine downstream of the flow control valve. This test works in the presence or absence of a check valve in the machine.
2) The master control switch is turned ON. The APL valve is closed and the patient port is occluded. The oxygen flush or a high flow from the flowmeter is used to fill the reservoir bag. As the bag begins to distend, the oxygen flush is released and the bag allowed to continue filling from the oxygen flowmeter while the pressure on the manometer in the breathing system is observed. The flow on the flowmeter is adjusted so that a pressure of 30 cm H_2O is maintained in the breathing system. If this pressure is overshot, the APL valve should be opened briefly. The flow necessary to maintain a steady pressure should be no greater than 350 mL/minute. If there is a continuing airway pressure alarm, it should be activated. The pressure should then be released by opening the APL valve (rather than removing the occlusion from the patient port at the Y-piece). This tests the APL valve function.
3) This test should also be performed with a vaporizer turned ON to determine whether a leak exists in the vaporizer.
4) Advantages of this test are that it can be performed quickly without accessory equipment, can check the breathing system as well as the low-pressure parts of the machine and allows the continuous airway pressure alarm to be checked. Disadvantages are that it is relatively insensitive to small leaks and does not provide information on whether the leak is in the breathing system or the machine.

3. **Turn the Machine Master Switch and All Other Necessary Equipment ON**

To continue the checkout, the machine master switch needs to be turned ON to enable the pneumatics and electronics. The machine should be allowed to complete its own diagnostic checks and any automated checking procedure. Any electrical equipment to be used during the case should be turned ON at this time with the exception of a diverting gas monitor, which should be turned ON only after the breathing system is checked for leaks and a heated humidifier.

4. **Flowmeters**

a. Each flowmeter should be examined with the flow control valve closed to make certain the indicator is at the zero position (or at the minimum mandatory flow if the machine is so equipped). Each flow control should be slowly opened and closed while observing the indicator. The indicator should move smoothly up and down and respond to small flow control adjustments. If the indicator is a rotameter or ball, it should rotate freely. An indicator that moves erratically or fails to return to zero may be displaying erroneous flow rates, and the machine should be taken out of service until the problem is corrected.

b. The oxygen/nitrous oxide proportioning system is checked by attempting to create a hypoxic mixture. Adjust the nitrous oxide flow up or the oxygen flow down while both are flowing. Turning the nitrous oxide flow up should cause the oxygen flow to increase or the nitrous oxide flow should not increase beyond the point where less than 25% oxygen would be delivered. If a high nitrous oxide flow is present and the oxygen flow is adjusted downward, the nitrous oxide flow should decrease. If the machine has a nitrous oxide:oxygen ratio alarm, it should be activated.

E. Adjustable Pressure-Limiting Valve

The APL valve and ventilator spill valve should be connected to the scavenging system interface. If an active disposal system is being used, the vacuum flow should be adjusted.

The APL valve is checked by closing it, occluding the patient port, and filling the system by using the oxygen flush so that the breathing system pressure gauge reads 50 cm H_2O. The APL valve is then opened. There should be a gradual pressure decrease. This establishes proper APL function and transfer tubing patency. If the scavenging system interface has a reservoir bag, it should inflate when the APL valve is opened and then deflate. If the pressure is released by removing the occlusion at the patient port, the APL valve and scavenging system patency will not be checked.

F. Scavenging System

1. **Closed System**

a. The valves in a closed scavenging system that let air into the scavenging system if the reservoir bag is empty and release excessive pressure if the bag is distended need to be checked. With minimal or no flow from the anesthesia machine, the APL valve should be fully opened and the patient port occluded. Vacuum to the scavenging interface should be turned ON. If there is a bag at the scavenging interface, it should collapse. The reservoir bag in the breathing system will likely also collapse. At this point, the breathing system pressure gauge should indicate a pressure of 0 to −2 cm H_2O. If the negative pressure is greater than this, the valve is not opening properly.

b. To test the positive-pressure relief valve on the scavenging interface, the vacuum to the interface is turned OFF, the patient port is occluded and the APL valve fully opened. The oxygen flush is then activated to fill both the reservoir bag in the breathing system and the bag on the scavenging interface. With the oxygen flush activated, the breathing system pressure indicator should read less than 10 cm H_2O.

c. An alternate pressure relief valve test can be used. The vacuum flow to the scavenging system is turned OFF, the patient port on the breathing system is occluded, and the APL valve is fully opened. The reservoir bag and the scavenging system bag are fully inflated by using the oxygen flush. A flow of 2 L/minute is then set on the oxygen flowmeter. The pressure gauge in the breathing system should read no more than 3 cm H_2O.

CLINICAL MOMENT If the air inlet or gas outlet valves in a closed scavenging system malfunction, there can be pressure problems in the breathing system. If the air inlet malfunctions, negative pressure could be applied to the breathing system. If the positive-pressure relief valve malfunctions, the patient could be exposed to continuous positive pressure.

2. **Open System**

   Open scavenging systems do not have valves because the system is open to atmosphere. Usually, there are two indicator lines on the scavenger flowmeter. The indicator should be between these lines.

CLINICAL MOMENT Frequently, the vacuum to an open interface is turned OFF and this is not recognized by the anesthesia provider. This will cause the excess gases from the breathing system or ventilator to be exhausted into the room.

G. Breathing System Checks

1. **Oxygen Monitor Calibration**

   a. Electrochemical oxygen analyzers usually require daily calibration. If calibration is required, the sensor should be removed from the breathing system and moved well away from sources of gas that might change the ambient oxygen concentration. It should be calibrated to 21% and the low-oxygen alarm checked by setting the lower limit above 21%. The sensor should then be placed securely in its mount in the breathing system, with the sensing end facing downward and the breathing system flushed with oxygen. This should result in a reading of more than 90%.

CLINICAL MOMENT Fuel cell oxygen analyzers have a life span measured in percent hours. Their service life can be extended by removing them from the breathing system and exposing them to room air when not in use.

   b. Paramagnetic oxygen analyzers do self-calibrations and do not need to be checked by the user.

2. **Initial Breathing System Status**

   a. The breathing system should be inspected to determine that no parts are damaged or missing and that all accessory equipment [e.g., humidifier, heat and moisture exchanger, filter, positive end-expiratory pressure (PEEP) valve] for the proposed anesthetic is in place. All connections should be made secure by "push and twist." If a diverting gas monitor is to be used, the sampling line should be checked for cuts, kinks, or occlusion and connected to the breathing system but the monitor should not be turned ON at this time. Transparent breathing tubes should be checked for foreign bodies. The bag-ventilator selector switch should be in the bag position. The pressure gauge should read zero. If the absorber is detachable, it should be checked to make certain that the attachment is secure.

   b. The absorbent color should be noted. If there is any color change, the absorbent should be discarded and replaced with fresh absorbent. If there is a dual-chamber absorber, both chambers should be changed at the same time Accumulated absorbent dust and water should be removed from the absorber dust cup, taking care not to spill either.

CLINICAL MOMENT If an absorbent containing sodium hydroxide is used, it should be changed at least once a week, regardless of the color. Monday morning is recommended. This will removed desiccated absorbent that might have been exposed to dry, fresh gas over the weekend.

CLINICAL MOMENT It is a good idea to put a date on the absorbent canister when it is changed so that it will not remain unnoticed in place indefinitely.

CLINICAL MOMENT If small detachable absorbent canisters that can be changed without interrupting circuit integrity are in use, they can be used until CO_2 appears in the inspired gas.

3. **Leaks in the Circle Breathing System**
   a. If the circle system has been checked for leaks in combination with low-pressure parts of the machine, this test does not need to be repeated.
   b. All gas flows should be at zero. If there is a minimum mandatory flow, the machine should be turned OFF. The APL valve is closed and the patient port is occluded. The breathing system should be pressurized to 30 cm H_2O using the oxygen flush (**Fig. 26.8**). If there is no leak, the pressure will remain near this level for at least 10 seconds. The APL valve is then opened. The pressure should decrease.

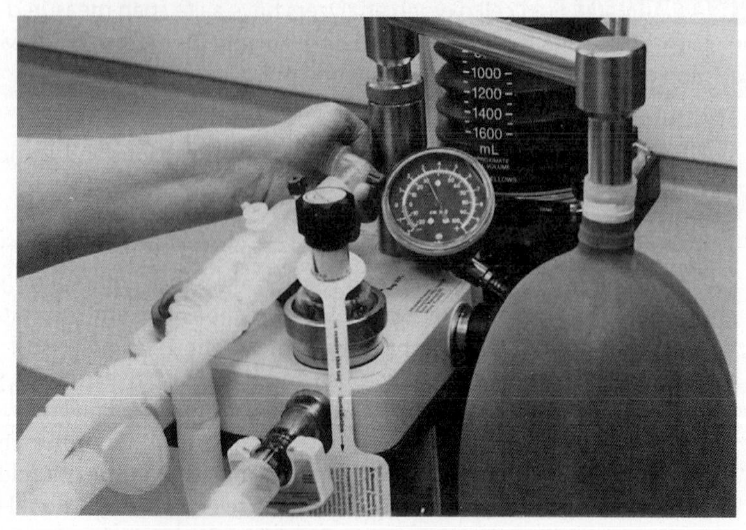

Figure 26.8 Test for leaks in the breathing system. With all gas flows set to zero or minimum, the adjustable pressure-limiting valve is closed and the patient port occluded. The reservoir bag is filled by using the oxygen flush until a pressure of 30 cm H_2O is displayed on the gauge. With no additional gas flow, the pressure should remain at this level for at least 10 seconds.

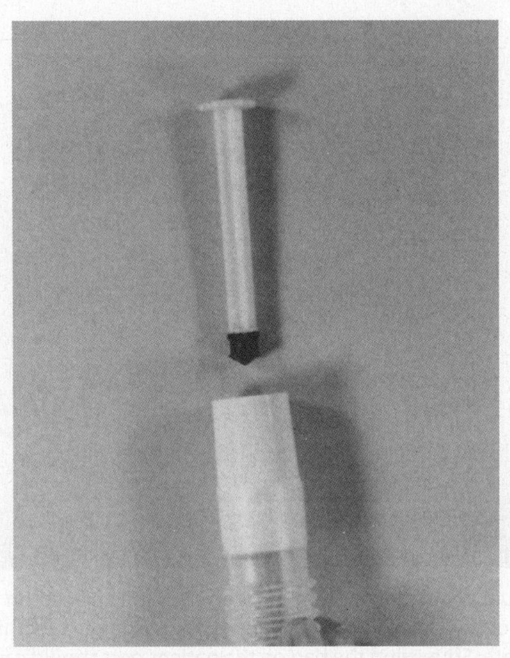

Figure 26.9 The Bain system inner tube test. The plunger from a small syringe is inserted into the patient end of the system over the end of the inner fresh gas delivery tubing. The flowmeter indicator should drop.

c. The leak can be quantified by adjusting the oxygen flowmeter to maintain a steady pressure of 30 cm H_2O in the breathing system (with the Y-piece occluded and the APL valve closed). The leak should not exceed 300 mL/minute.

4. **Leak in a Mapleson Breathing System**
A Mapleson breathing system should be connected to the fresh gas source with the APL valve closed. With the patient port occluded, the system should be pressurized using the oxygen flush. The system should maintain the pressure for at least 10 seconds. The pressure should be released by opening the APL valve.

5. **Bain System**
The integrity of the Bain breathing system inner tube (Chapter 5) is essential to avoid excessive dead space. Profound rebreathing and hypercarbia can occur if the inner tube has a hole, is detached at the machine end, or does not extend to the patient end of the outer tubing.

a. Inspection
The Bain system should first be inspected to determine whether the center tube is properly connected at both ends. Any retraction or disconnection from either end should cause the system to be rejected.

b. Inner Tube Occlusion Test
To perform this test, a 2-L/minute flow is set on one of the flowmeters. The plunger from a small syringe or a finger is inserted into the patient end, occluding the inner tube (**Fig. 26.9**). The flowmeter indicator should fall.

CLINICAL MOMENT If the Bain System has side holes or slots at the patient end, the inner tube occlusion test will not work.

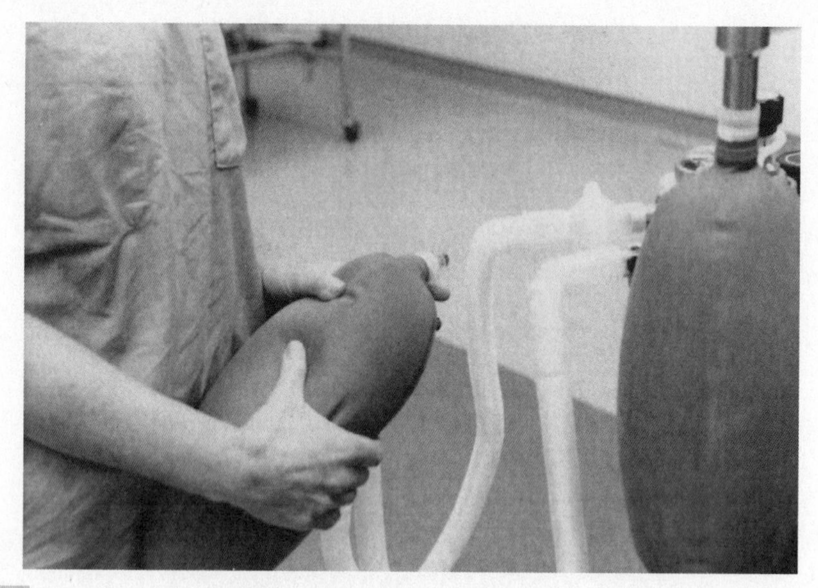

Figure 26.10 Test of manual ventilation system. A reservoir bag is placed on the patient port. The bag-ventilator switch is turned to the bag position. As the reservoir bag in the breathing system is squeezed, the bag on the port should inflate. Squeezing the bag on the patient port should cause the reservoir bag in the breathing system to inflate.

c. Oxygen Flush Test

To perform this test, the reservoir bag is filled. The patient port must be open to atmosphere. The oxygen flush valve on the machine is activated. The high gas flow through the inner tube will produce a Venturi effect, which lowers the pressure in the larger outer tube. If there are no problems with the inner tube, the bag should deflate. If the bag does not deflate or inflates, the inner tube should be checked. This test may fail to detect faults that can be detected by the inner tube occlusion test.

6. **Coaxial Circle System**

The system should be inspected to ensure that the breathing tubes are connected. If the inner tube has a break or is retracted, this can be detected by having the anesthesia provider or patient breathe through the system with the APL valve open and observing the capnograph. If there is a connection between the two limbs, the capnograph baseline will be elevated.

H. Manual and Automatic Ventilation Systems

1. A second reservoir bag is placed on the patient port (**Fig. 26.10**). The oxygen flowmeter should be set at the minimum flow or 300 mL/minute if there is no minimum flow. The bag-ventilator selector switch should be in the bag position and the APL valve closed. As the reservoir bag on the bag mount in the breathing system is squeezed, the bag on the patient port should inflate (**Fig. 26.10**). The bag on the patient port should then be squeezed. The reservoir bag on the bag mount should inflate.

CLINICAL MOMENT If a PEEP valve in the breathing system is set to a level other than zero, it may not be noticed but can be detected by feeling the bag and observing the pressure gauge when performing this test. PEEP should register on the pressure gauge.

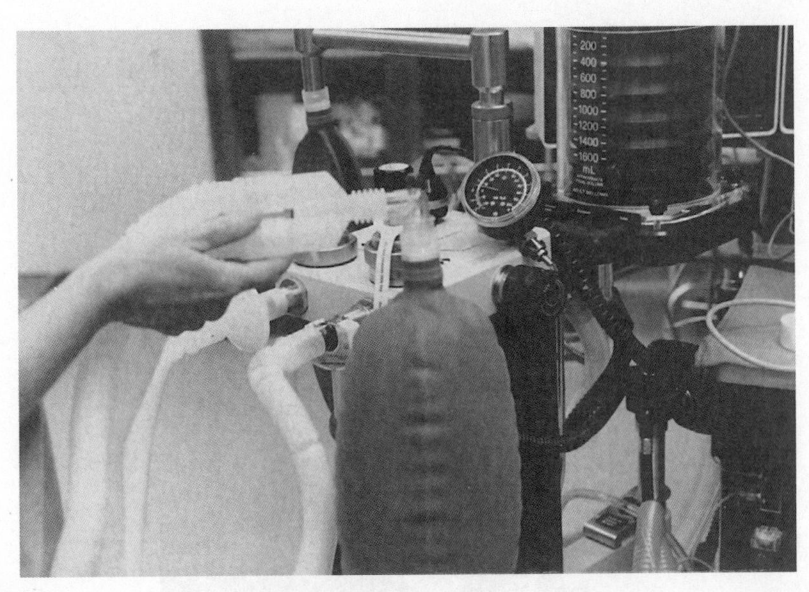

Figure 26.11 Test of ventilator. A reservoir bag is placed on the patient port. The oxygen flowmeter is set at a flow of 300 mL/minute. Ventilator parameters that are appropriate for the next patient are set. The bag-ventilator selector switch should be in the ventilator position. The bellows and the reservoir bag are filled, and the ventilator is turned on. The bellows should move freely and fill completely as the ventilator cycles. The unidirectional valves should be observed to make certain that the discs open properly.

2. Ventilator parameters appropriate for the patient should be set and the bag-ventilator selector switch placed in the ventilator mode. The oxygen flowmeter should be set at the minimum flow or OFF if there is no minimum flow. The bellows and reservoir bag on the patient port should be filled using the oxygen flush. The ventilator is then turned ON. The bag on the patient port should inflate and deflate (**Fig. 26.11**). The appropriate tidal volume should be delivered and the bellows should fill completely during exhalation. If the bellows does not completely fill, there is a serious leak. If using the PEEP valve is anticipated, it should be adjusted to different values and the breathing system pressure gauge observed to verify the correct pressure. The bag should be removed from the patient port and the ventilator allowed to continue cycling. The low airway pressure and tidal or minute volume alarms should annunciate after an appropriate delay. The PEEP valve should be returned to zero value.

CLINICAL MOMENT It is essential that the low airway pressure alarm be checked.

3. With the ventilator still cycling, the patient port should be occluded and the bellows filled using the oxygen flush. The breathing system pressure should rise no higher than that set on the high-pressure relief device. The high-pressure alarm should sound.
4. If a leak is found, it is important to determine whether it is in the breathing system or the ventilator. To check for a leak in ventilator with an upright bellows, the bellows should be filled, the patient port occluded, and the flowmeters turned OFF. Alternately, the bag-ventilator selector switch can be set to BAG. The bellows should stay inflated for at least 3 minutes. If it collapses, then there is a leak in the ventilator circuit.

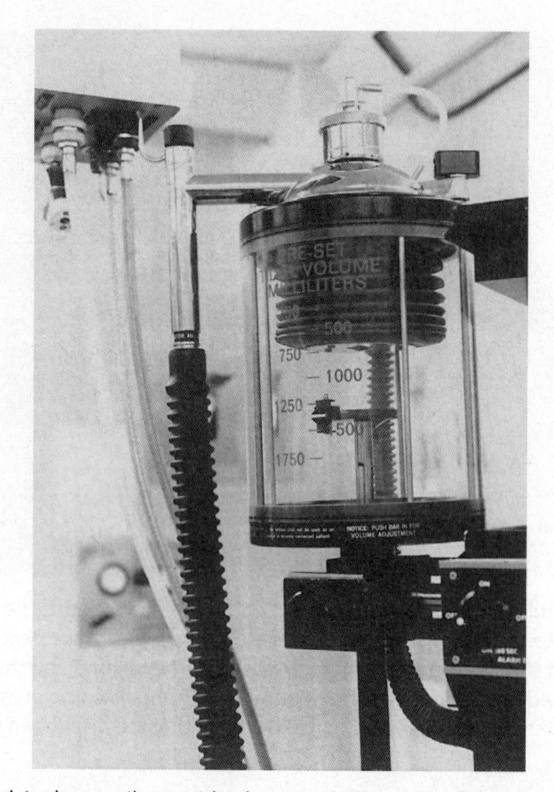

Figure 26.12 Test for leak in the ventilator with a hanging bellows. The flowmeters should be turned off or at minimum flow. The adjustable pressure-limiting valve is closed and the ventilator turned on. When the bellows is fully contracted against the head of the bellows assembly, the patient port is occluded (or the bag-ventilator selector switch is put in the bag position) and the ventilator is turned off. The bellows should remain at the top of the housing for at least 10 seconds.

5. To check for a leak in a ventilator with a hanging bellows (**Fig. 26.12**), all flowmeters should be turned OFF or set at the minimum flow and the ventilator turned ON. When the bellows is fully contracted, the ventilator is switched OFF and the patient port is occluded or the bag-ventilator selector switch is put in the bag position. The bellows should remain contracted at the top of the housing for at least 3 minutes. If it expands downward, a leak is present. Another way of performing this test is to occlude the patient port (or put the bag-ventilator selector switch in the bag position) with the ventilator turned OFF and lower the bellows stop (if present). The bellows should not expand downward.

I. Unidirectional Valve Tests

Many practitioners feel that observing the unidirectional valves rise and fall while the ventilator is cycling indicates proper functioning. This verifies that the valves open, but not that they close properly. During use, an incompetent unidirectional valve can often be detected by an inspired carbon dioxide level greater than zero when using a capnograph (Chapter 17). Some respirometers can detect reversed flow.

CLINICAL MOMENT The inspiratory valve may be incompetent without a rise in the inspired carbon dioxide level. Figure 17.15 shows the capnographic waveform associated with an incompetent inspiratory valve.

1. **Breathing Method**
   With the APL valve closed, the breathing system inspiratory limb is detached from the absorber and occluded. Wearing a mask, the tester tries to breath through the Y-piece (**Fig. 26.13A**). It should be possible to exhale freely but not inhale. Next, the exhalation tube is detached and occluded. The tester should be able to inhale but not exhale (**Fig. 26.13B**).
2. **Valve Tester**
   a. This method utilizes a device consisting of a bulb with a 22-mm female fitting that can attach to the inspiratory and exhalation ports. This device is available commercially but can be made from an irrigation bulb and a

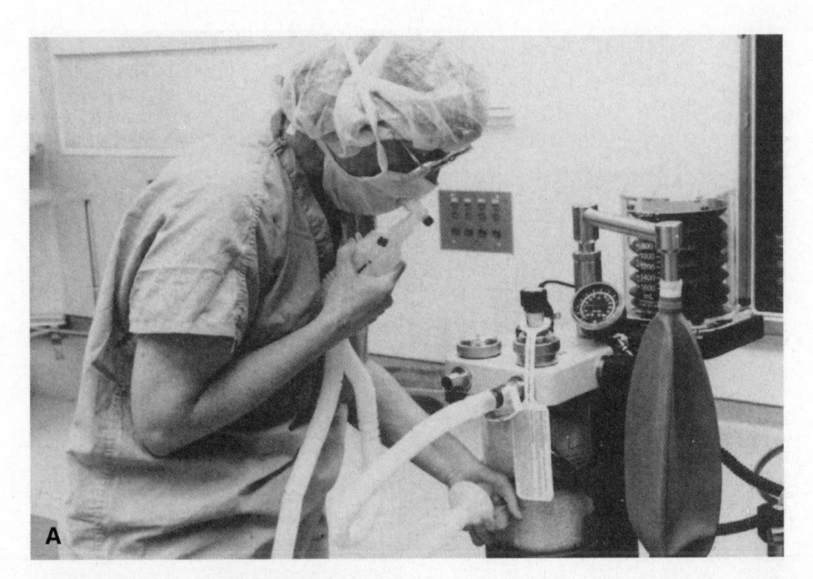

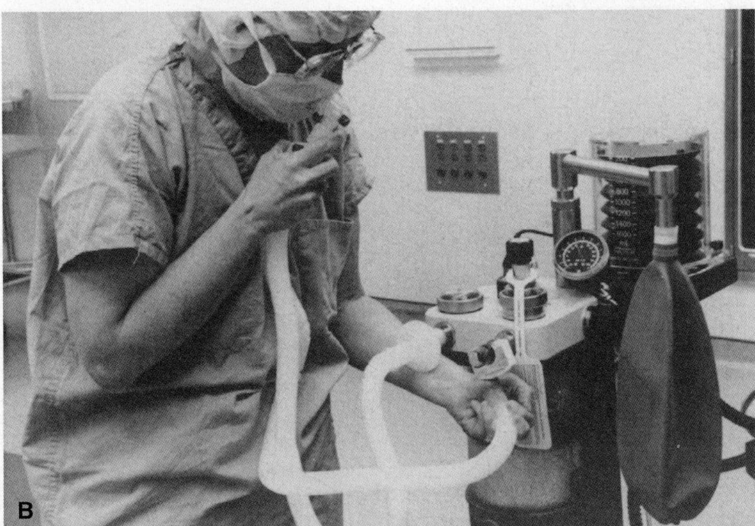

Figure 26.13 Checks for incompetent unidirectional valves. **A:** The inspiratory limb is detached and occluded. The tester tries to breathe through the Y-piece. It should be possible to exhale freely but not inhale. **B:** The exhalation tubing is detached and occluded. The tester should be able to inhale from the Y-piece but not exhale.

suitable connector. To test the inspiratory valve, the compressed bulb is attached to the inspiratory port. It should immediately reinflate. When the bulb is compressed, it should meet firm resistance (**Fig. 26.14A**).

b. To check the expiratory valve, the tester is attached to the expiratory port on the breathing system absorber with the bulb inflated. The bulb is squeezed, and it should remain compressed (**Fig. 26.14B**).

3. **Double-Bag Test**

a. Remove the breathing hose from the inspiratory limb and place a reservoir bag on that connection. Close the APL valve and activate the O_2 flush until

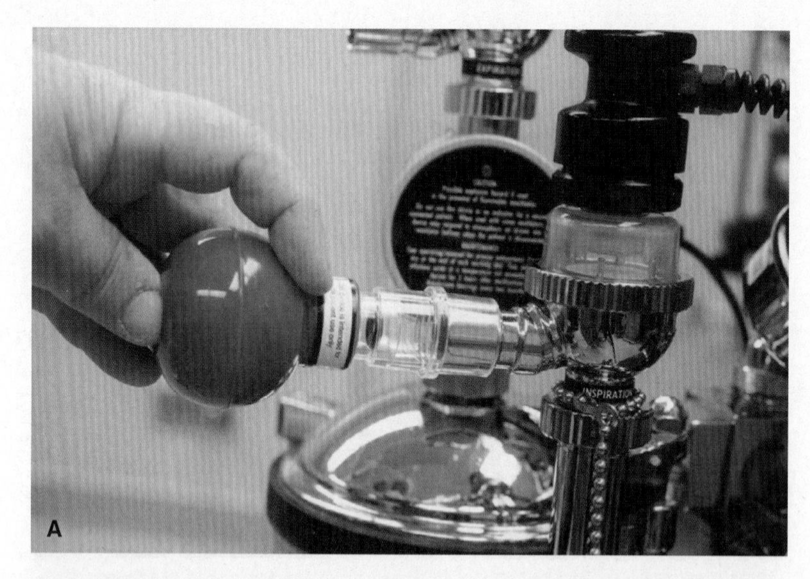

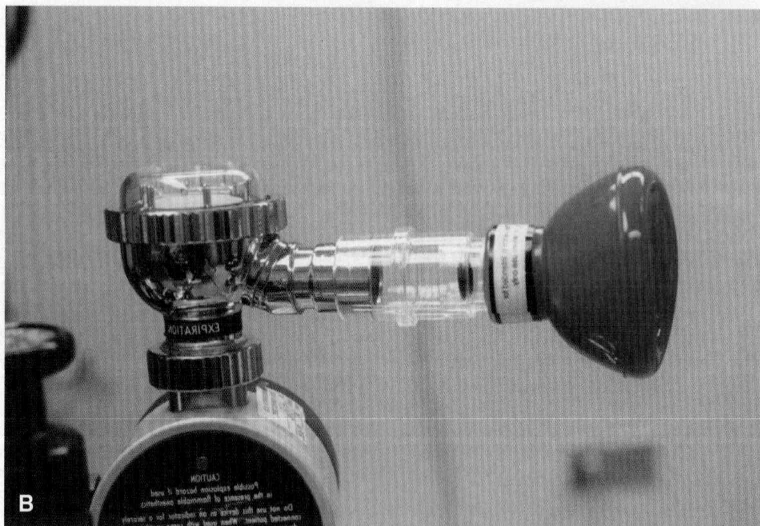

Figure 26.14 Checking the unidirectional valves using a valve tester. **A:** To test the inspiratory unidirectional valve, the bulb should be compressed and then attached to the inspiratory port. It should inflate. It should then not be possible to recompress the bulb. **B:** To test the expiratory unidirectional valve, the tester is attached just upstream of the valve. The bulb should compress easily and remain compressed.

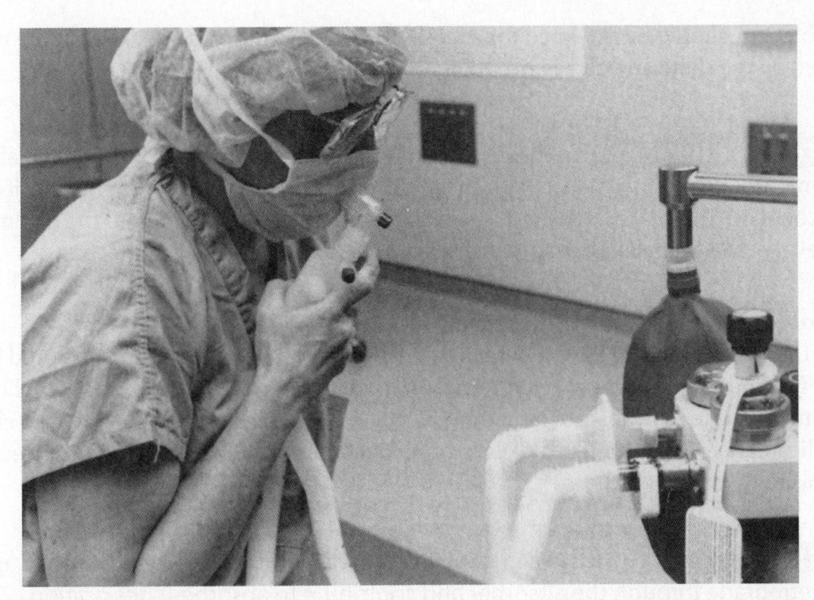

Figure 26.15 Breathing system patency can be confirmed by inhaling and exhaling through the patient port.

a system pressure of 30 cm H_2O is achieved. Both bags should be distended. The reservoir bag on the bag mount should remain inflated for at least 5 seconds. If it deflates the expiratory valve may be incompetent.

b. Open the APL valve and allow the circuit to decompress. If the bag in the inspiratory limb remains inflated, the inspiratory unidirectional valve is competent.

J. Final Configuration and Obstruction Check

At this point, all breathing system accessory equipment (e.g., PEEP valve, heated humidifier) should be in place and turned ON. Obstructions in the breathing system can be detected by having the patient breathe 100% oxygen through a mask, provided a tight mask fit is achieved. This can also be performed by the anesthesia provider wearing a mask (**Fig. 26.15**). The reservoir bag should inflate and deflate, and the breathing system pressure indicator should not show any PEEP. Negative pressure will reveal an obstruction in the inspiratory limb; positive pressure will reveal an obstruction in the expiratory limb. While this is being done, the capnograph should be checked to make certain that a normal waveform appears. The heated humidifier should only be turned ON after the anesthetic has begun and there is gas flow through the tubing.

K. Monitors and Controls

1. All monitors should be turned ON. Alarms should be tested by simulating alarm conditions and appropriate limits set.
2. The final status of all controls should be checked before the machine is put into use. This includes having all flow control valves closed, all flowmeters indicating zero flow (unless there is a minimum mandatory flow), all vaporizers turned OFF, the bag-ventilator switch set to BAG, the PEEP valve OFF, the APL valve open, and the scavenging system vacuum flow turned ON and adjusted.

V. Subsequent Checks on the Same Machine on the Same Day

If a thorough check is performed before the first case of the day, a less complete procedure can be used before subsequent cases. Those steps marked with an asterisk (*) in

Table 26.1 should be repeated for successive cases on the same day even if the machine is used by the same anesthesia provider.

CLINICAL MOMENT The absorbent is often changed between cases, but the absorber may not be properly reinstalled. The anesthesia provider may not even know if it was changed. This makes a breathing system leak check necessary before the beginning of every case. Some electronic machines provide a leak test between cases.

VI. Procedures at the End of the Case

At the conclusion of a case, flowmeters, vaporizers, and suction tubing should be turned OFF. Monitors that would need recalibration if turned OFF should be left ON or put in a standby mode. The absorbent should be checked for signs of exhaustion and changed, if indicated (see Chapter 5). The electronic machines usually have a way to determine that a case is over.

CLINICAL MOMENT If oxygen remains running and the flow is high, it may pass retrograde through the absorber and contribute to absorbent desiccation.

VII. Other Machine and Breathing System Checks

A. Oxygen Pressure Failure Alarm

1. Most anesthesia machines are equipped with an oxygen pressure failure alarm, which is activated if there is no or low oxygen pressure in the machine. The Association of Anaesthetists of Great Britain and Ireland recommend that this alarm be tested on a weekly basis.
2. To test this alarm, the oxygen pipeline hose is disconnected and all oxygen cylinders are closed. Any pressure remaining in the machine should be bled off by using the oxygen flush. The alarm should sound. The machine must be turned ON before this test is done.

B. Leaks at the Yoke

If a cylinder is not properly tightened in a yoke, there will be a gas leak when the cylinder is opened. A large leak will be apparent by the sound. A small leak may not be heard but could cause significant gas loss. If there is a minimum mandatory oxygen flow, the machine must be turned OFF. After the cylinder pressure for each gas has been checked and the valves closed, the cylinder pressure gauges should be observed for 2 to 5 minutes, with no flow on the flowmeters. A drop of more than 50 psig indicates significant leakage.

C. Oxygen Failure Safety Valve

The oxygen failure safety valve was included as a routine test in the first edition of the FDA checkout but was not made part of the later version because it rarely fails, and there are alarm systems that will detect low or absent oxygen pressure. To test this device, either the pipelines or the cylinders can be used. A cylinder of each gas on the machine is opened while the pipeline hoses are disconnected. If the pipeline is used as a gas source, the cylinders should be closed. Flows of 2 L/minute are established on the flowmeters for each gas. The oxygen cylinder is then turned OFF or the pipeline is disconnected. As the oxygen pressure falls, the nitrous oxide flow should decrease in proportion to the decrease in oxygen flow and eventually shut OFF before the oxygen pressure returns to zero. Restoring the oxygen pressure should cause the indicators to return to their previous positions. Air was controlled by the oxygen failure safety valve on some earlier anesthesia machines. Newer machines do not make the ability to deliver air dependent on oxygen pressure because the patient could be ventilated with air if the oxygen pressure failed.

D. Spare Components

Extra breathing system components should be immediately available. These include an additional disposable breathing system or individual components (Y-piece, breathing tubes, and reservoir bag) of reusable breathing systems.

E. Electrical System

Electrical system tests vary with the different makes and models of machines. Most have a means to test the reserve battery. In addition, there is usually an indication that the machine is working on the battery power. To check this, the machine is turned ON and then is disconnected from the mains power. The battery power indicator should illuminate. Electronic machines have an indicator of the battery charge level (see Chapter 3).

CLINICAL MOMENT If the electricity from the wall is not available, the caution on the machine may say "Loss of Mains Power." *Mains* refers to electricity from the electric company.

F. Vaporizer Exclusion System

Nearly all anesthesia machines with multiple direct-reading vaporizers have a mechanism that allows only one vaporizer to be turned ON at a time (Chapter 4). To test the vaporizer exclusion system, one vaporizer should be turned ON and an attempt made to turn each of the other vaporizers ON, one at a time.

VIII. Other Equipment

A. Tracheal Tubes

If it is planned to use a tracheal tube, a tube of appropriate size should be chosen for the patient. Lumen patency should be checked. With clear tubes, simple observation will suffice. With other tubes, it is necessary to look at both ends or insert a stylet. The cuff should be held inflated for at least 1 minute to verify that it does not leak. The cuff should inflate evenly and not stick to the tube wall or decrease the lumen size. A tube one size larger and one size smaller than the tracheal tube that is intended for use should be readily available but not necessarily opened.

B. Rigid Laryngoscopes

Laryngoscope malfunction is a frequent problem. At least two handles should be present, each fitted with the type of blade that the user anticipates will be best for the patient. The lights should be checked for adequate intensity. Blades of other sizes and shapes that may be needed should be immediately available and checked for proper function.

C. Accessory Intubation Equipment

A stylet and a bougie should be immediately available. If a rapid-sequence intubation is planned or a difficult intubation is anticipated, the stylet should be fitted into the tracheal tube. An intubating forceps should be immediately available. If a difficult intubation is anticipated, specialized equipment for difficult intubation should be in the operating room and checked for completeness, defects, and proper assembly.

D. Masks and Airways

An assortment of masks and airways in a variety of sizes should be readily available.

E. Other Equipment

Special equipment for particular cases, such as pipeline hose extensions, extensions breathing hoses, patient warming equipment, and infusion devices, should be present and checked before use.

IX. Procedures at the End of the Day

A. Following the last case of the day, the pipeline hoses should be disconnected at the wall or ceiling (not at the back of the machine) and coiled over the machine. If the hoses are disconnected at the back of the machine, they will continue to be pressurized and gas may be lost into the room through leaks. If the pipeline supply is connected to the machine and the oxygen flow control valve is open, dry gas can desiccate the absorbent, promoting the formation of carbon monoxide (Chapter 5). Cylinder valves should be closed. Each flow control valve should be opened until the cylinder and pipeline pressure gauges read zero and then closed.

B. Vaporizers should be filled at the conclusion of the day after most operating room personnel have vacated the room. This will decrease personnel exposure to anesthetic agents.

X. Checking New or Modified Equipment

A. Each new anesthesia machine, ventilator, or other complex piece of equipment should be checked for proper functioning before being put into use. This is best performed by a manufacturer's representative, who should also give in-service instructions. A document certifying that the equipment has been checked for proper assembly and function should be obtained and kept.

B. A user manual that contains assembly and installation instructions, maintenance requirements, checking procedures, and instructions for use is supplied with each piece of equipment. This must be read carefully and reviewed periodically. A copy should be kept in the central equipment files and with the equipment itself.

XI. Preventive Maintenance

Anesthetic equipment needs periodic maintenance to protect from failures caused by worn or deteriorating parts. Maintenance must be carried out by personnel specially trained to provide this service on this machine. Factory-certified parts should be used. Service records need to be kept to verify that the work was performed and who performed it. These records may be of value in the event of an equipment problem resulting in legal action. Accreditation organizations also need these records for audit purposes.

XII. Accident Investigation

A. Any time a patient has an unexplained problem, equipment malfunction or misuse should be suspected and the apparatus not used again until this has been disproved.

B. When there has been an injury to a patient, the healthcare facility safety officer (or risk manager) should be contacted at once to supervise or investigate the incident. An established protocol should be present and followed so that all important areas are covered systematically. All individuals involved in the incident should document their observations soon after the event while details are still fresh in their minds. This should be a simple statement of facts, without judgments about causality or responsibility.

C. The following questions need to be asked:

1. What was the date and time of the problem?
2. In what area did the problem occur?
3. What monitors were being used?
4. What were the set alarm limits?
5. What was the first indication that there was a problem?
6. At what time did this occur?
7. Who first noted the problem?
8. What changes attracted attention? Were any alarms activated?
9. What signs or symptoms did the patient exhibit?
10. Had there been any recent modifications to the electrical system or gas pipelines in that area?

11. Was anything altered shortly before the incident?
12. Was this the first case performed in that area that day?
13. Were there any problems during previous cases performed in that area on that day or the previous day?
14. Were there any unusual occurrences in other areas on that day or the previous day?
15. Had any equipment been moved into that area recently? Were there any problems noted in the room where it was previously used?
16. What preuse anesthesia equipment checks were made?
17. Who last filled the vaporizers on the anesthesia machine?
18. If a vaporizer was recently attached to the machine, were precautions taken to prevent liquid from being spilled into the outflow tract?
19. After the initial indication of a problem, what was the sequence of events?

D. An important step involves constructing a timeline, on which all events are listed chronologically. This will help to sort out events and may identify missing data.

E. Numerous photographs should be taken of the area from various angles, with all equipment situated where it was at the time of the incident. Each piece of equipment should be photographed separately.

F. After pictures have been taken, all supplies and equipment associated with the case should be saved and sequestered in a secure location and labeled "DO NOT DISTURB." Settings should not be changed. Relevant identifying information such as the manufacturer and lot and/or serial numbers should be recorded.

G. If after all this has been accomplished it appears possible that the equipment may be implicated in the problem, a thorough equipment inspection by an uninvolved third party who understands anesthesia equipment and has the necessary equipment to test the equipment should be conducted in the presence of anesthesia personnel, insurance carrier, healthcare facility safety officer, patient representative, and equipment manufacturers. The manufacturer's representative should not be relied on to inspect the equipment since a fault may be corrected during that inspection. The investigation should consist of an in-depth examination of the equipment similar to the checking procedures described earlier in this chapter. Vaporizers should be calibrated and checked to determine whether vapor is accurately delivered but not in the OFF position. An analysis should be made of the vaporizers' contents, if necessary. Following the investigation, a report that details all facts, analyses, and conclusions should be made.

H. If a problem with the equipment is found, an attempt should be made to reconstruct the accident, if this can be done without danger to anyone, and the equipment should again be locked up until any litigation is settled. If the investigation reveals no problems, the equipment can be returned to service with the consent of all parties.

I. The Safe Medical Devices Act of 1990 requires medical device user facilities to report incidents that reasonably suggest that there is a probability that a medical device has caused or contributed to the death, serious injury, or serious illness of a patient. The report is due as soon as possible but no later than 10 working days after the user facility becomes aware of the incident.

SUGGESTED READINGS

Abramovich A. Clinician recognizes importance of machine checkout response. APSF Newslett 2004–2005;19:51.

Carter JA. Checking anaesthetic equipment and the Expert Group on Blocked Anaesthetic Tubing (EGBAT). Anaesthesia 2004;59:105–107.

Cox M. Clinician recognizes importance of machine checkout. APSF Newslett 2004–2005;19:50.

Dorsch J, Dorsch S. Equipment checkout and maintenance. In: Understanding Anesthesia Equipment. Fifth edition. Philadelphia: Wolters Kluwer/Lippincott Williams & Wilkins, 2008:931–954.

Fasting S, Gisvold SE. Equipment problems during anaesthesia—are they a quality problem? Br J Anaesth 2002;89: 825–831.

Feldman JM, Olympio MA, Martin D, Striker A. New guidelines available for pre-anesthesia checkout. APSF Newslett Spring 2008;23:6–7.

Hart EM, Owen H. Errors and omissions in anesthesia: a pilot study using a pilot's checklist. Anesth Analg 2005;101: 246–250.

Ianchulev SA, Comunale ME. To do or not to do a preinduction check-up of the anesthesia machine. Anesth Analg 2005;101:774–776.

Katz J. Tips for pre-flighting your anesthesia workstation. Outpatient Surg Mag 2001;11:41–49.

Krimmer M, Lake A, Wray I. Covers for anaesthetic machines: an audit and standard. Eur J Anaesth 1997;14:505–513.

Lorraway PG, Savoldelli GL, Joo HS, et al. Management of simulated oxygen supply failure: is there a gap in the curriculum? Anesth Analg 2006;102:865–867.

Olympio M. Clinician recognizes importance of machine checkout Response. APSF Newslett 2004-2005;19:5051.

Sanchi O. Breathing system malfunction and the "extra circuit." Anaesthesia 2003;58:1131–1132.

Weigel WA, Murray WB. Detecting unidirectional valve incompetence by the modified pressure decline method. Anesth Analg 2005;100:1723–1727.

27 Cleaning, Disinfection, and Sterilization

ALL ANESTHESIA PRACTITIONERS SHOULD BE concerned with equipment cleanliness to prevent infection spread among patients and healthcare providers, including themselves. Nosocomial infections produce suffering and higher healthcare costs.

I. Definitions

A. *Antimicrobial*: A chemical or material capable of destroying or inhibiting the growth of microorganisms.

B. *Antiseptic*: A chemical germicide that has antimicrobial activity and that can be safely applied to living tissue. Antiseptics are regulated as drugs.

C. *Asepsis*: A scheme or process that prevents contact with microorganisms.

D. *Bacteria*: Microscopic unicellular organisms.

E. *Bactericide*: A chemical agent or compound that kills bacteria.
F. *Bacteriostat*: An agent that will prevent bacterial growth but does not necessarily kill the bacteria. Bacteriostatic action is reversible; when the agent is removed, the bacteria will resume normal growth.
G. *Bioburden* (*Bioload, Microbial Load*): The number and types of viable organisms contaminating an object. The bioburden level is related to the anatomic site where the device was used.
H. *Biological Indicator*: A sterilization process monitoring device consisting of a standardized, viable population of microorganisms (usually bacterial spores) that are known to be resistant to the mode of sterilization being monitored. Subsequent growth or failure of the microorganisms to grow under suitable conditions indicates whether or not conditions were adequate to achieve sterility.
I. *Ceiling Value*: Concentration of an airborne contaminant above which a person should not be exposed even momentarily.
J. *Chemical Indicator* (*Chemical Monitor, Sterilizer Control, Chemical Control Device, Sterilization Process Monitoring Device*): A sterilization process monitoring device designed to respond with a characteristic and visible chemical or physical change to one or more parameters of a sterilization process.
K. *Chemical Integrator*: Chemical indicator that reacts with a variety of sterilization parameters.
L. *Chemosterilizer* (*Chemical Sterilant*): Chemical used for the purpose of destroying all forms of microbiological life, including bacterial spores. The same chemical used for shorter exposure periods and/or at a lower concentration may be used for disinfection.
M. *Cleaning*: Removal of foreign material from an item.
N. *Contamination*: State of actually or potentially having been in contact with microorganisms.
O. *Critical Item*: Item that penetrates the skin or mucous membranes or is in contact with normally sterile areas of the body.
P. *Decontamination*: A process that renders contaminated inanimate items safe for handling by personnel who are not wearing protective attire (i.e., reasonably free of the probability of transmitting infection). Decontamination can range from simple cleaning to sterilization.
Q. *Disinfectant*: Chemical germicide formulated to be used on inanimate objects.
R. *Disinfection*: Process capable of destroying most microorganisms but, as ordinarily used, not bacterial spores. A disinfectant is usually a chemical agent, but some processes (such as pasteurization) are disinfecting. The Centers for Disease Control and Prevention (CDC) has adopted a classification that includes three levels of disinfection.
   1. *High-Level Disinfection*: A procedure that kills all organisms with the exception of bacterial spores and certain species, such as the Creutzfeldt-Jakob prion. Most high-level disinfectants can produce sterilization with sufficient contact time.
   2. *Intermediate-Level Disinfection*: A procedure that kills vegetative bacteria, including *Mycobacterium tuberculosis*, most fungi, and viruses but not bacterial spores.
   3. *Low-Level Disinfection*: A procedure that kills most vegetative bacteria (but not *M. tuberculosis*), some fungi, and viruses but no spores.
S. *Disposable*: Intended for use on one patient during a single procedure.
T. *Fungicide*: An agent or process that kills fungi.

U. *Germicide*: An agent that destroys microorganisms.
V. *Mechanical Monitor* (*Physical Monitor, Physical Indicator*): Sterilizer component that measures and records time, temperature, humidity, or pressure during a sterilization cycle.
W. *Noncritical Item*: An item that does not ordinarily touch the patient or touches only intact skin but not mucous membranes.
X. *Nosocomial*: Pertaining to a healthcare facility. A nosocomial infection is one acquired in a healthcare facility.
Y. *Permissible Exposure Limit* (*PEL*): The time-weighted average (TWA) maximum concentration of an air contaminant to which a worker can be exposed according to Occupational Safety and Health Administration (OSHA) standards.
Z. *Prions*: Proteinaceous infectious agents with no associated nucleic acids.
AA. *Processing*: All of the steps performed to make a contaminated device ready for patient use.
BB. *Pseudoinfection*: A positive culture without clinical infection.
CC. *Reprocessing*: Decontamination and repackaging of a device for reuse that has been used for its intended purpose and is labeled for single use.
DD. *Resterilization*: Sterilization of an "unopened" (i.e., inner wrap still intact and therefore the device is presumably "unused") sterile device or an unused wrapped sterile device that is past the expiration date.
EE. *Reusable*: Intended for repeated use either on the same patient or different patients, with appropriate reprocessing between subsequent uses.
FF. *Sanitization*: Process of reducing the number of microbial contaminants to a relatively safe level. In general, sanitation is used in reference to noncritical surfaces or applications in which stronger microbial agents may cause device materials to deteriorate.
GG. *Sanitizer:* A low-level disinfectant.
HH. *Semicritical Item*: A device that is intended to come in contact with mucous membranes or intact skin but will not normally come into contact with sterile tissues.
II. *Short-term Exposure Limit* (*STEL*): A 15-minute TWA exposure that should not be exceeded at any time during a workday.
JJ. *Spore*: The normal resting stage in the life cycle of certain bacteria.
KK. *Sporicide*: An agent that kills spores.
LL. *Standard Precautions*: Policies promulgated by the CDC that include universal precautions, airborne precautions, droplet precautions, and contact precautions. Standard precautions apply to all patients regardless of their diagnosis or known or presumed infection status.
MM. *Sterilant/Disinfectant*: Term applied by the Environmental Protection Agency (EPA) to a germicide that is capable of sterilization or high-level disinfection.
NN. *Sterile/Sterility*: State of being free from all living microorganisms. In practice, sterility is usually described in terms of the sterility assurance level (SAL). Before a manufacturer can label a product as sterile, it must have an SAL of 10^{-6}, which means that the possibility that microorganisms have survived on the item exists but is no greater than 1×10^{-6} or 1 in 1,000,000.
OO. *Sterility Assurance Level*: Probability that microorganisms will survive after a terminal sterilization process.
PP. *Sterilization*: Process capable of removing or destroying all viable forms of microbial life, including bacterial spores, to an acceptable SAL.
QQ. *Terminal Sterilization*: Sterilization process that is carried out after an item has been placed in its final packaging.

RR. *Threshold Limit Value Ceiling*: Concentration of an air contaminant to which it is believed that nearly all workers may be repeatedly exposed day after day without adverse effects.

SS. *Time-weighted Average*: Integration of all the concentrations of a chemical to which a worker has been exposed during as sampling period, reported as an average.

TT. *Transmission-Based Precautions*: Recommendations by the CDC for patients with known or suspected infection or colonization with highly transmissible or epidemiologically important pathogens that can be transmitted by airborne or droplet transmission or by contact with dry skin or contaminated surfaces.

UU. *Tuberculocide*: An agent or process that kills tubercle bacilli.

VV. *Universal Precautions*: Recommendations made by the CDC that healthcare workers use protective barriers and workplace practices to reduce the risk of exposure to blood and certain other body fluids. In 1996, universal precautions were incorporated into standard precautions, which expanded the coverage to any body fluid that may contain contagious microorganisms.

WW. *Vegetative*: Active growth phase of a microorganism.

XX. *Virucide*: Agent that inactivates viruses.

YY. *Virus*: Submicroscopic, noncellular particle composed of a protein shell and a nucleic acid core, and, in complex types, a surrounding envelope.

II. Resistance of Microorganisms to Disinfection and Sterilization

Microorganisms can be categorized into groups according to their innate resistance to a spectrum of physical processes or chemical germicidal agents. **Figure 27.1** shows a general order of microbial resistance levels. Resistance to disinfection and sterilization is not equivalent to resistance to antibiotics. For example, antibiotic-resistant strains of staphylococci do not appear to be more resistant to chemical germicides.

III. Cleaning

A. The first and most important step in decontamination is thorough cleaning. In some cases, cleaning may be sufficient to render an item suitable for reuse. If an article is not clean, retained salts and organic soil could inactivate chemical germicides or protect microorganisms during the disinfection or sterilization process. Even if the item is rendered sterile, the residues may interfere with the function of the device or cause an adverse patient reaction.

B. The cleaning area should be divided into dirty and clean areas. Signs showing where dirty equipment is to be placed should be prominently displayed. Personnel should wear a full complement of protective attire (hair covering, fluid-resistant mask, eyewear, waterproof gown or apron, appropriate gloves, and waterproof shoes or boots with nonskid soles). Personnel should be careful not to injure themselves with contaminated instruments.

C. Each device manufacturer's instructions should be followed to determine the appropriate cleaning methods and agents to remove soil without damaging the device. Tape should be removed and adhesive residue dissolved by using an appropriate solvent.

D. The next step is disassembly (if not done at the source). An initial water rinse or soaking with a specialized product (e.g., a protein-dissolving solution) can prevent blood coagulation and remove gross debris. The water temperature should not exceed 45°C, because higher temperatures cause proteinaceous soil to coagulate. An alternative is to use a spray-on precleaner to help to dissolve the soil.

E. After the equipment has soaked long enough to loosen organic matter, it should be thoroughly scrubbed inside and out. Particular attention should be paid to lumens, crevices, corners, grooves, and knurled or textured surfaces. It is important to have

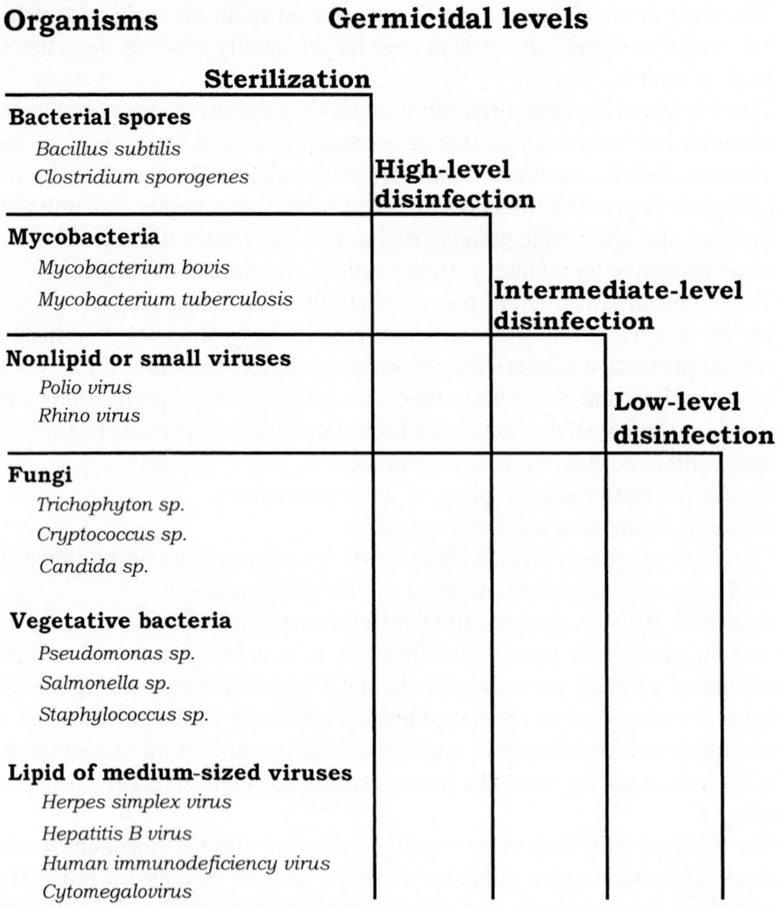

Organisms **Germicidal levels**

Sterilization

Bacterial spores
Bacillus subtilis
Clostridium sporogenes

High-level disinfection

Mycobacteria
Mycobacterium bovis
Mycobacterium tuberculosis

Intermediate-level disinfection

Nonlipid or small viruses
Polio virus
Rhino virus

Low-level disinfection

Fungi
Trichophyton sp.
Cryptococcus sp.
Candida sp.

Vegetative bacteria
Pseudomonas sp.
Salmonella sp.
Staphylococcus sp.

Lipid of medium-sized viruses
Herpes simplex virus
Hepatitis B virus
Human immunodeficiency virus
Cytomegalovirus

Figure 27.1 Descending order of resistance of organisms.

a variety of brushes. Brushes and other cleaning implements should be disposable or cleaned and sterilized or undergo high-level disinfection at least daily.

F. Immersible devices should be cleaned under water to prevent microorganisms from aerosolizing. A cloth soaked in detergent and water can be used to clean items that cannot be immersed. Detergents should be low sudsing and rinse off without leaving a residue. Detergent residues can lead to staining and may interfere with the action of some chemical disinfectants.

CLINICAL MOMENT Not all endoscopes containing eyepieces can be immersed. Consult the manufacturer's manual before immersing these instruments.

G. Some equipment that has joints, crevices, lumens, and other hard-to-reach areas can be treated in an ultrasonic cleaning system after gross soil has been removed. In an ultrasonic cleaner, high-frequency sound waves passing through a solvent produce submicroscopic bubbles. These bubbles collapse on themselves, generating tiny shock waves that knock debris off surfaces. A detergent is often added to the ultrasonic liquid. The water may be heated. Ultrasonic cleaning tanks are available in a variety of sizes and configurations. The equipment to be cleaned is placed in a basket or tray and into the ultrasonic tank for a preset period of time, usually 3 to 6 minutes. Ultrasonic cleaning monitors are available. Some manufacturers of delicate instruments, including laryngoscopes, recommend that they not be subjected to ultrasonic cleaning because the process may loosen fine screws and adversely affect alignment.

IV. Disinfection and Sterilization Methods

A. Pasteurization

With pasteurization (hot water disinfection), the equipment is immersed in water at an elevated temperature (but below 100°C) for a specified time. The time and temperature vary. A typical pattern is 30 minutes at a temperature of 70°C. Contact time is inversely related to temperature, that is, for equivalent microbial kill, a longer exposure time is required when the temperature is reduced. CDC guidelines refer to pasteurization as a high-level disinfection process, although some feel it is an intermediate-level process.

B. Steam Sterilization

1. Steam sterilization (autoclaving) utilizes saturated steam under pressure. It is the most widely used and inexpensive method of sterilization.
2. At sea level, water boils at 100°C. When it is boiled within a closed vessel at increased pressure, the temperature of the steam it forms will exceed 100°C. The temperature depends on the pressure within the chamber. Pressure per se has little or no sterilizing effect. It is the moist heat at a suitable temperature, as regulated by the pressure in the chamber, which brings about sterilization.
3. Increasing the temperature dramatically reduces the time needed to achieve sterilization. The minimum for sterilization is 121°C for 15 minutes. If the temperature is 126°C, the time is reduced to 10 minutes. It is 3.5 minutes at 134°C, and only a few seconds at 150°C.

CLINICAL MOMENT Manufacturers have specific recommendations about the temperature and time needed to sterilize their products. Consult their recommendations before autoclaving any specific device.

4. Autoclaving is effective because the steam transfers heat to materials rapidly on contact. Microbial destruction will be most effective at locations where saturated steam can contact the microorganisms. At locations inaccessible to steam penetration (as might occur with complex devices, improperly packaged items, or incorrect load configurations), some microbial destruction may occur, but dry heat sterilization is not as efficient as saturated steam.
5. Equipment to be sterilized is cleaned and then packaged in a material easily penetrated by steam. After sterilization, the packaging material prevents recontamination during subsequent handling and storage. An indicator that shows that an item has undergone steam sterilization is shown in **Figure 27.2**.

C. Dry Heat Sterilization

1. Dry heat is used for items that might be damaged by moisture. While slow, this technique penetrates well and does not corrode metal and sharp instruments. It is useful for nonaqueous liquids or semisolids such as talc, glycerin, oils, petroleum jelly, waxes, and powders.
2. Times and temperatures frequently used for dry heat sterilization include 170°C for 60 minutes, 160°C for 120 minutes, and 150°C for 150 minutes. Some dry heat sterilizers can reach temperatures up to 210°C. Convection hot air sterilizers

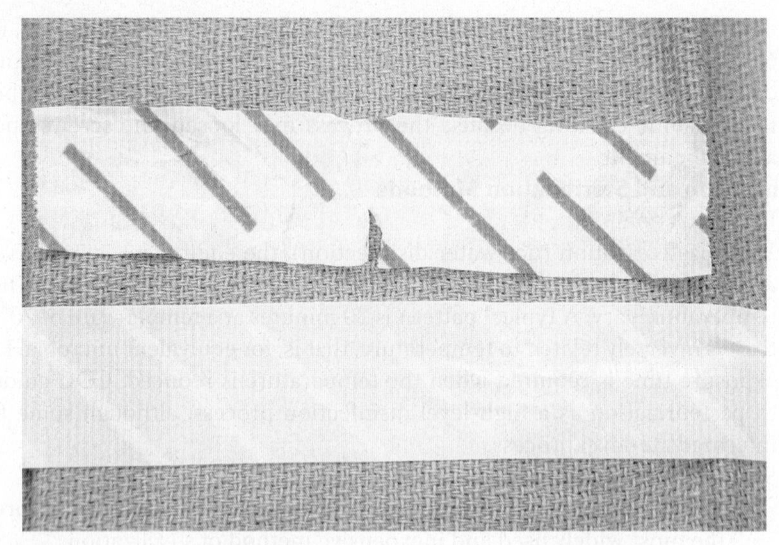

Figure 27.2 Autoclave tape is an example of an external process indicator. The exposed tape is at top.

improve heat transfer by using forced air. These units have comparatively fast cycle times.

> **CLINICAL MOMENT** Consult the manufacturer's user manual to determine which products are suitable for dry heat sterilization and the optimum recommended temperature.

D. Chemical Disinfection and Sterilization

Chemical (cold) disinfection/sterilization involves immersing an item in a solution that contains a disinfectant. This method is especially useful for heat-sensitive equipment. It can be accomplished using automated equipment, which typically provides a cycle of cleaning, rinsing, disinfection, rinsing, and sometimes drying.

1. **Factors Influencing Chemical Disinfection**

a. Chemical Concentration

In general, higher concentrations of the active ingredients increase the disinfectant's bactericidal ability. An exception is the alcohols. High chemical concentrations increase the potential for damage both to inanimate objects and to the skin and mucous membranes. For best results, products should be used according to the manufacturer's recommendations.

> **CLINICAL MOMENT** Water remaining on equipment that is immersed in a disinfectant solution will dilute the chemical agent. The equipment must be dried before it is disinfected.

b. Temperature

Higher temperatures usually increase the effectiveness of chemical agents. Special devices are available for heating some chemical solutions. Too high a temperature may cause the active ingredients to evaporate or degrade. The agent label should tell which temperature should be used.

Table 27.1 Capabilities of Disinfecting Agents[a]

Disinfectant	Gram-Positive Bacteria	Gram-Negative Bacteria	Tubercle Bacillus	Spores	Viruses	Fungi
Quaternary ammonium compounds	+	±	0	0	±	±
Alcohols	+	+	+	0	±	±
Glutaraldehydes	+	+	+	±	+	+
Hydrogen peroxide–based compounds	+	+	+	±	+	+
Formaldehyde and other agents	+	+	+	–	+	+
Phenolic compounds	+	+	±	0	±	±
Chlorine	+	+	+	–	+	+

Abbreviations: +, good; ±, fair, 0, little or none.
[a]From Chatbum RL. Decontamination of respiratory care equipment what can be done, what should be done. Respir Care 1989:34:98; and Berry AJ. Infection control in anesthesia. Anesth Clin North Am 1989;7:967–981.

c. Evaporation and Light Deactivation
If the solution is in an uncovered container, evaporation can occur. Usually, evaporation is not as serious as dilution. If the chemical agent is more volatile than the diluent, loss by evaporation can be very important. Chlorine products are especially susceptible to evaporation and deactivation from light exposure.

d. Bioburden
In general, the higher the level of microbial contamination, the longer the exposure to the chemical germicide necessary before the entire microbial population is killed. Items should be scrupulously cleaned. Liquid agents vary widely in their effectiveness against various types of microorganisms. **Table 27.1** shows the capabilities of some commonly used agents.

e. pH
The relative acidity or alkalinity of disinfectants can influence their activity. An increase in pH tends to decrease the efficacy of phenols, iodine, and hypochlorites. In contrast, increased pH will improve the antimicrobial activity of glutaraldehyde and quaternary ammonium compounds. Soluble calcium or magnesium in the water supply can react with detergents to form insoluble precipitates, which tend to neutralize some disinfectants.

f. Characteristics of the Item to Be Disinfected
A disinfectant solution will be effective only if it can contact both the inner and outer surfaces of the item being disinfected. Uneven or porous surfaces resist chemical disinfection. Entrapped air can prevent contact between the liquid and parts of the device.

g. Use Pattern, Use Life, and Storage Life
The disinfectant product label should be examined for information on the use pattern, use life, and storage life. *Use pattern* refers to how many times the solution can be used. Use life commonly applies to, but is not limited to, disinfectant products that require mixing two ingredients for activation. Once a disinfectant solution is mixed, there will be a limited period of time during which the solution is effective. The container should be marked with the date the solution was prepared and the date it expires. The storage life

is the time period after which the unused and/or unactivated disinfectant product is no longer deemed effective.

h. Time

The time required for different chemical agents to function effectively varies from seconds to hours and will depend on the factors just mentioned. Some microorganisms are killed faster than others. A lower disinfection level can be achieved in less time. Leaving devices in the disinfectant too long can make it hard to remove the chemical from the device.

2. **Agents**

No chemical germicide is suitable for all purposes. A number of factors should be considered in selecting the agent, including the degree of microbial death needed; the nature and composition of the item being treated; whether the item is critical, semicritical, or noncritical; cost; safety; and ease of use.

CLINICAL MOMENT Antiseptics are not appropriate for disinfecting inanimate surfaces or objects.

a. Glutaraldehyde

1) Glutaraldehyde-based solutions have been widely used because of their excellent germicidal properties, activity in the presence of organic matter, noncorrosiveness with most equipment, and lack of coagulation with proteinaceous material. Glutaraldehyde has an extensive shelf life. It may be used as long as 30 days after activation, provided in-use dilution and organic stress are properly controlled.

2) Local exhaust ventilation (either a ductless system or a ducted fume hood) should be installed to capture chemical vapors. A ducted fume hood should be connected to a nonrecirculating exhaust system that goes to the outside atmosphere at a location away from people and air intake ducts. Self-contained (ductless) fume hoods (**Fig. 27.3**) encapsulate the soaking container and have a blower that draws fumes away from the operator and delivers them to a system that chemically inactivates the germicide and returns clean filtered air to the room. This eliminates the need to install a duct.

3) Glutaraldehyde is effective against bacteria, fungi, and viruses at room temperature. High-level disinfection requires 20 to 30 minutes. Three to 10 hours are required to sterilize spores. Elevating the temperature can shorten these times. The manufacturer's instructions should always be consulted.

b. *ortho*-Phthalaldehyde

1) Orthophthalaldehyde (OPA or Cidex OPA) can achieve high-level disinfection at room temperature after a 12-minute exposure period and after a shorter time at an elevated temperature. It is sporicidal with prolonged exposure. It is often used in an automatic endoscope processing system, which reduces the processing time to 5 minutes. It is noncorrosive.

2) OPA has a number of advantages compared with glutaraldehyde. These include faster disinfection, minimal odor, no need for activation or mixing, and no OSHA vapor limit. It can be discarded down the drain. It is effective in the presence of organic soil. While more expensive per gallon than glutaraldehyde, it may be more economical at high-volume centers.

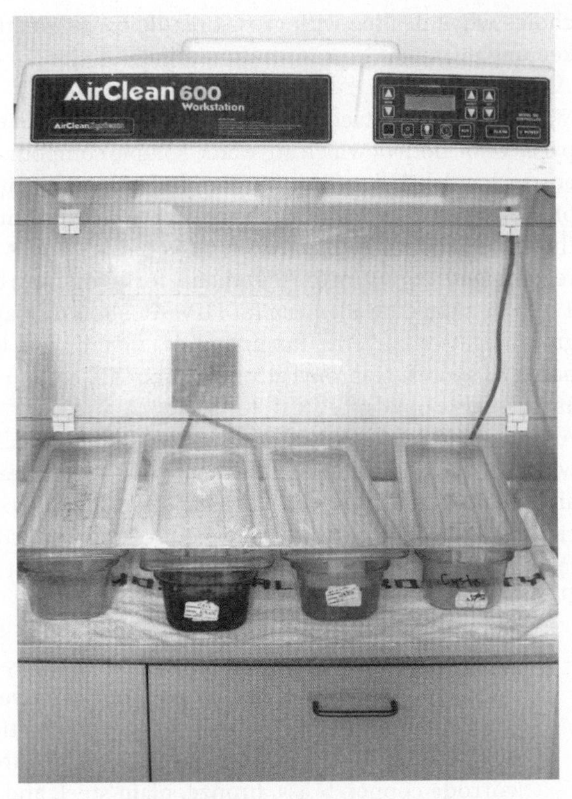

Figure 27.3 Glutaraldehyde user station. Fumes are drawn away from the operator and into a filter, where they are neutralized.

c. Quaternary Ammonium Compounds

Quaternary ammonium compounds (quats) are low-level disinfectants. They are bactericidal, fungicidal, and virucidal at room temperature within 10 minutes but have not demonstrated sporicidal effects. If a spore is coated with a quaternary ammonium compound, it will not develop into a vegetative cell as long as the germicide remains, but if the coating is removed, the spore can germinate. These compounds are more effective against gram-positive bacteria than gram-negative bacteria. Quats inactivate the human immunodeficiency virus (HIV), but some do not inactivate the hepatitis virus. They are ineffective against *M. tuberculosis* or hydrophilic viruses.

d. Phenolic Compounds

Phenolic compounds (phenolics, phenols) are derived from carbolic acid (phenol), one of the oldest germicides. They are sometimes combined with detergents to form detergent germicides. They are good bactericides and are active against fungi. They are active in the presence of organic matter and soap. Phenols are very stable and remain active after mild heating and prolonged drying. When moisture is applied to a surface that has been previously treated with a phenolic compound, it can redissolve the chemical so that it again becomes bactericidal. Phenolics remain active in contact with organic soil and for this reason are often the disinfectants of choice when dealing with gross organic contamination in general housekeeping.

e. Alcohols

Within healthcare facilities, alcohol usually refers to either ethyl or isopropyl alcohol, both of which are water-soluble compounds that are intermediate- or low-level disinfectants. The alcohols are best used at concentrations of 70% to 90% by volume. Both are effective against most viruses, including those for hepatitis B [hepatitis B virus (HBV)] and AIDS (HIV). The CDC recommends exposure to 70% ethanol for 15 minutes to inactivate HBV, but 1 minute should be adequate for HIV. Alcohols display high activity against gram-negative bacteria, fungi, and *M. tuberculosis* but cannot inactivate bacterial spores. Isopropyl alcohol cannot kill certain hydrophilic viruses.

f. Iodine Compounds

An iodophor is a combination of iodine and a solubilizing agent or carrier, with the resulting complex providing a sustained-release reservoir of iodine and releasing free iodine in aqueous solution. Iodophors are bactericidal, virucidal, and tuberculocidal but may require prolonged contact time to kill certain fungi and bacterial spores. Some iodophors do not kill *M. tuberculosis.*

g. Peracetic Acid

1) Peracetic (peroxyacetic) acid is bactericidal, fungicidal, virucidal, and sporicidal at low temperatures. It remains effective in the presence of organic material. It may be effective against prions. An important advantage is that its decomposition products (acetic acid, water, oxygen, and hydrogen peroxide) are not harmful. It can corrode copper, brass, bronze, plain steel, and galvanized iron, but these effects can be reduced by additives and pH modifications. A concentrated solution can cause eye and skin damage, but it has no OSHA exposure limit.
2) Steris 20 is a patented product that has been developed specifically for Steris processors. The active ingredient is a concentrate of 35% peracetic acid plus corrosion and degradation inhibitors contained in a sealed, single-use container. It should be used only in a Steris processing system.
3) The Steris 20 is a "just in time" system, meaning the items cannot stay in the processor until they are used. It is most commonly used for flexible endoscopes. The flexible scope tray must have the correct adapters for the scopes to be processed.
4) The Steris System 1 (SS1) was the subject of an FDA safety alert that stated that the current version of the SS1 has been significantly modified and had not received FDA approval and that the FDA had received reports of operational malfunctions that could cause serious injuries (1). The manufacturer has promised, with FDA approval, that the SS1 will be supported until August 2, 2011. At the time of writing, the manufacturer was working with the FDA on a 501K submission for an updated system 1. The reader is encouraged to check with the manufacturer for developments in this area.

h. Chlorine Compounds

1) Several chlorine compounds are available for use as disinfectants, including sodium and calcium hypochlorite (household bleach), chlorine dioxide, and chloramine T. The hypochlorites are the most

Table 27.2 Preparation of Household Bleach for Disinfection[a]

	Desired Chlorine Concentration			
	5000 ppm	**1000 ppm**	**500 ppm**	**100 ppm**
Dilution for use within 24 hours	1:10	1:50	1:100	1:500
Dilution for use for 1 to 30 days	1:5	1:25	1:50	1:250

[a]Starting with 5.25% NaOCl, which contains 50,000 ppm of free chlorine.

widely used compounds. They are inexpensive and fast acting. They are available in both liquid (sodium hypochlorite) and solid (calcium hypochlorite) forms. Relatively low concentrations of sodium hypochlorite (50 ppm) exhibit rapid activity against vegetative bacteria. One hundred ppm is effective against most fungi. Many viruses are inactivated at concentrations of 200 ppm, with HIV being susceptible at concentrations as low as 50 ppm. HBV exhibits marked inactivation at 500 ppm. Concentrations of 1000 ppm are considered adequate to achieve high-level disinfection. A 1:5 to 1:10 dilution will destroy the agent of Creutzfeldt-Jakob disease (CJD) after a 1-hour exposure period.

2) **Table 27.2** shows the dilution of 5.25% NaOCl (household bleach) needed to achieve the desired chlorine concentration. Solutions that will be used for extended periods (1 to 30 days) should have an initial concentration twice as high as actually desired and should be stored in an opaque container.

i. Hydrogen Peroxide

Hydrogen peroxide is an effective bactericide, fungicide, virucide, and sporicide. It is commercially available in several different concentrations. It is not inactivated by organic matter. There are no restrictions on disposal. It rapidly loses effectiveness when exposed to heat and light and requires careful storage. It can damage rubber and plastic and may corrode copper, zinc, and brass. It irritates skin and eyes. A 7.5% solution achieves high-level disinfection in 30 minutes. A 3% hydrogen peroxide solution provides effective low-level disinfection for work surfaces. Hydrogen peroxide is used for plasma sterilization (see in the following text).

j. Formaldehyde

Formaldehyde is a highly toxic and flammable gas that has been used as a disinfectant and a sterilant in both a water-based solution (formalin) and the gaseous state. It is noncorrosive and is not inactivated by organic matter. Although formalin is a high-level disinfectant, its uses are limited by its pungent fumes. Its toxicity requires that disinfected materials be thoroughly rinsed before use. The National Institute for Occupational Safety and Health (NIOSH) has indicated that formaldehyde should be handled as a potent sensitizer and probable carcinogen.

3. **Advantages and Disadvantages of Chemical Disinfection and Sterilization**

a. Advantages of liquid chemical disinfection include economy, speed, and simplicity. This is especially important in busy endoscopy suites because it enables equipment to be used several times a day. It is useful for equipment that requires high-level disinfection but not sterilization.

b. Chemical disinfection cannot be used for all types of equipment. Many devices cannot be soaked. Hinged instruments must be opened and those with sliding or multiple parts disassembled. Prepackaging is not possible, and the equipment will be wet. There is a risk of recontamination during subsequent rinsing, drying, or wrapping. With most agents, sterility cannot be guaranteed. The chemicals may be absorbed onto the treated items, causing harm to the patient. It is more expensive, less effective, and more prone to human error than steam sterilization.

CLINICAL MOMENT Some solutions are irritating to tissues and have unpleasant odors. Personnel who handle them must take precautions to avoid prolonged skin contact or vapor inhalation.

c. A significant disadvantage of cold sterilization is the lack of a good method for validation. The efficacy can be monitored only indirectly, through surveying patient outcomes, to identify subsequent infections that can be attributed to exposure to the reusable device.

E. Gas Sterilization

1. **Characteristics of Ethylene Oxide**

Ethylene oxide (EtO, EO) is a colorless, poisonous gas with a sweet odor. It is available in high-pressure tanks and unit-dose ampules and cartridges. It is flammable at concentrations of 3% or more. EO may be mixed with carbon dioxide or hydrochlorofluorocarbons. Mixtures containing up to 12% EO in these inert diluents are nonflammable but retain their sterilizing ability.

2. **The Sterilization Process**

EO concentrations between 450 and 750 mg/L are commonly used in processing medical products. EO solubility in the product and the diffusion rate through the product will influence the sterilant concentration. The operating pressure of the EO cycle will influence the gas diffusion rate. Packaging may also be critical. Devices that perform continuous EO monitoring in the sterilization chamber are available.

3. **Aeration**

EO not only comes in contact with an article's surface but also penetrates some items, which then retain varying amounts. These items need aeration (degassing, desorption, offgasing) to reduce EO to a level safe for both personnel and patient use. The acceptable level of residual EO depends on whether the item is to be used within or outside the body. Aeration may be accomplished passively in air (ambient aeration) or actively in a mechanical aerator.

a. Ambient Aeration

Ambient aeration is slower than mechanical aeration. Items that require between 8 and 12 hours of mechanical aeration may require 7 days of ambient aeration. Some items take between 5 and 6 weeks. The temperature in the aeration area should be at least 18°C.

CLINICAL MOMENT Because there is a wide range in the aeration times for various materials, it is important to determine what materials are present. Consult the user manual to determine the proper aeration time if EO is used.

b. Mechanical Aeration
   1) In mechanical aerators, a stream of filtered air is directed over the sterilized items. An EO sterilizer may be combined with an aerator so that one chamber is used for both processes.
   2) A number of factors affect mechanical aeration. These include the object and wrap thickness. The packaging material must allow fast gas transfer. Plastics cloth, paper, muslin, and rubber absorb significant quantities of EO. Items need to be packed loosely in the aerator to allow adequate airflow. Increased temperature accelerates desorption. The usual aeration temperature is between 50°C and 60°C. The usual aeration time is 12 hours at 50°C. If the temperature used is 60°C, the time is reduced to 8 hours.

4. **Complications of Ethylene Oxide Sterilization**
   a. Complications of EO sterilization that stem from failure to eliminate residual gas from sterilized items include skin reactions and laryngotracheal inflammation. Sensitization and anaphylaxis from exposure to products sterilized with EO have been reported.

CLINICAL MOMENT Products sterilized using EO may increase the risk of latex sensitization.

   b. Ethylene chlorhydrin is formed when EO comes into contact with chloride ions that may be present in previously γ-irradiated polyvinyl chloride (PVC) items. The American National Standards Institute at one time recommended that PVC items that have been γ-irradiated never be resterilized with EO, but very low levels of by-products in irradiated products treated with EO have cast doubt on this recommendation and EO sterilization of γ-irradiated PVC items may be acceptable if strict attention is paid to aeration.
   c. Perhaps, the greatest problem with using EO is the potential complications to workers who use the agent. The presence of gaseous EO in very high concentrations is easily detected because it is irritating to the eyes and mucous membranes, but odor is not a reliable way to detect its presence and does not provide adequate warning of hazardous concentrations.
   d. Acute exposure to significant levels of EO usually provokes an irritant response. Upper respiratory complaints, eye irritation, headache, blunting of taste or smell, a metallic taste, and coughing frequently occur. With higher concentrations, nausea, vomiting, diarrhea, increased fatigability, memory loss, drowsiness, weakness, dizziness, lack of coordination, chest discomfort, shortness of breath, difficulty swallowing, cramps, and convulsions may occur. Respiratory paralysis and peripheral nerve damage have been reported after massive exposure. The onset of neurological signs and symptoms may be delayed for 6 hours or more after exposure. EO gas is heavier than air and can cause asphyxiation in enclosed, poorly ventilated, or low-lying areas.
   e. Chronic EO exposure can affect the eyes (corneal burns, cataracts, epithelial keratitis), the central and peripheral nervous system, and skin (irritant and allergic reactions). Respiratory infections, anemia, and impaired cognitive function may occur. EO is a recognized mutagen and carcinogen and may adversely affect the reproductive system.

f. Once EO is emitted, it remains in the air without breaking down for long periods of time. People who live near facilities with sterilizers or aerators may be exposed to significant levels of airborne EO. Some state and local areas limit the amount of EO that can be emitted into the air. Catalytic converters that break EO down into carbon dioxide and water are available.

5. **Advantages and Disadvantages of Gas Sterilization**

a. EO sterilization is very reliable because the gas penetrates into crevices, narrow lumens, and regions blocked by liquids. It can be used on a wide variety of items, including those that would be damaged by heat or moisture. It is the only reliable and practical means for sterilizing many devices. Items can be packaged before sterilization and stored sterile for extended periods. Prepackaging eliminates the danger of recontamination that can occur during rinsing and packaging following cold sterilization and allows items to remain sterile during long-term storage. A large variety of equipment can be sterilized at one time.

b. EO has a number of disadvantages. Fires and explosions involving sterilizers have been reported. A major disadvantage is the long processing time required. This may make it necessary to have multiple sets of equipment. EO is more costly than most other types of sterilization. Personnel need to be highly trained and supervised. Measures to reduce employee exposure and monitor levels of EO must be taken. Some materials deteriorate after repeated EO sterilization, especially at elevated temperatures. It cannot be used to sterilize devices that have petroleum-based lubricants in or on them.

F. Radiation Sterilization

1. γ-Radiation uses an electromagnetic wave produced during the disintegration of certain radioactive elements. If the dosage applied to a product is large enough, all microorganisms, including bacterial spores and viruses, will be killed.
2. There are many advantages to γ-radiation. The product can be packaged in a wide variety of impermeable containers before treatment. The package will not interfere with the sterilization process. The treated items remain sterile indefinitely until the packaging seal is broken. Because there is virtually no temperature rise during treatment, thermolabile materials can be sterilized and thermolabile packaging can be used. Items may be used immediately after treatment, with no risk from retained radioactivity.
3. γ-Radiation is not practical for everyday use in healthcare facilities. It requires expensive equipment and is used only by large manufacturers to sterilize disposable equipment. Some healthcare facilities send their packs to outside facilities for treatment.

G. Gas Plasma Sterilization

1. Gas plasma is sometimes described as the fourth state of matter, consisting of a cloud of reactive ions, electrons, and neutral atomic and molecular particles. It is produced by applying energy to certain gases. Hydrogen peroxide vapor is most often used. The reactive species in the plasma interact with the molecules that are essential for the metabolism and reproduction of living cells.
2. Devices to be sterilized need to be thoroughly cleaned and dried. They can be unwrapped or enclosed in a nonwoven wrap. Cellulose-based materials such as cotton, paper, or gauze should not be used for wrapping because they absorb the sterilant vapors, reducing its concentration.

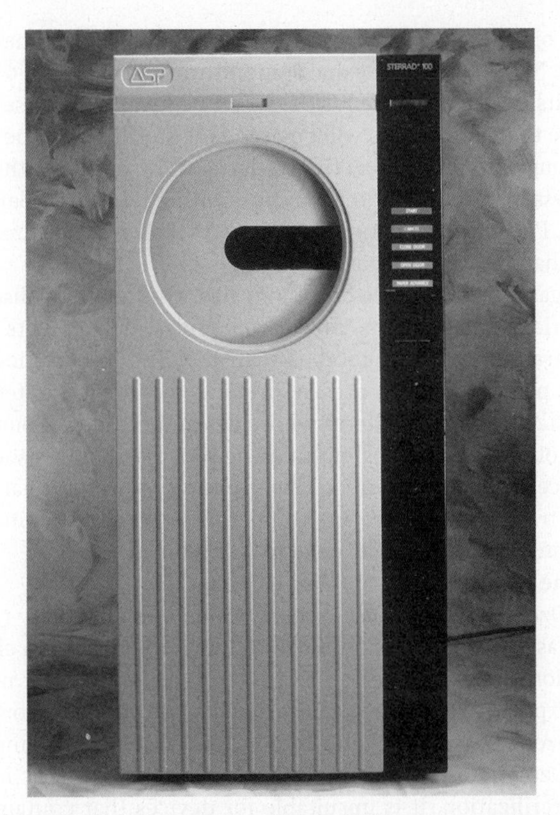

Figure 27.4 Gas plasma sterilizer. (Photograph courtesy of Sterrad, a division of Johnson & Johnson Company, Irvine, CA.)

CLINICAL MOMENT It is important that all items be clean and dry before placing them in a plasma sterilizer.

3. The sterilizer (**Fig. 27.4**) runs on an automatic, microprocessor-controlled cycle. The machine produces a printout for each load processed. If for any reason the process is outside the normal limits, the cycle is interrupted and the printout gives the reason. The hydrogen peroxide is contained in a sealed disposable cassette that is placed inside the sterilizer.

CLINICAL MOMENT It is important to read the instructions supplied with the sterilizer, especially when devices with small lumens are processed. Early models could not sterilize devices with long narrow lumens. Later models can sterilize most of these devices, although a longer cycle time may be required.

4. A gas plasma sterilizer is simple to operate. It uses relatively low concentrations of the sterilizing agent, does not leave toxic residuals, and has short processing times. The sterilized products are dry and immediately available for use or can be stored for later use. There is no need for cooling or aeration. There are no emissions or toxic by-products. The primary end products are oxygen and water.

5. Lack of worker exposure and environmental contamination are major advantages. No personnel or exhaust monitoring is needed. No water source, heating, or outside venting is required. It can be located in close proximity to the area where the instruments will be used. The sterilizer can be moved around easily.
6. Although gas plasma sterilizers have a low capacity, the volume of products processed per unit of time may be equivalent to that of large-capacity EO sterilizers. Plasma sterilization is less costly than EO sterilization but more expensive than steam sterilization.
7. The gas plasma sterilizer system has a number of disadvantages. Cellulose materials, paper, linens, powders, liquids, and implants cannot be processed. Penetration is not as good as with EO. The sterilization process is impaired when protein or salt is present. Devices that are to be sterilized must be able to withstand a vacuum. Items whose design permits the surfaces to collapse onto each other (e.g., bags) should not be processed unless some means to keep the surfaces separated is used. This process requires special supplies (e.g., indicators, trays, wraps) that are compatible with the system. Some wrapping and stacking techniques may need to be modified.
8. **Ozone Sterilization**
   a. Ozone sterilizers use oxygen, water, and electricity to produce ozone. The gas is humidified and dispersed into a sterilization chamber. The sterilization cycle includes air evacuation; air and ozone mixture admission; an exposure stage; and vacuum drying and ozone removal. After the cycle, the ozone passes through a catalytic converter that changes it back to oxygen.
   b. Ozone sterilization is useful for most items that need low-temperature sterilization. It is unsuitable for devices that contain natural gum rubber (latex) products, some plastics, textile fabrics, and some metals such as brass and copper.

CLINICAL MOMENT It is important to check the diameter and length of lumens on a device to be sterilized using ozone. The manufacturer's instructions need to be consulted.

V. A Program for Anesthesia Equipment

A. General Considerations

Those who are concerned with anesthesia equipment find themselves faced with a dilemma as to how much time, effort, and money should be expended to prevent infection transmission. With increased pressure to limit costs, there may be strong temptation and pressure to do less.

1. **Centers for Disease Control and Prevention Guidelines**

   The CDC has published guidelines on how to prevent or control nosocomial infections on the basis of a classification of instruments and other items by the risk of infection involved.

   a. Critical Items

   Critical items are items that penetrate the skin or mucous membranes or are in contact with normally sterile areas of the body. They include vascular and regional block needles and catheters. These items must be sterile because they bear a high risk of infection if they are contaminated.

   b. Semicritical Items

   Semicritical items do not pierce mucous membranes. Equipment that falls into this category includes endoscopes; laryngoscope blades; reusable rectal, nasopharyngeal, and esophageal temperature probes; face masks; oral and nasal airways; resuscitation bags; breathing tubes and connectors; oxygen masks; esophageal stethoscopes; and tracheal and double-lumen tubes. Ideally, semicritical items should be sterile. High-level disinfection is acceptable when sterilization is not practical.

c. Noncritical Items

Noncritical items do not touch the patient or touch only intact skin. Items in this category include stethoscopes (not esophageal); blood pressure cuffs and tubing; arm boards; pulse oximeter sensors and cables; electrocardiogram cables and electrodes; reusable skin temperature probes; temperature monitor cables; head straps; blood warmers; carbon dioxide absorber assemblies; adaptors for oxygen sensors; and the exteriors of the anesthesia machine, ventilator, humidifiers, scavenging system, resuscitation bags, intravenous fluid pumps, monitors, and equipment carts. Since intact skin normally acts as an effective barrier to most microorganisms, these items need only cleaning, followed by intermediate- or low-level disinfection.

d. Environmental Surfaces

Some experts add another category, environmental surfaces. These include surfaces that do not ordinarily come into direct contact with the patient, but if they do, it is only with intact skin. These surfaces may potentially contribute to secondary cross contamination by healthcare workers or medical instruments that subsequently come into contact with patients. These surfaces can be further divided into *medical equipment surfaces* such as adjustment knobs or handles and *housekeeping surfaces* such as floors, walls, and windowsills.

2. **The Anesthesia Work Area**

The anesthesia work area is usually the site where cleaning and other procedures are performed unless the equipment goes directly to a central reprocessing area. Procedures include disassembly, cleaning, disinfection, and sterilization. How much is done in the anesthesia workroom will depend on how much can be carried out by the operating room or central service department for the entire facility.

CLINICAL MOMENT When returning dirty equipment to the anesthesia work area, it should not be placed in an area where it can contaminate clean or sterile equipment. Areas should be well marked to determine where dirty equipment should be placed.

B. Individual Item Considerations

Choosing the proper decontamination method will depend on a number of factors, including whether the item is considered critical, semicritical, or noncritical; the nature of the contamination; the time required for processing; pressure, moisture, and chemical tolerance of the item; the availability of processing equipment; and the risks associated with the decontamination method. The manufacturer's instructions should be carefully studied and followed.

1. **Anesthesia Carts**

Equipment that is not kept sterile should be placed in drawers that are less frequently opened, that is, not in the same drawer as frequently used drugs. The top surface should be cleaned of visible material and disinfected with a germicide between subsequent cases and at the conclusion of the workday.

A clean covering should be placed on the top of the cart at the start of each case. Vertical surfaces should be cleaned at the end of the workday or if there is obvious contamination. At least once a month, all equipment should be removed and the drawers and containers cleaned and then wiped or sprayed with a germicide.

2. **Gas Cylinders**
Gas cylinders are transported to the facility in open trucks and are frequently stored outside. Before taking a gas cylinder into the operating room suite, the wrapper, if present, should be removed. The cylinder should be washed with water and detergent and wiped or sprayed with a germicide. After placing the cylinder on the anesthesia machine, it should be considered part of the machine and treated accordingly.
3. **Anesthesia Machines**
The same principles apply to cleaning anesthesia machines as to carts. The top surface should be supplied with a clean cover for each patient. The machine should be cleaned between subsequent cases and at the end of the workday with a detergent solution and then sprayed or wiped with a germicide. Particular attention should be paid to parts of the machine that are adjusted. This includes flow control valve and vaporizer adjustment knobs. Equipment should be removed from drawers and the drawers cleaned and disinfected regularly.

CLINICAL MOMENT Care must be taken not to get cleaning liquid in the vaporizer filling funnels. After the agent has dried, its residue can be washed into the vaporizing chamber when liquid agent is added.

4. **Anesthesia Ventilators**
The ventilator exterior should be treated in the same manner as the outside of an anesthesia machine. Many bellows and tubings can be sterilized using EO. An important feature of the newer generation of anesthesia ventilators is that most parts that come into contact with respiratory gases can be easily removed and steam autoclaved (**Fig. 27.5**). The manufacturer's recommendations should be followed.

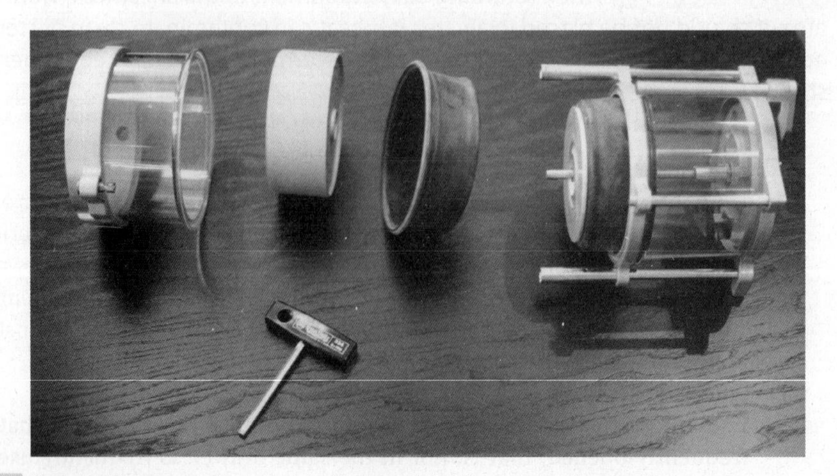

Figure 27.5 Drager Divan ventilator that is disassembled for steam autoclaving.

5. **Unidirectional Valves, Adjustable Pressure-Limiting Valve, and Water Traps**
The outside of adjustable pressure-limiting (APL) and unidirectional valves should be cleaned and disinfected periodically. Unidirectional valves are usually easily disassembled and cleaned by wiping the disc, the inside of the plastic dome, and the valve seat with alcohol or a detergent. Some APL valves may be autoclaved, and some can be pasteurized. Using glutaraldehyde on APL valves may cause stickiness and increase the opening pressure. Water traps should be cleaned and disinfected periodically and whenever water is visible. Refer to the manufacturer's recommendations.
6. **Absorbers**
   a. Studies suggest that patients rarely contaminate the absorbent with high levels of bacteria. The manufacturer's instructions should be followed with respect to disassembly, cleaning, and disinfection. Many of the newer anesthesia workstations have absorber assemblies that can be easily disassembled and steam autoclaved (**Fig. 27.6**). There is currently no consensus

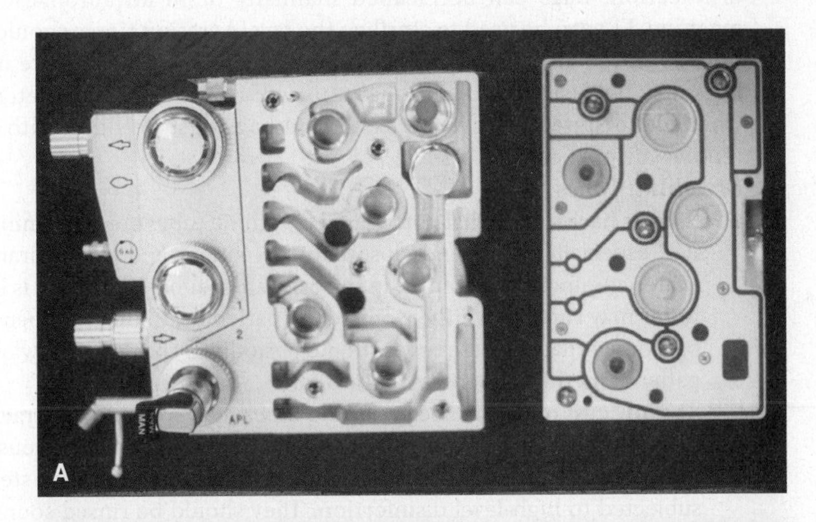

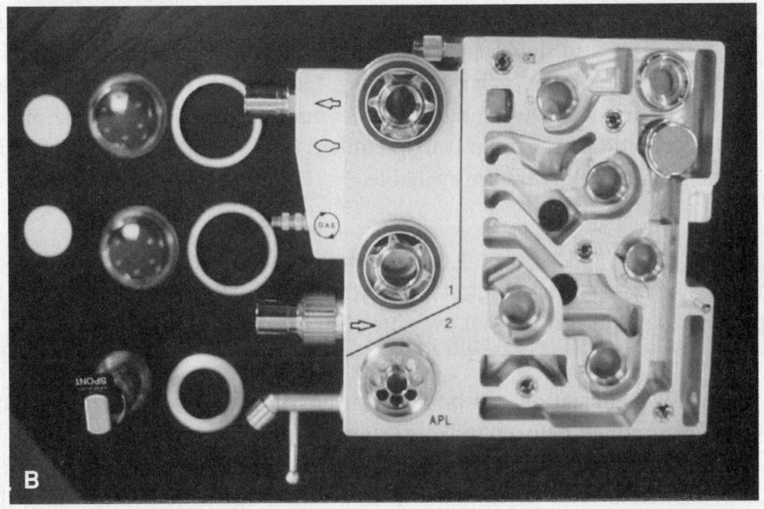

Figure 27.6 **A:** Absorber assembly that is partly disassembled. **B:** The adjustable pressure-limiting and unidirectional valves are also disassembled. The assembly can now be steam sterilized.

on whether the absorbent should be changed after use when the patient has methicillin-resistant *Staphylococcus auerus* infection (2).

b. Canisters should be cleaned when the absorbent is changed, with particular attention to screens because they are susceptible to obstruction. Some canisters can be steam autoclaved, and some can be sterilized using EO. Others can be disinfected by immersion in a liquid such as glutaraldehyde.

c. Newer absorbers use one or more disposable plastic receptacles. These are smaller than those used in older absorbers and are changed more frequently. Since they are disposable, they do not need to be cleaned. The user manual should be checked to determine whether the connections to the breathing system need regular cleaning.

7. **Reservoir Bag**

In most institutions, reservoir bags are supplied with the disposable breathing tubes as part of a set, so they do not need cleaning. Reusable reservoir bags should be cleaned and then sterilized or subjected to high-level disinfection. Bags can be cleaned manually or in an automatic washing machine. EO can be used to sterilize the bag. Aeration times should be carefully observed and the bag filled and emptied a few times before use. Some bags may be pasteurized, although this will result in gradual deterioration. Chemical disinfection can be used. The bag must be filled with liquid to remove air pockets.

8. **Breathing Tubes**

a. Studies have shown that corrugated breathing tubes are contaminated after use, especially at the end closest to the patient and the expiratory limb. Water commonly condenses in the expiratory tube. If the tube is lifted, this water may run down either toward the patient or to the absorber, reservoir bag, or ventilator. These tubes should periodically be drained away from the patient and the condensate discarded.

b. The low cost of disposable breathing tubes makes their use attractive, considering the cost and difficulty of cleaning and disinfecting reusable tubings. Reusable breathing tubings should be cleaned and then sterilized or subjected to high-level disinfection. They should be rinsed soon after use to prevent drying. They may then be soaked in a container that contains water and detergent. The long length and corrugations preclude a brush from being effective in cleaning. Ultrasonic cleaning can be used to remove debris, or a washing machine may be used. After washing, the tubings should be thoroughly dried unless they are to undergo pasteurization. Special tube dryers are available.

CLINICAL MOMENT Disposable tubings are usually supplied clean but not sterile. When it is necessary to include the breathing tubes in the surgical field, it is important to make certain that they are sterile.

c. Pasteurization can be used for corrugated tubings. The Y-piece should be removed beforehand; otherwise, a loose fit may result.

d. Chemical disinfection can be carried out by using an automatic washing machine or by immersion in a liquid agent. It is important that the tube be inserted vertically, making certain that it is filled on the inside and that there are no air pockets.

9. **Y-piece**
   a. The Y-piece is contaminated in a high percentage of cases. A contaminated Y-piece may cause patient-to-patient transmission of hepatitis C virus (HCV). Disposable Y-pieces that are permanently attached to disposable tubings are commonly used.
   b. A reusable Y-piece should be cleaned and sterilized or subjected to high-level disinfection. After use, it should be removed from the corrugated tubings and rinsed. It should then be soaked in a solution of water and detergent and then scrubbed manually or placed in a washing machine. If chemical disinfection or EO sterilization is to be used, it should be thoroughly dried. Y-pieces may be pasteurized, immersed in liquid agents, or sterilized using EO or plasma.
10. **Mapleson Systems**
    After use, a Mapleson system should be disassembled and the components cleaned. Metal components can undergo autoclaving. Rubber and plastic parts can undergo gas or plasma sterilization or a liquid chemical agent may be used. In many cases, disposable tubings are more cost-effective. A reusable APL valve may be difficult to sterilize.
11. **Adaptors**
    Adaptors that are used near the patient are contaminated in a high percentage of cases. After use, they should be rinsed and then soaked in a solution of detergent and water. They may be washed manually or in a washing machine. Rubber and plastic adaptors may be sterilized with EO, plasma, or a liquid such as glutaraldehyde. Metal adaptors may also be autoclaved or pasteurized.
12. **Scavenging Equipment**
    A satisfactory method of treating scavenging equipment is to wash the device in a detergent solution monthly and change the hoses that connect the device to the breathing system and ventilator at the same time. Lint may accumulate in the air intake valves on closed scavenging interfaces. These valves should be removed and cleaned frequently.
13. **Face Masks**
    a. Face masks are among the most heavily contaminated pieces of equipment. Because of their proximity to the patient, infection transmission is a definite possibility. For obviously contaminated cases, disposable masks should be used.
    b. Asepsis should be practiced when using face masks. A face mask should not be allowed to drop onto the floor or be exposed to obvious contamination. After use, the mask should be kept near the patient's head or with the dirty equipment. It should not be allowed to contaminate clean equipment.
    c. Reusable face masks should be cleaned and then sterilized or subjected to high-level disinfection. Immediately after use, the connector should be removed and the mask rinsed and then soaked and scrubbed. It may be cleaned automatically in a washing machine. Masks should always be thoroughly rinsed and dried.
    d. With gas sterilization, a mask can be kept sterile for long periods of time. Aeration must be adequate; otherwise, facial burns may result. Most automatic EO sterilizers employ a vacuum at least once during the sterilization cycle. This vacuum may cause the pneumatic cushion on the mask to be damaged. This can be prevented by removing the plug that seals the cushion or by using a sterilizer that does not have a vacuum phase.

e. Steam autoclaving is sometimes used for face masks. As with EO sterilization, it involves a vacuum phase that may damage the inflated cushion, so the plug should be removed beforehand. Pasteurization has been used for face masks.
f. Liquid chemical agents are often used to disinfect or sterilize face masks. Thorough rinsing is important to remove residual agent.

CLINICAL MOMENT Cracks in the reusable mask cushion can allow liquid agent to enter. When placed on a patient's face, the liquid can be squeezed out, possibly into the eyes.

14. **Head Straps**
After use, head straps should be subjected to cleaning with a detergent and then soaked in a disinfectant solution or sterilized using EO or plasma.
15. **Airways**
a. Airways should be treated as clean objects and not allowed to drop onto the floor. Most airways are now disposable.
b. As soon as possible after use, a reusable airway should be rinsed with cold water and placed in a solution of water and detergent. It can be washed manually or in a machine. It should be thoroughly rinsed to remove residual detergent.
c. Pasteurization, liquid chemical disinfection, and EO and plasma sterilization have been used for airways. Rubber airways may be autoclaved, but this will shorten their useful life.
16. **Rigid Laryngoscopes**
a. Disposable laryngoscopes are discussed in Chapter 14. Either the blade or the blade and handle may be disposable. While their light transmission is less than that of new reusable fiberoptic blades, the disposable blade may be brighter after the reusable blade is steam autoclaved numerous times.
b. Contaminated rigid laryngoscope blades and handles are common, and there are reported cases of serious cross infection arising from contaminated laryngoscopes. A particular concern is that the blade may be a vector for a variant of CJD.
c. Laryngoscopes should be stored under clean conditions. Disposable covers that fit over the handle and/or blade are available (**Fig. 27.7**), but may create difficulties during intubation.
d. After use, the handle and blade are considered contaminated and should not be placed on a clean surface. The glove that the operator is wearing may be inverted over the blade and the handle to prevent spreading contamination.
e. There is no consensus on what constitutes adequate blade or handle processing. The methods employed range from superficial cleaning to sterilization. If prion contamination is likely, a disposable blade should be used.
f. After use, the handle surface should first be wiped clean with water and detergent and then with alcohol. The batteries (and bulb chamber, if present) must be removed prior to disinfection or sterilization unless the handle is designed to be waterproof. The batteries must be removed if the method of sterilization includes a vacuum cycle, pressure, or heat. After the batteries are removed, the handle can be sterilized by using steam, plasma, or EO.

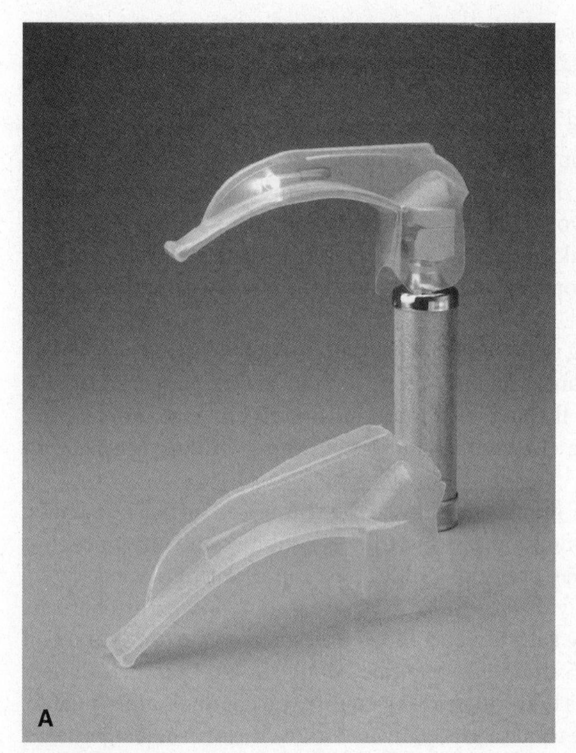

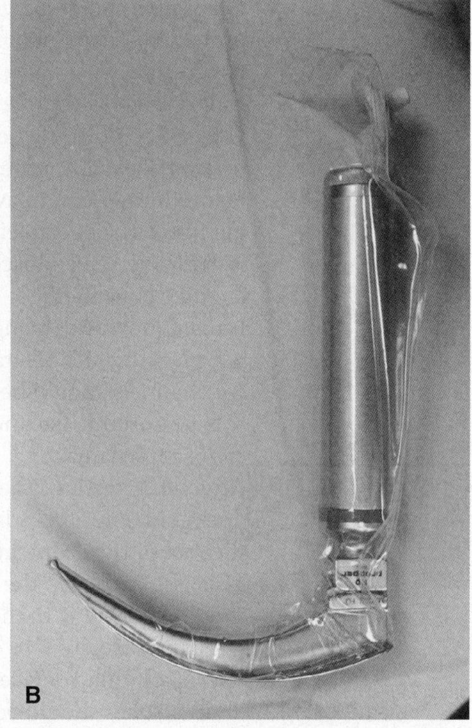

Figure 27.7 Disposable laryngoscope covers. **A:** Covering for blade only. (Photograph courtesy of Blue Ridge Medical, Inc., now part of Bound Tree Medical, Dublin, OH.) **B:** Covering for both the blade and the handle.

g. As soon as possible after use, the blade should be rinsed and immersed in water with an enzymatic detergent. It should be washed gently but thoroughly using a soft brush, with particular attention to the area around the bulb or light bundle. Cleaning is often inadequate. Ultrasonic cleaning is usually not recommended. After cleaning, the blade should be rinsed and dried.

h. Blades may undergo high-level disinfection or sterilization with EO, steam, plasma, or liquid chemicals. The Steris system can be used. EO is appropriate for most blades, provided a temperature of 180°F and pressure of 8 psi are not exceeded. No aeration is required. Some blades can be sterilized using steam. Flash sterilization is not recommended.

CLINICAL MOMENT Light transmission through fiber-optic laryngoscope blades will decrease after multiple steam sterilizations.

CLINICAL MOMENT Fiber-optic blades should not be immersed in cold water soon after autoclaving because the fiber-optic bundles may crack.

17. **Flexible Endoscopes**

a. Endoscopes are semicritical devices that carry a real risk of infection transmission to patients. Pseudoinfections have also been reported. A fiber-optic endoscope should be stored in a clean area, with the tip and flexible portion protected. Disposable suction valves may help to reduce the risk of cross infection.

b. A fiberscope is complex, fragile, and heat-sensitive, which makes it difficult to clean and disinfect or sterilize. It may be best to have it decontaminated in an endoscopy unit. Pressure (i.e., leak) testing should be performed before immersion to avoid costly damage that can occur during the cleaning process. Special leakage testers are available for this purpose. If a leak is detected, the endoscope should be removed from service and the manufacturer consulted.

c. Immediately after being removed from the patient, the fiberscope should be wiped with a disinfectant. The endoscope should not be squeezed tightly. All channels should be flushed with water and/or an enzymatic detergent. It is important that the enzymatic solution is properly diluted to prevent endoscope damage.

d. After leak testing, the fiberscope should be immersed in an enzymatic detergent solution. Some scopes do not have a submersible eyepiece, but the rest of the scope may be submersible. It is important to place a water-resistant cap over the video connector before submersion. All channels should be filled with the solution and allowed to soak for the time stated on the label (usually 2 to 5 minutes). The fiberscope should then be cleaned. Special cleaning devices that can be inserted into the channels are available. Short strokes should be used to gradually introduce the brush. If significant resistance is felt, proceed from the other direction rather than force the brush through a blocked channel. If a cleaning device cannot be passed easily through a channel, the scope should be sent for repair. The solution should be suctioned through all channels until they are free of debris. Suctioning fluid and air alternately removes more debris from lumens than suctioning only fluid. Special kits to check for blood residue in the channel are available.

e. Following cleaning, the fiberscope and all of its channels should be thoroughly rinsed with sterile water or rinsed with tap water and then alcohol. Tap water rinsing not followed by alcohol rinsing has been linked to contamination. The endoscope should be hung vertically to allow any remaining fluid to drain from the insertion tube.

f. Following cleaning, fiberscopes should be sterilized or undergo high-level disinfection. Current data suggest that high-level disinfection provides the same degree of safety as sterilization. If the scope is totally immersible, chemical disinfection can be used. Glutaraldehyde, hydrogen peroxide, and OPA are effective disinfectants. All lumens and/or channels must be filled. After disinfection, the device should be thoroughly rinsed with sterile water, followed by 70% alcohol. The Steris system can be employed, using special adaptors for the lumens.

g. Automated endoscope reprocessors that perform disinfection and rinsing are available, but some have been implicated in infections and pseudoinfections. All automatic reprocessing systems have filtration systems. It is important that the filters are changed regularly. The scope should be allowed to cool for at least 5 to 7 minutes after it has been processed.

h. Gas sterilization may also be used. It is effective but will keep the fiberscope out of service for a long period of time. Some suction valves can be autoclaved. Most fiberscopes have lumens that are too narrow and too long for plasma sterilization.

18. **Stylets and Bougies**
    a. Many believe that stylets and bougies should be kept sterile because they are placed inside a sterile tracheal tube. Reusable bougies are frequently contaminated. Sterile disposable stylets and bougies are available but may not work as well as multiple-use ones.
    b. As soon as possible after use, the stylet or bougie should be rinsed and then immersed in water and disinfectant. They may then be autoclaved, gas or plasma sterilized, or treated with liquid chemicals, depending on their construction. Of the liquid chemical agents, alcohol and glutaraldehyde are used most frequently. Plasma sterilization can also be used. If EO is used for sterilization, no aeration time is required unless the stylet or bougie is in a package.
19. **Tracheal and Double-Lumen Tubes and Connectors**
    a. A tracheal or double-lumen tube is placed in an area of the body that is normally sterile. It should be kept free of contamination until used. Disposable sterile tubes are available at such low cost that reusable ones are often not cost-effective. The tube should be kept in its package until just before use. The patient end should not be touched. Lubricants, stylets, and suction catheters used with these tubes should be free from contamination. If possible, the tube should not touch any part of the mouth or pharynx during insertion.

> **CLINICAL MOMENT** Studies indicate that tracheal tubes can be used for up to 28 days after being opened but not lubricated or removed from the package.

    b. The manufacturer's instructions should be followed for cleaning methods for reusable tubes.
20. **Suction Catheters**
    Suction catheters are disposable devices that are discarded after use unless used in a closed suction system. A contaminated suction catheter that may still be needed for a patient should be rinsed with sterile water and then returned to its packaging after use and not placed under the mattress of the operating room table or draped over the carbon dioxide absorber. At the end of each case, it must be discarded.
21. **Supraglottic Airway Devices**
    a. Up to 76% of laryngeal mask airways (LMAs) have been found to have occult blood on them after use. Contamination occurs after the first use and may continue to build up as the LMA is reused. There have been no reported cases of disease transmission between patients by a reusable LMA.
    b. Disposable supraglottic airway devices are available. They may be more economical to use than reusable devices when the costs of cleaning and sterilization are factored along with the number of reuses that a device will tolerate. The Association of Anaesthetists of Great Britain and Ireland recommends that a supraglottic airway used for tonsillectomy or adenoidectomy not be used again.
    c. The manufacturer's directions with regard to cleaning and sterilizing a supraglottic airway device should be followed. For reusable LMAs, the

following recommendations apply. Manufactures may alter their recommendations and for that reason they should be consulted. Soaking the device in a dilute (8% to 10%) solution of bicarbonate before cleaning will help to dissolve secretions. The inflation valve should not be exposed to any fluid. The device should be cleaned in dilute bicarbonate or mild detergent solution until all visible foreign material is removed. A pipe cleaner–type brush should be inserted through the distal aperture(s). Studies show that complete protein removal from an LMA is often not achieved. Ultrasonic cleaning may be more effective than other methods to remove proteinaceous material from the most inaccessible areas. Supplementary cleaning with potassium permanganate will significantly reduce or eliminate protein deposits. The supraglottic device should be rinsed with water and then dried.

d. Autoclaving is the only recommended sterilization method for reusable LMAs. Temperatures up to 134°C (273°F) may be used. Higher temperatures can cause the tube to become brittle and fragment. It may be preferable to use a sterilizer without a vacuum phase. As much air as possible should be removed from the cuff shortly before autoclaving. Residual air will expand in the heat and may damage the cuff, valve, or pilot balloon. After sterilization, the device should be left in its package until just prior to use.
e. Liquid chemical agents should not be used on an LMA because they are adsorbed onto the silicone and can cause pharyngitis and laryngitis as well as shorten the life of the LMA. Gas sterilization also must not be used.
f. The manufacturer's instructions should be followed for cleaning and sterilizing other reusable supraglottic devices.

22. **Resuscitation Bags**

Resuscitation bags have been implicated as the source of cross infection. Their relatively low cost probably makes disposable ones cost-effective. The primary source of contamination is the valve. This should be disassembled and cleaned and, if possible, disinfected or sterilized after each use or on a regular basis if dedicated to a single patient. The manufacturer's instructions should be followed.

23. **Blood Pressure Cuffs, Tubing, and Stethoscopes**

a. Blood pressure cuffs are frequently contaminated with blood and can be a reservoir of bacteria. Spraying cuffs with a topical disinfectant will reduce their bacterial load. Protective covers for cuffs are available. The arm can be wrapped with soft cotton before the cuff is applied to prevent skin contact. Reusable cuffs should be cleaned with a detergent at the end of the day and when visibly contaminated. Periodic disinfection or sterilization is advisable. Most cuffs can be washed after the bladder is removed. After drying, the cuff may be subjected to gas sterilization or chemical disinfection. Nonfabric cuffs can undergo plasma sterilization.
b. The stethoscope is a potential source for transmitting bacteria. Single-use covers are available. Stethoscopes can be washed with water and wiped with alcohol. Earplugs can be cleaned with an alcohol-saturated applicator.

24. **Pulse Oximeter Probes and Cables**

Pulse oximeter probes and cables are frequently contaminated with blood and organisms. Disposable probes may be reprocessed for reuse by pulse oximeter manufacturers and healthcare institutions. Reusable probes and cables should

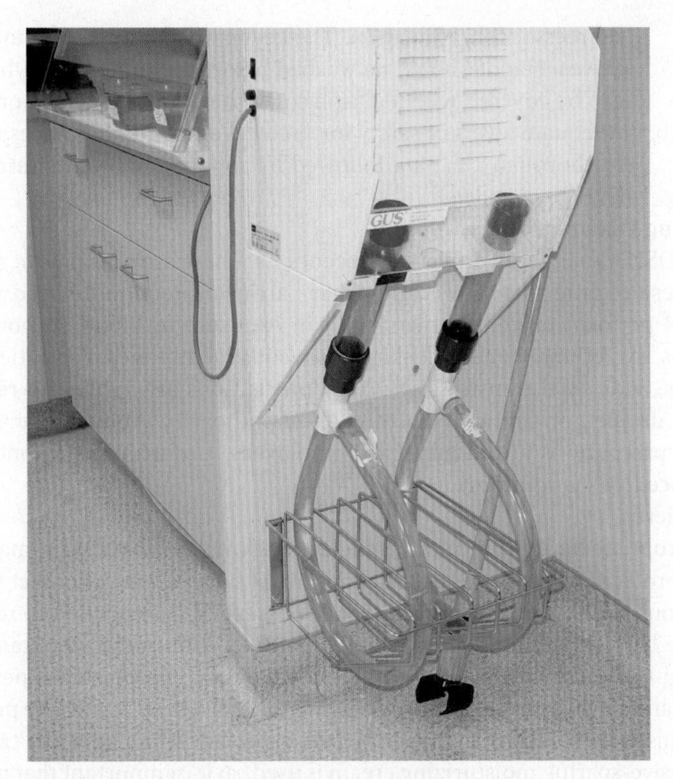

Figure 27.8 Soak station for transesophageal echocardiography probes.

be cleaned at the end of the day or when visibly contaminated by wiping with alcohol or the cleaning solution recommended by the manufacturer. Cables can undergo plasma sterilization.

25. **Temperature Monitors**

    Most temperature sensors are disposable or have disposable covers. Reusable temperature sensors should be cleaned with a disinfectant after use. Special soak stations for rectal probes are available.

26. **Transesophageal Echocardiography Probes**

    a. Transesophageal echocardiography probes are easily damaged. They should be cleaned carefully and then soaked in disinfectant. A soak station is shown in **Figure 27.8**. One container is for the disinfectant, and the second one is used for the initial rinse. Fumes are drawn away from the operator and into a special filter, where they are neutralized.

    b. An automated reprocessor for ultrasound probes that completes the disinfection and rinse cycles in less than 8 minutes is available. It uses a fresh bottle of a glutaraldehyde-based disinfectant for each cycle. This is pierced inside the reprocessor, avoiding splashes and spills. A vapor management system adsorbs chemical vapors.

    c. A chemical burn secondary to a probe that may not have been properly processed has been reported.

27. **Other**

    a. Objects that do not contact the patient but are contacted by the anesthesia provider's fingers (the pen used to record data, the computer keyboard, telephone, nerve stimulators, infusion devices, etc.) should be considered sources of contamination. The keyboard should not be touched with dirty gloves. Hands should be washed before touching the keyboard. Keyboards can be covered with a plastic cover that can be changed or cleaned.

b. Adequate levels of safety for medical equipment surfaces may be achieved by thorough cleaning followed by application of an intermediate- or low-level germicide.

VI. **Preventing Occupational Infection**

In 1991, OSHA mandated universal precautions. These are now part of standard precautions. These require that gloves and other barrier protection be used when healthcare personnel perform tasks that may result in exposure to blood and other body fluids, secretions, excretions, nonintact skin, or mucous membranes. For patients with specific infections, additional transmission-based precautions are applied to reduce the risk of airborne, droplet, or contact transmission of pathogens. Annual educational programs on these precautions are required for employees. Unfortunately, noncompliance with these procedures is common.

A. Barriers

Appropriate barrier precautions including gloves, fluid-resistant masks, face shields, eye protection, and gowns or lab coats must be used when contact with body fluids, mucous membranes, or broken skin is possible. It is important to remove or change these barriers immediately after use and before touching uncontaminated items or going to another patient. Using gloves can reduce needlesticks, percutaneous injuries, and surface contamination in the anesthesia workplace. Glove protection is compromised with each activity performed, especially when adhesive tape is torn unless adhesive-sparing moisturizing cream is used, so it is important that hand disinfection be performed immediately after removing gloves. A full-face disposable plastic shield is best for eye protection. Goggles or prescription glasses are less adequate. It should be noted that the edge of the face shield could be a source of injury to the patient.

B. Hand Hygiene

1. Anesthesia personnel can harbor high bacterial counts on their hands. Hand hygiene should be performed prior to and between patient contacts; after touching blood or other body fluids, secretions, excretions, mucous membranes, broken skin, wound dressings, or contaminated items; when the hands are visibly soiled; and at any other time when microorganisms might be transferred to other patients, staff, or environments. Using gloves does not preclude the need for proper hand hygiene.
2. Hand washing should be performed by first wetting the skin and then adding the soap or cleansing agent. Tepid water should be used. The hands should be rubbed together vigorously for at least 15 seconds, covering and generating friction on all surfaces, and then thoroughly dried.
3. If there is no visible soiling, rubbing with an alcohol-based gel or solution with persistent activity is more convenient and effective. When using an alcohol-based rub, rubbing should be continued until the hands are dry. If the hands dry in less than a minute, more of the waterless rub should be used. It is important to make certain that the rub is applied to all parts of the hand. Studies show that this is frequently not done. Some hand solution manufacturers recommend a soap-and-water hand wash after 8 to 10 consecutive applications of an alcohol-based gel or solution. A disadvantage of alcohol-based products is that they are flammable. However, a study published in 2003 found no fires attributable to hand sanitizers and the National Fire Protection Association now allows

alcohol-based hand sanitizer dispensers in corridors and other public areas, provided certain restrictions are observed.

C. Preventing Needlesticks

1. Percutaneous injury, especially a needlestick with a hollow needle, is associated with the risk of transmitting bloodborne infection. Used needles should not be recapped, bent, or broken by hand or otherwise manipulated using any technique that involves directing the point toward any part of the body. If it is necessary to recap a needle, a single-handed technique in which the needle is not directed toward an unprotected hand or a mechanical protective device should be used. Puncture-resistant sharps containers must be available in all work locations and should be located as close as possible to where sharps are used.
2. Routinely wearing gloves results in a significant reduction in needlestick and percutaneous injuries. Double gloving offers increased protection. Double-glove systems that use a colored inner glove make it easier to detect glove perforations.
3. Efforts to reduce needlesticks have resulted in a variety of new products. Protective devices such as shielded needles, protective lancets, and needleless intravenous line connectors can play an important role in preventing needlesticks. Straight needles that are used to suture central venous access and pulmonary artery catheters are associated with frequent injuries. The CDC recommends using curved, instrument-held suture needles.

D. Emergency Ventilation Devices

When resuscitation is performed, mouthpieces, resuscitation bags, or other ventilation devices should be used as an alternative to mouth-to-mouth ventilation.

VII. Personnel with Cutaneous Lesions

Healthcare workers with breaks in the skin or exudative lesions should refrain from direct patient contact and from handling patient care equipment unless the open area can be protected by a barrier that is impermeable to blood and body fluids.

VIII. Specific Disease States

A. Tuberculosis

1. *M. tuberculosis* is spread primarily via droplets. Because of their small size, droplets remain suspended in air currents and can spread over great distances. Tuberculosis (TB) is less infective after therapy has begun. Anesthesia providers are at risk of acquiring TB. The CDC recommends tuberculin screening of all healthcare workers, with retesting on a regular basis.
2. The CDC has published guidelines for preventing *M. tuberculosis* transmission in healthcare facilities, including the operating room suite. Respiratory isolation is required for all persons suspected or known to have active pulmonary TB until the diagnosis has been ruled out or therapy has been initiated and it can be demonstrated that the individual is no longer infectious.
3. If possible, elective procedures should be delayed until the patient is no longer infectious. A patient with TB who is undergoing surgery should be transported to the operating room wearing a surgical mask. Individuals caring for the infected patient, including those transporting the patient, should wear respiratory protection devices that meet CDC criteria for filtration and fit. Standard surgical masks are generally not suitable.
4. The operating room should have an anteroom that provides some isolation from outside hallways and negative air pressure relative to the corridor and

other operating rooms. Traffic in the room and opening and closing doors during surgery should be minimized. The patient should be the last case of the day or should have the procedure performed at a time when minimal personnel are present. Signs should be placed on the operating room doors to alert the staff to possible infection risks. Unnecessary or overstocked equipment should be removed from the room. A HEPA filter should be placed between the breathing system and the patient.

5. During postanesthesia recovery, the patient should be placed in a private room that meets the recommended standards for TB isolation rooms. Since most institutions do not have such an isolation room in the surgical suite, an alternative is to have postanesthesia care unit personnel provide postoperative care in the operating room or in the patient's isolation room. The isolation room should have negative pressure relative to the surrounding rooms, outside air exhaust, an anteroom to act as an airlock and ultraviolet lights to kill *M. tuberculosis* in infectious droplets. The caregiver in this area will need to have adequate supplies readily available so that it will not be necessary to make many trips into the main recovery area.
6. Equipment that has been used for a patient with TB should be sterilized or undergo high-level disinfection. In general, culturing anesthesia equipment for the presence of tubercle bacilli is not indicated.

B. Bloodborne Pathogens

1. HBV, HCV, and HIV can be transmitted through blood and other body fluids. The greatest risk of exposure is a needlestick. Large-gauge, hollow-bore needles with visible blood and deep penetration increase the risk. The risk of infection after a percutaneous exposure to blood-carrying HBV, HCV, and HIV is 10% to 30%, 2% to 4%, and 0.3%, respectively. Contaminated multidose vials and reusing needles and syringes have been implicated in nosocomial infections with HBV, HCV, and HIV. A breach in procedure by one person can place multiple patients at risk.

CLINICAL MOMENT Syringes and needles are sterile, single-use items and after entry or connection to a patient's vascular system or infusion must be considered contaminated and used only for that patient. Never use a syringe or medication from a container for more than one patient even if the needle has been changed.

2. Devices contaminated with blood from patients infected with a hepatitis virus or HIV should be thoroughly cleaned and sterilized or undergo high-level disinfection.
3. HBV can survive on inanimate objects for a long time. Fifty percent of surfaces from which hepatitis B antigen can be recovered do not have visible blood contamination. Multiple studies have shown that anesthesia providers are at risk for acquiring HBV. The primary strategy for preventing HBV infection is immunization with hepatitis B vaccine, which is recommended for all anesthesia personnel who do not have immunity. OSHA regulations require employers to provide the hepatitis B vaccine at no cost if occupational exposure is expected.
4. HCV is transmitted by respiratory secretions as well as blood. It can be transferred from anesthesia personnel to patients and patients to anesthesia providers.

HCV infection is a major cause of chronic liver disease and hepatocellular cancer and poses a considerable risk for anesthesia personnel. At present, there is no vaccine available to prevent infection, neither is there effective postexposure prophylaxis. Current recommendations from the CDC do not suggest that HCV-infected healthcare personnel be restricted from patient care duties as long as they follow strict aseptic techniques and standard precautions.

5. HIV is relatively unstable in the environment and is rapidly inactivated by a wide range of chemical germicides even those that are classified as low level.

C. Creutzfeldt-Jakob Disease

1. CJD is one of a group of neurodegenerative disorders known as transmissible spongiform encephalopathies and caused by prions. These diseases are characterized by incubation periods ranging from months to years, followed by rapidly progressive dementia. The disease is invariably fatal once clinical symptoms have appeared. Currently, there are no known treatments to inhibit its progression or outcome. There is no evidence that healthcare workers are at increased occupational risk for developing CJD.
2. The discovery that prions can lurk in body organs long before people exhibit signs of disease has the alarming implication that multiple-use devices used on infected individuals can transmit the disease. The extensive lymphoreticular involvement that is present in CJD raises the possibility that devices that come in contact with lymphoreticular tissues such as the tonsils could become contaminated. It has been recommended that laryngoscopes and supraglottic devices used on patients with suspected CJD be destroyed. Using disposable single-use devices, including laryngoscope blades, is recommended.
3. Prions are notoriously hardy and demonstrate resistance to normal sterilization methods. Standard washing techniques reduce the concentration of prions in an exponential fashion, but 10 to 20 cycles are required to produce negligible levels. Effective and ineffective methods of inactivation are listed in **Table 27.3**. Devices that are difficult or impossible to clean should be discarded.
4. The Creutzfeldt-Jakob prion requires a unique decontamination procedure. The preferred treatment of contaminated instruments after cleaning is steam sterilization for at least 30 minutes at a temperature of 132°C (121°C is ineffective). When a prevacuum sterilizer is used, 18 minutes between 134°C and 138°C has been found to be effective. Alternatively, items can be immersed in a 1N sodium hydroxide solution for 1 hour at room temperature and then steam sterilized at 121°C for 30 minutes. Noncritical patient care items or surfaces may be disinfected with either bleach (up to 1:10 dilution) or 1N sodium hydroxide at room temperature for 15 minutes.

CLINICAL MOMENT It may be necessary to discard some equipment after use with a patient at risk of transmitting CJD. Disposable equipment should be used as much as possible.

D. Severe Acute Respiratory Syndrome

1. Severe acute respiratory syndrome (SARS) is a viral disease that is transmitted by respiratory droplets or contact. Anesthesia providers are at high risk because of frequent exposure to patients' respiratory secretions. Traditional precautions may not afford adequate protection when handling SARS patients.

Table 27.3 Methods of Inactivation of Prions[a]

Effective Methods	Ineffective Methods
Incineration	Glutaraldehyde
Prolonged steam sterilization (132°C, 1 to 4 hours)	Formaldehyde
Others: 270°F for 18 minutes in a prevacuum sterilizer or at 250°F for 60 minutes in a gravity sterilizer	Hydrogen peroxide
Sodium hydroxide (1N, 1 hour)	Chlorine dioxide
Sodium hypochlorite (1:10 solution)	Phenolics
Proprietary phenolics	Iodophores
Peracetic acid in Steris system (possibly)	Alcohols Dry heat Boiling Desiccation Freezing Ultraviolet, ionizing, and microwave radiation Normally recommended autoclave cycles Ethylene oxide Gas plasma

[a]No method has currently been shown to be 100% effective against prions.
From Antloga K, Meszaros J, Malchesky PS, et al. Prion disease and medical devices. ASAIO J 2000;46:S69–S72.

2. Whenever possible, patients should have a private, negative-pressure room with at least 6 to 12 exchanges per hour. If this is unavailable, they should have a room with a HEPA filter.
3. A NIOSH-approved, fit-tested N-95 or greater respirator should be used when contact with these patients is necessary. Goggles or a face shield, a disposable gown and cap, and double gloves should be worn by the anesthesia provider and discarded when leaving the patient's room.
4. When surgery is required, efforts should be made to limit exposure to personnel and other patients. In addition to observing standard precautions, the anesthesia provider should use a respirator. Double gloves are recommended. The outer pair should be removed after direct patient contact and before touching equipment or furniture in other areas of the room. Hands should be washed immediately after the gloves are removed.

REFERENCES

1. O'Connor D. Inside the "Non-Recall Recall" of the SS1. Outpatient Surg Mag 2010;11(1):27–28.
2. Olympio M. Can soda lime canisters spread MRSA? APSF Newslett 2007;22:12–14.

SUGGESTED READINGS

Association of Anaesthetists of Great Britain and Ireland. Infection control in anaesthesia. Anaesthesia 2008;61: 1027–1036.

Berry AJ. Infection control recommendations; their importance to the practice of anesthesiology. ASA Newslett 2001;65:15.

Dorsch J, Dorsch S. Cleaning and sterilization. In: Understanding Anesthesia Equipment. Fifth edition. Philadelphia: Wolters Kluwer/Lippincott Williams & Wilkins, 2008:955–1002.

Farling P, Smith G. Anaesthesia for patients with Creutzfeldt-Jakob disease. A practical guide. Anaesthesia 2003;58: 627–629.

Katz JD. CDC guideline urges physicians to wash their hands of a dirty problem. ASA Newslett 2003;67:21.

Loftus BW, Koff MD, Burchman CC, Schwartzman D, et al. Transmission of pathogenic bacterial organisms in the anesthesia work area. Anesthesiology 1008;109:399–407.

Mauermann WJ, Nemergut EC. The anesthesiologist's role in the prevention of surgical site infections. Anesthesiology 2006;105:413–421.

Mayworm D. Expanding options for low-temperature sterilization. Outpatient Surg Mag 2004;5:82–84.

Nutty C. Double-dipping syringes is never OK. Outpatient Surg Mag 2009;10:66–67.

Rowley E, Dingwall R. The use of single-use devices in anaesthesia: balancing the risks to patient safety. Anaesthesia 2007;62:569–574.

Wilkes AR. Reducing the risk of prior transmission in anaesthesia. Anaesthesia 2005;60:527–529.

Index